T0289921

Assessment and Multimodal Management of Pain

Assessment and Multimodal Management of Pain

Editor: Lily Hunt

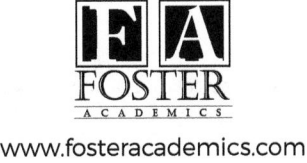

www.fosteracademics.com

www.fosteracademics.com

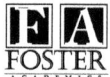

Cataloging-in-Publication Data

Assessment and multimodal management of pain / edited by Lily Hunt.
    p. cm.
Includes bibliographical references and index.
ISBN 978-1-64646-581-1
1. Pain--Treatment. 2. Pain. 3. Pain--Physiological aspects. 4. Pain medicine. I. Hunt, Lily.
RB127 .P35 2023
616.047 2--dc23

Foster Academics,
118-35 Queens Blvd., Suite 400,
Forest Hills, NY 11375, USA

ISBN 978-1-64646-581-1 (Hardback)

Contents

Preface

In my initial years as a student, I used to run to the library at every possible instance to grab a book and learn something new. Books were my primary source of knowledge and I would not have come such a long way without all that I learnt from them. Thus, when I was approached to edit this book; I became understandably nostalgic. It was an absolute honor to be considered worthy of guiding the current generation as well as those to come. I put all my knowledge and hard work into making this book most beneficial for its readers.

Pain refers to an emotional experience and unpleasant sensation commonly caused by tissue damage. It enables the body to respond and prevent any further damage. Acute pain and chronic pain are the two primary types of pain. Acute pain is a typical reaction to an illness or injury. It usually begins abruptly and is short-lived. Chronic pain lasts longer than the anticipated period for recovery. It usually lasts longer than three months. The initial assessment of pain generally starts with a physical examination. Pain is measured by determining its impact on activities like work, mood, sleep and relationships. Complementary therapies, pain medications, and physical therapy are major therapies for the effective management of pain. The multimodal management of pain includes relying on multiple therapies and medications for pain management. Some of the groups of medications, which are used in combination for managing pain are alpha-2 agonists, local anaesthetics, NSAIDs, opioids and acetaminophen. This book is a detailed explanation of pain assessment and multimodal management. It is a resource guide for experts as well as students.

I wish to thank my publisher for supporting me at every step. I would also like to thank all the authors who have contributed their researches in this book. I hope this book will be a valuable contribution to the progress of the field.

Editor

Single and double pain responses to individually titrated ultra-short laser stimulation in humans

Anna Sellgren Engskov[1]*[iD], Agneta Troilius Rubin[2] and Jonas Åkeson[1]

Abstract

Background: This preclinical study in humans was designed to selectively induce delayed nociceptive pain responses to individually titrated laser stimulation, enabling separate bedside intensity scoring of both immediate and delayed pain.

Methods: Forty-four (fourteen female) healthy volunteers were subjected to repeated nociceptive dermal stimulation in the plantar arc, based on ultra-short carbon dioxide laser with individually titrated energy levels associated with mild pain.

Results: Data was analysed in 42 (12 female) subjects, and 29 of them (11 females) consistently reported immediate and delayed pain responses at second-long intervals to each nociceptive stimulus. All single pain responses were delayed and associated with lower levels ($p = 0.003$) of laser energy density (median 61; IQR 54–71 mJ/mm^2), compared with double pain responses (88; 64–110 mJ/mm^2). Pain intensity levels associated with either kind of response were readily assessable at bedside.

Conclusions: This study is the first one to show in humans that individually titrated ultra-short pulses of laser stimulation, enabling separate pain intensity scoring of immediate and delayed responses at bedside, can be used to selectively induce and evaluate delayed nociceptive pain, most likely reflecting C-fibre-mediated transmission. These findings might facilitate future research on perception and management of C-fibre-mediated pain in humans.

Keywords: Humans, Lasers, Nerve fibers, Nociceptors, Nociceptive pain, Pain measurement, Visual analog scale

Background

Nociceptive pain in man, peripherally transmitted by myelinized Aδ- and non-myelinized C-fibres, is characterized by immediate, mainly pricking [1], and more well-confined sensations, and by delayed, dull or pressing [1], and less well-confined sensations, respectively.

Selective activation of C-fibres is important considering that chronic pain is associated with C-fibre-mediated activity [2], and being able to induce and evaluate selective activation of C-fibres might have clinical implications for individually tailored management of pain. To be useful, techniques for experimental induction of nociceptive pain in humans should convey non-inflammatory and rapidly transient pain, be reproducible, and preferably also be individually adjustable. Ultra-short laser stimulation with a carbon dioxide (CO_2) laser meets these criteria and has been used to induce selective activation of C-fibres in humans [3–5], mainly based on different thermal thresholds of Aδ- and C-fibre nociceptors. It has also been used to evoke separate pain responses mediated by Aδ- and C-fibres [3, 5–9], based on differences in nociceptive response latency and neuronal conduction velocity, and assessed by visual analogue scale (VAS) scoring [8, 10], in humans.

This explorative study in humans, based on the use of individually titrated ultra-short laser stimulation enabling separation in time of immediate and delayed pain responses – interpreted, based on their time characteristics, to reflect Aδ- and C-fibre-mediated transmission – was primarily

* Correspondence: anna.sellgren_engskov@med.lu.se
[1]Department of Clinical Sciences Malmö, Anaesthesiology and Intensive Care Medicine, Lund University, Skåne University Hospital, Carl Bertil Laurells gata 9, 3rd floor, SE-20502 Malmö, Sweden

designed for selective induction of delayed nociceptive pain responses, readily assessable by bedside scoring.

Methods
Study setting
This prospective preclinical study, approved by the regional Human Research Ethics Review Board (Approval No. LU 337–02, LU 697–03, and LU 2010/160), Lund, Sweden, was carried out in a study setting at Skåne University Hospital, Malmö, Sweden, by three study investigators, one 32-year-old female junior resident physician, and two male senior undergraduate medical students aged 27 and 38 years.

Subjects
Forty-four (fourteen female) healthy adult volunteers with no current history of pain, reduced sensibility in their lower extremities, or current use of analgesics or other drugs affecting pain perception, were included after normal physical examination. Informed written and verbal consent was obtained from all study participants. The study participants were not allowed to use ethanol or any drug affecting pain perception within 24 h before the study interventions.

Induction of pain
Nociceptive pain was thermally induced by ultra-short pulsed CO_2 laser stimulation (10 W effect, 3 mm beam diameter) with a Coherent Ultrapulse 2500C w CPG Laser (Coherent Inc., Santa Clara, California, USA). Each study participant was familiar with the technique of nociceptive stimulation at the time of evaluation, since the laser energy to be consistently used in each participant was determined at least 48 h in advance by incremental five-millisecond increases in pulse duration, starting at 10 ms, until mild intensity levels [11] of immediate and/or delayed pain were consistently induced. Individual levels of laser energy density were calculated from laser effect, pulse duration, and beam diameter. Each participant was subjected to four complete series of nociceptive stimulation by the same study investigator. A series comprised three stimuli, at least one minute apart, located at slightly different skin areas of the plantar arc. The study participants were not informed about their pulse duration, and hence blinded to their individually titrated levels of laser energy density.

Evaluation of pain
Before individual titration of laser energy density, each participant was carefully instructed how to assess pain intensity levels of immediate (first) and/or delayed (second) pain, following each nociceptive stimulus, on a horizontal 100 mm VAS ruler. Single pain was defined as one reported sensation of mild pain intensity (either immediate or delayed), and double pain defined as two sensations of mild pain intensity, i.e. one immediate and one delayed.

Statistics
Based on data previously obtained in 35 volunteers evaluating experimentally induced pain by VAS scoring [12], at least 40 study participants had been estimated to be required for analysis of single and double pain responses in the present study.

Parametric data is presented as mean ± standard deviation (SD). Non-parametric data is reported as median with interquartile range (IQR) in parenthesis.

Individual median values with 95% confidence intervals (CI) of immediate and delayed pain intensity during the four series of laser stimuli were calculated from corresponding individual mean values of each series of three. Individual mean values were also tested for order effect with Friedman's test, and linear regression with a mixed model approach.

The Mann-Whitney U-test was used to compare titrated levels of laser energy density between subjects reporting immediate or delayed pain intensity. The same test was also used to compare female and male subjects with respect to laser energy density and reported pain intensity levels, and in a subanalysis, to compare levels of energy density between subgroups of pain-matched males evaluated by a female or a male investigator.

Levels of probability (p) below 0.05 were considered to indicate statistical significance.

Results
Subjects
Two female study participants, considered unable to reliably assess the intensity of pain, were excluded. Results were obtained and analysed in the remaining 42 (twelve female) subjects, aged 27 ± 3.4 years and weighing 72 ± 12 kg.

Induction of pain
There was a tendency towards higher laser energy levels for consistent induction of mild pain in male (median 85 (IQR 60–110) mJ/mm^2) than in female (median 68 (IQR 51–82) mJ/mm^2) study participants ($p = 0.06$). Significantly higher titrated levels of energy density ($p = 0.008$) were used in those five males evaluated by a female study investigator (median 224 (IQR 160–253) mJ/mm^2) than in five males, matched for pain intensity, evaluated by a male investigator (median 74 (IQR 60–81) mJ/mm^2).

Transient dyschromic spots at the site of dermal stimulation, corresponding to the diameter of the laser beam, disappeared within few days. No other adverse effects were observed or reported.

Evaluation of pain
The first and second components of double pain responses appeared immediately and at least one second

after the laser pulse, and single pain responses were consistently delayed. Twenty-nine (eleven female) study participants consistently reported double pain responses to each nociceptive stimulus, four (one female) reported single pain responses once or twice, and nine (no female) consistently reported single pain responses only.

Significantly lower ($p = 0.003$) levels of laser energy density were used in subjects with single pain responses than in those with double pain responses (median 61 (IQR 54–71) vs. 88 (64–110) mJ/mm^2), as shown in Fig. 1.

Individually assessed intensity levels of immediate and delayed pain are shown in Fig. 2. There was no difference ($p > 0.300$) in reported levels of pain intensity between female and male study participants (median 2.6 (2.0–3.1) vs. 2.3 (IQR 2.0–2.8) VAS units).

Immediate pain intensity did not differ significantly ($p > 0.300$) between the four series of stimulation (second vs. first – 0.119 (CI -0.374–0.136); third vs. first – 0.144 (– 0.400–0.111); fourth vs. first – 0.245 (– 0.500–0.010)), whereas the intensity of delayed pain was significantly higher ($p < 0.001$) during the first series (second vs. first – 0.445 (– 0.728–-0.163); third vs. first – 0.381 (– 0.663–-0.098), fourth vs. first – 0.567 (– 0.850–-0.285)).

Discussion

In this study – based on individually titrated ultra-short laser stimulation for induction, and on bedside scoring with VAS for evaluation, of pain – we were able to evoke isolated delayed single pain responses at lower, and

separately assessable immediate and delayed pain responses at higher, levels of stimulation intensity.

Influence on peripheral sensitisation and central habituation of pain perception during individual titration, was reduced by gradually increasing the duration of each laser pulse, in agreement with previous recommendations [13, 14]. To avoid epidermal overheating and tissue damage during the study intervention, and to consistently compare pain responses to the same individual level of nociceptive stimulation, we considered it important to use individually titrated, instead of predefined [3, 5, 8, 15, 16], energy levels of laser stimulation, found to induce mild pain intensity, and also to stimulate slightly different skin areas at minute-long intervals.

Thermal induction of pain mediated by Aδ- and C-fibres in humans requires skin temperature levels exceeding activation thresholds of their nociceptors, corresponding to 44.3–46.5 °C versus 41.8–42.4 °C at foot level, i.e. to a difference in heating of two to four degrees centigrade [3]. Those physiological differences at nociceptive receptor level – consistent with our main finding of single pain responses being induced by lower levels of laser energy than double pain responses – enable selective thermal activation of C-fibre nociceptors at temperature levels above their nociceptive threshold and still below that of Aδ-fibre nociceptors [3–5]. Moreover, they most likely explain why all single pain responses in the present study were delayed, i.e. C-fibre mediated.

Our findings of significantly higher laser energy for induction of mild pain in males studied by a female than

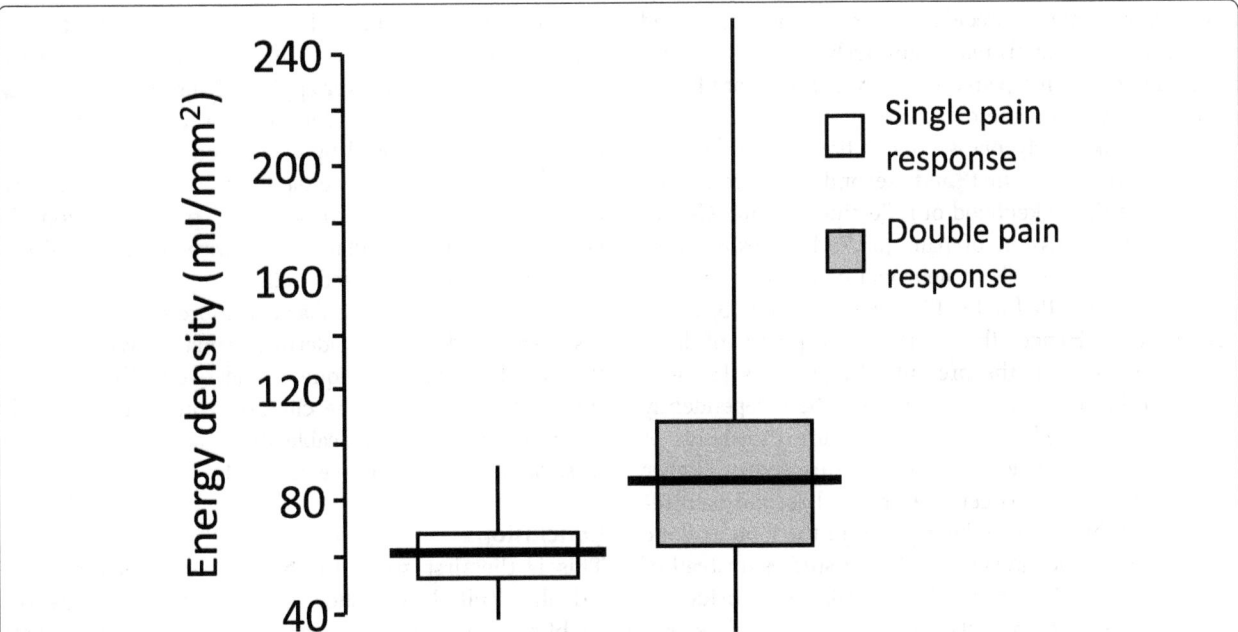

Fig. 1 Energy density levels used to induce nociceptive pain by ultra-short CO_2 laser stimulation in the arc of the foot in 13 (one female) subjects not consistently reporting double pain responses, and in 29 (eleven female) subjects reporting double pain responses of mild intensity. All single pain responses were delayed. Median values are indicated by bold horizontal lines, interquartile range by boxes, and range by vertical lines

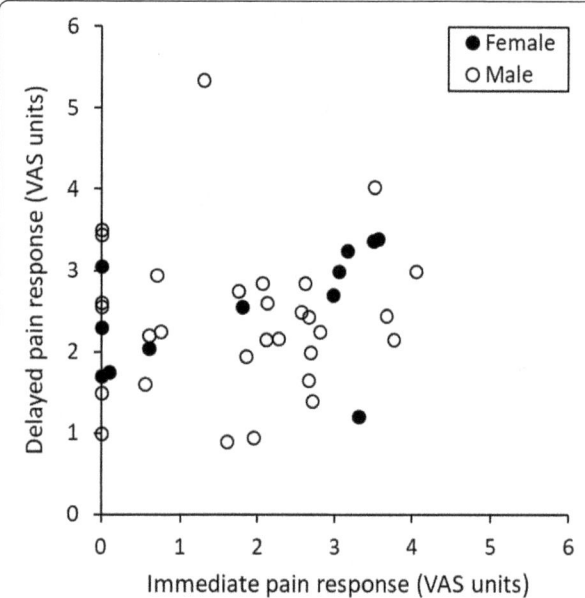

Fig. 2 Median intensity levels of immediate and delayed pain induced by ultra-short CO_2 laser stimulation in the arc of the foot, assessed by individual visual analogue scale (VAS) scoring, in 13 (one female) subjects not consistently reporting double pain responses, and in 29 (eleven female) subjects reporting double pain responses of mild intensity. All single pain responses were delayed

by a male – enabled by involving more than one study investigator and interpreted to reflect corresponding differences in pain sensitivity – might indicate potential impact of experimenter gender on pain perception. However, this finding in a limited number of study participants was not a predefined aim of this study and should hence be interpreted cautiously. Follow-up studies, preferably with a paired cross-over design, are highly desirable to confirm these findings.

Our approximately one-second difference in time latency between the first and second pain responses strengthens their likelihood of reflecting Aδ- and C-fibre mediated transmission of pain [3, 7, 16], respectively, corresponding to levels of neuronal conduction velocity estimated at 11–19 [3, 15–17] versus 0.7–1.5 [3, 6, 13, 15, 16] m/s. Hence, the short-lasting pulses of laser stimulation used in the present and previous [3, 5–9] studies allow both pain components to be independently evaluated, provided that the temperature thresholds of Aδ- and C-fibre nociceptors are both exceeded. Higher separation in time between the first and second pain responses is achieved by inducing pain in the foot, as done in the present and previous [3, 7, 16] studies, instead of in the hand [1, 4–6, 8–10, 14, 15, 18, 19], considering the up to 35% more delayed transmission of second (C-fibre mediated) pain along the estimated 80–100 cm axonal distance between the plantar arc and the lumbosacral spinal cord [3, 7, 16].

Despite being widely used in research and clinical practice, established bedside tools for pain scoring have been used in few previous studies on nociceptive pain induced by laser stimulation [4, 8, 10, 14, 19], and mainly with assessment of pain intensity on eleven-level visual analogue [10] or numeric rating [4, 14, 19] scales, i.e. with lower resolution than in the present study.

We did not use neuronal or cerebrocortical electrophysiological measurements – in addition to individual pain scoring – to distinguish between first (Aδ-fibre mediated) and second (C-fibre mediated) pain responses, based on differences in their nociceptive response latency and neuronal transmission properties. Nevertheless, the approximately one-second delay of each reported single pain, and second double pain, sensation – interpreted to reflect C-fibre mediated transmission – is consistent with recent neurophysiological findings [10]. Moreover, the induction of two pain responses, consistently well separated in time at bedside, by a single nociceptive stimulus, conforms to simultaneous activation of Aδ- and C-fibre fibres.

Although we did not measure plantar skin temperature – neither before nor after pain stimulation – we do not believe potential individual differences in baseline skin temperature to have considerably influenced our results, since CO_2 laser stimuli have been shown to induce similar local heating patterns at skin temperatures between 27 °C and 32 °C [3, 14].

Results reported here were obtained in more study participants compared with most previous studies based on laser-induced pain [1, 3–10, 14], except for two previous [16, 18] and one recent [19] studies in similar numbers of subjects. The risk for carry-over effects was reduced by allowing minute-long time intervals between stimulations to avoid overlapping of subsequent pain responses. Furthermore, order effects were diminished and data accuracy improved by using median values of individually calculated average data obtained under identical conditions from repeated series of pain induction. In contrast to earlier similar studies with standardized energy levels (2–4), we used individually titrated levels of laser energy to induce similar and more predictable pain responses and avoid epidermal damage. We consider this readily usable technique of selective C-fibre stimulation and evaluation to be clinically, but not necessarily scientifically, more applicable than spatial filter [20] or dissociating Aδ-fibre nerve block [21] techniques.

Conclusions

This is the first study to show in humans that individually titrated ultra-short pulses of laser stimulation, enabling separate pain intensity scoring of immediate and delayed responses at bedside, can be used to selectively induce delayed nociceptive pain, most likely reflecting transmission by C-fibres, considering their lower nociceptive thermal threshold, longer nociceptor latency and lower axonal conduction velocity. These findings might promote future research on C-fibre-mediated pain in humans, and possibly also enable more specific evaluation of various analgesic interventions primarily in a research context.

Abbreviations
CO_2: Carbon dioxide; IQR: Interquartile range; LU: Lund University; P: Level of statistical probability; SD: Standard deviation; VAS: Visual analogue scale

Acknowledgements
The authors thank Peter Persson, Fredrik Persson and Jenny Friberg Törnquist for valuable assistance.

Authors' contributions
This study was designed by ASE, ATR and JÅ, and was ethically applied for by ASE and JÅ. The study participants were recruited and included by ASE and JÅ, and the study was carried out by ASE and JÅ. Study data was recorded by ASE and JÅ, compiled by ASE and analysed by ASE, ATR and JÅ. The first draft of the manuscript was prepared by ASE, and ASE, ATR and JÅ contributed to, read and approved the final version.

Authors' information
Anna Sellgren Engskov, MD, PhD student and resident in anaesthesiology and intensive care medicine, Agneta Troilius Rubin, MD, PhD, associate professor and senior consultant in dermatology, and Jonas Åkeson, MD, PhD, EDAIC, ETP, professor and senior consultant in anaesthesiology and intensive care medicine, Lund University, Skåne University Hospital, Malmö, Sweden.

Author details
[1]Department of Clinical Sciences Malmö, Anaesthesiology and Intensive Care Medicine, Lund University, Skåne University Hospital, Carl Bertil Laurells gata 9, 3rd floor, SE-20502 Malmö, Sweden. [2]Dermatology, Lund University, Skåne University Hospital, Malmö, Sweden.

References
1. Beissner F, Brandau A, Henke C, Felden L, Baumgartner U, Treede RD, et al. Quick discrimination of Adelta and C fiber mediated pain based on three verbal descriptors. PLoS One. 2010;5(9):e12944.
2. Orstavik K. Pathological C-fibres in patients with a chronic painful condition. Brain. 2003;126(3):567–78.
3. Plaghki L, Decruynaere C, Van Dooren P, Le Bars D. The fine tuning of pain thresholds: a sophisticated double alarm system. PLoS One. 2010;5(4):e10269.
4. Tzabazis AZ, Klukinov M, Crottaz-Herbette S, Nemenov MI, Angst MS, Yeomans DC. Selective nociceptor activation in volunteers by infrared diode laser. Mol Pain. 2011;7(18):1–7.
5. Churyukanov M, Plaghki L, Legrain V, Mouraux A. Thermal detection thresholds of Adelta- and C-fibre afferents activated by brief CO2 laser pulses applied onto the human hairy skin. PLoS One. 2012;7(4):e35817.
6. Bromm B, Treede RD. Nerve fibre discharges, cerebral potentials and sensations induced by CO2 laser stimulation. Hum Neurobiol. 1984;3(1):33–40.
7. Arendt-Nielsen L. Second pain event related potentials to argon laser stimuli: recording and quantification. J Neurol Neurosurg Psychiatry. 1990; 53(5):405–10.
8. Nahra H, Plaghki L. Innocuous skin cooling modulates perception and neurophysiological correlates of brief CO2 laser stimuli in humans. Eur J Pain. 2005;9(5):521–30.
9. Ploner M, Gross J, Timmermann L, Schnitzler A. Cortical representation of first and second pain sensation in humans. Proc Natl Acad Sci U S A. 2002; 99(19):12444–8.
10. Azevedo E, Silva A, Martins R, Andersen ML, Tufik S, Manzano GM. Activation of C-fiber nociceptors by low-power diode laser. Arq Neuropsiquiatr. 2016; 74(3):223–7.
11. Jensen M. Interpretation of visual analog scale ratings and change scores: a reanalysis of two clinical trials of postoperative pain. J Pain. 2003;4(7):407–14.
12. Chen CC, Johnson MI. A comparison of transcutaneous electrical nerve stimulation (TENS) at 3 and 80 pulses per second on cold-pressor pain in healthy human participants. Clin Physiol Funct Imaging. 2010;30(4):260–8.
13. Cruccu G, Pennisi E, Truini A, Iannetti GD, Romaniello A, Le Pera D, et al. Unmyelinated trigeminal pathways as assessed by laser stimuli in humans. Brain. 2003;126(Pt 10):2246–56.
14. Iannetti GD, Leandri M, Truini A, Zambreanu L, Cruccu G, Tracey I. Adelta nociceptor response to laser stimuli: selective effect of stimulus duration on skin temperature, brain potentials and pain perception. Clin Neurophysiol. 2004;115(11):2629–37.
15. Tran TD, Lam K, Hoshiyama M, Kakigi R. A new method for measuring the conduction velocities of Abeta-, Adelta- and C-fibers following electric and CO(2) laser stimulation in humans. Neurosci Lett. 2001;301(3):187–90.
16. Obi T, Takatsu M, Yamazaki K, Kuroda R, Terada T, Mizoguchi K. Conduction velocities of Adelta-fibers and C-fibers in human peripheral nerves and spinal cord after CO2 laser stimulation. J Clin Neurophysiol. 2007;24(3):294–7.
17. Iannetti GD, Truini A, Romaniello A, Galeotti F, Rizzo C, Manfredi M, et al. Evidence of a specific spinal pathway for the sense of warmth in humans. J Neurophysiol. 2003;89(1):562–70.
18. Arendt-Nielsen L, Bjerring P. Sensory and pain threshold characteristics to laser stimuli. J Neurol Neurosurg Psychiatry. 1988;51(1):35–42.
19. Staikou C, Kokotis P, Kyrozis A, Rallis D, Makrydakis G, Manoli D, et al. Differences in pain perception between men and women of reproductive age: a laser-evoked potentials study. Pain Med. 2017;18(2):316–21.
20. Hoeben RM, Krabbenbos IP, van Dongen EPA, Tromp SC, Boezeman EHJF, van Swol CFP. Selective laser stimulation of Aδ- or C-fibers through application of a spatial filter: a study in healthy volunteers. Journal of Neurology Research. 2016;6(1):1–7.
21. Magerl W, Ali Z, Ellrichä J, Meyer RA, Treede R-D. C- and Aδ-fiber components of heat-evoked cerebral potentials in healthy human subjects. Pain. 1999;82:127–37.

2

The effect of ultrasound-guided erector spinae plane block on postsurgical pain

Mark C. Kendall*, Lucas Alves, Lauren L. Traill and Gildasio S. De Oliveira

Abstract

Background: The effect of erector spinae plane block has been evaluated by clinical trials leading to a diversity of results. The main objective of the current investigation is to compare the analgesic efficacy of erector spinae plane block to no block intervention in patients undergoing surgical procedures.

Methods: We performed a quantitative systematic review of randomized controlled trials in PubMed, Embase, Cochrane Library, and Google Scholar electronic databases from their inception through July 2019. Included trials reported either on opioid consumption or pain scores as postoperative pain outcomes. Methodological quality of included studies was evaluated using Cochrane Collaboration's tool.

Results: Thirteen randomized controlled trials evaluating 679 patients across different surgical procedures were included. The aggregated effect of erector spinae plane block on postoperative opioid consumption revealed a significant effect, weighted mean difference of − 8.84 (95% CI: − 12.54 to − 5.14), (P < 0.001) IV mg morphine equivalents. The effect of erector spinae plane block on post surgical pain at 6 h compared to control revealed a significant effect weighted mean difference of − 1.31 (95% CI: − 2.40 to − 0.23), P < 0.02. At 12 h, the weighted mean difference was of − 0.46 (95% CI: − 1.01 to 0.09), P = 0.10. No block related complications were reported.

Conclusions: Our results provide moderate quality evidence that erector spinae plane block is an effective strategy to improve postsurgical analgesia.

Keywords: Erector spinae plane block, Postoperative pain, GRADE criteria, Meta-analysis

Background

The misuse of prescribed opioids leading to the current opioid epidemic crisis has put greater emphasis on the development of non-opioid analgesic techniques to manage postoperative pain [1–3]. A large variety of regional anesthesia techniques have been commonly used to minimize postoperative pain [4–6]. In addition, several techniques (e.g., transverse abdominis plane blocks, pectoral nerve blocks, brachial plexus blocks) have been evaluated in quantitative systematic reviews [7–9]. These techniques have emerged as effective non-opioid strategies to reduce post-surgical pain.

The erector spinae plane block has been used clinically by anesthesiologists as a potential non-opioid analgesic strategy across multiple surgical procedures [10–14]. The block is considered easy to perform and can be easily implemented in the perioperative period [15, 16]. Recent clinical trials have assessed the efficacy of the erector spinae plane block on postoperative analgesia

* Correspondence: mark.kendall@lifespan.org
Department of Anesthesiology, The Warren Alpert Medical School of Brown University, Providence, Rhode Island, USA

with inconsistent results. Nonetheless, to the best of our knowledge, no quantitative systematic review has evaluated the effectiveness of the erector spinae plane block to improve postoperative analgesia.

The objective of our study was to examine the analgesic efficacy of erector spinae plane block for postoperative analgesia outcomes in patients undergoing surgical procedures. In addition, we also investigated the potential side effects related to the use of the erector spinae plane block.

Methods

We performed a quantitative systematic review according to the PRISMA guidelines [17]. The study was registered with the PROSPERO international database (CRD42020148072; registered August 2019). We followed similar methods as previously published by our group [18, 19].

Systematic search and inclusion criteria

A comprehensive search of randomized trials investigating the effects of erector spinae plane block to control (i.e. no block or sham block) on postoperative surgical analgesia was performed using web-based electronic databases PubMed, Google Scholar, the Cochrane Database of Systematic Reviews, and Embase from inception up to July 2019. The search words 'erector spine block', 'erector spinae plane block', or "ESPB" were used in various combinations using Boolean operators. Search strategy is shown in Additional file 1. The search was limited to adults older than 18 years of age and there were no language restrictions. The bibliographies of the identified studies were evaluated and reviewed for additional studies. There was no search performed for unpublished or non-peer reviewed studies. Included trials reported either opioid consumption or pain scores as postoperative pain outcomes. No minimum sample size was required for inclusion in the quantitative analysis.

Exclusion criteria

Studies were excluded if a direct comparison of erector spinae plane block and no block could not be determined. Non-randomized controlled trials, anatomical or cadaver studies, case reports, or editorials were not considered for inclusion.

Selection of included studies and data extraction

Two investigators (MCK and LA) independently reviewed the abstracts obtained from the initial search using the predetermined inclusion and exclusion criteria. The trials that were not relevant based on the inclusion criteria were omitted. Any discrepancies encountered during the selection process were resolved by discussion among the evaluators (MCK and LA). If there was a

disagreement then the final decision was determined by the senior investigator (GDO). Data extraction was carried out by using a pre-designed data collection form. The primary source of data extraction was from either the text or tables. If the data could not be found in either location, we extracted the data manually from available figures or plots. The extracted data obtained from studies included the sample size, number of study participants in treatment/control groups, surgery description, type of local anesthetic dose, single-shot or bilateral block placement, use of ultrasonography for block placement, postoperative opioid consumption, postoperative pain scores, postoperative nausea and vomiting, and adverse events. Postoperative opioid consumption was converted to intravenous morphine milligram equivalents assuming no cross-tolerance (morEq) [20]. Continuous data was recorded using mean and standard deviation. Data variables presented as median, interquartile range, or mean ± 95% confidence interval (CI) were transformed to mean and standard deviation [21, 22]. For studies that did not provide standard deviation, the standard deviation was estimated using the most extreme values. If the same outcome variable was reported more than once then the most conservative value was used.

Risk of bias assessment

The validity of the included studies was evaluated in accordance with Cochrane risk-of-bias tool (RoB-2) [23]. This recently new assessment tool consists of five domains focusing on where bias might be introduced into a trial. The domains consist of: bias arising from the randomization process, bias due to deviations from the intended interventions, bias due to missing outcome data, bias in measurement of the outcome, and bias in the selection of the reported result. Each category was recorded as "low risk of bias", "some concerns", or "high risk of bias." Two investigators (MCK and LA) independently assessed the risk of bias of included studies and any inconsistencies were resolved by discussion with senior author (GDO).

Primary outcome

Postoperative opioid consumption (IV morEq) reported at 24 h following surgery.

Secondary outcomes

Postoperative pain scores (numeric pain rating score, 0 = no pain, 10 = extreme pain) at rest and with activity at 6 h, at 12 h, and at 24 h after surgery, block complications, and postoperative nausea and vomiting displayed as (n).

Meta-analysis

The weighted mean differences (WMD) with 95% confidence interval (CI) were calculated and reported for continuous data for total opioid consumption up to 24 h and pain scores (NRS) at 6 h, 12 h and at 24 h. Statistical significance required that the 95% CI for continuous data did not include zero and for dichotomous data, the 95% confidence interval did not include 1.0. Due to the variety of surgical procedures, we chose to use the random-effects model in an attempt to generalize our findings to studies not included in our meta-analysis [24]. Asymmetric funnel plots were analyzed for publication bias using Egger's regression test [25]. A one sided $P < 0.05$ was considered as an indication of an asymmetric funnel plot. In the presence of an asymmetric funnel plot, a file drawer analysis was performed, which estimates the lowest number of additional studies that if they would become available, it would reduce the combined effect to non-significance assuming the average z-value of the combined P values of these missing studies would be 0. Heterogeneity was considered to be high if the I^2 statistic was greater than 50%. If heterogeneity was high, we performed a sensitivity analysis by removing individual studies and investigated surgical procedures by examining its effect on the overall heterogeneity. A P value < 0.05 was required to reject the null hypothesis. Analyses was performed using Stata

version 15 (College Station, Texas) and Comprehensive Meta-analysis software version 3 (Biostat, Englewood, NJ).

Results

A flow diagram of the literature search and reasons for exclusion are shown in Fig. 1.

The initial query identified 903 articles and 884 articles were excluded after review of the study abstracts. A total of 19 articles were evaluated and after full-text review 6 articles were omitted. Thirteen studies involving 679 subjects fulfilled the inclusion criteria and were included in the final analysis [26–38]. The median number of patients was 50 (IQR, 40 to 60). All included studies reported on opioid consumption and/or pain scores at rest or during activity. Table 1 provides details of the study characteristics of the included trials.

Quality assessment

All included trials reported inclusion and exclusion criteria and described baseline characteristics. The risk of bias assessment according to the Cochrane Handbook using the Cochrane risk-of-bias assessment tool (RoB-2) is presented in Table 2. The quality of evidence of the included studies was summarized using the Grading of Recommendations, Assessment, Development, and Evaluation (GRADE) criteria and is presented in Table 3.

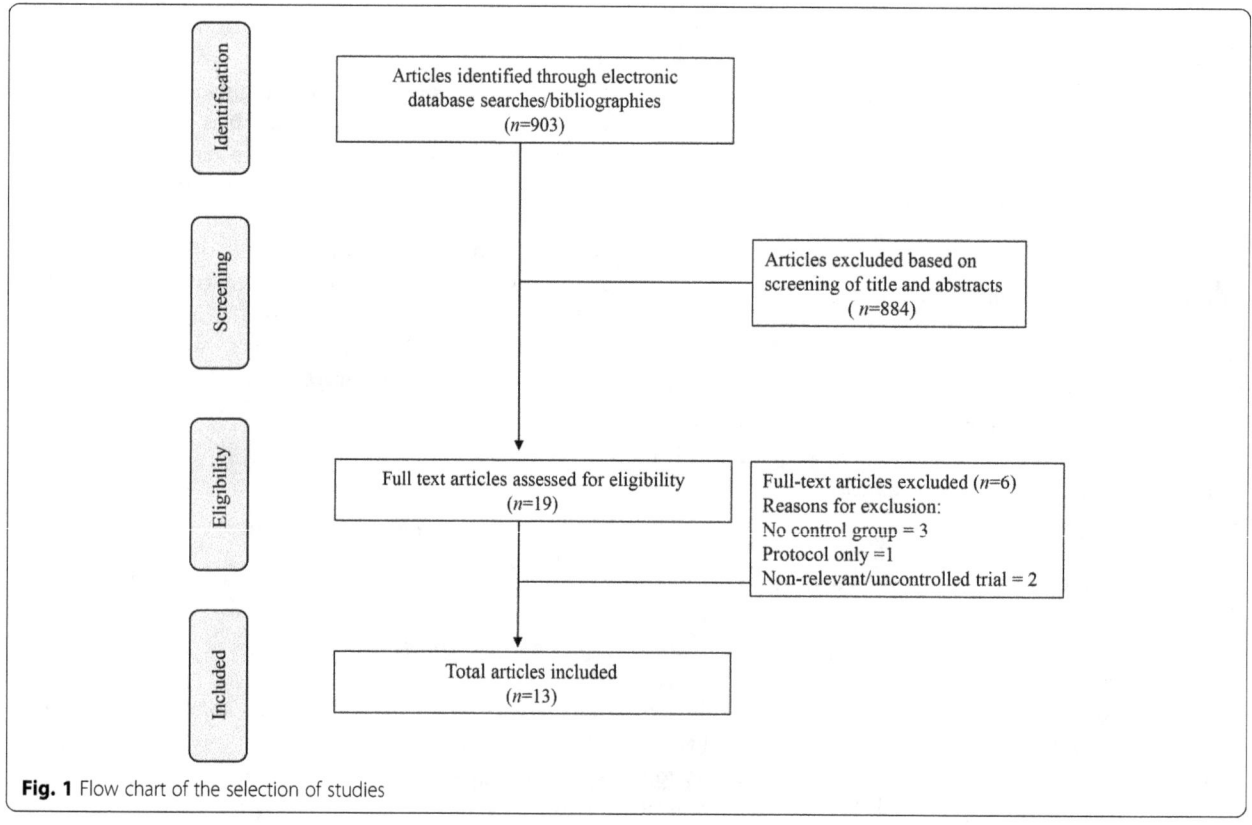

Fig. 1 Flow chart of the selection of studies

Table 1 Cochrane risk-of-bias assessment for included studies (RoB 2)

Authors/Year	Bias arising from the randomization process	Effect of assignment to intervention	Effect of adhering to intervention	Bias due to missing outcome data	Bias in measurement of outcomes	Bias in the selection of the reported result	Overall risk of bias
Abu Elyazed et al. [26] 2019	Low	Low	Low	Low	Low	Low	Low
Aksu et al. [27] 2019	Low	Some concerns	Low	Low	Low	Low	Some concerns
Ciftci et al. [28] 2018	Low	Some concerns	Low	Low	Some concerns	Low	High
Gurkan et al. [29] 2018	Low	Some concerns	Low	Low	Low	Low	Some concerns
Hamed et al. [30] 2019	Low	Low	Low	Low	Low	Low	Low
Krishna et al. [31] 2019	Low	Low	Low	Low	Low	Low	Low
Oksuz et al. [32] 2019	Low	Some concerns	Low	Low	Low	Low	Some concerns
Singh et al. [33] 2019	Low	Some concerns	Low	Low	Some concerns	Low	High
Singh et al. [34] 2019	Low	Some concerns	Low	Low	Low	Low	Some concerns
Tulgar et al. [35] 2018	Low	Low	Low	Low	Low	Low	Low
Tulgar et al. [36] 2018	Low	Low	Low	Low	Low	Low	Low
Tulgar et al. [37] 2019	Low	Low	Low	Low	Low	Low	Low
Yayik et al. [38] 2019	Some concerns	Some concerns	Low	Low	Low	Low	High

Postoperative opioid consumption reported up to 24 h following surgery

The pooled effect of twelve studies [26–30, 32–38] examining the effect of erector spinae plane block on postoperative opioid consumption compared to control at 24 h after surgery revealed a significant effect, weighted mean difference (WMD) of – 8.84 (95% CI: – 12.54 to – 5.14), ($P < 0.001$) mg IV morEq (Fig. 2). The heterogeneity was high ($I^2 = 98\%$) and could be partially explained by whether the block was placed bilaterally or as a single-shot procedure ($I^2 = 91\%$). The type of surgery did not substantially reduce the heterogeneity any further ($I^2 = 86\%$). Potential sources of heterogeneity were further tested by a sensitivity analysis by removing individual studies which did not significantly reduce the heterogeneity among the studies.

A subgroup analysis of surgery type revealed the reduction of opioid consumption compared to control was statistically significant in patients who underwent chest surgical procedures WMD of – 9.04 (95% CI: – 11.37 to – 6.70), $P < 0.001$ and in patients who underwent spine or orthopedic procedures WMD of – 4.13 (95% CI: – 5.78 to – 2.48), $P < 0.001$. Patients who had abdominal surgery did not experience statistical significance, WMD of – 12.05 (95% CI: – 25.88 to 1.79), $P = 0.09$. Visual examination of the funnel plot and Egger's regression test ($P = 0.06$) revealed no apparent publication bias.

Postoperative pain at rest 6 h after surgery

The combined effect of nine studies [26, 27, 29–31, 33–35, 37] evaluating erector spinae plane block on postsurgical pain compared to control at 6 h following surgery displayed a significant effect, WMD of – 1.31 (95% CI: –

2.40 to – 0.23) (0–10 numerical scale), $P < 0.02$ (Fig. 3a). Heterogeneity was high ($I^2 = 96\%$) and could be partially explained by the type of block placement in which the heterogeneity decreased to $I^2 = 89\%$ for studies utilizing single-shot blocks. When investigating the type of surgical procedure the heterogeneity decreased to 10% for studies of spine/orthopedic procedures.

A subgroup analysis looking at type of surgery indicated that the reduction in postsurgical pain compared to control was statistically different in patients who underwent abdominal surgical procedures WMD of – 1.35 (95% CI: – 2.25 to – 0.45), $P = 0.003$, or spine/orthopedic procedures WMD of – 0.95 (95% CI: – 1.60 to – 0.31), $P = 0.004$. However, postsurgical pain compared to control was not different in patients who had chest surgical procedures WMD of – 1.34 (95% CI: – 3.56 to 0.88), $P = 0.24$. A sensitivity analysis was performed by omitting individual studies which did not considerably reduce heterogeneity. An examination of the funnel plot to test publication bias did reveal asymmetry. The Egger's regression test result was $P = < 0.001$.

Postoperative pain at activity 6 h after surgery

One study reported the effect of erector spinae plane block on postsurgical pain during movement compared to control at 6 h after surgery and demonstrated a mean difference of – 0.55 (95% CI) -1.21 to 0.11, $P = 0.01$ [37].

Postoperative pain at rest 12 h following surgery

The effect of ten studies [26, 27, 29–31, 33–35, 37, 38] investigating erector spinae plane block on postoperative surgical pain compared to no block or sham block at 12 h after surgery did not show a significant effect WMD of

Table 2 Summary of study characteristics included in analysis

Authors	Year of Publication	Procedures	Treatment/Control	UG	Treatment	Anesthesia	Method of extraction
Abu Elyazed et al. [26]	2019	Open epigastic hernia repair	30/30	Y	Bilateral 20 ml 0.25% bupivacaine Sham block (1 ml NS)	General	Text Table
Aksu et al. [27]	2019	Breast surgery	25/25	Y	Single-shot 20 ml 0.25% bupivacaine No block	General	Text Table
Ciftci et al. [28]	2019	Video assisted thoracic surgery	30/30	Y	Single-shot 20 ml 0.25% bupivacaine No block	General	Text Table
Gurkan et al. [29]	2018	Breast cancer surgery	25/25	Y	Single-shot 20 ml 0.25% bupivacaine Sham block (NS)	General	Text Table
Hamed et al. [30]	2019	Abdominal hysterectomy	30/30	Y	Bilateral 20 ml 0.5% bupivacaine Sham block (NS)	General	Text Table
Krishna et al. [31]	2018	Cardiac surgery	53/53	Y	Bilateral 3 mg/kg 0.375% Ropivacaine No block	General	Text Table
Oksuz et al. [32]	2019	Reduction mammoplasty	21/22	Y	Bilateral 20 ml 0.25% bupivacaine No block	General	Text
Singh et al. [33]	2019	Radical mastectomy	20/20	Y	Single-shot 20 ml 0.5% bupivacaine No block	General	Text
Singh et al. [34]	2019	Lumbar spine surgery	20/20	Y	Bilateral 20 ml 0.5% bupivacaine No block	General	Text Table
Tulgar et al. [35]	2019	Laparoscopic Cholecystectomy	20/20	Y	Bilateral 20 ml 0.5% bupivacaine No block	General	Text Table
Tulgar et al. [36]	2018	Orthopedic surgery	20/20	Y	Single-shot 20 ml 0.5% bupivacine No block	General	Text Table
Tulgar et al. [37]	2018	Laparoscopic Cholecystectomy	15/15	Y	Bilateral 20 ml 0.375% bupivacaine No block	General	Text Table
Yayik et al. [38]	2019	Lumbar decompression surgery	30/30	Y	Bilateral 20 ml 0.25% bupivacaine No block	General	Text Table

UG ultrasound guided, *NS* normal saline

− 0.46 (95% CI: − 1.01 to 0.09), (0–10 numerical scale), $P = 0.10$, (Fig. 3b). Heterogeneity was found to be high ($I^2 = 87\%$) and was slightly decreased to $I^2 = 62\%$ for studies using single-shot block placement. The heterogeneity decreased to $I^2 = 0\%$ for studies involving only abdominal surgical procedures. A sensitivity analysis was performed by omitting individual studies which did not significantly reduce heterogeneity.

A subgroup analysis involving the type of surgery revealed that the reduction in postsurgical pain compared to control was statistically different in patients who underwent abdominal surgical procedures WMD of − 0.57 (95% CI: − 0.95 to − 0.19), $P = 0.003$. However, postsurgical pain at rest compared to control was not different in patients 12 h after chest surgical procedures WMD of − 0.70 (95% CI: − 1.51 to 0.12), $P = 0.09$ or spine/orthopedic procedures WMD of − 0.11 (95% CI: − 1.22 to 0.99), $P = 0.84$. An examination of the funnel plot to test publication bias did not reveal asymmetry. The Egger's test result was $P = 0.47$.

Postoperative pain at activity 12 h after surgery
There were two studies that reported on postoperative surgical pain at activity 12 h after surgery. Tulgar et al. [37] reported the effect of erector spinae plane block on postsurgical pain during movement compared to control at 12 h after surgery and demonstrated a weighted mean difference of − 0.60 (95% CI: − 1.09 to − 0.11), $P = 0.02$.

Table 3 Summary of the quality of evidence (GRADE) for comparing erector spinae plane block to a control group for the primary and secondary outcomes of the included studies

# studies in design (n)	Risk of bias	Inconsistency	Indirectness	Imprecision	Publication bias	Overall quality of evidence[e]	Importance
Postoperative opioid consumption at 24 h							
12 (573)	None serious[a]	Serious[b]	None serious	None serious	Undetected	⊕⊕⊕○ Moderate	Important
Postoperative pain at rest at 6 h							
9 (486)	None serious[a]	Serious[b]	None serious	None serious	Detected[c]	⊕⊕⊕○ Moderate	Important
Postoperative pain at rest at 12 h							
10 (546)	None serious[a]	Serious[b]	None serious	None serious	Undetected	⊕⊕⊕○ Moderate	Important
Postoperative pain at rest at 24 h							
10 (500)	None serious[a]	Serious[d]	None serious	None serious	Undetected	⊕⊕⊕○ Moderate	Important
Postoperative nausea and vomiting							
11 (596)	None serious[a]	None serious	None serious	None serious	Undetected	⊕⊕⊕⊕ High	Important

[a]Majority of studies had allocation concealment and used blinded outcome assessments; lost to follow up was very low; the overall risk of bias was felt to be none serious
[b]There is high heterogeneity among the included studies; sensitivity analysis did not significantly reduce heterogeneity
[c]Funnel plot did reveal asymmetry; Egger's test, $P = < 0.05$
[d]There is high heterogeneity among the included studies; subgroup analysis of type of block placement did significantly reduce heterogeneity
[e]Grade Workshop Group grades of evidence: high quality: further research very unlikely to change confidence in estimate of effect; moderate quality; further research likely to have important impact on confidence in estimate of effect and may change estimate; low quality; further research very likely to have important impact on confidence in estimate of effect and likely to change estimate; very low quality: very uncertain about estimate

Postoperative opioid consumption at 24 hours

Study name	Lower limit	Upper limit	Z-Value	p-Value	Difference in means
Hamed 2019	-6.605	-1.395	-3.009	0.003	-4.000
Tulgar 2019	-33.907	-29.853	-30.821	0.000	-31.880
Singh 2019 1	-8.709	-5.991	-10.603	0.000	-7.350
Tulgar 2018 1	-4.112	-2.288	-6.877	0.000	-3.200
Abu Elyazed 2019	-11.981	-7.839	-9.377	0.000	-9.910
Gurkan 2018	-13.935	-7.745	-6.865	0.000	-10.840
Singh 2019 2	-6.896	-4.704	-10.375	0.000	-5.800
Aksu 2019	-12.293	-8.067	-9.445	0.000	-10.180
Oksuz 2019	-7.193	-4.467	-8.385	0.000	-5.830
Yayik 2019	-4.620	-2.180	-5.464	0.000	-3.400
Ciftli 2019	-13.264	-9.936	-13.667	0.000	-11.600
Tulgar 2018 2	-4.352	-0.388	-2.343	0.019	-2.370
	-12.537	-5.141	-4.685	0.000	-8.839

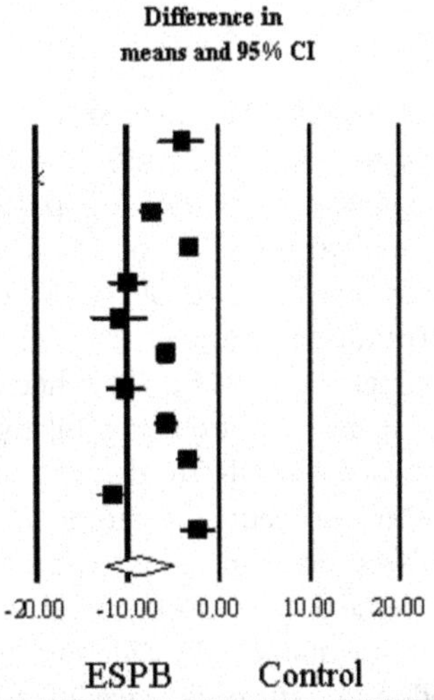

Fig. 2 Postoperative opioid consumption at 24 h. Meta-analysis evaluating the effect of erector spinae plane block on opioid consumption compared to control at 24 h following surgery. The overall effect of the erector spinae plane block versus control was estimated as a random effect. The point estimate for the overall effect was − 8.84 (95%CI: − 12.54 to − 5.14), ($P < 0.001$) mg IV morphine equivalents. The weighted mean difference for individual studies is represented by the square symbol on Forrest plot, with 95% CI of the difference shown as a solid line

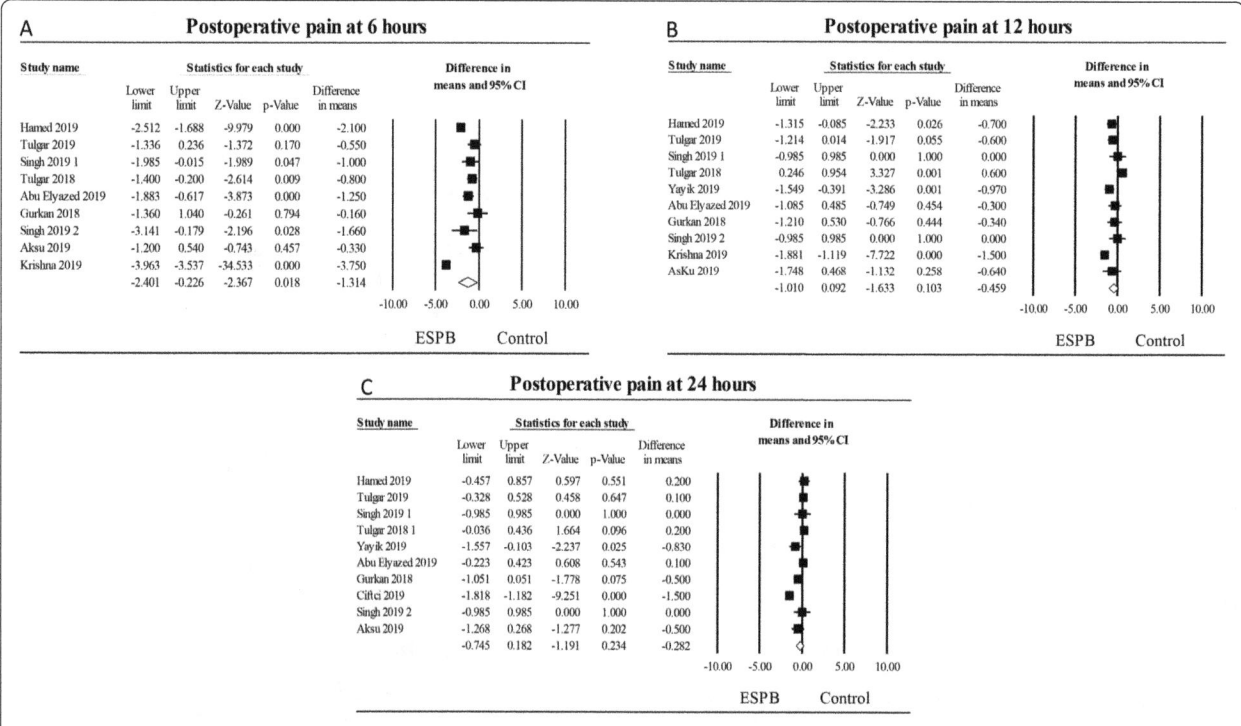

Fig. 3 Postoperative pain at rest at 6 h, 12 h and at 24 h. The meta-analysis evaluating the effect of erector spinae plane block on pain scores at 6 h (**a**), at 12 h (**b**), and at 24 h (**c**) compared to control was estimated as a random effect. The point estimate for the overall effect on postoperative pain scores at 6 h following surgery was − 1.31 (95% CI: − 2.40 to − 0.23), $P < 0.02$, (0–10 numerical scale). The point estimate for the overall effect on postoperative pain at 12 h following surgery was − 0.46 (95% CI: − 1.01 to 0.09), $P = 0.10$. The point estimate for the overall effect on postoperative pain scores at 24 h following surgery was − 0.28 (95% CI: − 0.75 to 0.18), $P = 0.23$. The weighted mean difference for individual studies is represented by the square symbol on Forrest plot, with 95% CI of the difference shown as a solid line

Yayik et al. [38] reported the effect of erector spinae plane block on postsurgical pain during movement compared to control at 12 h after surgery and demonstrated a weighted mean difference of − 1.14 (95% CI: − 1.50 to − 0.78), $P < 0.01$.

Postoperative pain at rest 24 h following surgery

The pooled effect of ten studies [26–30, 33–35, 37, 38] examining erector spinae plane block on postoperative surgical pain compared to no block or sham block did not reveal a significant effect WMD of − 0.28 (95% CI: − 0.75 to 0.18), (0–10 numerical scale), $P = 0.23$, (Fig. 3c). Heterogeneity was high ($I^2 = 89\%$). The heterogeneity decreased to $I^2 = 30\%$ for studies using bilateral block placement. A sensitivity analysis by deleting individual studies did not substantially reduce heterogeneity.

A subgroup analysis involving the type of surgery demonstrated that reduction in postsurgical pain compared to control was not statistically different in patients who underwent abdominal surgical procedures WMD of 0.11 (95% CI: − 0.13 to 0.35), $P = 0.35$, spine/orthopedic surgical procedures WMD of − 0.17 (95% CI: − 0.85 to 0.51), $P = 0.63$, or after chest procedures WMD of − 0.70 (95% CI: − 1.43 to 0.03), $P < 0.06$. An examination of the

funnel plot did not reveal asymmetry; Egger's regression test result was $P = 0.40$.

Postoperative pain at activity 24 h after surgery

The pooled effect of three studies evaluating the effect of erector spinae plane block on postoperative surgical pain during activity compared to control did not show a significant effect, weighted mean difference of − 0.65 (95% CI: − 1.40 to 0.11), $P = 0.09$. Heterogeneity was $I^2 = 89\%$ [28, 37, 38].

Postoperative nausea and vomiting (PONV)

The pooled effect of eleven studies [26–29, 31, 33–38] that examined erector spinae plane block on postoperative nausea and vomiting compared to no block or sham block showed a significant effect, OR of 0.29 (95% CI: 0.14 to 0.63) ($P = 0.001$), (Fig. 4). Heterogeneity was moderate, $I^2 = 40\%$. Heterogeneity was decreased to $I^2 = 0\%$ when investigating either abdominal or spine/orthopedic procedures. A sensitivity analysis by omitting individual studies did not significantly reduce heterogeneity.

A subgroup analysis involving the type of surgery revealed that postoperative nausea and vomiting compared to control was reduced in spine/orthopedic surgical procedures WMD of 0.29 (95% CI: 0.09 to 0.91), $P =$

0.03. In contrast, the postoperative nausea and vomiting compared to no block or sham block was not different in patients who had chest surgery, WMD of 0.22 (95% CI: 0.05 to 1.04), $P = 0.06$ or abdominal surgery WMD of 0.39 (95% CI: 0.10 to 0.1.47), $P = 0.16$.

Adverse events

All thirteen studies reported either no adverse events (i.e. respiratory depression, local systemic toxicity, hematoma) or did not report any adverse events. One study [26] reported two patients who received erector spinae plane block who experienced intraoperative hypotension compared to one patient in the control group to an estimated incidence of 0.2% (95% CI: 0.3 to 1).

Discussion

The most important finding of the current investigation was the reduction of postoperative pain in patients who received an erector spinae plane block compared to a control group across multiple surgical procedures. Patients in the erector spinae plane group reported substantially less pain in the immediate postoperative phase (e.g., 6 h after surgery). Our results suggest that the erector spinae plane block is an effective strategy to reduce postsurgical pain.

Our results are important as pain continues to be poorly controlled after surgery. A recent study by Herbst et al. showed that 23.3% of postsurgical readmissions were related to poor postoperative pain control [39]. Appropriate postoperative analgesia control has been associated with improved patient satisfaction, and it is utilized in the HCAPS survey used to evaluate quality of care in hospitals [40, 41]. Thus, by using the erector spinae plane block, clinical practitioners may reduce pain-related readmissions and improve patient satisfaction after surgery.

Another important finding of our current investigation was the effect of the erector spinae plane block on the reduction of postoperative nausea and vomiting. This is interesting as not all analgesic interventions have been shown to reduce opioid-related side effects [42–44]. In addition, the effect was large and comparable to other first line pharmacological agents for postoperative nausea and vomiting prophylaxis. Based on our results, one could argue that the effect of the erector spinae plane block on PONV was likely due to the reduction of postoperative pain rather than the estimated opioid sparing effects.

One of the main advantages of the erector spinae plane block is that the block is considered easy to be performed, especially when compared to paravertebral

Incidence of nausea and vomiting during hospital stay

Study name	Lower limit	Upper limit	Z-Value	p-Value	Odds ratio	Odds ratio and 95% CI
Tulgar 2019	0.012	8.260	-0.691	0.490	0.317	
Singh 2019 1	0.004	1.339	-1.767	0.077	0.069	
Tulgar 2018 1	0.072	2.760	-0.870	0.384	0.444	
Abu Elyazed 2019	0.100	4.153	-0.464	0.643	0.643	
Gurkan 2018	0.221	2.252	-0.588	0.556	0.706	
Singh 2019 2	0.008	4.009	-1.082	0.279	0.180	
Aksu 2019	0.347	4.371	0.322	0.747	1.231	
Oksuz 2019	0.005	1.896	-1.540	0.123	0.096	
Yayik 2019	0.044	1.241	-1.706	0.088	0.235	
Ciftci 2019	0.007	0.161	-4.261	0.000	0.034	
Tulgar 2018 2	0.019	2.017	-1.369	0.171	0.196	
	0.137	0.625	-3.177	0.001	0.293	

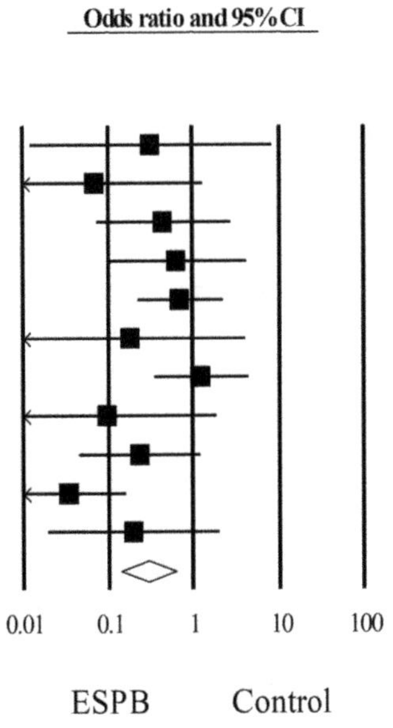

0.01   0.1   1   10   100

ESPB   Control

Fig. 4 Incidence of postoperative nausea and vomiting at 24 h after surgery. Random-effects meta-analysis evaluating the effect of erector spinae plane block on nausea and vomiting compared to control. Squares to the right of the middle vertical line indicates that erector spinae plane block was associated with increased odds of nausea, whereas squares to the left of the middle vertical line show that erector spinae plane block was associated with decreased odds of nausea. The horizontal lines represent the 95% CI and the diamond shape represents the overall effect of erector spinae plane block on postoperative nausea and vomiting compared to control. CI = confidence interval

blocks or thoracic epidurals. This is important because it not only maximizes efficacy of the block, but also allows its implementation across multiple surgical procedures. The injection is performed deep in the erector spinae muscle and superficial to the tips of the thoracic transverse processes. The block has an excellent safety profile since the local anesthetic injection is distant from the pleura, major blood vessels, and spinal cord.

The anatomical localization of the spinal nerves and the different anatomy of the vertebral column may be a major factor for the various postoperative outcomes following the placement of an erector spinae plane block. Recent literature has reported that different volumes of local anesthetic injectate and its corresponding spread are influenced by the site of injection. For example, a 5 mL of injectate was needed to cover one vertebral level in the lumbar region, whereas only 3.3 (radiological imaging studies) to 3.5 (cadaveric dissections studies) mL are needed in thoracic region [45]. In our study, we found that patients who underwent spine or orthopedic surgeries compared to control experienced clinical pain relief at 6 h which dissipated by 12 h after surgery. In contrast, studies investigating erector spinae plane block to control in patients undergoing chest surgical procedures reported no significant pain relief at any three of the study time periods in the postoperative period. Nonetheless, patients who underwent chest or spine/orthopedic procedures reported opioid sparing effects at 24 h after surgery. Future clinical trials investigating the optimal volume of local anesthetics in different anatomical regions and different types of surgeries to determine analgesic adequacy is warranted.

The findings of our study should only be interpreted within the context of its limitations. First, in order to minimize heterogeneity, we compared erector spinae plane block to an "inactive" control group. More recently, studies have compared the erector spinae plane blocks to other commonly performed blocks (e.g., transversus abdominis plane block, paravertebral blocks) [46–48]. Nonetheless, the number of randomized trials are not yet adequate to perform a quantitative analysis comparing the erector spinae plane blocks to other regional blocks. Secondly, we limited our comparison to acute postoperative pain. Some recent reports have highlighted the potential use of the erector spinae plane block for chronic pain conditions [49, 50]. It is conceivable that the erector spinae plane block may reduce opioid consumption among chronic pain patients. Third, we did not include studies investigating continuous catheter infusions of local anesthetics in the erector spine plane as most investigations are limited to case reports. The use of a continuous catheter erector spinae block can prolong the local anesthetic blockade extending the postoperative pain relief beyond 12 h [51, 52]. Randomized

trials confirming the efficacy of continuous catheter erector spinae blocks are warranted due to the limited analgesic duration of single-shot blocks. Last, we included a large multitude of surgical procedures with various anatomical differences in an attempt to improve the generalizability of our findings, which may account for the significant heterogeneity present in the current studies. Nonetheless, we used the random effect model for all of the analyses and were able to explain some of the heterogeneity based on the utilization of either unilateral or bilateral placement of the block or by the category of surgical location. However, the high levels of heterogeneity among the studies makes publication bias concerning in the studies published to date. Further investigations of erector spinae plane block for postoperative analgesia with larger sample sizes are needed to address the wide variability of the effect sizes seen in our analysis.

Conclusion

In summary, our results provide moderate-quality evidence the erector spinae plane block may be an effective analgesic strategy to minimize postoperative pain and reduce postoperative opioid consumption across several types of surgeries. In addition, a high quality of evidence demonstrated that erector spinae plane block also reduced postoperative nausea and vomiting. More studies are necessary to confirm our findings of a possible short-term analgesic benefit of the erector spinae plane block.

Abbreviations
CI: Confidence interval; ESPB: Erector spinae plane block; GRADE: Grading of Recommendations, Assessment, Development, and Evaluation; HCAPS: Hospital Consumer Assessment of Healthcare Providers and Systems; I²: Heterogeneity; IQR: Interquartile range; IV: Intravenous; NRS: Numrical rating scale; WMD: Weighted mean differences

Acknowledgements
None.

Authors' contributions
MCK, LA, LT, and GDO contributed to the design and implementation of the manuscript, to the analysis of the results, writing of the manuscript, editing and approving the final version of the manuscript. All authors agree on the accuracy and integrity of the manuscript.

References
1. Neuman MD, Bateman BT, Wunsch H. Inappropriate opioid prescription after surgery. Lancet. 2019;393:1547–57.
2. Beloeil H, Albaladejo P, Sion A, et al. Multicentre, prospective, double-blind, randomised controlled clinical trial comparing different non-opioid analgesic combinations with morphine for postoperative analgesia: the OCTOPUS study. Br J Anaesth. 2019;122(6):e98–e106.
3. Soffin EM, Lee BH, Kumar KK, Wu CL. The prescription opioid crisis: role of the anesthesiologist in reducing opioid use and misuse. Br J Anaesth. 2019; 122:e198–208.
4. Yao Y, Li J, Hu H, Xu T, Chen Y. Ultrasound-guided serratus plane block enhances pain relief and quality of recovery after breast cancer surgery: A

randomised controlled trial. Eur J Anaesthesiol. 2019;36:436–41.

5. Rao Kadam V, Ludbrook G, van Wijk RM, et al. Comparison of ultrasound-guided transmuscular quadratus lumborum block catheter technique with surgical pre-peritoneal catheter for postoperative analgesia in abdominal surgery: a randomised controlled trial. Anaesthesia. 2019;74(11):1381–8.

6. Clement JC, Besch G, Puyraveau M, et al. Clinical Effectiveness of single dose of intravenous dexamethasone on the duration of ropivacaine axillary brachial plexus block: the randomized placebo-controlled ADEXA trial. Reg Anesth Pain Med. 2019;44:370-4. https://doi.org/10.1136/rapm-2018-100035.

7. Lovett-Carter D, Kendall MC, McCormick ZL, et al. Pectoral nerve blocks and postoperative pain outcomes after mastectomy: a meta-analysis of randomized controlled trials. Reg Anesth Pain Med. 2019. https://doi.org/10.1136/rapm-2019-100658.

8. Schnabel A, Reichl SU, Weibel S, et al. Efficacy and safety of dexmedetomidine in peripheral nerve blocks: A meta-analysis and trial sequential analysis. Eur J Anaesthesiol. 2018;35:745–58.

9. Mayhew D, Sahgal N, Khirwadkar R, Hunter JM, Banerjee A. Analgesic efficacy of bilateral superficial cervical plexus block for thyroid surgery: meta-analysis and systematic review. Br J Anaesth. 2018;120:241–51.

10. Taketa Y, Irisawa Y, Fujitani T. Comparison of ultrasound-guided erector spinae plane block and thoracic paravertebral block for postoperative analgesia after video-assisted thoracic surgery: a randomized controlled non-inferiority clinical trial. Reg Anesth Pain Med. 2019. https://doi.org/10.1136/rapm-2019-100827.

11. Adhikary SD, Liu WM, Fuller E, Cruz-Eng H, Chin KJ. The effect of erector spinae plane block on respiratory and analgesic outcomes in multiple rib fractures: a retrospective cohort study. Anaesthesia. 2019;74(5):585–93.

12. Moore RP, Liu CJ, George P, et al. Early experiences with the use of continuous erector spinae plane blockade for the provision of perioperative analgesia for pediatric liver transplant recipients. Reg Anesth Pain Med. 2019. https://doi.org/10.1136/rapm-2018-100253.

13. Hamadnalla H, Elsharkawy H, Shimada T, Maheshwari K, Esa WAS, Tsui BCH. Cervical erector spinae plane block catheter for shoulder disarticulation surgery. Can J Anaesth. 2019;66(9):1129–31.

14. Tulgar S, Selvi O, Kapakl MS. Erector spinae plane block for different laparoscopic abdominal surgeries: case series. Case Rep Anesthesiol. 2018;2018:3947281.

15. Forero M, Adhikary SD, Lopez H, Tsui C, Chin KJ. The Erector Spinae Plane Block: A Novel Analgesic Technique in Thoracic Neuropathic Pain. Reg Anesth Pain Med. 2016;41:621–7.

16. Chin KJ, Malhas L, Perlas A. The Erector Spinae Plane Block Provides Visceral Abdominal Analgesia in Bariatric Surgery: A Report of 3 Cases. Reg Anesth Pain Med. 2017;42:372–6.

17. Moher D, Liberati A, Tetzlaff J, Altman DG, PRISMA Group. Preferred reporting items for systematic reviews and meta-analyses: the PRISMA statement. PLoS Med. 2009;6:e1000097.

18. Kendall MC, Castro Alves LJ, De Oliveira G Jr. Liposome bupivacaine compared to plain local anesthetics to reduce postsurgical pain: an updated meta-analysis of randomized controlled trials. Pain Res Treat. 2018;2018:5710169.

19. Kendall MC, Alves LJ, Pence K, Mukhdomi T, Croxford D, De Oliveira GS. The effect of intraoperative methadone compared to morphine on postsurgical pain: a meta-analysis of randomized controlled trials. Anesthesiol Res Pract. 2020;2020:6974321. https://doi.org/10.1155/2020/6974321.

20. Available: http://www.globalrph.com/narcoticonv.htm [Accessed Last accessed 7/2019]..

21. Wan X, Wenqian W, Liu J, Tong T. Estimating the sample mean and standard deviation from the sample size, median, Range And/or Interquartile Range. BMC Med Res Methodol. 2014;14:135.

22. Hozo SP, Djulbegovic B, Hozo I. Estimating the mean and variance from the median, range, and the size of a sample. BMC Med Res Methodol. 2005;5:13.

23. Sterne JAC, Savović J, Page MJ, et al. RoB 2: a revised tool for assessing risk of bias in randomised trials. BMJ. 2019;366:l4898.

24. DerSimonian R, Laird N. Meta-analysis in clinical trials. Control Clin Trials. 1986;7:177–88.

25. Egger M, Davey Smith G, Schneider M, et al. Bias in meta-analysis detected by a simple, graphical test. BMJ. 1997;315(7109):629–34.

26. Abu Elyazed MM, Mostafa SF, Abdelghany MS, Eid GM. Ultrasound-guided erector spinae plane block in patients undergoing open epigastric hernia repair: a prospective randomized controlled study. Anesth Analg. 2019;129:235–40.

27. Aksu C, Kus A, Yorukoglu HU, Kilic CT, Gurkan Y. Analgesic effect of the bi-level injection erector spinae plane block after breast surgery: a randomized controlled trial. Agri. 2019;31:132–7.

28. Ciftci B, Aksoy M, Ince I, Ahıskalıoglu A, Yılmazel UE. The effects of positive end-expiratory pressure at different levels on postoperative respiration parameters in patients undergoing laparoscopic cholecystectomy. J Investig Surg. 2018;31:114–20.

29. Gürkan Y, Aksu C, Kuş A, Yörükoğlu UH, Kılıç CT. Ultrasound guided erector spinae plane block reduces postoperative opioid consumption following breast surgery: a randomized controlled study. J Clin Anesth. 2018;50:65–8.

30. Hamed MA, Goda AS, Basiony MM, Fargaly OS, Abdelhady MA. Erector spinae plane block for postoperative analgesia in patients undergoing total abdominal hysterectomy: a randomized controlled study original study. J Pain Res. 2019;12:1393–8.

31. Krishna SN, Chauhan S, Bhoi D, et al. Bilateral erector spinae plane block for acute post-surgical pain in adult cardiac surgical patients: a randomized controlled trial. J Cardiothorac Vasc Anesth. 2019;33:368–75.

32. Oksuz G, Bilgen F, Arslan M, Duman Y, Urfalıoglu A, Bilal B. Ultrasound-guided bilateral erector spinae block versus tumescent anesthesia for postoperative analgesia in patients undergoing reduction mammoplasty: a randomized controlled study. Aesthet Plast Surg. 2019;43:291–6.

33. Singh S, Kumar G, Akhileshwar. Ultrasound-guided erector spinae plane block for postoperative analgesia in modified radical mastectomy: A randomised control study. Indian J Anaesth. 2019;63:200–4.

34. Singh S, Choudhary NK, Lalin D, Verma VK. Bilateral ultrasound-guided erector spinae plane block for postoperative analgesia in lumbar spine surgery: a randomized control trial. J Neurosurg Anesthesiol. 2019. https://doi.org/10.1097/ANA.0000000000000603.

35. Tulgar S, Kapakli MS, Senturk O, Selvi O, Serifsoy TE, Ozer Z. Evaluation of ultrasound-guided erector spinae plane block for postoperative analgesia in laparoscopic cholecystectomy: a prospective, randomized, controlled clinical trial. J Clin Anesth. 2018;49:101–6.

36. Tulgar S, Kose HC, Selvi O, et al. Comparison of ultrasound-guided lumbar erector spinae plane block and Transmuscular Quadratus Lumborum block for postoperative analgesia in hip and proximal femur surgery: a prospective randomized feasibility study. Anesth Essays Res. 2018;12:825–31.

37. Tulgar S, Kapakli MS, Kose HC, et al. Evaluation of ultrasound-guided erector spinae plane block and oblique subcostal transversus abdominis plane block in laparoscopic cholecystectomy: randomized, controlled, Prospective Study. Anesth Essays Res. 2019;13:50–6.

38. Yayik AM, Cesur S, Ozturk F, et al. Postoperative analgesic efficacy of the ultrasound-guided erector spinae plane block in patients undergoing lumbar spinal decompression surgery: a randomized controlled study. World Neurosurg. 2019;126:e779–85.

39. Herbst MO, Price MD, Soto RG. Pain related readmissions /revisits following same-day surgery: Have they decreased over a decade? J Clin Anesth. 2017;42:15.

40. Shanthanna H, Paul J, Lovrics P, et al. Satisfactory analgesia with minimal emesis in day surgeries: a randomised controlled trial of morphine versus hydromorphone. Br J Anaesth. 2019;122:e107–13.

41. Smith GA, Chirieleison S, Levin J, et al. Impact of length of stay on HCAPS scores following lumbar spine surgery. J Neurosurg Spine. 2019;31(3):366–71.

42. Fujii T, Shibata Y, Akane A, et al. A randomised controlled trial of pectoral nerve-2 (PECS 2) block vs. serratus plane block for chronic pain after mastectomy. Anaesthesia. 2019;74(12):1558–62.

43. De Oliveira GS, Castro Alves LJ, Nader A, Kendall MC, Rahangdale R, McCarthy RJ. Perineural dexamethasone to improve postoperative analgesia with peripheral nerve blocks: a meta-analysis of randomized controlled trials. Pain Res Treat. 2014;2014:179029.

44. Gasanova I, Alexander JC, Estrera K, et al. Ultrasound-guided suprainguinal fascia iliaca compartment block versus periarticular infiltration for pain management after total hip arthroplasty: a randomized controlled trial. Reg Anesth Pain Med. 2019;44(2):206–11.

45. De Cassai A, Andreatta G, Bonvicini D, Boscolo A, Munari M, Navalesi P. Injectate spread in ESP block: a review of anatomical investigations. J Clin Anesth. 2020;61:109669.

46. Nagaraja PS, Ragavendran S, Singh NG, et al. Comparison of continuous thoracic epidural analgesia with bilateral erector spinae plane block for perioperative pain management in cardiac surgery. Ann Card Anaesth. 2018;21:323 7.

47. Heinink T. Erector spinae block or paravertebral block or thoracic epidural for analgesia after rib fracture? Anaesthesia. 2019;74(8):1066.

48. Wang HJ, Liu Y, Ge WW, et al. Comparison of ultrasound-guided serratus anterior plane block and erector spinae plane block perioperatively in radical mastectomy. Zhonghua Yi Xue Za Zhi. 2019;99(23):1809–13.

49. Tulgar S, Selvi O, Senturk O, Serifsoy TE, Thomas DT. Ultrasound-guided erector spinae plane block : Indications, Complications, and Effects on Acute and Chronic Pain Based on a Single-center Experience. Cureus. 2019;11:e3815.

50. Kot Baixauli P, Rodriguez Gimillo P, Baldo Gosalvez J, De Andrés Ibáñez J. The erector spinae plane block (ESPB) in the management of chronic thoracic pain. Correlation of pain/analgesia areas and long-term effect of the treatment in three cases. Rev Esp Anestesiol Reanim. 2019;66(8):443–6.

51. Forero M, Rajarathinam M, Adhikary S, Chin KJ. Continuous erector spinae plane block for rescue analgesia in thoracotomy after epidural failure: a case report. A Case Rep. 2017;8(10):254–6.

52. Scimia P, Basso Ricci E, Droghetti A, Fusco P. The ultrasound-guided continuous erector spinae plane block for postoperative analgesia in video-assisted thoracoscopic lobectomy. Reg Anesth Pain Med. 2017;42(4):537.

3

Effect of magnesium supplementation on emergence delirium and postoperative pain in children undergoing strabismus surgery

Ji-Hyun Lee, Seungeun Choi, Minkyoo Lee, Young-Eun Jang, Eun-Hee Kim, Jin-Tae Kim and Hee-Soo Kim[*]

Abstract

Background: The benefits of intraoperative magnesium supplementation have been reported. In this prospective, randomized study, the effects of magnesium supplementation during general anaesthesia on emergence delirium and postoperative pain in children were evaluated.

Methods: A total of 66 children aged 2 to 5 years who underwent strabismus surgery were assigned to the magnesium or to the control group. Preoperative anxiety was assessed using the modified Yale Preoperative Anxiety Scale. After anaesthesia induction, the magnesium group received an initial loading dose of 30 mg/kg magnesium sulphate over 10 min and, then, continuous infusion of 10 mg/kg per h until 10 min before the end of the surgery. The control group received an equal volume of normal saline via the same regimen. The Paediatric Anaesthesia Emergence Delirium (PAED) score, pain score, and respiratory events were assessed at the postanaesthetic care unit.

Results: Data obtained from 65 children were analyzed. The PAED and pain scores of the two groups did not differ significantly. There were 26 of 33 (78.8%) and 27 of 32 (84.4%) children with emergence delirium in the control and the magnesium groups, respectively (odds ratio 0.69, 95% CI 0.19–2.44; $p = 0.561$). The preoperative anxiety score was not significantly correlated with the PAED score. The incidence of respiratory events during the emergence period did not differ significantly between the two groups.

Conclusions: Magnesium supplementation during anaesthesia had no significant effects on the incidence of emergence delirium or postoperative pain in children undergoing strabismus surgery.

Keywords: Emergence delirium, Magnesium, Ophthalmologic surgical procedure, Paediatrics, Pain

* Correspondence: dami0605@snu.ac.kr
Department of Anaesthesiology and Pain Medicine, Seoul National University Hospital, Seoul National University College of Medicine, # 101 Daehakno, Jongnogu, Seoul 03080, Republic of Korea

Background

Emergence delirium after general anaesthesia is a common phenomenon, and rates > 80% have been reported in children [1]. It has been associated with fast-acting inhalation anaesthetics, such as sevoflurane or desflurane, male sex, ophthalmology and otolaryngology procedures, younger age, and preoperative anxiety, and its incidence has been shown to be reduced by intraoperative opioids, benzodiazepine, and alpha 2 adrenergic agonists [2].

Magnesium is the fourth most common cation in the human body and known to be a modulator of transmembrane ion transport and energy metabolism [3]. Magnesium sulphate is an N-methyl-D-aspartate receptor antagonist that is used to treat hypomagnesemia, preeclampsia and polymorphic ventricular arrhythmia, and also used as an anti-convulsive agent. Additionally, the use of magnesium during the perioperative period has been associated with increased sedation, analgesia, reduced administration of neuromuscular blockade agents, and the prevention of ischemic-reperfusion injury [4, 5]. In children, intraoperative infusion of magnesium may reduce emergence delirium after adenotonsillectomy [6] and hernia repair [7]. However, Apan et al. [8] reported that magnesium supplementation had no influence on the incidence of emergence delirium in paediatric patients.

Perioperative hypomagnesemia is common because some intravenous fluid solutions administered during fasting, including Hartman solution and normal saline, do not contain magnesium [9]. Therefore, magnesium supplementation during anaesthesia can reduce the required amounts of sedatives, analgesics, or neuromuscular blocking agents, and contribute to improved postoperative outcomes [10]. We hypothesised that magnesium supplementation in paediatric patients may also be associated with reductions in the amounts of anaesthetics and analgesics required, and reduced postoperative emergence delirium. Our aim was to evaluate the effects of magnesium supplementation during general anaesthesia on emergence delirium and postoperative pain in children undergoing strabismus surgery. Other post-anaesthesia recovery parameters, including nausea, vomiting, and respiratory complications, were also assessed.

Methods

Study population

This single-centre study was performed at the Seoul National University Children's Hospital, a tertiary children's hospital in South Korea. Sixty-six children aged 2–5 years (American Society of Anesthesiologists physical status I or II) who were scheduled for elective strabismus surgery under general anaesthesia were included. The exclusion criteria were as follows: history of hypersensitivity and malignant hyperthermia, currently taking an anti-epileptic drug, known myasthenia gravis, myasthenic syndrome, neuromuscular disease, arrhythmia,

moderate cardiovascular, pulmonary, hepatobiliary, or renal disease, or overweight (body mass index > 85 percentile). The study protocol was approved by the Institutional Review Board of the Seoul National University Hospital (approval number: H1703–110-840; date of approval: May 8, 2017) and was registered at https://clinicaltrials.gov (number: NCT03132701; principal investigator: Hee-Soo Kim; date of registration: April 9, 2017). The anaesthesiologists involved in the study obtained written informed consent from the parents or their guardians after explaining the study protocol to them.

Group allocation

This study was a randomised, controlled, parallel-designed trial. Following a simple randomisation procedure (computerised random number; https://www.randomizer.org), the children were allocated to the magnesium or the control group. An anaesthetic nurse who was not involved in the study prepared coded and sealed, opaque envelopes, and the allocation ratio was 1:1. Immediately before induction of anaesthesia, she prepared the study drug, either magnesium or normal saline, according to group allocation. The patients, attending anaesthesiologists, and two researchers (LJH and CSE) who assessed the preoperative anxiety and outcomes including delirium scale and pain score were blinded to group allocations.

Anaesthesia and study protocol

All strabismus surgeries were performed as day surgeries, and started before 11 am according to the day-surgery policy of our centre. All patients had the following minimum fasting time; 8 h for heavy meal, 6 h for light meal and non-human milk, and 2 h for clear fluid. An intravenous line was established in all children before anaesthetic induction, and Ringer's lactate solution was administered before and during anaesthesia.

The extent of preoperative anxiety was assessed using the modified Yale Preoperative Anxiety Scale (m-YPAS) [11] when patients and their parents arrived at the reception area of the operating room. Anaesthesia induction was commenced with atropine 0.02 mg/kg, propofol 2.5 mg/kg after electrocardiography monitoring, pulse oximetry, and non-invasive blood pressure determination. No other systemic or local analgesics, such as opioids or eye drops, were used during the induction period. Facemask ventilation was performed with sevoflurane and 100% oxygen and, then, a flexible laryngeal mask airway (Marshall flexible LAD®, Marshall Airway Products Ltd., Radstock, UK) was inserted. The intracuff pressure of the laryngeal mask airway was adjusted within 30–40 cmH_2O using a cuff manometer (VBM Medizintechnik GmbH, Sulz am Neckar, Germany). Neuromuscular blocking agents were not used basically, but allowed as needed for the maintenance of anaesthesia. Mechanical ventilation was commenced using volume-controlled mode with tidal volume of 8 ml/kg without positive end-expiratory pressure. During anaesthesia, sevoflurane concentration was controlled to maintain a bispectral index target between 40 and 60.

At the beginning of anaesthesia induction, the children in the magnesium group received an initial intravenous loading dose of 30 mg/kg magnesium sulphate over 10 min (0.3 ml/kg), then continuous infusion of 10 mg/kg (0.1 ml/kg) per h until 10 min before the end of surgery. The control group received an equal volume of normal saline via the same infusion regimen. Preparations of ephedrine and atropine were readied for possible complications such as hypotension and bradycardia.

At the end of surgery, propacetamol 30 mg/kg was administered to all patients. After gentle pharyngeal suction, the laryngeal mask airway was removed and the patient was transferred to the postanaesthetic care unit (PACU). Complications during the emergence period, such as laryngospasm, bronchospasm, desaturation, breath holding, and coughing were recorded.

At the PACU, all patients' vital signs, including heart rate, noninvasive blood pressure, respiratory rate, and peripheral oxygen saturation, were continuously monitored and recorded every 5 min. The Paediatric Anaesthesia Emergence Delirium (PAED) score (Fig. 1a) [12] and other complications were assessed on arrival in the PACU and every 10 min until discharge from the PACU. The pain score (Children's Hospital of Eastern Ontario Pain scale; CHEOPS, Fig. 1b [13]) was also assessed on arrival in the PACU, at 30 min after arrival, and at discharge. When the PAED score was greater than 12, which was considered as the presence of emergence derlirium [14], nalbuphine 0.1 mg/kg was administered intravenously. When the CHEOPS score was more than 7, ketorolac 0.5 mg/kg was administered intravenously if the patients did not receive nalbuphine. Patients were discharged from the PACU when they had a modified Aldrete score greater than 9. The patients were continuously monitored for complications, including nausea, vomiting and respiratory concerns. Symptoms of hypermagnesaemia, such as hypotension, bradycardia, lethargy, paralysis and headache, were also monitored until

A. PAED score

Behaviour	Not at all	Just a little	Quite a bit	Very much	Extremely
Makes eye contact with caregiver	4	3	2	1	0
Actions are purposeful	4	3	2	1	0
Aware of surroundings	4	3	2	1	0
Restless	0	1	2	3	4
Inconsolable	0	1	2	3	4

B. CHEOP scale

Points	Crying	Facial expressions	Child verbal	Torso	Touch	Legs
0	Smiling	Smiling	Positive			
1	No cry	Composed	None, complaints other than pain	Neutral	Not touching	Neutral
2	Moaning, crying	Grimace	Pain-related complaints, both pain and nonpain-related complaint	Shifting, tense, shivering, upright, restrained	Reach, touch, grab, restrained	Squirming kicking, drawn up, tensed, standing, restrained
3	Screaming					

Fig. 1 Pediatric Anaesthesia Emergence Delirium score (**a**) and Children's Hospital of Eastern Ontario Pain scale (**b**)

the patients were discharged from the ambulatory surgery centre.

Statistical analysis

The primary outcome of this study was the PAED score in both groups. The occurrence of emergence delirium was defined when the PAED scores were ≥ 12 at any time point in the PACU. The secondary outcomes included the incidence of emergence delirium during PACU stay, CHEOPS score, incidence of nausea, vomiting and respiratory complications, and length of PACU stay.

The sample size was calculated based on a previous study [6] that investigated the effects of intra-operative magnesium sulphate administration on the incidence of emergence delirium in children who had undergone adenotonsillectomy. In that study, the respective rates of emergence delirium in the magnesium and the control group were 36 and 72%, respectively. Thus, the sample size required for our study was calculated to be approximately 30 patients per group, with an alpha error of 0.05 and a power of 0.8, as determined via PASS software 2008 (version 8.0.16; NCSS statistical software, Kaysville, UT, USA). Based on an attrition rate of up to 10%, a total of 66 patients were enrolled.

All data were analysed using SPSS for Windows (version 23.0; IBM Corp., Armonk, NY, USA). Data normality was assessed using the Kolmogorov–Smirnov test. Categorical variables are expressed as numbers and percentages, and continuous variables as means and standard deviations or medians and interquartile ranges. The Chi-square test was used to assess the significance of categorical data comparisons, and the Fisher's exact test was used when the expected count of > 20% cells was less than five. The Pearson's correlational analysis was performed to assess the correlation between the preoperative anxiety and PAED scores. The Student's t-test or the Mann–Whitney rank-sum test were used to examine the significance of continuous data comparisons. Repeated measures data were analysed by the analysis of variance, and the Bonferroni's correction was used for post-hoc analysis. All p values < 0.05 were considered statistically significant.

Results

A total of 66 paediatric patients were initially enrolled from June to December 2017, and randomised into two groups. One patient in the magnesium group was subsequently excluded due to a lack of PAED and pain score assessment. Therefore, data from 65 children (33 and 32 in the control and the magnesium group, respectively) were analysed (Fig. 2).

Table 1 shows the demographic data of patients in the magnesium and the control groups. There were no significant differences in baseline characteristics including

the preoperative m-YPAS scores between the two groups.

Table 2 shows the postoperative PAED and the CHEOPS scores in both groups. The median PAED scores over time did not differ significantly (p = 0.806) between the two groups. Figure 3a shows the PAED scores over time in both groups. The incidences of emergence delirium were 26 (78.8%) and 27 (84.4%) in the control and the magnesium groups, respectively (OR 0.69, 95% CI 0.19–2.44, p = 0.56).

The CHEOPS scores over time did not differ significantly between the two groups (Fig. 3b). No rescue analgesics were administered in the PACU in either group. The m-YPAS score was not significantly correlated with the PAED score at any time-point (PACU entry, r = 0.1, p = 0.438; after 10 min, r = 0.12, p = 0.336; after 20 min, r = 0.04, p = 0.750; after 30 min, r = 0.07, p = 0.599; exiting PACU, r = 0.13, p = 0.343).

Table 3 shows the intraoperative variable data in both groups. The peak inspiratory pressure, the mean sevoflurane concentration, and mean bispectral index value during surgery did not differ significantly in the two groups. There were no differences in the intraoperative mean heart rate and blood pressures between the two groups. During emergence, the diastolic and mean blood pressures were higher in the control group than in the magnesium group (diastolic blood pressure: 68 [15] vs 60 [11] mmHg, mean differences [95% CI], 8 [3–13] mmHg, p = 0.004; mean blood pressure: 84 [13] vs 76 [10] mmHg, mean differences [95% CI], 7 [1–13] mmHg, p = 0.015).

In the PACU, no patient experienced nausea and vomiting. There were no significant complications during the PACU stay in both groups. Moreover, the length of stay at the PACU was similar between the two groups.

Discussion

In this study, we found that magnesium supplementation during strabismus surgery had no significant effect on the incidence of emergence delirium and postoperative pain in children. In addition, there was no significant difference in respiratory complications, length of PACU stay, and other intraoperative parameters between the magnesium and control groups. Lastly, there were no complications associated with intraoperative magnesium supplementation.

Although the mechanism of emergence delirium after general anaesthesia has not been clearly defined, there are some well-known risk factors including young age, no previous surgery, ophthalmology procedures, otorhinolaryngology procedures, volatile anaesthetics such as sevoflurane, and preoperative anxiety [2, 15]. In addition, postoperative pain evidently may have a role in emergence delirium because the administration of

Table 1 Demographic characteristics of the study population

	Control (n = 33)	Magnesium (n = 32)	P value
Age (years)	4.4 ± 0.9	4.0 ± 1.2	0.218
Sex (M/F, %)	14/19 (42.4/57.6)	14/18 (43.8/56.3)	0.914
Height (cm)	108.6 ± 8.0	105.4 ± 9.0	0.135
Weight (kg)	18.4 ± 3.0	17.4 ± 3.1	0.176
Operation time (min)	25 (20–35)	20 (15–28.75)	0.138
Anesthesia time (min)	44.8 ± 2.6	40.8 ± 10.9	0.180
Size of laryngeal mask airway (2/2.5, %)	26/7 (78.8/21.2)	28/4 (87.5/12.5)	0.511
m-YPAS			
Activity	2.0 (1.0–2.0)	2.0 (1.0–2.0)	0.281
Vocalization	2.0 (1.0–3.0)	2.0 (1.0–3.0)	0.781
Emotional expressivity	2.0 (1.25–3.0)	2.0 (1.0–3.0)	0.300
State of apparent arousal	2.0 (1.0–2.75)	1.0 (1.0–2.0)	0.534
Use of parents	2.0 (1.25–3.0)	2.0 (1.0–3.0)	0.501
Total score	47.5 (30.4–58.0)	41.7 (28.3–60.0)	0.465

Data are presented as mean ± standard deviations, median (interquartile ranges) or number (percentage)
m-YPAS Modified Yale Preoperative Anxiety Scale

analgesics, including opioids, has been reported to prevent the emergence delirium in children [16, 17].

In this report, the term 'emergence delirium' was used to describe the behavioural change following general anaesthesia to maintain consistency with the referenced reports. However, there have been inconsistent use of the terms 'delirium' and 'agitation' in the literature. Emergence delirium refers to an altered state of consciousness, which begins with emergence from anaesthesia and continues through the early recovery period. On the other hand, emergence agitation is an umbrella term, and is affected by emergence delirium, pain, and several

Table 2 Postoperative PAED and CHEOPS scores in both groups

	Control (n = 33)	Magnesium (n = 32)	P value
PAED score			0.806*
PACU in	15.0 (0–18.0)	16.5 (0–19.0)	0.417
10 min	12.0 (0–15.0)	14.0 (0–17.0)	0.313
20 min	10.0 (0–14.0)	11.0 (0–15.0)	0.253
30 min	4.5 (0–12.25)	8.0 (0–15.0)	0.171
PACU out	7.5 (0–12.0)	5 (0–15.0)	0.967
CHEOPS score			0.623*
PACU in	9.0 (4.0–11.0)	10.0 (4.0–12.0)	0.390
30 min	7.0 (4.0–8.0)	7.0 (4.0–9.75)	0.199
PACU out	7.0 (4.0–8.0)	7.0 (4.0–10.0)	0.664

Data are presented as median (interquartile ranges)
*P value from repeated measures ANOVA
CHEOPS Children's Hospital of Eastern Ontario Pain scale, *PACU* Postanaesthetic are unit, *PAED* Pediatric anesthesia emergence delirium

other factors [12, 18]. In this study, PAED scores were used to assess 'delirium' apart from pain.

The activation of N-methyl-D-aspartate (NMDA) receptor changes the excitatory properties of neurons that can induce seizures, and as magnesium is an NMDA receptor antagonist it can have sedative and anticonvulsive effects. In addition, magnesium has analgesic effects and can lead to a reduction in perioperative opioid consumption by blocking the NMDA receptors, which are involved in nociception [9]. Therefore, considering the effect of magnesium and the mechanism of emergence delirium, it is reasonable to expect that magnesium may reduce emergence delirium.

There are limited data pertaining to the association between magnesium supplementation and reduced emergence delirium [6, 7]. According to Abdulatif et al. [6], 30 mg/kg bolus intravenous magnesium sulphate followed by 10 mg/kg per h during sevoflurane anaesthesia reduced the incidence of emergence delirium with a relative risk of 0.51 in children undergoing adenotonsillectomy [6]. Bondok et al. [7] reported that no emergence delirium occurred in male children who received magnesium supplementation undergoing elective inguinal herniorrhaphy.

To the best of our knowledge, this is the first study that evaluated the effect of magnesium supplementation in children undergoing ophthalmic surgery. There were some differences between the present study and previous studies. In two studies demonstrating the beneficial effect of magnesium, combination analgesic therapy was used with opioids, non-steroidal anti-inflammatory drugs, and regional block [6, 7]. In our study, we used

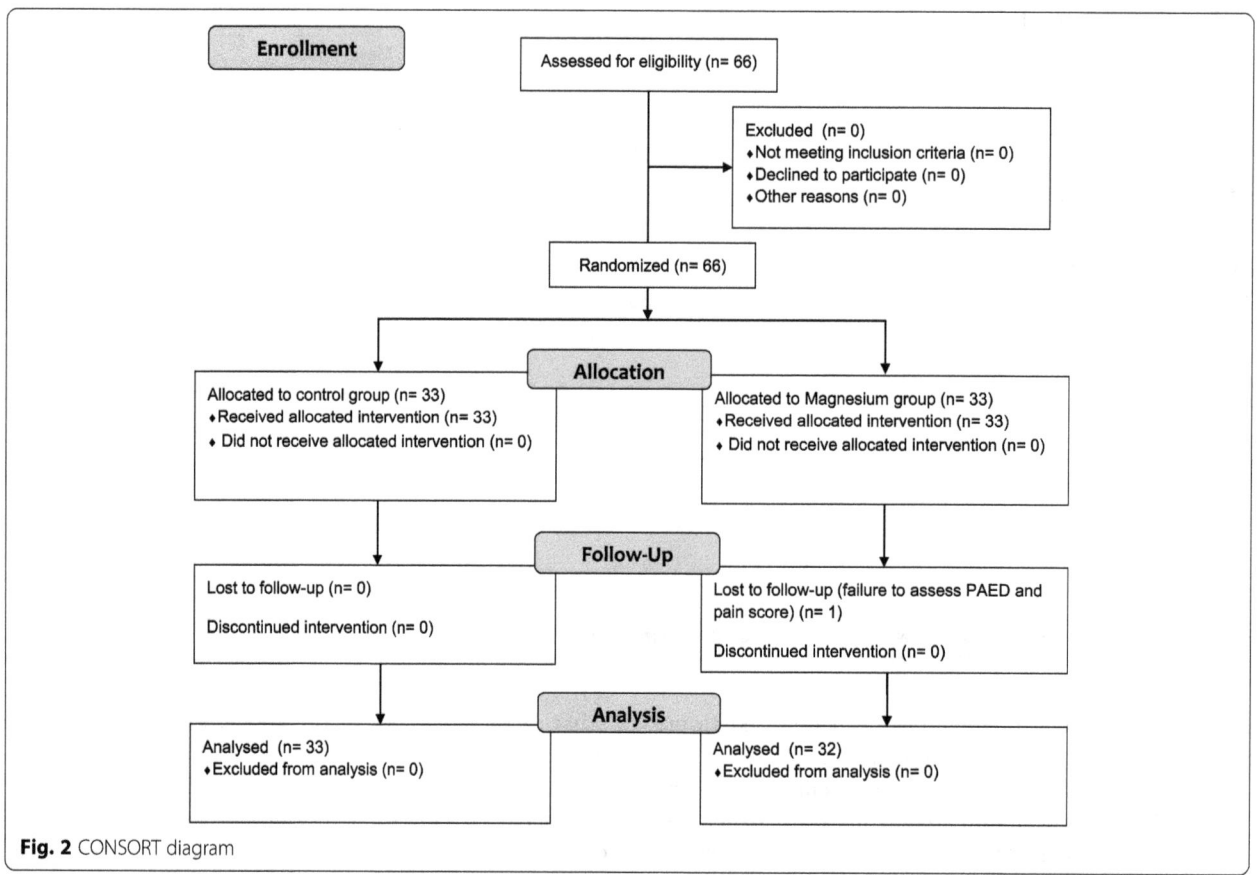

Fig. 2 CONSORT diagram

propacetamol only for pain control to minimise the confounding effects of analgesics. The differences in the analgesic use and type of surgery might contribute to the higher incidence of emergence delirium in this study (approximately 80%) compared to that in previous studies (35% [6] and 50% [7]).

There are several possible reasons for the nonsignificant association between magnesium and emergence delirium observed in this study. Magnesium concentrations may have been within the normal range even in the control group, as it was reported by Apan et al. [8] Therefore, the additional increase in magnesium concentration may not have functioned to reduce emergence delirium or pain. In addition, genetic factors may also be relevant. Genetic differences in pain sensitivity [19], responses to analgesics due to alterations of pharmacokinetic and pharmacodynamic parameters [20, 21], and emergence delirium [22] have been reported. Additionally, there may be differences associated with race. Finally, there might be other factors that influenced the occurrence of emergence delirium. According to Joo et al., emergence delirium was associated with the level of invasiveness of the procedure in children undergoing ophthalmic surgery [23]. There were wide variations in operating time in this study, and we speculated that complexity of surgery, surgical skill, or operation time

might be potential factors affecting the recovery characteristics.

Preoperative anxiety can affect emergence delirium [2, 24], and several studies have reported their association [25, 26]. However, in this study, we could not find a correlation between the m-YPAS and PAED scale. Our result was similar to that of a previous study, suggesting that visual disturbances might play a greater role in emergence delirium compared with preoperative anxiety [23].

Previous studies concluded that perioperative adjuvant magnesium sulphate administration reduced the requirements for nondepolarizing neuromuscular blockers [27–29]. We also expected that intraoperative magnesium supplementation could reduce the peak inspiratory pressure and spontaneous respiratory effort, as magnesium has property for potentiation of muscle relaxation and, thus, no neuromuscular blockade was used in the present study [10]. However, we could not find the group difference in the peak inspiratory pressure and incidence of spontaneous respiratory effort.

On the other hand, the control group showed higher diastolic and mean blood pressure during the emergence period when compared to the magnesium group. Magnesium has vasodilatory effects, and is known to reduce the need for alpha-beta blockers [9]. Hypotension is one of the complications of magnesium administration,

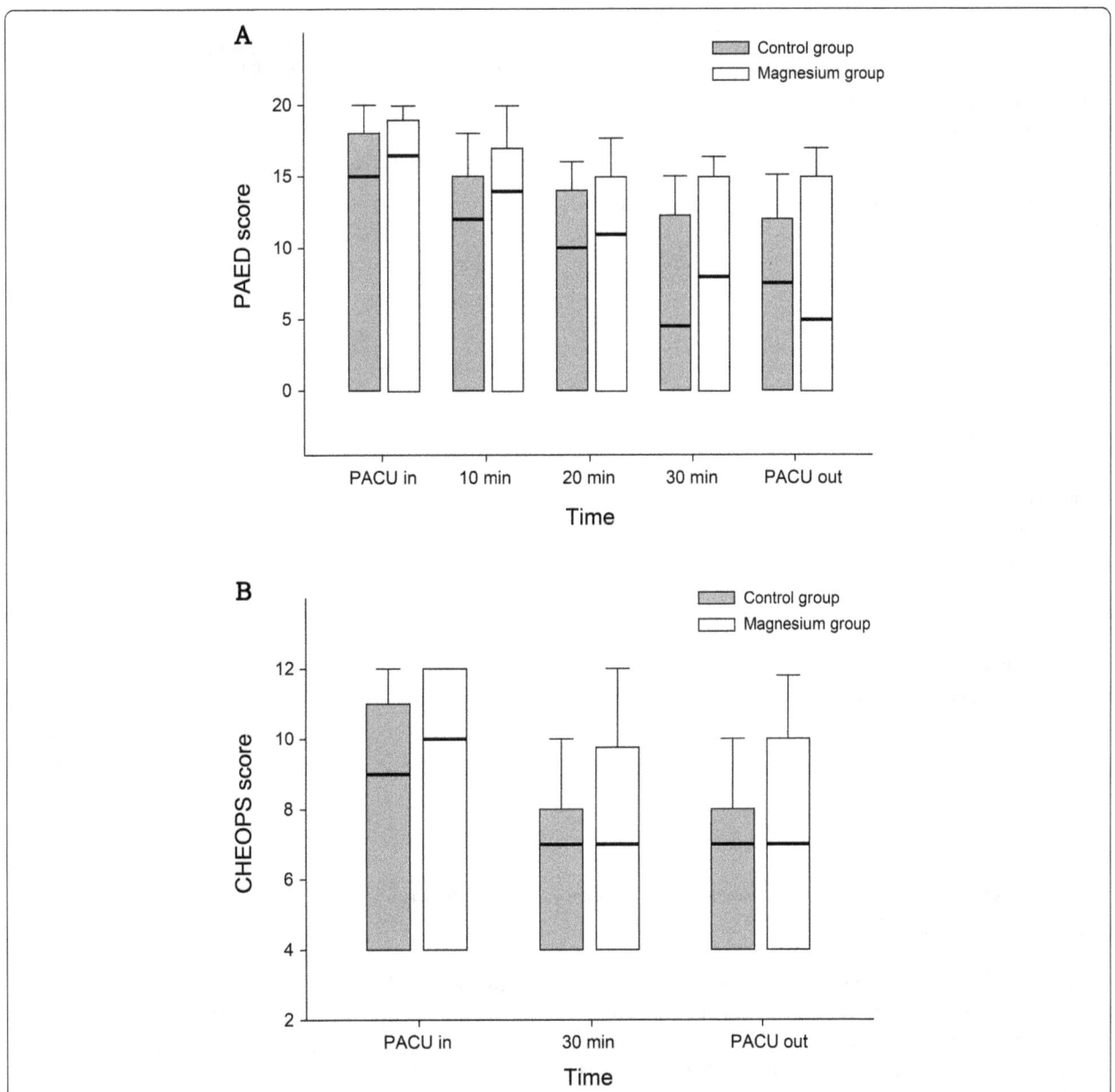

Fig. 3 The PAED score (**a**) and the CHEOPS score (**b**) over time in both groups. The boundary of the box indicates the 25th and 75th percentile, and a bold line within the box marks the median. The error bars indicate the 10th and 90th percentiles. PAED, Pediatric Anaesthesia Emergence Delirium; CHEOPS, Children's Hospital of Eastern Ontario Pain Scale

which can occur when the serum magnesium level exceeds 3–4 mg/dl [9]. Although we could not assess the serum magnesium level, there were no patients with significant hypotension. Sympathetic tone usually increases during the emergence period, and we speculated that magnesium may prevent the further increase in blood pressure in the magnesium group.

Our study had some limitations. The sample size was too small with regard to the statistical power, as it was calculated based on previous studies, in which there were significant differences between the control and magnesium groups [6]. Additionally, the serum magnesium levels were not evaluated before and after the administration of magnesium sulphate in all patients. Magnesium supplementation can be helpful when hypomagnesemia is obvious, but hypomagnesemia may not be commonly associated with short operations and minimal fasting times [8]. Second, there might be a possibility of hypermagnesemia and safety issue should be considered. The possible adverse effects of hypermagnesemia are bradycardia and hypotension. However, there were no cases of clinical consequences and no need for

Table 3 Intraoperative and postoperative variables of both groups

	Control (n = 33)	Magnesium (n = 32)	P value
Number of attempts for laryngeal mask airway insertion	1 (1–1)	1 (1–1)	0.965
Number of cases for laryngeal mask repositioning	0	0	.
Mean sevoflurane concentration (vol%)	2.7 ± 0.3	2.5 ± 0.4	0.707
Intraoperative mean BIS value	50 ± 4	49 ± 3	0.192
Peak inspiratory pressure (cmH₂O)			
Maximum pressure	15.2 ± 4.6	15.6 ± 4.8	0.790
Minimum pressure	12.7 ± 2.2	13.3 ± 2.4	0.359
Intraoperative hemodynamic parameters			
Heart rate (bpm)	129 ± 18	134 ± 13	0.219
Systolic blood pressure (mmHg)	92 ± 7	93 ± 10	0.611
Diastolic blood pressure (mmHg)	49 ± 8	48 ± 8	0.391
Mean blood pressure (mmHg)	66 ± 9	63 ± 7	0.231
Hemodynamic parameters during emergence			
Heart rate (bpm)	122 ± 19	124 ± 14	0.628
Systolic blood pressure (mmHg)	107 ± 15	101 ± 11	0.087
Diastolic blood pressure (mmHg)	68 ± 15	60 ± 11	0.004*
Mean blood pressure (mmHg)	84 ± 13	76 ± 10	0.015*
Time from surgery end to PACU admission (min)	5.9 ± 2.2	6.1 ± 2.8	0.733
Respiratory event during emergence	8 (24.2%)	8 (25.0%)	1.0
Laryngospasm	0	1 (3.1%)	1.0
Desaturation	4 (12.1%)	2 (6.3%)	0.672
Breath holding	2 (6.1%)	0	0.492
Coughing	4 (12.1%)	5 (15.6%)	1.0
Length of PACU stay	34.2 (3.1)	34.5 (5.4)	0.771

Data are presented as median (interquartile ranges), mean ± standard deviations or number (percentages)
*P < 0.05 between the control and magnesium groups
BIS Bispectral index, PACU Postanaesthetic care unit

treatment withdrawal in paediatric population [9]. In addition, there were no critical incidents related to magnesium supplementation in the present study. Third, the incidence of emergence delirium was higher than expected when calculating the sample size. This may be associated with the relatively high pain scores in our patients. When preschool children with emergence delirium have pain, pain-related behaviour could be assessed as emergence delirium [30]. Additionally, postoperative nausea and vomiting may present as agitation. Finally, the PAED and pain scores were assessed only in the PACU. The data would have been more informative and valuable if the patients were followed up for emergence delirium and pain in the first 24 h postoperatively.

In conclusion, in our study magnesium supplementation had no significant effect on emergence agitation or postoperative pain in children who had undergone strabismus surgery. Other strategies to minimise emergence agitation in children should also be investigated.

Abbreviations
BIS: Bispectral index; CHEOPS: Children's Hospital of Eastern Ontario Pain scale; m-YPAS: Modified Yale Preoperative Anxiety Scale; NMDA: N-methyl-D-aspartate; PACU: Postanaesthetic care unit; PAED: Paediatric Anaesthesia Emergence Delirium

Acknowledgments
None.

Authors' contributions
KHS, LJH and KJT designed the study, performed the statistical analysis, and drafted the manuscript. CSE, LMK and JYE interpreted the data, revised the manuscript, collected the data and assisted in drafting the manuscript. KEH revised the manuscript and approved the version to be published. All authors read and approved the final submitted version of the manuscript.

References
1. Cole JW, Murray DJ, McAllister JD, Hirshberg GE. Emergence behaviour in children: defining the incidence of excitement and agitation following anaesthesia. Paediatr Anaesth. 2002;12(5):442–7.
2. Mason KP. Paediatric emergence delirium: a comprehensive review and interpretation of the literature. BJA. 2017;118(3):335–43.
3. de Baaij JH, Hoenderop JG, Bindels RJ. Magnesium in man: implications for health and disease. Physiol Rev. 2015;95(1):1–46.

4. Lysakowski C, Dumont L, Czarnetzki C, Tramer MR. Magnesium as an adjuvant to postoperative analgesia: a systematic review of randomized trials. Anesth Analg. 2007;104(6):1532–9.

5. Albrecht E, Kirkham KR, Liu SS, Brull R. Peri-operative intravenous administration of magnesium sulphate and postoperative pain: a meta-analysis. Anaesthesia. 2013;68(1):79–90.

6. Abdulatif M, Ahmed A, Mukhtar A, Badawy S. The effect of magnesium sulphate infusion on the incidence and severity of emergence agitation in children undergoing adenotonsillectomy using sevoflurane anaesthesia. Anaesthesia. 2013;68(10):1045–52.

7. Bondok R, Ali R. Magnesium sulfate reduces sevoflurane-induced emergence agitation in pediatric patients. Ain Shams J Anaesthesiol. 2014; 7(3):282–8.

8. Apan A, Aykac E, Kazkayasi M, Doganci N, Tahran FD. Magnesium sulphate infusion is not effective on discomfort or emergence phenomenon in paediatric adenoidectomy/tonsillectomy. Int J Pediatr Otorhinolaryngol. 2010;74(12):1367–71.

9. Eizaga Rebollar R, Garcia Palacios MV, Morales Guerrero J, Torres LM. Magnesium sulfate in pediatric anesthesia: the super adjuvant. Paediatr Anaesth. 2017;27(5):480–9.

10. Do S-H. Magnesium: a versatile drug for anesthesiologists. Korean J Anesthesiol. 2013;65(1):4–8.

11. Kain ZN, Mayes LC, Cicchetti DV, Bagnall AL, Finley JD, Hofstadter MB. The Yale preoperative anxiety scale: how does it compare with a "gold standard"? Anesth Analg. 1997;85(4).783–8.

12. Sikich N, Lerman J. Development and psychometric evaluation of the pediatric anesthesia emergence delirium scale. Anesthesiology. 2004;100(5): 1138–45.

13. McGrath PA. The multidimensional assessment and management of recurrent pain syndromes in children. Behav Res Ther. 1987;25(4):251–62.

14. Driscoll JN, Bender BM, Archilla CA, Klim CM, Hossain MJ, Mychaskiw GN, Wei JL. Comparing incidence of emergence delirium between sevoflurane and desflurane in children following routine otolaryngology procedures. Minerva Anestesiol. 2017;83(4):383–91.

15. Voepel-Lewis T, Malviya S, Tait AR. A prospective cohort study of emergence agitation in the pediatric postanesthesia care unit. Anesth Analg. 2003;96(6):1625–30.

16. Fan KT, Lee TH, Yu KL, Tang CS, Lu DV, Chen PY, Soo LY. Influences of tramadol on emergence characteristics from sevoflurane anesthesia in pediatric ambulatory surgery. Kaohsiung J Med Sci. 2000;16(5):255–60.

17. Dahmani S, Stany I, Brasher C, Lejeune C, Bruneau B, Wood C, Nivoche Y, Constant I, Murat I. Pharmacological prevention of sevoflurane- and desflurane-related emergence agitation in children: a meta-analysis of published studies. Br J Anaesth. 2010;104(2):216–23.

18. Bajwa SA, Costi D, Cyna AM. A comparison of emergence delirium scales following general anesthesia in children. Paediatr Anaesth. 2010;20(8):704–11.

19. Crews KR, Gaedigk A, Dunnenberger HM, Leeder JS, Klein TE, Caudle KE, Haidar CE, Shen DD, Callaghan JT, Sadhasivam S, et al. Clinical Pharmacogenetics implementation consortium guidelines for cytochrome P450 2D6 genotype and codeine therapy: 2014 update. Clin Pharmacol Ther. 2014;95(4):376–82.

20. Manworren RC, Jeffries L, Pantaleao A, Seip R, Zempsky WT, Ruano G. Pharmacogenetic testing for analgesic adverse effects: pediatric case series. Clin J Pain. 2016;32(2):109–15.

21. Kolesnikov Y, Gabovits B, Levin A, Voiko E, Veske A. Combined catechol-O-methyltransferase and mu-opioid receptor gene polymorphisms affect morphine postoperative analgesia and central side effects. Anesth Analg. 2011;112(2):448–53.

22. Kim JH. Mechanism of emergence agitation induced by sevoflurane anesthesia. Korean J Anesthesiol. 2011;60(2):73–4.

23. Joo J, Lee S, Lee Y. Emergence delirium is related to the invasiveness of strabismus surgery in preschool-age children. J Int Med Res. 2014;42(6): 1311–22.

24. Kain ZN, Caldwell-Andrews AA, Maranets I, McClain B, Gaal D, Mayes LC, Feng R, Zhang H. Preoperative anxiety and emergence delirium and postoperative maladaptive behaviors. Anesth Analg. 2004;99(6):1648–54.

25. Weldon BC, Bell M, Craddock T. The effect of caudal analgesia on emergence agitation in children after sevoflurane versus halothane anesthesia. Anesth Analg. 2004;98(2):321–6.

26. Konig MW, Varughese AM, Brennen KA, Barclay S, Shackleford TM, Samuels PJ, Gorman K, Ellis J, Wang Y, Nick TG. Quality of recovery from two types of general anesthesia for ambulatory dental surgery in children: a double-blind, randomized trial. Paediatr Anaesth. 2009;19(8):748–55.

27. Na HS, Lee JH, Hwang JY, Ryu JH, Han SH, Jeon YT, Do SH. Effects of magnesium sulphate on intraoperative neuromuscular blocking agent requirements and postoperative analgesia in children with cerebral palsy. Br J Anaesth. 2010;104(3):344–50.

28. Lee DH, Kwon IC. Magnesium sulphate has beneficial effects as an adjuvant during general anaesthesia for caesarean section. Br J Anaesth. 2009;103(6): 861–6.

29. Ryu JH, Kang MH, Park KS, Do SH. Effects of magnesium sulphate on intraoperative anaesthetic requirements and postoperative analgesia in gynaecology patients receiving total intravenous anaesthesia. Br J Anaesth. 2008;100(3):397–403.

30. Aroke EN, Crawford SL, Dungan JR. Pharmacogenetics of ketamine-induced emergence phenomena: a pilot study. Nurs Res. 2017;66(2):105–14.

4

Postoperative pain treatment with erector spinae plane block and pectoralis nerve blocks in patients undergoing mitral/tricuspid valve repair

Bogusław Gawęda[1], Michał Borys[2*] ⓘ, Bartłomiej Belina[3], Janusz Bąk[1], Miroslaw Czuczwar[2],
Bogumiła Wołoszczuk-Gębicka[3], Maciej Kolowca[1] and Kazimierz Widenka[1]

Abstract

Background: Effective postoperative pain control remains a challenge for patients undergoing cardiac surgery. Novel regional blocks may improve pain management for such patients and can shorten their length of stay in the hospital.

To compare postoperative pain intensity in patients undergoing cardiac surgery with either erector spinae plane (ESP) block or combined ESP and pectoralis nerve (PECS) blocks.

Methods: This was a prospective, randomized, controlled, double-blinded study done in a tertiary hospital. Thirty patients undergoing mitral/tricuspid valve repair via mini-thoracotomy were included. Patients were randomly allocated to one of two groups: ESP or PECS + ESP group (1:1 randomization). Patients in both groups received a single-shot, ultrasound-guided ESP block. Participants in PECS + ESP group received additional PECS blocks. Each patient had to be extubated within 2 h from the end of the surgery. Pain was treated via a patient-controlled analgesia (PCA) pump. The primary outcome was the total oxycodone consumption via PCA during the first postoperative day. The secondary outcomes included pain intensity measured on the visual analog scale (VAS), patient satisfaction, Prince Henry Hospital Pain Score (PHHPS), and spirometry.

Results: Patients in the PECS + ESP group used significantly less oxycodone than those in the ESP group: median 12 [interquartile range (IQR): 6–16] mg vs. 20 [IQR: 18–29] mg ($p = 0.0004$). Moreover, pain intensity was significantly lower in the PECS + ESP group at each of the five measurements during the first postoperative day. Patients in the PECS + ESP group were more satisfied with pain management. No difference was noticed between both groups in PHHPS and spirometry.

Conclusions: The addition of PECS blocks to ESP reduced consumption of oxycodone via PCA, reduced pain intensity on the VAS, and increased patient satisfaction with pain management in patients undergoing mitral/tricuspid valve repair via mini-thoracotomy.

Keywords: Erector spinae plane (ESP) block, Pectoralis nerve (PECS) blocks, Patient-controlled analgesia (PCA), Visual analog scale (VAS)

* Correspondence: michalborys1@gmail.com
[2]Second Department of Anesthesia and Intensive Care, Medical University of Lublin, ul. Staszica 16, 20-081 Lublin, Poland

Background

Postoperative pain remains a primary challenge in patients undergoing thoracotomy [1]. Poorly managed postoperative pain is associated with an increased number of postoperative complications, including prolonged mechanical ventilation and pulmonary infections [2, 3]. Well-established pain management is an essential aspect of the Enhanced Recovery After Surgery (ERAS) protocol [4]. Recently, we have attempted to institute the ERAS protocol for cardiac surgery procedures performed in our department. Thus, an effective and safe analgesic technique was needed, which was compatible with the ERAS concept.

Among many regional anesthesia techniques for patients undergoing cardiac surgery, thoracic epidural analgesia (TEA) is associated with reduced incidences of cardiovascular events and infections, lower cost, and shortened length of hospital stay [5–7]. Thoracic paravertebral block (PVB) exhibits similar effectiveness to that of TEA for analgesia after cardiothoracic surgery [8, 9]. Other regional anesthesia techniques are not well-established in cardiothoracic surgery [10]. Novel fascial blocks, including the erector spinae plane (ESP) block and pectoralis nerve (PECS) block, have been recently proposed as effective methods of pain management for patients undergoing cardiac surgery [11, 12].

Our previous, prospective, cohort study demonstrated that the ESP block combined with low-dose intravenous oxycodone was an effective analgesic technique for patients who had undergone mitral or/and tricuspid valve repair via right mini-thoracotomy [13]. In that study, all patients could be weaned from mechanical ventilation within 2 h postoperatively and were transferred to the general ward on the second postoperative day. However, an abrupt reduction in pain intensity was observed at the 24th postoperative hour; this was clearly associated with the removal of chest drains. We hypothesized that an additional regional block, covering the area of the anterior part of the chest wall, might improve postoperative pain management [14, 15].

The objective of this study was to compare postoperative pain intensity in patients undergoing cardiac surgery with either ESP block or combined ESP and PECS blocks by assessing oxycodone consumption during the first operative day (primary objective), as well as by comparing patients' subjective pain intensity by using the visual-analogue scale (VAS, secondary objective).

Methods

This was a randomized, controlled, double-blind trial conducted in a tertiary cardiac surgery department. Before patient recruitment, the study protocol was approved by the Bioethics Committee of the Medical University of Lublin, Lublin, Poland (permit number KE-0254/127/2018), and registered at ClinicalTrials.gov (NCT03592485). Written informed consent was obtained from each patient, and the study was conducted in accordance with the tenets of the Declaration of Helsinki for medical research involving human subjects.

Participants

The inclusion criteria were as follows: patients who (1) required mitral and/or tricuspid valve repair; (2) underwent surgery via right mini-thoracotomy approach; (3) were more than 18 years of age; and (4) were less than 80 years of age. The exclusion criteria included: (1) coagulopathy, defined as known bleeding disorder; (2) allergy to local anaesthetics; (3) depression, which could significantly influence pain perception; (4) epilepsy; (5) antidepressant or epileptic drug treatment; (6) chronic usage of analgesic drugs; (7) addiction to alcohol or recreational drugs. Data from patients who required endotracheal intubation and respiratory support for > 2 h from the end of surgery were also excluded from the analysis.

Intervention

Patients were randomly allocated to one of two groups (1:1 ratio, parallel randomization) via computer-generated randomization conducted by a team member who was not involved in the surgery or patient assessment. The same team member prepared opaque envelopes in which the intervention type was concealed. These envelopes were opened a few minutes before attempting the regional block. Patients were randomly assigned to the ESP or PECS + ESP group.

In the ESP group, ultrasound-guided ESP block at the fourth thoracic level was performed before the surgery and induction of general anesthesia with Ropivacaine (0.375%; Ropimol, Molteni, Italy, 0.2 mL/kg) as described in our previous study (Fig. 1) [13]. The maximum dosage of ropivacaine could not exceed 20 mL in this group. In the PECS + ESP group, in addition to ESP block, ultrasound-guided PECS blocks type I and II were performed. Local anesthetic (6–8 ml) was deposited in the fascial plane between the pectoralis major and minor muscles (PECS I, Fig. 2); 12–14 ml was deposited between the pectoralis minor and serratus anterior muscles (PECS II, Fig. 3). The total dose of local anesthetic could not exceed 40 mL (150 mg of ropivacaine) in this group.

Anesthesia

Etomidate (Hypnomidate, Janssen-Cilag International NV, Belgium), remifentanil (0.5–1.0 mcg kg^{-1} min^{-1}) (Ultiva, GlaxoSmithKline, UK), and rocuronium (0.6 mg kg^{-1}) (Esmeron, N.V. Organon, Holland) were used for the induction of general anesthesia. Maintenance was provided with 0.5 minimum alveolar concentration of sevoflurane (age-adjusted, Sevorane, Abbvie, USA), remifentanil, and

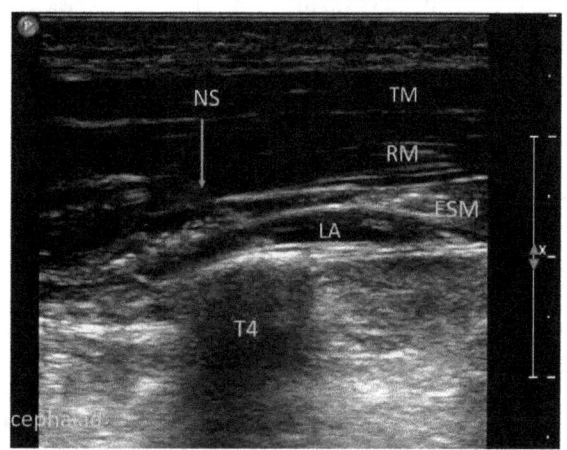

Fig. 1 Erector spinae plane block. ESM – erector spinae muscle, LA – local anesthetic, NS- needle shaft, RM- rhomboid muscle, T4 – the transverse process of the fourth thoracic vertebra, TM – trapezius muscle

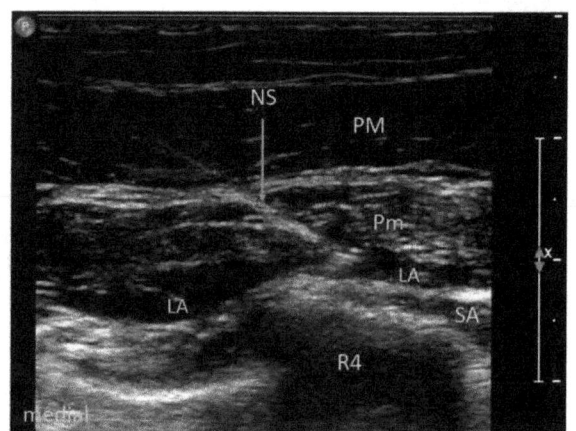

Fig. 3 Pectoralis nerves block type II. LA – local anesthetic, NS – needle shaft, PM – pectoralis major muscle, Pm – pectoralis minor muscle, R4 – fourth rib, SA – serratus anterior muscle

incremental doses of rocuronium. Remifentanil was continued to achieve a target plasma concentration of 4–8 ng ml^{-1} and adjusted to the patient's heart rate and blood pressure. During the procedure, the right lung was deflated, and the left lung was ventilated with a mixture of air and O_2. Residual neuromuscular block was reversed with sugammadex (BridionN.V. Organon, Holland) at the end of surgery.

An intravenous bolus of oxycodone (0.1 mg kg^{-1}) was administered 30 min prior to the surgery end. Patients were transferred to the intensive care unit where target plasma concentration of remifentanil was reduced to 0.5–2 ng ml^{-1}. Ventilation was continued for 60–120 min and patients were observed for occurrence of excessive postoperative

bleeding and hemodynamic instability. If no problems were recognized, remifentanil infusion was discontinued, and the patient's trachea was extubated. Postoperative pain treatment was continued with a patient-controlled analgesia (PCA) pump which supplied oxycodone (1 mg per dose, at 7-min intervals, without basal infusion) during the first 24 postoperative hours.

Moreover, intravenous paracetamol, 1 g per 6 h, was administered routinely. Postoperative pain was evaluated by nurses using the VAS at 2, 4, 6, 8, 12, and 24 h postoperatively. Patients could evaluate their pain severity from 0 (no pain) to 100 mm (maximum pain) on the VAS. If pain intensity exceeding 40 mm on the VAS, up to two extra doses of oxycodone (5 mg each, rescue analgesia) could be administered intravenously by the nurse. Patients were transferred to the surgery ward by the end of the first postoperative day if no complications were present.

Surgery

For mini-invasive mitral and/or tricuspid valve surgery, the patient was placed in the supine position with elevated right hemithorax, and the right upper arm was flexed anteriorly with the forearm in front of the face. Transoesophageal echocardiographic (TEE) monitoring was performed for all patients to confirm the appropriate establishment of cardiopulmonary bypass (CPB), valvular repair, and heart de-airing. The chest was prepared and draped, and the right lung was deflated; a thoracotomy (5 to 7 cm in length) was then performed in the fourth intercostal space in the submammary fold, from the anterior to the medial axillary line. Small accessory incisions were made for the endoscope, aortic clamp, venting tube, CO_2 line, and atrial retractor.

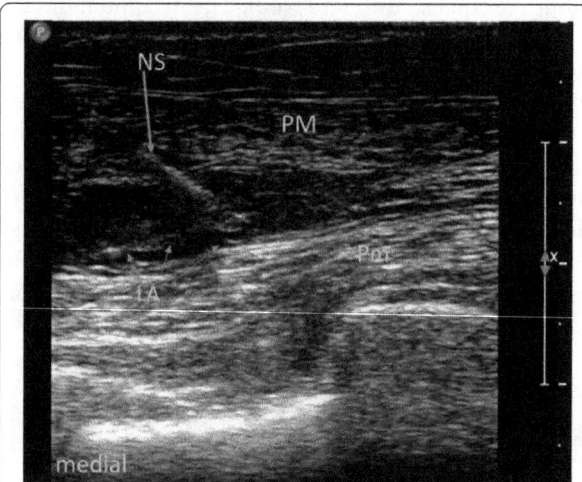

Fig. 2 Pectoralis nerves block type I. LA – local anesthetic, NS – needle shaft, PM – pectoralis major muscle, Pm – pectoralis minor muscle

CPB was established via femoral vessel cannulation; if tricuspid valve surgery was also planned, the right jugular vein was cannulated percutaneously. Patients were cooled to 34 °C, the pericardium was opened, and cardioplegia was administered to the aortic root after cross-clamping of the aorta. The mitral and tricuspid valve (if required) was repaired using valvular rings and artificial Gore-Tex chordae, if required. After completion of the repair, patients were rewarmed and weaned from CPB and TEE examination was performed to assure the quality of the repair. The surgery site and the postoperative drain position are presented in Fig. 4.

Outcomes
Primary outcome
The total consumption of oxycodone during the first 24 postoperative hours. This outcome was presented also as morphine equivalence (ME, 1 mg of oxycodone = 1.5 mg of morphine [16]). Secondary outcome: Pain intensity assessed on the VAS at the 2, 4, 6, 8, 12, and 24 h after surgery by nurses who were blinded to the type of treatment.

Other outcomes
The other measured variables were pain intensity (assessed by patients using the Prince Henry Hospital Pain Score (PHHPS)), patient satisfaction with pain management, and assessment of pulmonary function. PHHPS was used to assess the effect of analgesia provided by regional block and intravenously administered painkillers on deep breathing and coughing. Patients could describe their pain severity using a five-grade scoring system from 0 to 4, in which 0 indicated 'no pain on coughing', 1 indicated 'pain

on coughing, but not on deep breathing', 2 indicated 'pain on deep breathing, but not at rest', 3 indicated 'slight pain at rest', and indicated 4 'severe pain at rest'. PHHPS was assessed at the time of admission, as well as at 1 day and 4 days after surgery. Patient satisfaction with pain management was assessed at the time of discharge from the hospital. Patients could describe their satisfaction with pain management as perfect (5), good (4), moderate (3), poor (2), or very poor (1).

Pulmonary function tests were performed by a physician who was not involved in anesthesia or surgery. The physician assessed each study participant by using the SP10W spirometer (Contec Medical Systems Co., Ltd., People's Republic of China) before surgery, as well as 1 day and 4 days after surgery.

Statistical analysis
Data are presented as medians [interquartile ranges (IQRs)]. The Mann–Whitney U test was used for nonparametric data. If normal distribution was confirmed, Student's t-test was used. Parametric data are presented as means with 95% confidence intervals (95% CIs). All analyses were performed in Statistica 13.1 software (Stat Soft. Inc., Tulsa, OK, USA).

Power analysis
The sample size was calculated based on our preliminary results. The mean consumption of oxycodone was 22 mg per day in patients who had the ESP block alone, and 10 mg in patients who had ESP, PECS I, and PECS II blocks. The calculated sample size was 12 individuals per group ($\alpha = 0.05$; power = 0.8). Thus, we decided to recruit 15 patients in each group.

Results
This study was conducted from July 2018 to August 2018. Overall, 30 patients were analyzed, 15 per group (Fig. 5). Patient demographics and surgery times are presented in Table 1. No differences were found between the groups regarding patient demographics, surgery times, or American Society of Anesthesiologist Physical Status Classifications. We did not notice any relevant complications among the study participants.

Oxycodone consumption
The primary outcome of our study was the oxycodone consumption via PCA during the first 24 postoperative hours. Patients in the PECS + ESP group used significantly less oxycodone than individuals in the ESP group: 12 [IQR: 6–16] mg vs. 20 [IQR: 18–29] mg or 18 [9–24] vs. 30 [27–43.5] ME ($p = 0.0004$) (Fig. 6). Six patients required rescue dosages of oxycodone; all were in the ESP group.

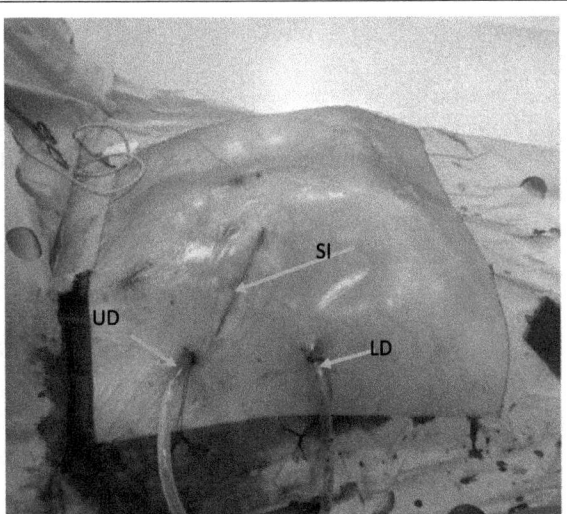

Fig. 4 Postoperative drain positions. The figure presents the positions of chest drains and the site of the incision. UD—upper drain, the proximal end in the apex of the lung, LD—lower drain, inserted horizontally ("lying on the diaphragm"), SI—surgical incision

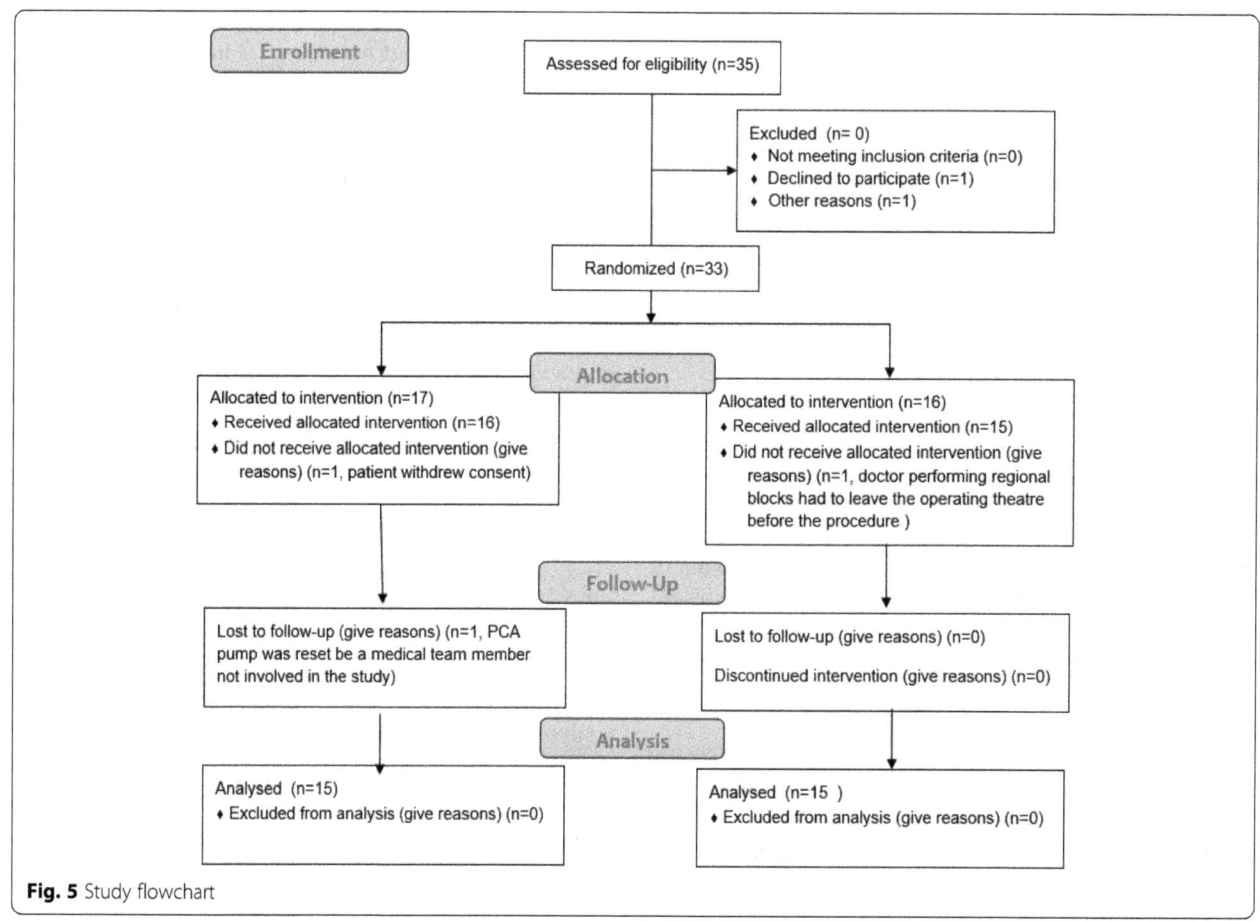

Fig. 5 Study flowchart

Pain intensity

Pain intensity was significantly lower in patients in the PECS group, compared with those in the ESP group, at the time of each clinical evaluation (Fig. 7, Table 2).

Prince Henry hospital pain score

No difference was found between the ESP and PECS + ESP groups regarding pain severity measured on PHHPS. None of the patients reported any pain at the time of admission. In both groups, pain severity was 1 [IQR: 1–1] on the first postoperative day and 1 [IQR: 0–1] on the fourth postoperative day.

Patient satisfaction with pain management

Patients in the PECS + ESP group were more satisfied with pain management, compared with patients in the ESP group: 4 [IQR: 4–4] vs. 3 [IQR: 1–4] ($p = 0.0007$).

Table 1 Patient demographics

Group	ESP	PECS + ESP	p-value
Age (years)	60. 7 (53.9–67.6)	53.9 (45.7–62.0)	0.18
Weight (kg)	82.3 (75.7–88.9)	79.3 (71.1–87.5)	0.55
Height (m)	175.5 (170.5–180.5)	172.6 (167.1–178.1)	0.41
BMI (kg/m2)	26.9 (24.4–29.4)	26.5 (24.7–28.2)	0.78
Males N (%)	12 (80)	10 (67)	0.68
Surgery time (minutes)	226.7 (207.3–246)	213.7 (189.5–237.8)	0.38
ASA	2 [2–2]	2 [2–2]	0.63

Age, weight, height, body mass index (BMI), and surgery time are shown as means and 95% confidence intervals. American Society of Anesthesiologists Physical Status Classification (ASA) is shown as median and interquartile range. Patient sex is shown as the number (percent) of males in each group. P-values were calculated with Student's t-test (normally distributed continuous data), the Mann–Whitney U test (non-normally distributed data), and the Fisher exact test (frequency data). ESP – erector spinae plane, PECS –pectoralis nerve

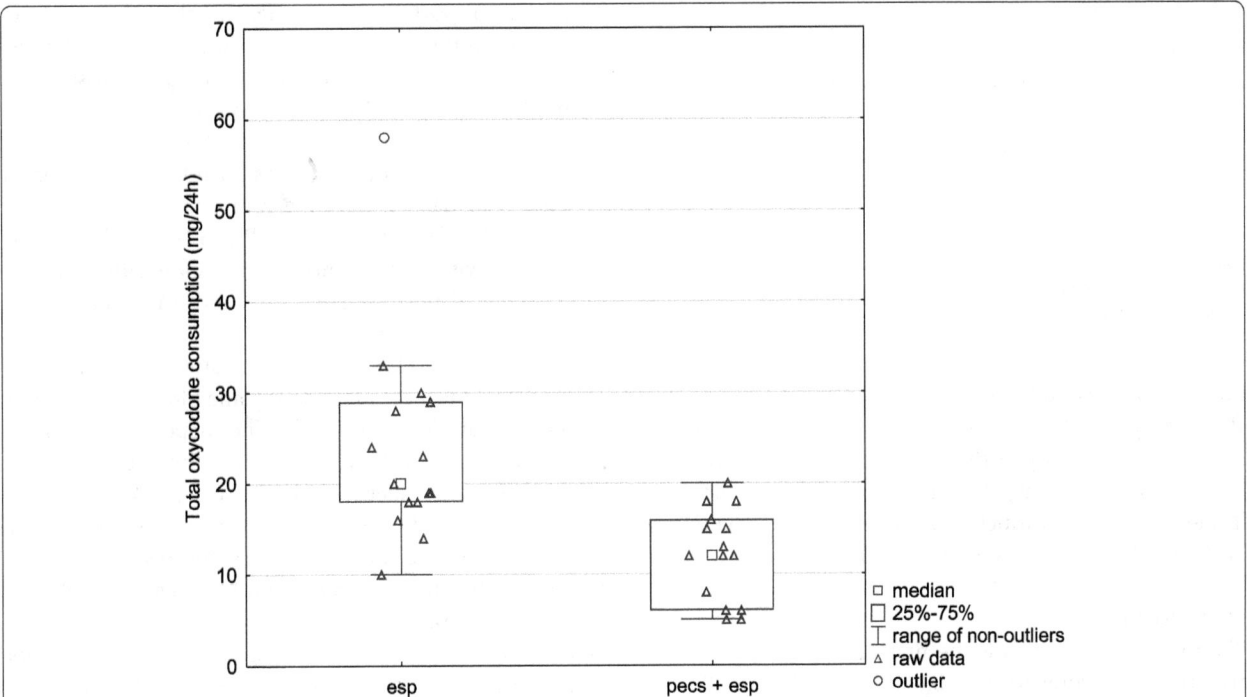

Fig. 6 Total oxycodone consumption during the first postoperative day was significantly lower in patients who had PECS I + PECS II + ESP block (PECS + ESP group) than in patients who had ESP block alone. Results are presented as medians and interquartile ranges. ESP – erector spinae plane, PECS – pectoralis nerve

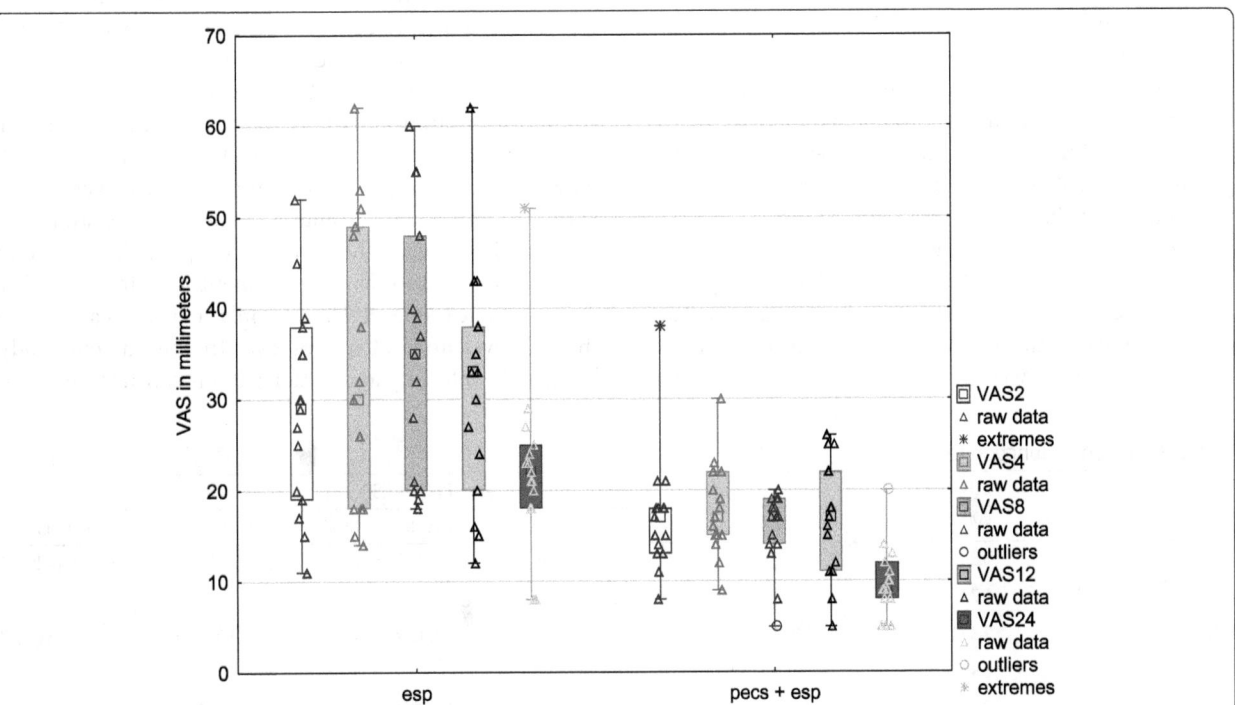

Fig. 7 Pain intensities reported by individual patients (triangles) and by groups of patients (boxes and whiskers) using the VAS. Results are presented as medians, 25th–75th percentile ranges (interquartile ranges - boxes), and 1st-99th percentile ranges (whiskers). VAS2, VAS4, VAS8, VAS12, and VAS24 denote pain intensity measurements at the second, fourth, eighth, 12th, and 24th hours postoperatively. ESP – erector spinae plane, PECS – pectoralis nerve, VAS – visual analog scale

Table 2 Pain intensity

Pain evaluation	ESP	PECS + ESP	p value
2 h	29 [19–38]	17 [13–18]	0.004
4 h	30 [18–49]	17 [15–22]	0.005
8 h	35 [18–49]	17 [14–19]	< 0.001
12 h	33 [20–38]	17 [11–22]	0.002
24 h	22 [18–25]	9 [8–12]	<0.001

Pain intensity reported by patients and presented as medians and interquartile ranges. P-values were calculated with the Mann–Whitney U test. ESP – erector spinae plane, PECS – pectoralis nerve

Pulmonary function tests

Pulmonary function tests did not differ between the study groups for any of the evaluations. Selected parameters from pulmonary function tests are presented in Table 3. Pulmonary function decreased by approximately 30% from baseline but was similar in both groups.

Discussion

To our knowledge, this is the first randomized controlled trial (RCT) to compare ESP block with ESP plus PECS I and II blocks in patients undergoing cardiac surgery comprising valve surgery via right mini-thoracotomy. The results of the current study showed that the inclusion of an additional regional anesthesia technique (PECS I + PECS II blocks) with the ESP block significantly reduced oxycodone consumption and alleviated postoperative pain severity measured on the VAS (Figs. 6 and 7). Moreover, patients in the PECS + ESP group were more satisfied with pain management. However, pain management, as measured using the PHHPS, was good in both groups, and there was no difference in pulmonary function tests between the study groups. Of 30 patients, all could be weaned from mechanical ventilation in accordance with the study protocol (within 2 h from the end of the surgery).

ESP block provides satisfactory analgesia in patients after mini-thoracotomy procedures. In the current study, of 15 patients in the ESP group, 12 reported that their pain management was perfect or good; only a single

participant reported pain management as poor. However, a continuing obstacle to the improvement of postoperative analgesia remains chest pain associated primarily with chest drains. We considered two regional techniques for additional analgesia: PECS and the serratus anterior block. Both methods have been described in patients who have undergone mini-thoracotomy procedures [15, 17]. We chose to use PECS blocks due to our experience with this method. This modification significantly reduced postoperative pain and improved patient satisfaction in the PECS group.

Both ESP and PECS blocks are relatively new analgesic techniques. ESP is an interfascial plane block developed by Ferrero et al. in 2016 [18]. The deposition of local anesthetic in a location anterior to the erector spinae muscle causes multidermatomal sensory block on the ipsilateral side [19]. PECS blocks require an injection of local anesthetic into two planes: between the pectoralis major and pectoralis minor muscles; and between the pectoralis minor and serratus anterior muscles [15]. These techniques block branches of the brachial plexus (anterior thoracic nerves). Recently, new studies have shown further use of ESP and PECS block in cardiac surgery [11, 12].

Although PECS and ESP blocks appear to cover similar areas, their clinical efficacy is still under investigation. The results presented in cadaveric studies showed some unpredictably of ESP block [19, 20]. In the study by Adhikary et al., the dye spread to the intercostal space was between 5 to 10 spaces, to the epidural space from 2 to 5, and the intercostal foramina from 2 to 3. Thus, the spread of dye in the ESP block was changeable and could differ significantly between only three cadavers. In a very recent study by Choi et al., 14 cadavers were evaluated (7 per group). Two volumes of dye were compared, 10 and 30 mL. Similarly to the previous study, the dye was injected at the level of T5 [20].. Interestingly, the superior costotransverse ligament was stained in 3 of 7 cadavers at the level T3, and only in 1 of 7 cadavers at the T2 level after 30 mL of dye. In the current study, lower pain intensity and better patient satisfaction in the

Table 3 Pulmonary function tests

Time of assessment	ESP			PECS + ESP		
	FVC (L)	FEV1 (L/s)	PEF (L/s)	FVC (L)	FEV1 (L/s)	PEF (L/s)
Admission	3.3 (2.5–4.0)	2.7 (2.1–3.3)	6.4 (4.9–7.9)	3.4 (3.0–3.8)	2.7 (2.5–3.0)	5.6 (4.8–6.4)
p-value	0.73	1.0	0.32			
POD1	2.3 (1.8–2.9)	1.8 (1.4–2.2)	4.7 (3.7–5.6)	2.6 (2.2–3.0)	2.0 (1.7–2.3)	4.8 (3.9–5.7)
p-value	0.47	0.35	0.87			
POD4	2.6 (2.1–3.1)	2.1 (1.7–2.5)	6.2 (5.1–7.3)	2.8 (2.4–3.2)	2.2 (1.8–2.6)	5.4 (4.4–6.3)
p-value	0.50	0.81	0.21			

Selected results of pulmonary function tests in both groups of patients. Spirometry was performed 1 day before surgery (admission), 1 day after surgery (POD1), and 4 days after surgery (POD4). Data are presented as means and 95% confidence intervals. P-values were calculated with Student's t-test was. ESP – erector spinae plane, PECS – pectoralis nerve, FVC – forced vital capacity, FEV1 – forced expiratory volume in 1 s, PEF – peak expiratory flow

PECS + ESP group could be caused by the covering area not fully supplied by ESP block in some patients. It appears that pain intensity alleviation and improved patient satisfaction could be caused by only PECS II block. PECS I block which covers a small area of the anterior chest wall could be an unnecessary procedure in our trial. However, we cannot fully exclude its usefulness in this case. More evidence is necessary.

Other potential techniques that could be used in patients after mitral and/or tricuspid valve repair via mini-thoracotomy include PVB and TEA. PVB seems superior to TEA for this type of surgery because its analgesic area is limited to the operated side [1, 21]. Data to compare pain relief between ESP and PVB are lacking, but we suspect that their efficacy is similar. However, we hypothesized that PVB could be associated with an increased risk of pleural puncture, relative to that of ESP block [22]. Further RCTs are needed to investigate whether ESP and PVB are equivalent with respect to pain management, complication rate, and patient satisfaction.

The other regional anesthesia method which could be effective after mini-thoracotomy procedures are the intercostal blockade. This procedure could be performed at the end of surgery by the surgeon under direct vision. However, the intercostal blockade provides the highest plasma ropivacaine concentration of all anesthetic techniques, with the peak plasma concentration at 21 ± 9 min from injection and sensory blockade (measured by pinprick) lasting of 6.0 ± 2.5 h only [23].

Our study had some limitations. Although statistical significance was demonstrated for primary and secondary outcomes, the sample size was relatively small. Thus, the lack of complications could be the result of a low number of participants. The current study showed that the addition of PECS block to ESP block improved postoperative pain control and increased patient satisfaction. However, PECS blocks may be sufficient as a single regional analgesia technique for pain management in patients undergoing valve repair via right mini-thoracotomy. Moreover, PECS blocks could be superior to ESP block for this type of surgery. The current study did not exclude this alternative. Neither ESP nor PECS blocks effectiveness was confirmed in the operating theatre with the loss of sensation technique before the surgery.

Conclusion

In conclusion, the current study demonstrated that the addition of PECS blocks to ESP block led to reduced consumption of oxycodone via PCA, reduced pain intensity on VAS, and increased patient satisfaction with pain management in patients undergoing mitral/tricuspid valve repair via mini-thoracotomy. However, there were no differences between the study groups regarding pulmonary function tests.

Abbreviations
CBP: Cardiopulmonary bypass; CI: Confidence interval; ERAS: Enhanced Recovery After Surgery; ESP: Erector spinae plane; IQR: Interquartile range; ME: Morphine equivalence; PCA: Patient-controlled analgesia; PECS: Pectoralis nerve; PHHPS: Prince Henry Hospital Pain Score; PVB: Paravertebral block; TEA: Thoracic epidural analgesia; TEE: Transoesophageal echocardiography; VAS: Visual analog scale

Acknowledgments
None.

Authors' contributions
BG, MB, BB, JB, MC, BWG, MK, KW: conceived and designed the study. BG, BB, MK, KW: conducted the study. MB, BG, BWG: analyzed the data. MB, BWG, and BG: prepared the first draft of the manuscript. BB, JB, MC, MK, KW: contributed to the major revision of the manuscript. All authors contributed to the final manuscript revisions and approved the final version.

Author details
[1]Division of Cardiovascular Surgery, St. Jadwiga Provincial Clinical Hospital, ul. Lwowska 60, 35-301 Rzeszów, Poland. [2]Second Department of Anesthesia and Intensive Care, Medical University of Lublin, ul. Staszica 16, 20-081 Lublin, Poland. [3]Anesthesiology and Intensive Care Department with the Center for Acute Poisoning, St. Jadwiga Provincial Clinical Hospital, ul. Lwowska 60, 35-301 Rzeszów, Poland.

References
1. Mesbah A, Yeung J, Gao F. Pain after thoracotomy. BJA Education. 2016; 16(1):1–7. https://doi.org/10.1093/bjaceaccp/mkv005.
2. Agostini P, Cieslik H, Rathinam S, et al. Postoperative pulmonary complications following thoracic surgery: are there any modifiable risk factors? Thorax. 2010;65:815–8.
3. Szelkowski LA, Puri NK, Singh R, Massimiano PS. Current trends in preoperative, intraoperative, and postoperative care of the adult cardiac surgery patient. Curr Probl Surg. 2015;52:531–69. https://doi.org/10.1067/j.cpsurg.2014.10.001 Epub 2014 Oct 28.
4. Noss C, Prusinkiewicz C, Nelson G, Patel PA, Augoustides JG, Gregory AJ. Enhanced Recovery for Cardiac Surgery. J Cardiothorac Vasc Anesth. 2018; S1053–0770(18):30049–1. https://doi.org/10.1053/j.jvca.2018.01.045.
5. Landoni G, Isella F, Greco M, Zangrillo A, Royse CF. Benefits and risks of epidural analgesia in cardiac surgery. Br J Anaesth. 2015;115:25–32. https://doi.org/10.1093/bja/aev201.
6. Scott NB, Turfrey DJ, Ray DA, Nzewi O, Sutcliffe NP, Lal AB, Norrie J, Nagels WJ, Ramayya GP. A prospective randomized study of the potential benefits of thoracic epidural anesthesia and analgesia in patients undergoing coronary artery bypass grafting. Anesth Analg. 2001;93(3):528–35.
7. Bignami E, Landoni G, Biondi-Zoccai GG, et al. Epidural analgesia improves outcome in cardiac surgery: a meta-analysis of randomized controlled trials. J Cardiothorac Vasc Anesth. 2010;24:586–97.
8. Scarfe AJ, Schuhmann-Hingel S, Duncan JK, Ma N, Atukorale YN, Alun L. Cameron; Continuous paravertebral block for post-cardiothoracic surgery analgesia: a systematic review and meta-analysis. Eur J Cardio-Thoracic Surg. 2016;50(6):1010–8. https://doi.org/10.1093/ejcts/ezw168.
9. Tahara S, Inoue A, Sakamoto H, et al. A case series of continuous paravertebral block in minimally invasive cardiac surgery. JA Clin Rep. 2017; 3:45.
10. Chakravarthy M. Regional analgesia in cardiothoracic surgery: a changing paradigm toward opioid-free anesthesia? Ann Card Anaesth. 2018;21:225–7.
11. Kumar KN, Kalyane RN, Singh NG, Nagaraja PS, Krishna M, Babu B, Varadaraju R, Sathish N, Manjunatha N. Efficacy of bilateral pectoralis nerve block for ultrafast tracking and postoperative pain management in cardiac surgery. Ann Card Anaesth. 2018;21:333–8.
12. Nagaraja PS, Ragavendran S, Singh NG, Asai O, Bhavya G, Manjunath N. Rajesh K comparison of continuous thoracic epidural analgesia with bilateral erector spinae plane block for perioperative pain management in cardiac surgery. Ann Card Anaesth. 2018;21:323–7.
13. Borys M, Gawęda B, Horeczy B, et al. Erector spinae-plane block as an analgesic alternative in patients undergoing mitral and/or tricuspid valve repair through a right mini-thoracotomy – an observational cohort study. Videosurgery and Other Miniinvasive Techniques/Wideochirurgia i inne

techniki małoinwazyjne. 2019. https://doi.org/10.5114/wiitm.2019.85396.

14. Blanco R. The 'pecs block': a novel technique for providing analgaesia after breast surgery. Anesthesia. 2011;66:847–8.

15. Yalamuri S, Klinger RY, Bullock WM, Glower DD, Bottiger BA, Gadsden JC. Pectoral Fascial (PECS) I and II blocks as rescue analgesia in a patient undergoing minimally invasive cardiac surgery. Reg Anesth Pain Med. 2017; 42:764–6. https://doi.org/10.1097/AAP.0000000000000661.

16. Kalso E, Pöyhiä R, Onnela P, Linko K, Tigerstedt I, Tammisto T. Intravenous morphine and oxycodone for pain after abdominal surgery. Acta Anaesthesiol Scand. 1991;35:642–6. https://doi.org/10.1111/j.1399-6576.1991. tb03364.

17. Costa F, Nenna A, Barbato R, Benedetto M, Del Buono R, Agrò FE. Serratus anterior plane block for right minithoracotomy revision after mitral valve repair. Minerva Anestesiol. 2017;83:1333–4. https://doi.org/10.23736/S0375-9393.17.12186-3.

18. Forero M, Adhikary SD, Lopez H, et al. The erector Spinae plane block: a novel analgesic technique in thoracic neuropathic pain. Reg Anesth Pain Med. 2016;41:621–7.

19. Adhikary S, Bernard S, Lopez H, et al. Erector Spinae Plane Block Versus RetrolaminarBlock: A Magnetic Resonance Imaging and Anatomical Study. Reg Anesth Pain Med. 2018;23:756–62. https://doi.org/10.1097/AAP. 0000000000000798.

20. Choi YJ, Kwon HJ, O J, et al. Influence of injectate volume on the paravertebral spread in erector spinae plane block: An endoscopic and anatomical evaluation. PLoS One. 2019;14:e0224487. https://doi.org/10.1371/journal.pone.022448.

21. Carmona P, Llagunes J, Casanova I, Mateo E, Cánovas S, Martín E, Marqués JI, Peña JJ, de Andrés J. Continuous paravertebral analgesia versus intravenous analgesia in minimally invasive cardiac surgery by mini-thoracotomy. Rev Esp Anestesiol Reanim. 2012;59:476–82. https://doi.org/10.1016/j.redar.2012.04.014.

22. Kus A, Gurkan Y, Gul Akgul A, Solak M, Toker K. Pleural puncture and intrathoracic catheter placement during ultrasound guided paravertebral block. J Cardiothorac Vasc Anesth. 2013;27:e11–2. https://doi.org/10.1053/j.jvca.2012.10.018.

23. Kopacz DJ, Emmanuelsson BM, Thompson GE, et al. Pharmacokinetics of ropivacaine and bupivacaine for bilateral intercostal blockade in healthy male volunteers. Anesthesiology. 1994;81:1139–48. https://doi.org/10.1097/00000542.

5

The efficacy of antipyretic analgesics administration intravenously for preventing rocuronium-associated pain/withdrawal response

Jia Wang[1], Yu Cui[2], Bin Liu[1*] and Jianfeng Chen[1]

Abstract

Background: Rocuronium-associated injection pain/withdrawal response (RAIPWR) was non-ideal but occurred frequently when injection intravenously during anesthesia induction. Many studies had reported that pretreating with antipyretic analgesics (AAs) could reduce the occurrence of RAIPWR, but there was no consensus yet. Therefore, this meta-analysis was designed to systematically evaluate the benefits of AAs on RAIPWR in patients.

Methods: PubMed, Cochrane Library, Ovid, EMbase, Chinese National Knowledge Infrastructure (CNKI), Wan Fang Data were searched by January 1st 2019 for randomized controlled trials (RCTs) applying AAs to alleviate RAIPWR in patients who underwent elective surgery under general anesthesia. Two investigators assessed quality of RCTs and extracted data respectively and the meta-analysis was carried on Revman 5.3 software. Moreover, we compared AAs in pros and cons directly with lidocaine, the most reported medicine to prevent RAIPWR.

Results: Data were analyzed from 9 RCTs totaling 819 patients. The results of Meta-analysis showed that compared to the control group, pretreating with AAs could prevent the total occurrence of RAIPWR [Risk ratio (RR), 0.52; 95% confidence interval (CI), 0.42 to 0.66; $P < 0.0001$], and took effect on moderate (RR, 0.56; 95%CI, 0.43 to 0.73; $P < 0.0001$) and severe RAIPWR (RR = 0.14; 95%CI, 0.08 to 0.24; $P < 0.00001$). When compared to lidocaine, the preventive effect was not so excellent as the latter but injection pain induced by prophylactic occurred less.

Conclusion: The currently available evidence suggested that pretreating with AAs intravenously could alleviate RAIPWR.

Keywords: Rocuronium, Injection pain, Withdrawal response, Antipyretic analgesics, Meta-analysis

Background

Rocuronium, a timely nondepolarizing muscle relaxant, is routinely applied in clinical anesthesia practice, and also an alternative to succinylcholine in rapid sequence induction [1] without side effects such as cardiovascular response, elevating blood potassium, or inducing myoclonus [2]. However, without preventive measures, about 50–80% [3–5] of patients experienced injection pain, and even in anesthetized patients, withdrawal movement of the arm which may soon extend to the whole body

* Correspondence: liubinhxyy@163.com
[1]West China Hospital of Sichuan University, No. 37th, Guoxue Lane, Wuhou District, Chengdu City, Sichuan Province, P.R. China

could be motivated by rocuronium injection. How to re-duce the side effect of rocuronium is of significant im-portance of its clinical application.

Antipyretic analgesics (AAs) are a well-known cat-egory of drugs that have long been identified safe and ef-fective to control acute postoperative pain and long-term chronic pain [6–8]. In recent years, some clinical trials reported the preventive effect of AAs on rocuronium-associated injection pain/withdrawal re-sponse (RAIPWR), but systematic review regarding the efficacy as yet has not been addressed. Thus, we aimed to assess the effectiveness of several widely used AAs of eliminating RAIPWR by conducting a Meta-analysis.

Methods

Source of data and search strategy

The study was conducted and presented in accordance with the systematic review guideline [9], and the study protocol was registered with the International Prospect-ive Register of Systematic Reviews (https://www.crd.york.ac.uk/prospero/#recordDetails) with the ID of CRD42019129776. Two investigators independently searched PubMed, Cochrane Library, Ovid, EMbase, Chinese National Knowledge Infrastructure (CNKI) and Wan Fang data electronically for randomized controlled trials (RCTs) published by January 1st 2019 applying AAs to alleviate RAIPWR. Search terms included: anti-pyretic analgesics, acetaminophen, paracetamol, pare-coxib, ketorolac, flurbiprofen, lornoxicam, rocuronium, injection pain, withdrawal. To identify all available evi-dence, we scanned the references cited in RCTs revolved and reviews with similar subject for eligible studies manually.

Study selection

This system review and meta- analysis recruited RCTs meting the following criteria only:

(1) Surgical patients involved in were at ASA physical status I to II and aged 2 to 75 years old.
(2) Rocuronium was utilized during general anesthesia induction, and AAs were applied intravenously to prevent RAIPWR while placebo or normal saline was used in the controlled group.
(3) The first outcomes of interest were the total incidence of RAIPWR and the occurrence of three degrees of RAIPWR (mild, moderate and severe). The secondary outcomes were the incidence of RAIPWR and adverse reactions of medicines used for pretreatment (AAs and lidocaine). Besides, quantitative data of outcomes were reported.
(4) Outcome measurement methods: a) severity of injection pain from rocuronium was graded as follows: none, negative response to questioning;

mild, pain reported in response to questioning only, without any behavioral signs; moderate, pain reported in response to questioning and accompanied by a behavioral sign, or pain reported spontaneously without questioning; severe, strong vocal response or response accompanied by facial grimacing, arm withdrawal, or tears. b) The severity of rocuronium-induced withdrawal response was rated as follows: none, no response; mild, move-ment at the wrist only; moderate, movement/with-drawal involving arm only (elbow/shoulder); severe, generalized response, withdrawal or movement in more than one extremity, coughing, or breath hold-ing [5]. c) Adverse reactions of preventative medi-cine were evaluated by systemic (mainly cardiovascular reaction, such as hypertension, hypotension, tachycardia, bradycardia, etc.) and local reactions (the condition of injection site, such as edema, flushing or allergic reaction).

Initially, titles and abstracts were screened to discard unrelated studies and the full text of potentially eligible studies were carefully read. Then, data on the following items would be extracted: author, published year, location of trial, type of surgery, ASA status, sample size, patient age range, type and dosage of AAs, the outcome assessment and so on. Study screening and data export were finished by two researchers respectively (Jia Wang, Jianfeng Chen), and then the works were exchanged for rationality and accuracy. If any disagreements, the third researcher (Yu Cui) would interpose and make the final decision when necessary.

Risk of bias assessment

When an RCT met the aforementioned selection criteria, its methodological quality was assessed on the basis of the suggestions in the *Cochrane Handbook for System-atic Reviews of Interventions* [9], and the evaluation con-tents contained seven domains: random sequence generation(selection bias), allocation concealment (selec-tion bias), blinding of participants and personnel (per-formance bias), blinding of outcome assessment (detection bias), incomplete outcome data (attrition bias), selective reporting (reporting bias) and other bias. In each special aspect of risk was graded as "yes" for low risk, "unclear" and "no" for high risk. We included a 'Risk of bias' detailing all of the judgements made for all included studies in the review.

Statistical methods

Meta-analyses were carried out by Review Manager soft-ware (RevMan, version 5.3 for Windows, Oxford, UK; The Cochrane Collaboration, 2008). The categorical variable was expressed in relative risk (RR) with its 95% confidence interval (95%CI), and the continuous variable was expressed in weighted mean deviation (WMD) with 95%CI. We considered $P < 0.05$ and RR not crossing the identity line as statistically significant. Heterogeneity among studies was assessed using both the χ^2 test and the I^2 statistic. If $I^2 \leq 50\%$, we considered there was no homogeneity among studies and the fixed-effects model was eligible; On the contrary, when $I^2 > 50\%$, indicating significant heterogeneity, and the random-effects model was applied for meta-analysis. In terms of outcomes with heterogeneity, an effort was made to explore the source, mainly via conducting meta-analysis stratified by patients' characters, severity of RAIPWR and administration route of AAs, etc. We also conducted sensitivity analysis by removing studies in sequence.

Results

Description of studies

We initially identified 84 records according to the retrieval strategy aforementioned, and 9 [10–18] of them involving 819 patients were included eventually according to the inclusion and exclusion criteria (Fig. 1 PRISMA diagram showing article selection for this review). Six kinds of AAs (acetaminophen/paracetamol, parecoxib, ketorolac, flurbiprofen, lornoxicam and propacetamol) were reported to be used for preventing RAIPWR through two routes of intravenous administration. One was intravenous directly (IV), the other was injecting with venous occlusion (IVVO) by tourniquet. The basic characteristics of enrolled studies were listed in Table 1 (Table 1 Characteristics of studies included in Meta-analysis).

Evaluation of methodological quality

Meticulous details regarding the risk of bias in each aspect of included studies were presented in the Risk of bias graph (Fig. 2 Risk of bias graph). Moreover, a summary of judgements about each methodological quality domain for each included RCT was shown in Fig. 3 (Fig. 3 Risk of bias summary). In general, most of studies were assessed to be of low to moderate risk of bias, and reporting bias and selective bias turned out to be the main risk of bias in this study.

The incidence of RAIPWR

In this meta-analysis, 9 RCTs [10–18] with 819 patients were included and reported the incidence of total and different severities of RAIPWR. Statistical heterogeneity ($P < 0.00001$, $I^2 = 73\%$) was found among them, thus a random-effects model was adopted to conduct meta-analysis and the result showed the preventive effect of AAs on total RAIPWR was significant [Risk ratio (RR), 0.52; 95% confidence interval (95%CI), 0.42 to 0.66; $P < 0.0001$; $I^2 = 73\%$] (Fig. 4 AAs vs. control-the total incidence of RAIPWR). We further conducted subgroup analysis stratified by severity of RAIPWR and method of administration of AAs. The results which operated under fixed-effects model showed that AAs were able to drop down the incidence of moderate RAIPWR notably (RR, 0.56; 95%CI, 0.43 to 0.73; $P < 0.0001$; $I^2 = 39\%$) and the occurrence of severe RAIPWR (RR, 0.14; 95%CI, 0.08 to 0.24; $P < 0.00001$; $I^2 = 0\%$). In terms of the mild RAIPWR, AAs hadn't shown significant effect (RR, 0.88; 95%CI, 0.69 to 1.13; $P = 0.32$; $I^2 = 43\%$). Generally, the results seemed to reveal that the more serious the degree of RAIPWR was, the more obvious the effect of AAs was (Fig. 5 AAs vs. control-the incidence of different severities RAIPWR). In addition, the results stratified by administration method of AAs indicated that AAs could reduce the incidence of RAIPWR no matter with (RR, 0.56; 95%CI, 0.43 to 0.72; $P < 0.0001$; $I^2 = 72\%$) or without tourniquet (RR, 0.46; 95%CI, 0.35 to 0.60; $P < 0.00001$; $I^2 = 9\%$) under the random-effects model (Fig. 6 Incidence of RAIPWR-subgroup analysis of different administration methods).

Comparison of AAs and lidocaine (Fig. 7 AAs vs. lidocaine- **a**. the incidence of RAIPWR; **b**. the incidence of injection pain from preventive drugs).

The incidence of RAIPWR

There were 6 studies [10–14, 16] which reported the effect of AAs and lidocaine on preventing RAIPWR. The result in the fixed-effects model showed that RAIPWR

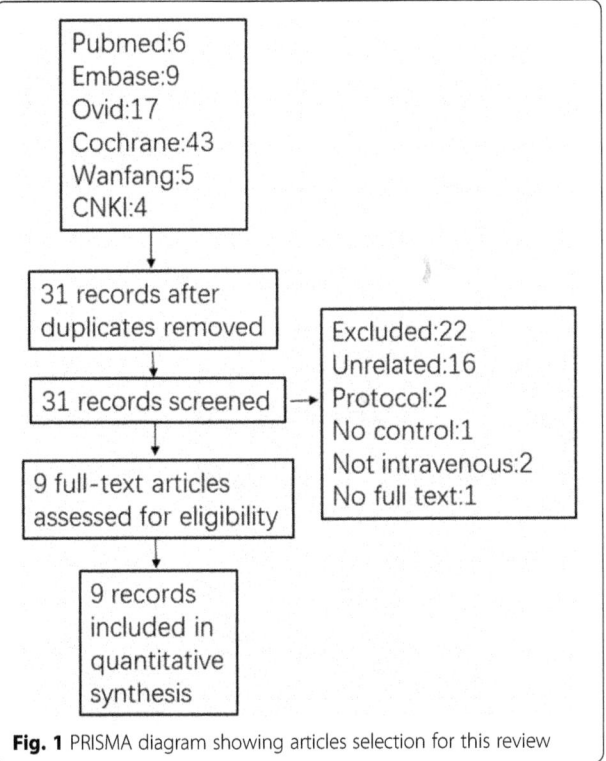

Fig. 1 PRISMA diagram showing articles selection for this review

Table 1 Characteristics of studies included in Meta-analysis

Study	Country	Surgical setting	Age (yr)	ASA	Administration method	Group (n, patients)	Outcomes
Younghoon Jeon 2010	Korea	Elective surgery	45.4 ± 11.1 45.9 ± 14.2 50.1 ± 10.6	I-II	IVVO	N S (n = 39) lidocaine 40 mg (n = 39) paracetamol 50 mg (n = 40)	A/B/C/D
Yonghong Zhang 2012	China	Elective surgery	45.18 ± 12.44 41.28 ± 14.12 45.24 ± 14.36 43.54 ± 15.01	I-II	IVVO	N S (n = 40) lidocaine 40 mg(n = 40) parecoxib 20 mg(n = 40) parecoxib 40 mg(n = 40)	A/B/C/D
Younghoon Jeon 2013	Korea	Elective surgery	46.8 ± 11.5 48.5 ± 13.1 46.2 ± 16.3	I-II	IVVO	placebo(n = 35) lidocaine 20 mg(n = 35) ketorolac 10 mg(n = 35)	A/B/C/D
Gülnaz Ateş 2014	Turkey	Elective surgery	36.45 ± 12.94 35.58 ± 11.9 39.27 ± 11.81	I-II	IVVO	N S (n = 60) lidocaine 40 mg(n = 60) paracetamol 50 mg(n = 60)	A/B/C/D
Sennur Uzun 2014	Turkey	3 kinds of elective surgeries	41.8 ± 13.9 42.7 ± 11.9 41.7 ± 13.3	I-II	IVVO	N S(n = 50) lidocaine 40 mg(n = 50) aracetamol 50 mg(n = 50)	A/B/C/D
Cheng Yuan 2014	China	Elective surgery	45.8 ± 10.3 46.9 ± 9.6 44.3 ± 9.8 43.7 ± 10.6	I-II	IV IVVO IV IVVO	N S (n = 20) N S (n = 20) flurbiprofen 50 mg(n = 20) flurbiprofen 50 mg(n = 20)	A/B/D
Li Sha 2014	China	Elective surgery	46.7 ± 11.1 48.4 ± 13.2 46.2 ± 14.6	I-II	IVVO	N S (n = 35) lidocaine 40 mg (n = 35) flurbiprofen 50 mg(n = 35)	A/B/C/D
Ma Qingjie 2016	China	Elective surgery	39.2 ± 3.7 38.5 ± 4.1 40.3 ± 5.2	I	IV	N S (n = 40) parecoxib20mg (n = 40) parecoxib40mg (n = 40)	A/B
Yu Liang 2018	China	Elective surgery	40.7 ± 8.7 42.7 ± 7.7 43.7 ± 7.3	I-II	IV	N S (n = 20) lornoxicam 4 mg(n = 20) lornoxicam 8 mg(n = 20)	A/B

NS normal saline, *A* the incidence of rocuronium-associated injection pain/withdrawal response, *B* the incidence of different severities rocuronium-associated injection pain/withdrawal response, *C* occurrence of injection pain caused by antipyretic analgesics (AAs and lidocaine), *D* local reaction of injection site, *IVVO* injection intravenously with venous occlusion, *IV* intravenous directedly

occurred more frequently in patients pretreated with AAs than lidocaine, indicating AAs were not so efficient as lidocaine on preventing RAIPWR (RR = 1.43, 95%CI (1.16, 1.77), P = 0.001; I^2 = 21%). (Fig. 7a the incidence of RAIPWR).

The side effect of AAs and lidocaine

There were 3 studies [10, 13, 14] which reported the occurrence of injection pain of prevention drugs which were used with the purpose of reducing the RAIPWR when administrated via intravenous, and no statistically

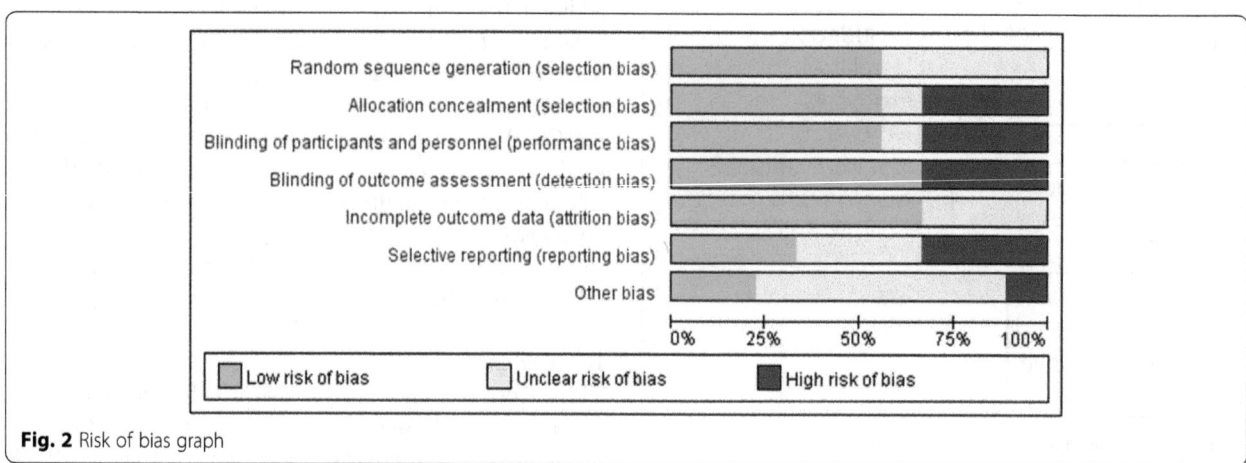

Fig. 2 Risk of bias graph

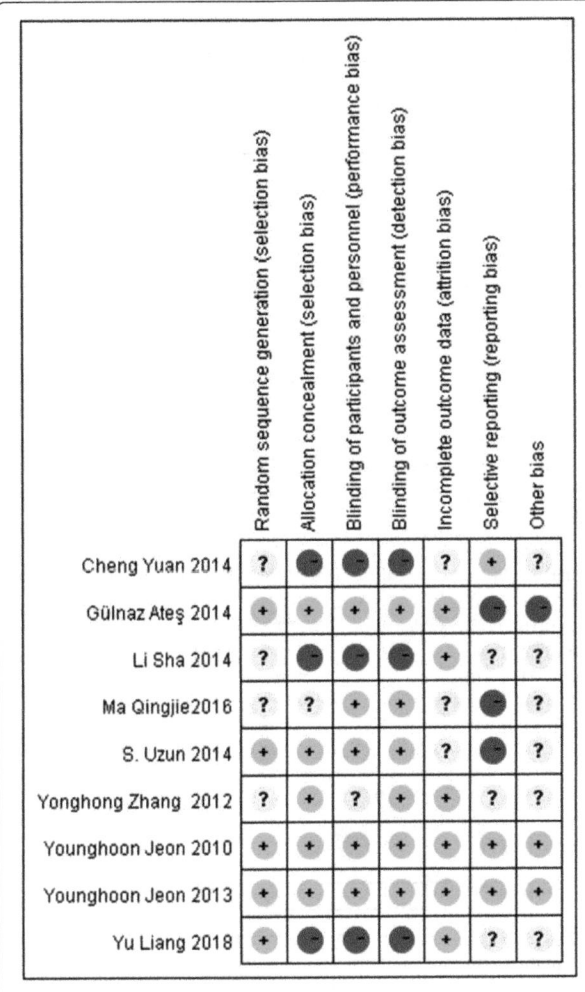

Fig. 3 Risk of bias summary

heterogeneity among them ($P = 0.99$, $I^2 = 0\%$), so the fixed-effects model was utilized. The result suggested the incidence of injection pain of AAs was lower than that of lidocaine, and the difference was of statistically

significance (RR,0.43; 95%CI, 0.23 to 0.80; $P = 0.008$; $I^2 = 0\%$). (Fig. 7 b the incidence of injection pain from preventive drugs).

No systemic adverse effect and skin reactions at injection site was reported.

Sensitivity analysis

High levels of heterogeneities arose when exploring the effect of AAs on total incidence of RAIPWR and the subgroup analysis stratified by administration methods of AAs (73 and 70% respectively), and both of them disappeared when excluded one of studies [14]. Whereas, the results were consistent with that before excluding the given study in the fixed-effects model, indicating that the evaluation of corresponding effect size was stable and reliable in our Meta-analysis. (Table 2 Sensitivity analysis).

Discussion

During anesthesia induction period, injection pain/withdrawal response from rocuronium occurred frequently. This meta-analysis included 9 RCTs involving 819 patients, and the observable endpoints were the incidence of total and different severities of rocuronium-induced injection pain/withdrawal response. The results indicated that AAs were effective in preventing, especially for moderate and severe RAIPWR, though not as effective as lidocaine. Our secondary outcome, pain generated by preventative medicines themselves was reported in 3 RCTs [10, 13, 14], and the result suggested the injection pain induced by AAs occurred less than that of lidocaine.

Previous studies revealed AAs were capable of alleviating injection pain from propofol [19, 20], and some studies were designed to identify the prophylactic effect of AAs on rocuronium-induced injection pain/withdrawal response under the assumption that the mechanisms of injection pain generated by propofol and

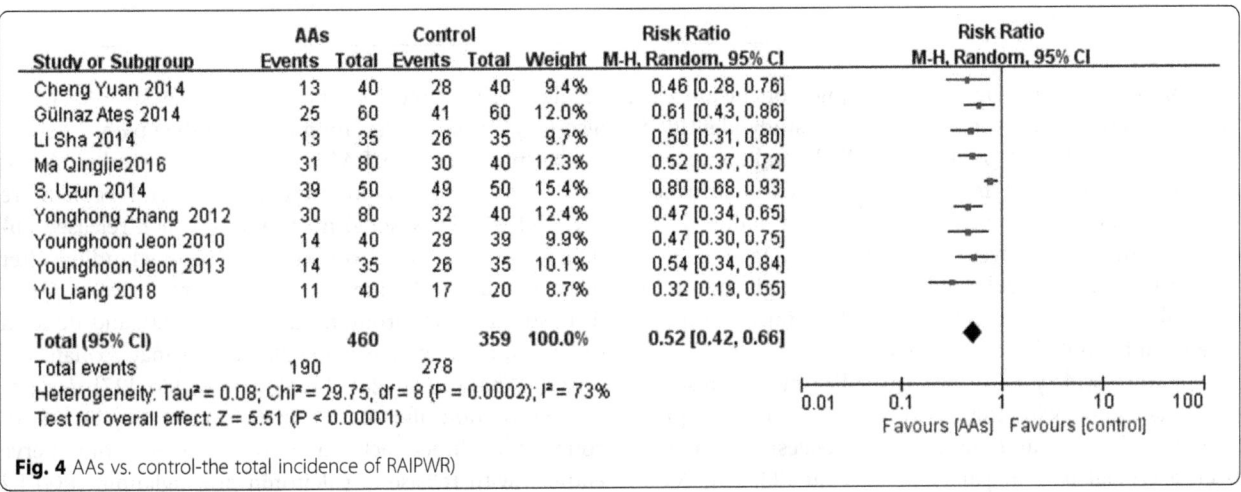

Fig. 4 AAs vs. control-the total incidence of RAIPWR)

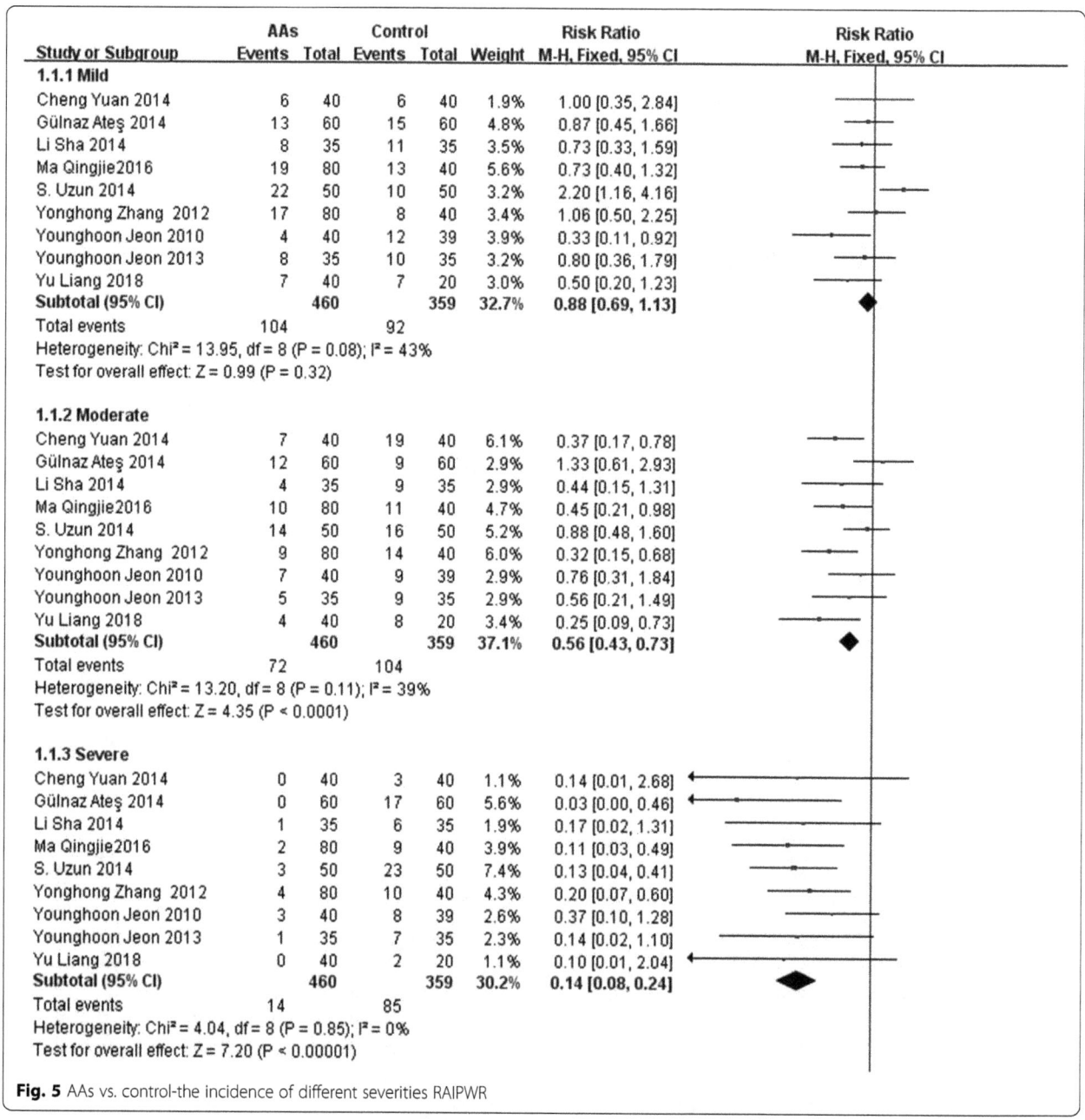

Fig. 5 AAs vs. control-the incidence of different severities RAIPWR

rocuronium were the same. However, no conclusion has been reached on the benefit to date. Our study identified the preventive effect of AAs on RAIPWR, and compared it with lidocaine, the most widely applied pharmacological method to prevent injection pain induced by rocuronium [21], in advantages and disadvantages simultaneously, and the results indicated AAs might be more desirable for pretreatment due to less injection pain when administrated intravenously.

AAs were widely used to treat inflammatory disease for decades and with the emergence of concept of preemptive analgesia and multimodal analgesia, AAs had been a crucial part in pain management [22, 23]. As a result, when applied to prevent RAIPWR, AAs could also play a role in alleviating postoperative pain.

The mechanism of RAIPWR is still unrevealed. Arndt and Klement [24] reported that peripheral veins were invested with polymodal nociceptors, which released endogenous pain mediators such as prostaglandins after being stimulated by unphysiological osmolarity or pH of drug solution. Rocuronium has a PH of 4.0, and dilution could reduce injection pain [25], which may explain the injection pain of it [26]. Blunk and Seifert [27] demonstrated the dolorific effect of rocuronium may be on account for direct activation of C-nociceptors nerve endings with release of calcitonin prostaglandin (PG) E2

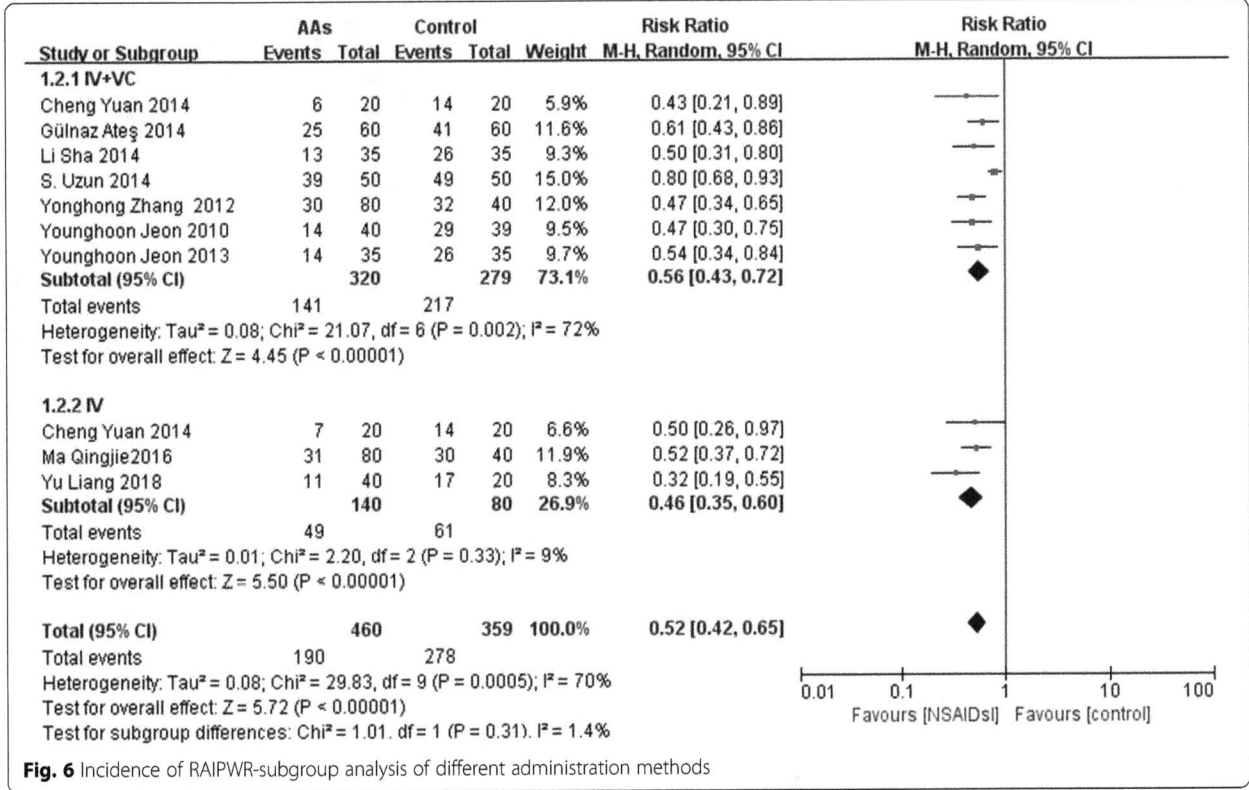

Fig. 6 Incidence of RAIPWR-subgroup analysis of different administration methods

and gene-related peptide (CGRP). In animal experiments, Baek and his colleagues [28] found that rocuronium was able to suppress nitric oxide production and enhance prostaglandin E2 synthesis in calf pulmonary artery endothelial cells, inducing inflammation and pain.

Antipyretic analgesics, containing nonsteroidal anti-inflammatory drugs (NSAIDs) and the most widely used analgesic in the world, acetaminophen [29], are cyclooxygenase (COX) enzyme blockers which may exert their analgesic effects via inhibiting the synthesis of

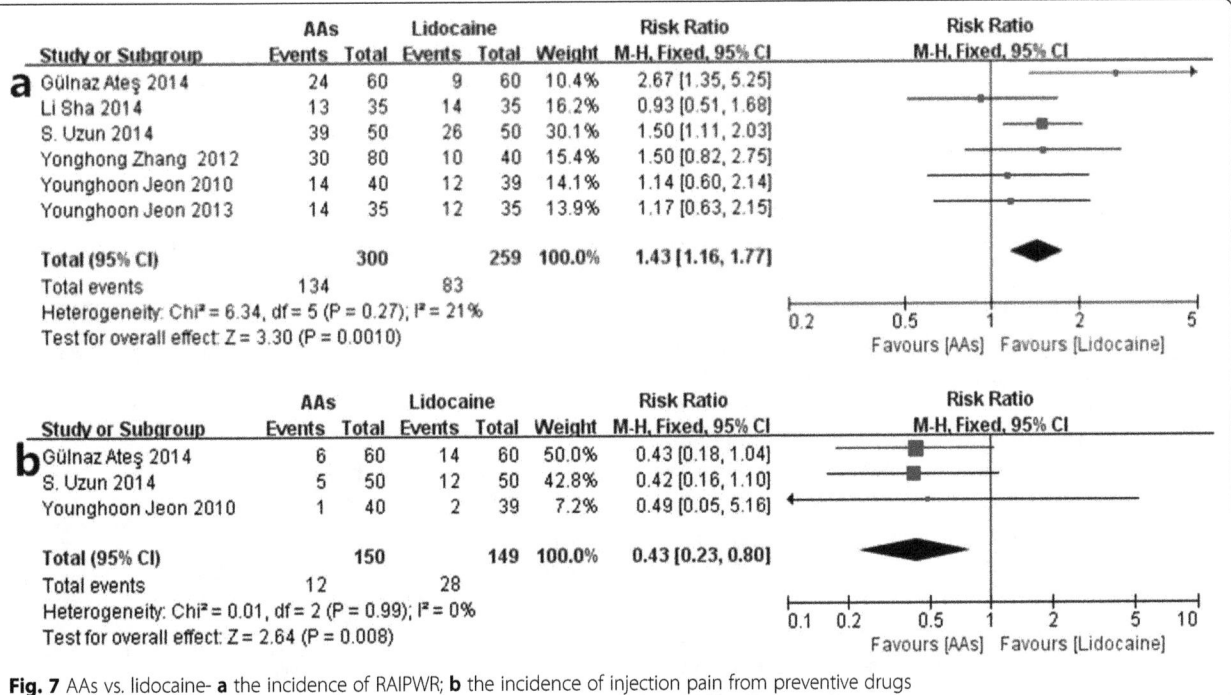

Fig. 7 AAs vs. lidocaine- **a** the incidence of RAIPWR; **b** the incidence of injection pain from preventive drugs

Table 2 Sensitivity analysis

Comparison		RR (95%CI)	P	I^2	Effect model
Total incidence of RAIPWR	Primary analysis	0.52 (0.42,0.66)	$P < 0.00001$	73%	Random-effects
	Exclude "Uzun 2014" [14]	0.5 (0.43,0.57)	$P < 0.00001$	0%	Fixed-effects
Administration by IV + VC	Primary analysis	0.56(0.43,0.72)	$P < 0.00001$	72%	Random-effects
	Exclude "Uzun 2014" [14]	0.51(0.43,0.61)	$P < 0.00001$	0%	Fixed-effects

prostaglandins peripherally and preventing the release of PGE2 together with activating medullary and cortical regions involved in the descending inhibitory pain cascade centrally [30].

Injecting lidocaine was reported the best intervention to prevent RAIPWR [21], and we found AAs also took effect. Though were not so effective as lidocaine, the injection pain caused by preventive medicine itself occurred less when AAs were acting as pretreatments in our review, namely, AAs may be more acceptable and suitable for patients regarding the side effect of prophylactic itself.

Limitations of our review. Firstly, our study recruited literatures published in only Chinese and English, which may lead to bias caused by the publication language. Secondly, the injection sites, dosage, injection speed of drugs and other details of pretreatment varied among enrolled studies, which may influence the results. However, all RCTs illustrated the details of the intervention: prophylactic or placebo was injected 2 to 5 min before intravenous rocuronium, and after assessment finished, other anesthetics (such as opioids and propofol) for induction were administrated, guaranteeing that the injection pain or withdrawal movement was merely caused by rocuronium, and the prophylactic effect, if any, was the result of pretreatment. Thirdly, some of studies included didn't depict details of random sequence generation [11,15–17,] and allocation concealment [15, 16, 18], and 3 of them didn't mention the blind method [15, 16, 18], all of above may lead to high risk of bias, so the power of this review was confined. We discovered Uzun's study [14] was the main source of heterogeneity when carried out sensitive analysis, so we rechecked this study, and found that methodology it abided by resembled to others but they enrolled patients who underwent elective orthopedic, gastrointestinal, and gynecological procedures while other studies recruited all kinds of elective surgeries. Given the impossible task of conducting subgroup analysis stratified by operation types, and the results were homogeneous when excluded the particular study or not, we didn't do further analysis.

Conclusion

In this meta-analysis, current evidence suggested that pretreating with AAs was effective in dropping the occurrence of the RAIPWR, and especially in term of moderate and severe degree of it. However, comparing to pretreating with lidocaine, AAs were not so efficient as the latter, while caused less injection pain and might be more suitable for pretreatment. Considering the quality and quantity of studies involved in this review, it was recommended that more multicenter, randomized, and double-blind controlled trials with larger samples size were needed to confirm the above conclusions.

Abbreviations

RAIPWR: Rocuronium-associated injection pain/withdrawal response; AAS: Antipyretic analgesics; ASA: American Society of Anesthesiology; RCT: Randomize control trial; CI: Confidence interval; NSAIDs: Nonsteroidal anti-inflammatory drugs; COX: Cyclooxygenase; GRP: Gene-related peptide; NS: Normal saline; IVVO: Injection intravenously with venous occlusion; IV: Injection intravenously

Acknowledgements

Not applicable.

Authors' contributions

The literature search was performed by JW and all hits were screened and reviewed for eligibility by JW and JFC independently. Disagreement was resolved by consulting YC and BL. The data extraction and reexamination of the accuracy of data was executed by WJ and YC. The analysis was carried out and the manuscript was drafted by JW and critically reviewed and edited by YC and BL. All authors read and approved the final manuscript.

Author details

¹West China Hospital of Sichuan University, No. 37th, Guoxue Lane, Wuhou District, Chengdu City, Sichuan Province, P.R. China. ²Chengdu Women's & Children's Central Hospital, Chengdu 610000, P.R. China.

References

1. Magorian T, Flannery KB, Miller RD. Comparison of rocuronium, succinylcholine, and vecuronium for rapid-sequence induction of anesthesia in adult patients. Anesthesiology. 1993;79(5):913–8.
2. Martin R, Carrier J, Pirlet M, Claprood Y, Tétrault JP. Rocuronium is the best non-depolarizing relaxant to prevent succinylcholine fasciculations and myalgia. Can J Anaesth. 1998;45(6):521–5.
3. Steegers MA, Robertson EN. Pain on injection of rocuronium bromide. Anesth Analg. 1996;83(1):203.
4. Borgeat A, Kwiatkowski D, Ruetsch YA. Spontaneous movements associated with rocuronium injection: the effects of prior administration of fentanyl. J Clin Anesth. 1997;9(8):650–2.
5. Shevchenko Y, Jocson JC, McRae VA, et al. The use of lidocaine for preventing the withdrawal associated with the injection of rocuronium in children and adolescents. Anesth Analg. 1999;88(4):746–8.
6. Hillstrom C, Jakobsson JG. Lornoxicam : pharmacology and usefulness to treat acute postoperative and musculoskeletal pain a narrative review. Expert Opin Pharmacother. 2013;14(12):1679–94.
7. Smith SR, Deshpande BR, Collins JE, et al. Comparative pain reduction of oral non-steroidal anti-inflammatory drugs and opioids for knee osteoarthritis: systematic analytic review. Osteoarthr Cartil. 2016;24(6):962–72.
8. Machado GC, Maher CG, Ferreira PH, et al. Non-steroidal anti-inflammatory drugs for spinal pain: a systematic review and meta-analysis. Ann Rheum Dis. 2017;76(7):1269–78.
9. Higgins JPT, Green S (editors). Cochrane Handbook for Systematic Reviews

of Interventions Version 5.1.0 [updated March 2011]. Cochrane Collaboration, 2011. Available from www.cochrane-handbook.org.

10. Jeon Y, Baek SU, Park SS, et al. Effect of pretreatment with acetaminophen on withdrawal movements associated with injection of rocuronium: a prospective, randomized, double-blind, placebo controlled study. Korean J Anesthesiol. 2010;59(1):13–6.

11. Zhang Y, Xiang Y, Liu J. Prevention of pain on injection of rocuronium: a comparison of lidocaine with different doses of parecoxib. J Clin Anesth. 2012;24(6):456–9.

12. Jeon Y, Ha JH, Lee JE, et al. Rocuronium-induced withdrawal movement: influence ketorolac or a combination of lidocaine and ketorolac pretreatment. Korean J Anesthesiol. 2013;64(1):25–8.

13. Ates G, Kose EA, Oz G, et al. Effect of paracetamol pretreatment on rocuronium-induced injection pain: a randomized, double-blind, placebo-controlled comparison with lidocaine. J Clin Anal Med. 2014;5(6):508–10.

14. Uzun S, Erden IA, Canbay O, et al. The effect of intravenous paracetamol for the prevention of rocuronium injection pain. Kaohsiung J Med Sci. 2014; 30(11):566–9.

15. Cheng Y, Chen S, Zheng J. The preventive effect of flurbiprofen axeti on rocuronium induced withdrawal response. Zhejiang Clin Med. 2014;16(7): 1157–8.

16. Sha LI, Wei-qian T, Fang-bing JI, et al. Effect of combination of flurbiprofen axetil and lidocaine with tourniquet on rocuronium injection-induced pain. J Clin Anesth. 2014;30(5):469–71.

17. Ma Q, Na L. Effect of pretreatment with Parecoxib sodium on injection pain of rocuronium bromide. Chin Med Guide. 2016;14(13):23.

18. Yu L. Effect of pretreatment with lornoxicam on rocuronium bromide induced injection pain. Mod Pract Med. 2018;30(02):157–9.

19. Zhang L, Zhu J, Xu L, et al. Efficacy and safety of flurbiprofen axetil in the prevention of pain on propofol injection: a systematic review and meta-analysis. Med Sci Monit. 2014;20:995–1002.

20. Canbay O, Celebi N, Arun O, et al. Efficacy of intravenous acetaminophen and lidocaine on propofol injection pain. Br J Anaesth. 2008;100(1):95–8.

21. Hemanshu P, Pal SG, Zulfiqar A, et al. Pharmacological and non-pharmacological interventions for reducing rocuronium bromide induced pain on injection in children and adults. Cochrane Database Syst Rev. 2016; 2:CD009346.

22. Ong Cliff K-S, Philipp L, Seymour Robin A, et al. The efficacy of preemptive analgesia for acute postoperative pain management: a meta-analysis. Anesth Analg. 2005;100:757–73 table of contents.

23. Araki Y, Kaibori M, Matsumura S, et al. Novel strategy for the control of postoperative pain: long-lasting effect of an implanted analgesic hydrogel in a rat model of postoperative pain. Anesth Analg. 2012;114(6):1338–45.

24. Arndt JO, Klement W. Pain evoked by polymodal stimulation of hand veins in humans. Physiol (Lond). 1991;440:467–78.

25. Shin YH, Kim CS, Lee JH, et al. Dilution and slow injection reduces the incidence of rocuronium-induced withdrawal movements in children. Korean J Anesthesiol. 2011;61(6):465–9.

26. Woo HD, Nyeo KB, Ho CS, et al. Neutralized rocuronium (pH 7.4) before administration prevents injection pain in awake patients: a randomized prospective trial. J Clin Anesth. 2007;19:418–23.

27. Blunk JA, Seifert F, Schmelz M, et al. Injection pain of rocuronium and vecuronium is evoked by direct activation of nociceptive nerve endings. Eur J Anaesthesiol. 2003;20:245–53.

28. Bin BS, Soon SM, Hee HJ, et al. Rocuronium bromide inhibits inflammation and pain by suppressing nitric oxide production and enhancing prostaglandin E synthesis in endothelial cells. Int Neurourol J. 2016;20:296–303.

29. Richette P, Latourte A, Frazier A. Safety and efficacy of paracetamol and NSAIDs in osteoarthritis: which drug to recommend? Expert Opin Drug Saf. 2015;14(8):1259–68.

30. Cashman JN. The mechanisms of action of NSAIDs in analgesia. Drugs. 1996;5:13–23.

6

Continuous block at the proximal end of the adductor canal provides better analgesia compared to that at the middle of the canal after total knee arthroplasty

Yuda Fei[1], Xulei Cui[1]* , Shaohui Chen[1], Huiming Peng[2], Bin Feng[2], Wenwei Qian[2], Jin Lin[2], Xisheng Weng[2] and Yuguang Huang[1]

Abstract

Background: The optimal position for continuous adductor canal block (ACB) for analgesia after total knee anthroplasty (TKA) remains controversial, mainly due to high variability in the localization of the the adductor canal (AC). Latest neuroanatomy studies show that the nerve to vastus medialis plays an important role in innervating the anteromedial aspect of the knee and dives outside of the exact AC at the proximal end of the AC. Therefore, we hypothesized that continuous ACB at the proximal end of the exact AC could provide a better analgesic effect after TKA compared with that at the middle of the AC (which appeared to only block the saphenous nerve).

Methods: Sixty-two adult patients who were scheduled for a unilateral TKA were randomized to receive continuous ACB at the proximal end or middle of the AC. All patients received patient-controlled intravenous analgesia with sufentanil postoperatively. The primary outcome measure was cumulative sufentanil consumption within 24 h after the surgery, which was analyzed using Mann-Whitney U tests. P-values < 0.05 (two-sided) were considered statistically significant. The secondary outcomes included postoperative sufentanil consumption at other time points, pain at rest and during passive knee flexion, quadriceps motor strength, and other recovery related paramaters.

Results: Sixty patients eventually completed the study (30/group). The 24-h sufentanil consumption was 0.22 µg/kg (interquartile range [IQR]: 0.15–0.40 µg/kg) and 0.39 µg/kg (IQR: 0.23–0.52 µg/kg) in the proximal end and middle groups ($P = 0.026$), respectively. There were no significant inter-group differences in sufentanil consumption at other time points, pain at rest and during passive knee flexion, quadriceps motor strength, and other recovery related paramaters.

(Continued on next page)

* Correspondence: cui.xulei@aliyun.com
[1]Anesthesiology Department, Peking Union Medical College Hospital, Chinese Academy of Medical Sciences, and Peking Union Medical College, Shuaifuyuan 1#, Dongcheng District, Beijing 100730, China

(Continued from previous page)

Conclusions: Continuous ACB at the proximal end of the AC has a better opioid-sparing effect without a significant influence on quadriceps motor strength compared to that at the middle of the AC after TKA. These findings indicates that a true ACB may not produce the effective analgesia, instead, the proximal end AC might be a more suitable block to alleviate pain after TKA.

Keywords: Opioid-sparing, Total knee anthroplasty, Adductor canal block, Analgesia, Sufentanil

Background

Severe pain is common after total knee anthroplasty (TKA), especially in the first 24 h postoperatively and during active range of motion [1], which may span from 2 ~ 3 days and significantly limit early mobilization, rehabilitation, and recovery [2, 3]. Continuous adductor canal block (ACB) is recommended as an analgesic method for early postoperative pain treatment after TKA as it preserves quadriceps strength compared with continuous femoral nerve block. Continuous ACB also provides better analgesia compared with single ACB [4].

The optimal location for continuous ACB for TKA has been investigated by previous randomized clinical trials (RCTs) [5–8]. However, identification of the adductor canal (AC) was not consistent [5–8], and the results differed. The AC is a musculoaponeurotic tunnel that runs proximally from the apex of the femoral triangle (FT)/proximal end (entrance opening) of the AC where the medial borders of the sartorius muscle (SM) and adductor longors muscle (ALM) align, to the adductor hiatus distally where the femoral artery (FA) diverges from the SM and becomes deep [9]. The internal landmarks defined above can be easily identified via ultrasound, which has recently been deemed to be a more accurate and reliable method to identify the exact location of the AC [10–12]. However, to the best of our knowledge, the ideal continuous ACB location (for analgesia after TKA) of the true AC identified with these sonographic landmarks has not been investigated in a clinical setting.

Inside the AC, the neurovascular bundle is situated between the adductor muscles (longus and magnus) posteromedially, the medial vastus muscle anterolaterally, and the vastoaddutor membrane anteromedially [10–12]. Studies which have investigated the relevant neuroanatomy of the thigh and knee found that the saphenous nerve (SN) that innervates the anteriomedia of the knee is the only nerve that is consistently found in the AC [10, 13, 14]. The nerve to vastus medialis (NVM), a femoral nerve branch which also plays an important role in the inervation of the anteromedial aspect of the knee [10, 15–17], though described in anatomical textbooks as being within the AC, has been recently shown to dive into a fascial tunnel, proximal to the entrance of the AC, between the medial vastus muscle and the ALM outside the AC in 90% of humans [13, 18, 19]. Indeed, previous cadaveric studies by Andersen et al. and, more recently, by Johnston et al. found that injectates administered into the AC or the distal AC could only capture the SN [18, 20]. In contrast, when the injectates were administered into the distal FT, both the SN and NVM were stained [19, 20]. Other investigators speculated that "a true ACB may not produce effective analgesia after TKA if the NVM is an important contributor to knee innervation" [12].

We therefore conducted this clinical trial to test the hypothesis that during continuous ACB, postoperative analgesia after TKA would improve with the catheter tip inserted at the less studied proximal end of the true AC, compared with a more distal locaion at the middle of the AC. The primary outcome was the median sufentanil consumption 24 h after surgery.

Methods
Enrollment

This study was approved by the Institutional Review Board of Peking Union Medical College Hospital in Beijing, China (#ZS-1030) and was registered at Clinical-Trials.gov (NCT03942133; date of registration: May 06, 2019; date of patient enrollment: May 11, 2019). Written informed consent was obtained from all participants before taking part. This manuscript adheres to the applicable Consolidated Standards of Reporting Trials guidelines and was conducted in accordance with the Declaration of Helsinki. Adult (≥18 years of age) patients with an American Society of Anesthesiologists (ASA) physical status classification of I to III who were scheduled for unilateral, primary TKA were approached for inclusion. Exclusion criteria were a body mass index (BMI) > 40, contraindications to peripheral nerve blocks, known daily intake of opioids (morphine, oxycodone, methadone, ketobemidone, fentanyl), alcohol or drug abuse, intolerance of nonsteroidal anti-inflammatory drugs, diabetes, lower limb neuropathy, and the inability to accurately describe postoperative pain to the investigators (e.g., a language barrier or a neuropsychiatric disorder).

Randomization and blinding

Participants were randomized to either the proximal end or middle group with a ratio of 1:1 using a computer-generated sequence given by a professional statistician who was not otherwise involved in the study. Allocation concealment was ensured by the use of sealed, opaque, sequentially numbered envelopes which remained concealed until the block was performed.

All the ultrasound-guided continuous ACBs were conducted by a single senior experienced staff anesthesiologist (C.X.) in a dedicated procedure room, where all other surgeons, nurses (except the assistant research nurse in the procedure room), and study participants were not presented at the time of performing the block. Surgeries were conducted by the same surgical team blinded to subject allocation using a standardized approach.

Perioperative management

All recruited subjects were interviewed on the day before surgery. Baseline pain severity and quadriceps strength of the operative leg were recorded. Subjects were informed of the postoperative continuous ACB and patient-controlled intravenous analgesia (PCIA) schedule, with a goal of maintaining pain scores < 4 on an 11-point numerical rating scale (NRS, 0: no pain; 10: maximum pain imaginable). No preoperative medications were administered.

Catheter insertion procedure

All perineural catheter insertions were performed 40 min before surgery in a dedicated procedure room. Standard monitoring and peripheral venous access were established. Patients were placed in a supine position with the operative knee slightly flexed and externally rotated. With the ultrasound screen facing away from the patient, an ultrasound scan was carried out with a 13–6 MHz linear probe (Sonosite X-port, SonoSite Inc., Bothell, WA) which was positioned perpendicular to the skin in the medial upper-thigh region. The entire procedure was performed after strict aseptic precautions were taken and skin infiltration (2 ~ 3 mL of 1% lidocaine) was performed with a 100 mm, 17 gauge, insulated nerve block needle and a 19 gauge perineural catheter (SonoPlex Stim cannula; Pajunk, Geisingen, Germany).

For subjects randomized to the proximal end group, a short-axis dynamic scan was performed (Fig. 1A). The insertion site was defined by the ultrasound image as the location where the medial margins of the SM and ALM intersected [13] (Fig. 1a). Then, the needle was inserted in-plane in a short-axis lateral-to-medial orientation, through the SM with the final needle tip positioned between the FA and SN (Fig. 1A, a). If the SN could not be

well visualized, the needle tip was placed at a 5 o'clock position relative to the FA within the AC [21]. For subjects randomized to the middle group, we used a slightly modified method described by Koscielniak-Nielsen [22]. After identifying the proximal end of the AC in the short-axis view, the ultrasound transducer was rotated 90° to image the SN in the long-axis with the cranial end of the transducer aligned with the proximal end of the AC (Fig. 1B, b). To ensure adequate blinding of the block type to all research personnel performing follow-up evaluations, we choose a needle puncture site at a similar level as in the proximal end group (Fig. 1B). The needle was inserted in-plane in a long-axis with cranial-to-caudal orientation toward the location, 3 ~ 5 cm caudal to the proximal end of the canal, and with the needle tip placed deep into the SM and just superficial to the SN (Fig. 1B, b). If the SN could not be well visualized, the needle tip was placed lateral to the FA within the AC [21].

In both groups, after hydro-dissection with 0.9% saline to confirm proper needle-tip placement within the AC, the perineural catheter was advanced 1 ~ 1.5 cm into the AC under direct ultrasound visualization. After withdrawing the needle, the perineural catheter was tunneled subcutaneously and secured to the upper part of the thigh with surgical glue and an occlusive dressing with an anchoring device. The time between needle skin entry to needle removal was recorded as the block performance time. Ten milliliters of 0.2% ropivacaine was injected as the loading dose via the catheter after negative aspiration. Catheter insertion success was defined as a decrease in the cutaneous sensation to pinprick in the SN distribution area over the ipsilateral medial calf within 30 min after injection. Subjects with a failed catheter insertion or misplaced catheter indicated by a lack of sensory change had their catheter replaced or were withdrawn from the study.

Intraoperative management

A bispectral index (BIS) monitor was connected for all patients. General anesthesia was induced with intravenous midazolam (1 mg), fentanyl (2 µg/kg), propofol (1.5 ~ 2.0 mg/kg), and rocuronium (0.6 mg/kg). All patients received laryngeal mask airway intubation. Anesthesia was maintained with a sevoflurane and O_2-N_2O mixture to keep the BIS within 40 ~ 60. Intravenous fentanyl (1 µg /kg) and rocuronium bromide (0.6–0.9 mg/kg) were administered intraoperatively as needed. On completion of surgery, sevoflurane and N_2O were discontinued and the neuromuscular blockade was reversed using neostigmine (50 µg/kg) and atropine (20 µg/kg). Extubation was carried out when patients were fully awake.

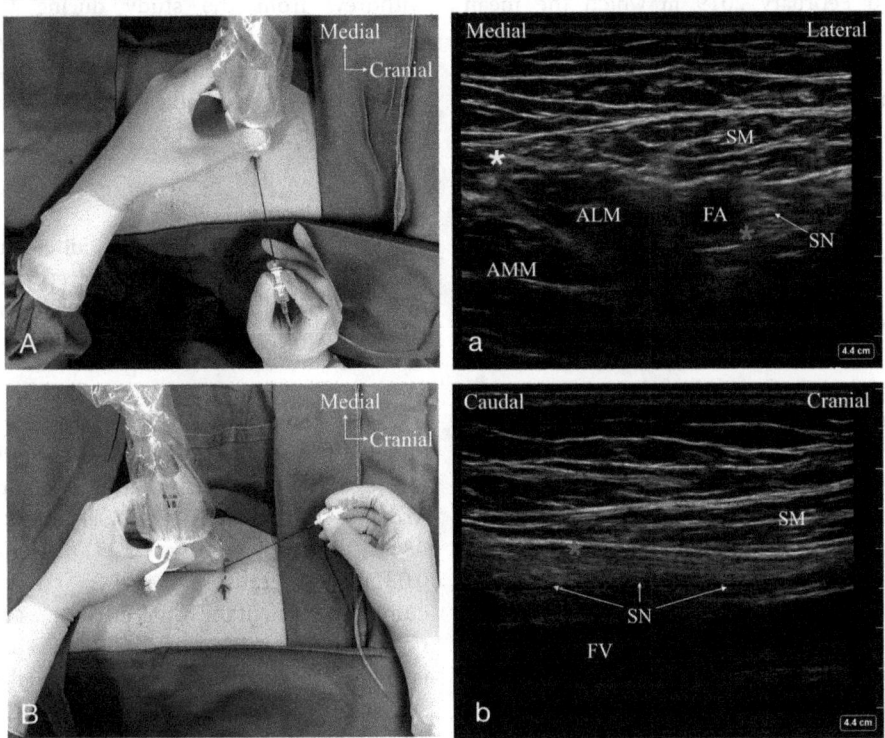

Fig. 1 Ultrasound-guided proximal end adductor canal block (ACB) (A/a) and middle ACB (B/b) techniques. (A) Ultrasound probe position of short-axis scanning at the proximal end of the AC and needle orientation for proximal end ACB. (a) Short-axis ultrasound scan image at the proximal end of the AC. (B) Ultrasound probe position of long-axis scanning with the cranial end of the probe aligned with the proximal end of the AC and needle orientation for middle ACB. (b) Long-axis ultrasound scan image with the cranial end of the probe aligned with the proximal end of the AC (at the cranial side in the image). The purple arrow indicates the skin mark of the puncture point for proximal end ACB; the purple dotted line indicates the skin mark of the proximal end of the AC; the red asterisk indicates the endpoint target for the needle tip; the yellow asterisk indicates the alignment of the medial borders of the SM and ALM. ALM, adductor longus muscle; AMM, adductor magnus muscle; FA, femoral artery; FV, femoral venous; SM, sartorius muscle

Postoperative analgesia

Continuous ACB was initiated immediately after surgery in both groups using an electronic pump (Gemstar, Hospiria Inc., USA) to administer 0.2% ropivacaine at a rate of 6 ml/h through the catheter. PCIA was commenced using a pump set (Gemstar, Hospiria Inc., USA) to deliver boluses of 1.5 ~ 2 μg sufentanil with a 5-min lockout interval and no background infusion. The maximum permitted dosage of sufentanil was set at 8 μg/h. Continuous ACB and PCIA were continued until 48 h after the surgery in both groups. Intravenous parecoxib sodium (40 mg), Q12 h, was administered for 3 days postoperatively.

Outcomes and data collection

Patients were evaluated postoperatively at 0, 2, 4, 8, 12, 24, and 48 h. The primary outcome measure was the 24 h sufentanil consumption after surgery. The secondary outcome measures included sufentanil consumption at other postoperative time points; pain intensity both at rest and upon passive knee extension to 60° assessed with the NRS score; quadriceps motor strength assessed

by a physiotherapist using Lovett's 6-point scale (0 = no voluntary contraction possible, 1 = muscle flicker, but no movement of limb, 2 = active movement only with gravity eliminated, 3 = movement against gravity but without resistance, 4 = movement possible against some resistance and 5 = normal motor strength against resistance) preoperatively and postoperatively [23]; time to ambulation after surgery defined as the time from the end of surgery until ambulation assisted by a walker or ward nurse; episodes of PONV within 48 h after surgery; patient's satisfaction with anesthesia and analgesia, which were separately assessed at 48 h using a 5-point scale (5, very satisfied; 4, satisfied; 3, neither satisfied nor dissatisfied; 2, dissatisfied; 1, very dissatisfied); and block-related complications including puncture point infection, leakage, catheter dislodgment, and falling down. The durations of postoperative length of stay were also retrieved from electronic medical records.

Sample size

The sample size requirement was calculated based on a pilot study (*n* = 10) performed at our institution between

January 2019 and February 2019 in which the mean (standard deviation, SD) cumulative 24 h sufentanil consumption after TKA was 0.235 (0.172) µg/kg in the proximal end group and 0.376 (0.188) µg/kg in the middle group. A sample size of 28 patients would be needed for a power (1-beta) of 0.80 and a significance level (alpha) of 0.05. Since it is presumed that 24 h sufentanil consumption may not follow a normal distribution, and since a calculation which assumes a normal distribution might underestimate the sample size, we planned to enroll 31 patients per group.

Statistical analysis

The statistical analyses were performed using SPSS version 15.0 (SPSS Inc., Chicago, IL, USA). Variables and demographics that followed a normal distribution are expressed as the mean (standard deviation) and were analyzed using a Student's t-test. Variables that did not follow a normal distribution are presented as the median (interquartile range, IQR) and were analyzed using the Mann-Whitney U test. Categorical data are reported as the proportion or percentage and were analyzed using the Chi-squared test. P-values < 0.05 (two-sided) were considered statistically significant.

Results

Of the 66 subjects who were approached, 2 (3.03%) did not meet the inclusion criteria (1 patient's BMI was > 40 kg/m^2, and 1 patient received tramadol tablets for osteoarthritic knee pain); additionally, 2 (3.03%) patients refused to participate. The remaining 62 subjects were randomly assigned to one of the study groups. One subject who was randomized to the proximal end group unexpectedly needed to undergo bilateral TKA and 1 subject who was randomized to the middle group

withdrew from the study during the postoperative follow-up period. Sixty subjects, including 30 in each group with no clinically relevant differences noted between the groups (Table 1) were included in the final analysis (Fig. 2).

Primary outcome

The median (IQR) 24 h sufentanil consumption was significantly lower in the proximal end group than in the middle group [0.22 (0.15–0.40) vs. 0.39 (0.23–0.52) µg/kg, $P = 0.026$] (Table 2).

Secondary outcomes

Sufentanil consumption was also significantly lower in the proximal end group than in the middle group at 8 h [0.06 (0–0.18) vs. 0.21 (0.10–0.44) µg/kg, $P = 0.001$] and 48 h [0.43(0.23–0.74) vs. 0.59 (0.41–0.89) µg/kg, $P = 0.031$] postoperatively (Table 2). To clarify whether the cumulative sufentanil difference at 24 h and 48 h could be the representation of the initial 8 h difference which is carried forwardly, we also compared the difference of sufentanil consumption during the 8 h -to-24 h, 8 h -to-48 h and 24 h-to 48 h time intervals (Table 3), and the result did not show significant difference between groups ($Ps > 0.05$). There were no significant differences in median NRS scores (at rest/upon passive flexion of the operated knee) or quadriceps strength scores assessed at 0, 2, 4, 8, 24, and 48 h postoperatively ($Ps > 0.05$) between groups (Table 3, Table 4). The two treatment groups also did not differ significantly in terms of episodes of PONV within 48 h after surgery, time to ambulation, satisfaction scores with anesthesia and analgesia assessed 48 h after surgery, or postoperative length of hospital stay ($Ps > 0.05$) (Table 4).

Table 1 Demographics, preoperative, and intraoperative data

	Proximal end ($n = 30$)	Middle ($n = 30$)
Demographic data		
Age (years), mean (SD)	68.60 (6.20)	67.47 (6.37)
Female Sex, n (%)	26 (86.67%)	25 (83.33%)
BMI (kg/m^2), mean (SD)	25.27 (3.50)	25.80 (2.28)
ASA-PS class (I/II/III), n	5/24/1	5/25/0
Preoperative data		
NRS score at rest, median (IQR)	0 (0–3)	0 (0–3)
NRS score with activity, median (IQR)	5 (3–6)	5 (4–6)
Quadriceps strength score, median (IQR)	5 (5–5)	5 (5–5)
Time to complete the block and catheter insertion (sec), mean (SD)	144.00 (69.86)	136.37 (84.74)
Intraoperative data		
Operation duration (min), mean (SD)	86.57 (28.71)	93.73 (19.90)
Intraoperative fentanyl (µg/kg), mean (SD)	3.32 (1.21)	3.46 (1.20)

ASA-PS American Society of Anesthesiologists-physical status, *SD* Standard deviation, *IQR* Interquartile range

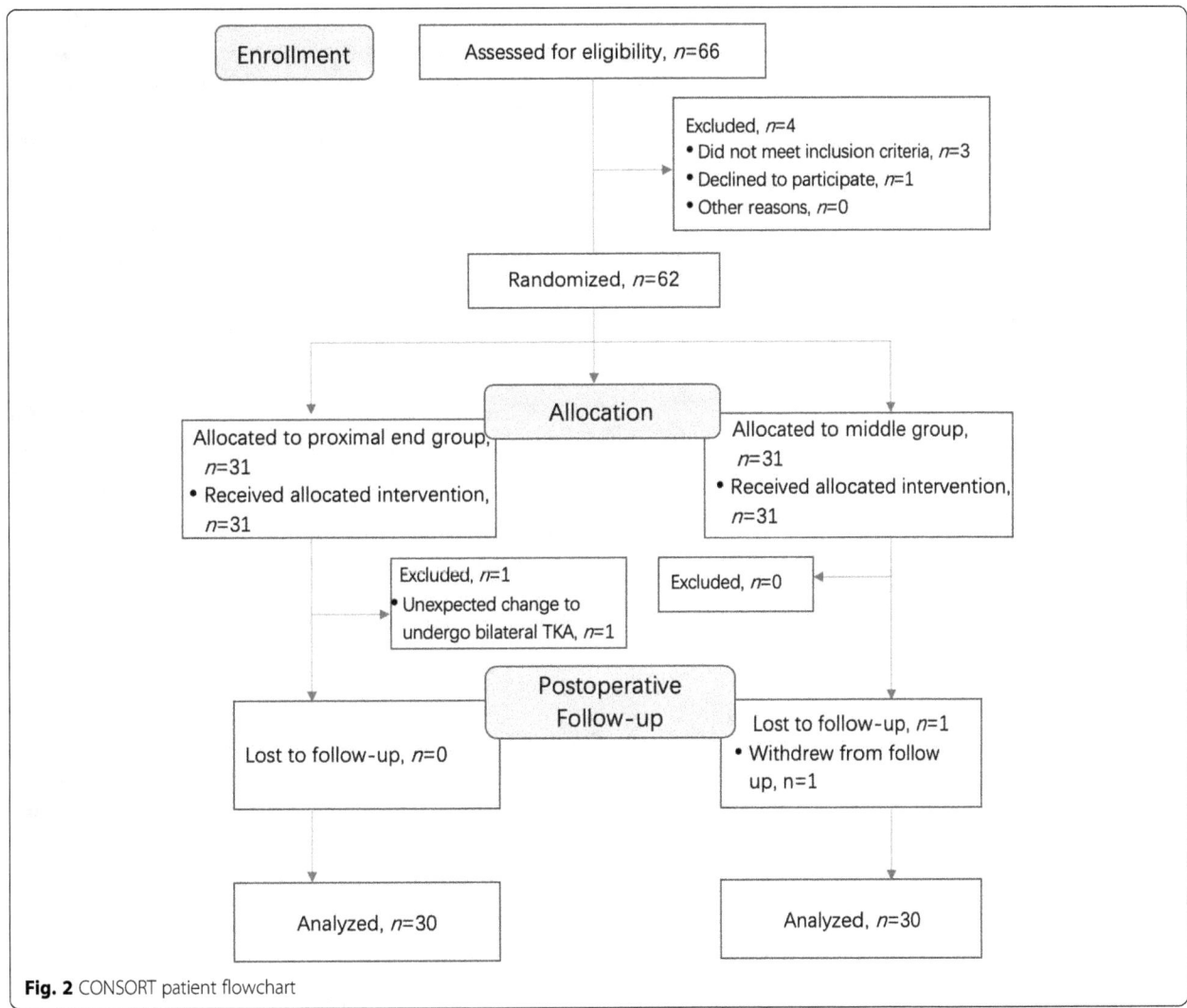

Fig. 2 CONSORT patient flowchart

Table 2 Cumulative sufentanil consumption (µg/kg) after surgery for both groups

	Proximal end (n = 30)	Middle (n = 30)	P value
Cumulative sufentanil consumption (µg/kg) at different time points			
Primary outcome			
24 h	0.22 (0.15–0.40)	0.39 (0.23–0.52)	0.026
Secondary outcomes			
2 h	0 (0–0.04)	0.02 (0–0.07)	0.222
4 h	0.03 (0–0.08)	0.07 (0–0.21)	0.143
8 h	0.06 (0–0.18)	0.21 (0.10–0.44)	0.001
48 h	0.43 (0.23–0.74)	0.59 (0.41–0.89)	0.031
Cumulative sufentanil consumption (µg/kg) at different time intervals			
8 h-to-24 h	0.13 (0.07–0.17)	0.10 (0.05–0.19)	0.525
8 h-to-48 h	0.38 (0.22–0.50)	0.38 (0.19–0.52)	0.842
24 h-to-48 h	0.17 (0.08–0.36)	0.21 (0.11–0.46)	0.280

Data are presented as the median (interquartile range)

All continuous ACBs were successful. No infection at the catheter insertion sites or dislodgment of the catheter were reported. Only one case of insertion site leakage was found in the proximal end group. There were also no reported falls secondary to quadriceps weakness.

Discussion

The main finding of this study was that continuous ACBs performed at the proximal end of the AC in comparison to that at the middle of the AC showed a superior opioid-sparing effect 24 h after TKA; in addition, both ACB locations had a similar influence on the strength of the quadriceps.

To our best knowledge, this is the first clinical RCT compares a continuous ACB performed at the proximal end of the AC (where the medial border of the SM intersects the medial border of the ALM) with a middle AC injection. The underlying mechanism of the current result could be explained by a more recent anatomical study by Tran published after the initiation of the

Table 3 Postoperative pain NRS scores at each time point for both groups

	Proximal end (n = 30)	Middle (n = 30)	P value
NRS at rest, median (IQR)			
0 h	0 (0–3)	0.5 (0–3)	0.753
2 h	0.5 (0–3)	1.5 (0–3)	0.906
4 h	0.5 (0–2.63)	1.5 (0–3)	0.488
8 h	0 (0–2.0)	1 (0–2.0)	0.567
24 h	0.5 (0–3.25)	1 (0–3)	0.798
48 h	0 (0–2)	0 (0–1)	0.165
NRS upon passive flexion of the operated knee to 60°, median (IQR)			
0 h	2 (0–5)	2.5 (0–4.25)	0.861
2 h	3 (0–6)	3 (2–5)	0.625
4 h	2 (0–4)	2 (1.75–4.25)	0.447
8 h	2 (0–4)	2.5 (0–4)	0.815
24 h	3 (0.75–5)	3 (2–5)	0.788
48 h	2.5 (1–4)	3 (1–3.25)	0.845

IQR Interquartile range, *NRS* Numerical rating scale

present trial [24]. In his study, following a proximal end AC injection with 10 ml of dye in seven lightly embalmed specimens, they found that the dye spread consistently stained the SN, posteromedial branch of the VMN, superior medial genicular nerve and the genicular branch of the obturator nerve, which are sensory nerves that innervate the knee joint [24]. Instead, cadaveric studies using a distal AC injection failed to report staining of the posteromedial branch of NVM and/or its

distal branch, the superomedial genicular nerve [19, 20]. We also found the superior analgesic effect of proximal end AC block could only be obviously observed till 8 h after surgery. We suppose this could be due to the effect of the initial loading dose of ropivacaine. A 10 ml injection of 0.2% ropivacaine at the middle of the AC may spread cephalad toward the proximal end of the AC and as a result provide similar analgesia at least during the first 4 h after surgery. Following that, when the analgesic effect of the initial dose wore off, 'rebound pain' may have occurred and induced 'rebound' opioid consumption requirements [25, 26], as shown at the 8 h time point in the middle ACB group in this study. The initial 8 h difference might have also carried forwardly till 48 h after surgery in the current study, since the difference of opioid consumption during the 8 h -to-24 h, 8 h-to-48 h and 24 h-to 48 h time interval did not show significance. This phenomenon indicates that a high volume of single injection at the middle AC may produce similar analgesia at the early period immediately after TKA, while a continuous low volume infusion at the proximal end of AC could provide consistent and prolonged pain relieve during the following period.

In studies aiming to clarify the optimal location to maintain ACB after TKA, three previously published RCTs by Mariano [5], Romano [6] and Meier [7] had investigated the "proximal AC" and "distal AC" and failed to detect significant differences in regard to 24 h postoperative opioid consumption, as well as in quadriceps strength or motor function. The discrepancies between

Table 4 Postoperative recovery related data for both groups

	Proximal end (n = 30)	Middle (n = 30)	P
Quadriceps motor strength scores, median (IQR)			
0 h	3 (1–3)	3 (2–3)	0.513
2 h	3 (2–4)	3.25 (1.75–4)	0.477
4 h	3.5 (2–4)	3.75 (3–4)	0.486
8 h	4 (3–4)	4 (3–5)	0.684
24 h	4 (3–5)	4.5 (3.88–5)	0.332
48 h	4.75 (4–5)	5 (4–5)	0.356
Incidence of PONV within 48 h, median (IQR)	0 (0–0)	0 (0–1)	0.412
Time to ambulation (h), mean (SD)	39.53 (13.11)	42.01 (17.13)	0.532
Satisfaction score with anesthesia assessed at 48 h, median (IQR)	5 (5–5)	5 (4.75–5)	0.629
Satisfaction score with analgesia assessed at 48 h, median (IQR)	5 (5–5)	5 (4–5)	0.412
Block related complications			
Puncture point infection, n	0	0	–
Leakage, n	1	0	–
Catheter dislodgment, n	0	0	–
Falling down, n	0	0	–
Postoperative LOS (days), mean (SD)	5.46 (2.76)	5.72 (1.94)	0.680

IQR Interquartile range, *LOS* Length of stay, *PONV* Postoperative nausea and vomiting, *SD* Standard deviation

the present study and these three RCTs can likely be attributed to the different definitions of the AC [5–7]. Base on their description, these studies actually compared the distal FT [5, 6] or the proximal AC [7] with a more cephalad injection in the FT [5–7], instead of the distal AC with the proximal AC. In another study with the similar purposes, Sztain8 compared the analgesic effect of continuous ACB at the mid-thigh level (termed "proximal AC" in their study), defined as the midpoint between the anterior superior iliac spine and the patella [12, 27, 28] which recently has been proved to actually indicate a cranial location to the proximal end of AC and inside the distal FT in most subjects [11], with a more distal insertion closer to the adductor hiatus. The result showed the mid-thigh level block provide improved analgesic effect after TKA. Both the study by Sztain [8] and the current study provided clinical evidence supporting previous speculation that, instead of a true AC, a distal TF or a proximal end AC block would be more suitable to alleviate pain after knee surgery [10, 13, 20].

The ideal location for continuous ACB after TKA is supposed to be where it achieves maximum analgesia with minimal quadriceps weakness. The current study did not show a significant difference in the effect of catheter locations on quadriceps strength measured manually by a physiotherapist on a Lovett's scale. This could also be explained by the finding of the latest cadaveric study by Tran [24], where the proximal end AC injection (10 ml, which is the same volume as the loading dose in the present study) was found to spare the anterior branches of the NVM which would likely preserve greater vastus medialis activation, contributing to the quadriceps motor sparing characteristic of the proximal ACB. Another non-negligible contributor could be the following blockade infusion (at a rate of 6 ml/h) regimen adopted in the current study which may avoid further cephalad spread of the local anesthetic following the initial dose to the motor component of the femoral nerve [29]. A further study powered to explore the effect of catheter location on quadriceps motor function is needed.

The current study had some limitations. First, the quadriceps muscle strength was only evaluated manually by a physiotherapist on a Lovett's scale, which is not as precise as by using the force dynamometer such as the measurement of maximum voluntary isometric contraction [7, 29]. In addition, we did not implement a validated test to measure patient mobilization ability, such as the Timed "Up and Go" measurement [30], which could directly reflect the balance between "pain-control during movement" and "preserving strength" that is important for effective pain management after TKA [31]. The current study is unable to show whether continuous

infusion will increase blockade related side effects. Comparing the analgesic effect and safety of the single shot ACB, continuous ACB without single shot initiation, and single shot initiation followed by continuous infusion is not the primary interests of the present work, but clearly warrants further studies. Finally, as this is a single-center study with a small sample size which is limited to TKA patients, the results may not be generalizable to other types of knee procedures.

Conclusions
In conclusion, this study demonstrates that continuous ACB at the proximal end of the AC—the location on ultrasound where the medial margins of the SM and ALM intersect—provides a better analgesic effect without significantly compromising quadriceps motor strength compared to that at the middle of the AC after TKA. These results confirm the findings reported by the latest cadaveric study on the neuroanatomy of the AC. Moreover, it also indicates that a true ACB may not produce the effective analgesia, instead, a proximal end AC might be a more suitable block to alleviate pain after TKA, which enables informed choices for further RCTs.

Abbreviations
AC: Abbductor canal; ACB: Adductor canal block; ALM: Adductor longors muscle; ASA: American Society of Anesthesiologists; BIS: Bispectral index; BMI: Body mass index; FA: Femoral artery; FT: Femoral triangle; IQR: Interquartile range; NRS: Numerical rating scale; NVM: Nerve to vastus medialis; PCIA: Patient-controlled intravenous analgesia; RCT: Randomized clinical trial; SD: Standard deviation; SM: Sartorius muscle; SN: Saphenous nerve; TKA: Total knee anthroplasty

Acknowledgements
We thank the Department of Orthopedic team at Peking Union Medical College Hospital for supporting this research.

Authors' contributions
XC and YF conceived and designed the experiment. YF, XC, HP, and BF performed the experiment. SC collected and assembled the data. HP, BF, WQ, JL and XW provided the study material or patients. YF and XC analyzed and interpreted the data. YF contributed to the writing of the manuscript. XW and YH were responsible for clinical coordination. All authors read and approved the final manuscript.

Author details
[1]Anesthesiology Department, Peking Union Medical College Hospital, Chinese Academy of Medical Sciences, and Peking Union Medical College, Shuaifuyuan 1#, Dongcheng District, Beijing 100730, China. [2]Orthopaedic Department, Peking Union Medical College Hospital, Chinese Academy of Medical Sciences, and Peking Union Medical College, Shuaifuyuan 1#, Dongcheng District, Beijing 100730, China.

References
1. Fischer HB, Simanski CJ, Sharp C, Bonnet F, Camu F, Neugebauer EA, et al. A procedure-specific systematic review and consensus recommendations for postoperative analgesia following total knee arthroplasty. Anaesthesia. 2008; 63:1105–23.
2. Andersen LØ, Husted H, Kristensen BB, Otte KS, Gaarn-Larsen L, Kehlet H. Analgesic efficacy of intracapsular and intra-articular local anaesthesia for knee arthroplasty. Anaesthesia. 2010;65:904–12.

3. Gerbershagen HJ, Aduckathil S, van Wijck AJ, Peelen LM, Kalkman CJ, Meissner W. Pain intensity on the first day after surgery: a prospective cohort study comparing 179 surgical procedures. Anesthesiology. 2013;118: 934–44.

4. Wang C, Chen Z, Ma X. Continuous adductor canal block is a better choice compared to single shot after primary total knee arthroplasty: a meta-analysis of randomized controlled trials. Int J Surg. 2019;72:16–24.

5. Mariano ER, Kim TE, Wagner MJ, Funck N, Harrison TK, Walters T, et al. A randomized comparison of proximal and distal ultrasound-guided adductor canal catheter insertion sites for knee arthroplasty. J Ultrasound Med. 2014; 33:1653–62.

6. Romano C, Lloyd A, Nair S, Wang JY, Viswanathan S, Vydyanathan A, et al. A randomized comparison of pain control and functional mobility between proximal and distal adductor canal blocks for total knee replacement. Anesth Essays Res. 2018;12:452–8.

7. Meier AW, Auyong DB, Yuan SC, Lin SE, Flaherty JM, Hanson NA. Comparison of continuous proximal versus distal adductor canal blocks for total knee arthroplasty. Reg Anesth Pain Med. 2018;43:36–42.

8. Sztain JF, Khatibi B, Monahan AM, Said ET, Abramson WB, Gabriel RA, et al. Proximal versus distal continuous adductor canal blocks: does varying perineural catheter location influence analgesia? A randomized, subject-masked, controlled clinical trial. Anesth Analg. 2018;127:240–6.

9. Hussain N, Ferreri TG, Prusick PJ, Banfield L, Long B, Prusick VR, et al. Adductor canal block versus femoral canal block for total knee arthroplasty: a meta-analysis: what does the evidence suggest? Reg Anesth Pain Med. 2016;41:314–20.

10. Laurant DB, Peng P, Arango LG, Niazi AU, Chan VW, Agur A, et al. The nerves of the adductor canal and the innervation of the knee: an anatomic study. Reg Anesth Pain Med. 2016;41:321–7.

11. Bendtsen TF, Moriggl B, Chan V, Børglum J. Basic topography of the saphenous nerve in the femoral triangle and the adductor canal. Reg Anesth Pain Med. 2015;40:391–2.

12. Wong WY, Bjørn S, Strid JM, Børglum J, Bendtsen TF. Defining the location of the adductor canal using ultrasound. Reg Anesth Pain Med. 2017;42:241–5.

13. Bendtsen TF, Moriggl B, Chan V, Børglum J. The optimal analgesic block for total knee arthroplasty. Reg Anesth Pain Med. 2016;41:711–9.

14. Manickam B, Perlas A, Duggan E, Brull R, Chan VW, Ramlogan R. Feasibility and efficacy of ultrasound-guided block of the saphenous nerve in the adductor canal. Reg Anesth Pain Med. 2009;34:578–80.

15. Baccarani G, Zanotti G. The innervation of the skin on the antero-medial region of the knee. Ital J Orthop Traumatol. 1984;10:521–55.

16. Andrikoula S, Tokis A, Vasiliadis HS, Georgoulis A. The extensor mechanism of the knee joint: an anatomical study. Knee Surg Sports Traumatol Arthrosc. 2006;14:214–20.

17. Tubbs RS, Loukas M, Shoja MM, Apaydin N, Oakes WJ, Salter EG. Anatomy and potential clinical significance of the vastoadductor membrane. Surg Radiol Anat. 2007;29:569–73.

18. Andersen HL, Andersen SK, Tranum-Jensen J. The spread of injectate during saphenous nerve block at the adductor canal: a cadaver study. Acta Anaesthesiol Scand. 2015;59:238–45.

19. Runge C, Moriggl B, Børglum J, Bendtsen TF. The spread of ultrasound-guided injectate from the adductor canal to the genicular branch of the posterior obturator nerve and the popliteal plexus: a cadaveric study. Reg Anesth Pain Med. 2017;42:725–30.

20. Johnston DF, Black ND, Cowden R, Turbitt L, Taylor S. Spread of dye injectate in the distal femoral triangle versus the distal adductor canal: a cadaveric study. Reg Anesth Pain Med. 2019;44:39–45.

21. Kwofie MK, Shastri UD, Gadsden JC, Sinha SK, Abrams JH, Xu D, et al. The effects of ultrasound-guided adductor canal block versus femoral nerve lock on quadriceps strength and fall risk: a blinded, randomized trial of volunteers. Reg Anesth Pain Med. 2013;38:321–5.

22. Koscielniak-Nielsen ZJ, Rasmussen H, Hesselbjerg L. Long-axis ultra- sound imaging of the nerves and advancement of perineural catheters under direct vision: a preliminary report of four cases. Reg Anesth Pain Med. 2008; 33:477–82.

23. Compston A. Aids to the investigation of peripheral nerve injuries. Medical Research Council: nerve injuries research committee. His Majesty's stationery office: 1942; pp 48 (iii) and 74 figures and 7 diagrams; with aids to the examination of the peripheral nervous system. By Michael O'Brien for the Guarantors of Brain. Saunders Elsevier. 2010:[8] 64–94. Brain. 2010;133:2838–44.

24. Tran J, Chan VWS, Peng PWH, Agur AMR. Evaluation of the proximal adductor canal block injectate spread: a cadaveric study. Reg Anesth Pain Med. 2020;45:124–30.

25. Abdallah FW, Halpern SH, Aoyama K, Brull R. Will the real benefits of single-shot interscalene block please stand up? A systematic review and meta-analysis. Anesth Analg. 2015;120:1114–29.

26. Lavand'homme P. Rebound pain after regional anesthesia in the ambulatory patient. Curr Opin Anaesthesiol. 2018;31:679–84.

27. Bendtsen TF, Moriggl B, Chan V, Pedersen EM, Børglum J. Redefining the adductor canal block. Reg Anesth Pain Med. 2014;39:442–3.

28. Anagnostopoulou S. Saphenous and infrapatellar nerves at the adductor canal: anatomy and implications in regional anesthesia. Orthopedics. 2016; 39:e259–62.

29. Jæger P, Zaric D, Fomsgaard JS, Hilsted KL, Bjerregaard J, Gyrn J, et al. Adductor canal block versus femoral nerve block for analgesia after total knee arthroplasty: a randomized, double-blind study. Reg Anesth Pain Med. 2013;38:526–32.

30. Yeung TS, Wessel J, Stratford PW, MacDermid JC. The timed up and go test for use on an inpatient orthopaedic rehabilitation ward. J Orthop Sports Phys Ther. 2008;38:410–7.

31. Shumway-Cook A, Brauer S, Woollacott M. Predicting the probability for falls in community-dwelling older adults using the timed up & amp; amp; go test. Phys Ther. 2000;80:896–903.

7

Pain management after ambulatory surgery: A prospective, multicenter, randomized, double-blinded parallel controlled trial comparing nalbuphine and tramadol

Yu-jiao Guan[1], Lai Wei[2], Qin Liao[3], Qi-wu Fang[4], Nong He[5], Chong-fang Han[6], Chang-hong Miao[7], Gang-jian Luo[8], Han-bing Wang[9], Hao Cheng[10], Qu-lian Guo[1*] and Zhi-gang Cheng[1*]

Abstract

Background: Postoperative pain in ambulatory surgery is a multifactorial issue affecting patient satisfaction, time of discharge, and rehospitalization. This study evaluated the efficacy and safety of nalbuphine for the treatment of postoperative pain after ambulatory surgery, relative to tramadol.

Methods: This multi-center, randomized, double blind, and controlled study was conducted at 10 centers. In accordance with the inclusion criteria, 492 ambulatory surgery patients were recruited. These patients had moderate to severe pain after ambulatory surgery, with a visual analogue scale (VAS) score > 3 cm. They were randomly divided into an experimental ($n = 248$) or control ($n = 244$) group and treated for analgesia with 0.2 mg/kg of nalbuphine or 2 mg/kg of tramadol, respectively. VAS scores, adverse events, and vital signs of the patients were recorded before administration (baseline; T_1); and 30 min (T_2), 2 h (T_3), 4 h (T_4), and 6 h (T_5) after administration of analgesia. A decrease in pain intensity of more than 25% compared with the baseline was used as an indicator of analgesic efficacy. The experimental and control groups were compared with regard to this indicator of efficacy at each timepoint.

Results: The VAS scores of the experimental and control groups were statistically comparable at timepoints T_1-T_4. At T_5, the VAS scores of the experimental group were significantly lower than that of the control. The pain intensity was significantly higher in the experimental group compared with the control at T_2 and T_3. Adverse events and vital signs were similar for the two groups at each timepoint.

Conclusions: Nalbuphine can provide effective and safe pain relief in patients after ambulatory surgery.

Keywords: Nalbuphine, Tramadol, Ambulatory surgery, Postoperative analgesia, Anesthesia, Pain

* Correspondence: qulianguo@hotmail.com; chengzg2004@hotmail.com
[1]Department of Anesthesiology, Xiangya Hospital of Central South University, No. 87 Xiangya Road, Changsha, Hunan, China

Background

Postoperative pain is a multifactorial issue that may result in patient dissatisfaction, delayed discharge, and unanticipated hospital admission after ambulatory surgery [1]. Both delayed discharge and unanticipated hospital admission have the undesirable effect of increasing healthcare costs [2]. In the postoperative period, moderate to severe pain are frequently observed during the first 24 to 48 h after ambulatory surgery [3].

Patient recovery after ambulatory surgery has improved since the introduction of the concept of enhanced recovery after surgery, a multimodal perioperative care pathway designed to achieve early recovery after surgery [4]. Ambulatory surgery has significantly shortened hospitalization, accelerated turnover, and reduced hospital costs and rates of nosocomial infections [5]. However, the shortened hospitalization and increased mobility of surgical patients have necessitated the need to improve the efficacy of anesthesia and perioperative management. Therefore, postoperative pain and the complications arising from its treatment are important considerations for patients undergoing ambulatory surgery.

Various drugs have been used to prolong postoperative analgesia, such as tramadol [6], ketorolac [7], dexmedetomidine [8], ketamine [9], and nalbuphine [10]. Nalbuphine, a synthetic opioid agonist-antagonist analgesic, is primarily a kappa (κ) agonist and a partial mu (μ) antagonist. It has a better safety profile with fewer side effects compared with other opioids, because of its agonist and antagonist activities [11]. Nalbuphine [12] exerts its analgesic and hypnotic effects through its κ opioid receptor, which may reduce μ opioid receptor-related adverse events. Numerous studies [13, 14] have reported its advantages in pain management.

There have been few studies in China of nalbuphine for the treatment of postoperative pain after ambulatory surgery. The present study evaluated the analgesic efficacy and safety of intravenous nalbuphine hydrochloride, relative to tramadol, for the treatment of postoperative pain after ambulatory surgery, including a noninferiority control trial.

Methods

Participants

This study was approved by the Ethics Committee of Xiangya Hospital of Central South University (IRB 201608066). Written informed consent was obtained from all subjects participating in the trial. The trial was registered prior to patient enrollment at chictr.org.cn (ChiCTR-IOR-16010032, Principal investigator: Qulian Guo, Date of registration: 2016-11-26).

A multicenter, prospective, randomized, parallel-controlled, double-blinded study for pain management after ambulatory surgery in adult patients was undertaken in 10 hospitals. Patients were screened at each center. The study was reported in accordance with the guidelines of the Consolidated Standards of Reporting Trials (CONSORT).

The patient inclusion criteria were as follows: 18 to 65 years old; ASA (American Society of Anesthesiologists) I-II; with postoperative pain after surgeries of the breast (except radical surgery for mastocarcinoma) or thyroid, or hysteroscopy, or laparoscopic cholecystectomy; operative time < 2 h; visual analog scale (VAS) score < 3 cm before the surgery, and VAS score > 3 cm after recovery from anesthesia; body mass index (BMI) 18–29 kg/m^2, and signed informed consent.

Patients were excluded from this study if they were allergic to the medication or any of the excipients in the product. Patients with current or histories of any of the following were also excluded: opioid allergy; acute or chronic alcoholism or drug addiction; neurological disease; opioid used within the last 3 months; paralytic ileus; increased intracranial pressure or head injury; chronic opioid use (taking opioids for more than 3 months); hypotension; hypothyroidism, asthma (to be avoided during seizure); hypertrophy of the prostate; epilepsy; coronary heart disease; bronchial asthma; respiratory insufficiency; or respiratory failure. Patients taking or who had taken monoamine oxidase inhibitor or antidepressants within the past 15 days were excluded. Patients with abnormal preoperative liver and kidney function were also excluded, defined as abnormal alanine aminotransferase (ALT), aspartic aminotransferase (AST), blood urea nitrogen (BUN) or creatinine (Cr) (ALT and AST > 1.5 times the normal limit, and BUN and Cr higher than the normal limit); coronary heart disease; bronchial asthma; respiratory insufficiency or respiratory failure; or poorly controlled or difficult hypertension. The latter was defined as systolic blood pressure (SBP) ≥ 160 mmHg or diastolic pressure (DBP) ≥ 100 mmHg. In addition, patients with any of the following were excluded: pregnancy; abnormal coagulation function; participation in another medication trial within the previous 30 days; unable to express their intention correctly; poor compliance; unable to complete the study program; or anyone the researchers considered inappropriate to participate.

Trial design

Patients were randomly assigned to receive either the experimental (group E) or control (group C) treatment in the postoperative period. Group E was treated with nalbuphine hydrochloride (1,161,101 Yichang Humanwell Pharmaceutical) diluted with saline to 1 mg/L. Group C was administered tramadol hydrochloride diluted with saline to 10 mg/L.

The study medication was selected and prepared according to a random number list (nalbuphine hydrochloride or tramadol hydrochloride). The study was blinded, by excluding the researcher who prepared the postoperative medications from participating in test observations and follow-ups. The researchers involved in observation and evaluation of the experiment, and patients and doctors, were blinded throughout the study.

Interventions

All patients were administered intravenously with 5 mg of dexamethasone before induction of general anesthesia, and 8 mg of ondansetron at the time of surgery completion, to prevent postoperative nausea and vomiting. The bispectral index (BIS) value was maintained between 40 and 60 during the operation. Anesthesia induction was performed using sufentanil (0.5 µg/kg) and propofol (2–2.5 mg/kg), with cisatracurium (0.1–0.2 mg/kg) given when necessary. Anesthesia was maintained by simultaneous infusion of propofol and remifentanil (0.1–0.15 µg/kg/min). An additional 0.1 mg/kg of cisatracurium was added intraoperatively when required. Intraoperative fluid infusion and other anesthetic management were performed routinely.

After the surgery, patients who were fully awake and feeling pain for the first time were assessed for pain while at rest, using the VAS. If the VAS score was > 3 cm, the patients were included in the study and the pain score was used as the baseline (T_1). The test medications (nalbuphine hydrochloride or tramadol hydrochloride) were administered at 0.2 mL/kg. The VAS at rest was used to evaluate the efficacy of the medications and was recorded before administration (T_1), and after administration at 30 min (T_2), 2 h (T_3), 4 h (T_4), and 6 h (T_5). The following vital signs were recorded at each timepoint: SBP, DBP, mean arterial pressure (MAP), heart rate, and respiratory rate. Adverse events and any medications used were also recorded.

Within 2 h after administration of the medications, if the VAS score was > 3 cm, it was deemed that the analgesic effect was invalid, and the patient was discontinued from the trial. One hundred milligrams of flurbiprofen axetil was infused intravenously as a rescue analgesia, and the name and dose were recorded. The use of other analgesics aside from those involved in the study, such as opioids, tranquilizers, anesthetics and antiemetics, were prohibited during the study period. If other analgesics were required to control the pain, the patient was discontinued.

Outcomes

Primary outcome

The pain intensity was measured using the VAS. A decrease in VAS score of more than 25% compared with the baseline was used as an indicator of analgesic efficacy [15]. The VAS score was also compared between groups E and C at all timepoints to determine any differences in the efficacy and duration of the analgesic effects.

Secondary outcome

The vital signs (SBP, DBP, respiratory rate and heart rate) were measured and used as safety indicators. The vital signs were also compared between groups E and C, and within each group, at each timepoint. Any differences observed could be used as a secondary indicator to determine analgesic efficacy.

Adverse events

Adverse events such as medication extravasation, dizziness, nausea, vomiting, and hidrosis were recorded during the study. The rates of adverse events was compared between groups E and C to determine the effects of the treatments.

Sample size

Sample size was calculated by VAS at rest at each timepoint. Based on a previous report [16], a single intravenous injection of tramadol was administered to patients with postoperative pain after day surgery, and the VAS score was ~ 2.43 cm at 30 min after administration. Assuming that the analgesic effect of nalbuphine was better than tramadol, with α = 0.05 and β = 0.2, the VAS score difference between the two groups ($\mu_A - \mu_B$) would be 0.5 and the standard deviation σ = 1.7. The sample size(n) was calculated using the formula [17]:

$$n = 2\left[\alpha\left(z_{1-\alpha/2} + z_{1-\beta}\right)/(\mu_A - \mu_B)\right]^2$$

Each group required 182 subjects and with consideration of the estimated dropout rate, 250 patients were included in each group. Therefore, 500 patients were recruited in this study, with 50 patients in each center.

Statistical methods

Descriptive statistics were used to describe all demographic data. The t-test was applied to analyze the changes in VAS scores between the two treatment groups at each timepoint, and at different timepoints relative to the baseline. The Wilcoxon test was used to analyze the pain classification of patients at each observation timepoint. The pain intensity between the two groups was compared using the chi-squared (χ^2) test. $P < 0.05$ was considered statistically significant. The incidence of adverse events, changes in blood pressure, respiratory rate, and heart rate relative to the baseline at each timepoint, and differences between the groups, were analyzed using the *t*-test.

Results

Participants

The study population comprised 492 randomly coded patients recruited from 10 centers (Fig. 1). However, 55 patients were excluded as they did not meet the eligibility criteria of a VAS score < 4 cm. Thus, the trial consisted of 437 patients: 209 in group E, and 228 in group C.

Baseline data

The differences in age and gender between groups E and C were not statistically significant (Table 1). The results of the preoperative test, physical examination, and medical histories of the two groups were relatively similar, with no statistical difference. There were no statistically significant differences in the types of surgery between the two groups (Table 2). There were also no differences in the use of opioids including sufentanil and remifentanil between the two groups, during surgery.

During the observation period, 14 (6.3%) and 20 (9.0%) patients in groups E and C, respectively, were treated with rescue analgesic medication consisting of 100 mg of flurbiprofen axetil. There was no statistically significant difference between the two groups

with regard to the percentage using rescue analgesic medication ($\chi^2 = 1.206$; $P = 0.272$). There was no significant deviation from the regimen for all concomitant and combination medications and no statistically significant difference between the two groups.

Table 1 Patient demographics of groups E and C[a]

	Group E	Group C	P
Subjects, n	209	228	
Gender, n (%)			
Male	52 (25.0)	48 (21.1)	0.340
Female	156 (75.0)	179 (78.9)	
Age, y	40.66 ± 12.04	40.67 ± 11.81	0.994
BMI, kg/m²	23.15 ± 2.84	23.20 ± 2.87	0.847
Respiration, rpm	17.09 ± 1.81	17.04 ± 2.18	0.808
Heart rate, bpm	74.45 ± 8.43	74.48 ± 9.75	0.978
Heart rhythm, n (%)			
Normal	207 (99.0)	225 (99.1)	1.000
Abnormal	2 (1.0)	2 (0.9)	
SBP, mmHg	121.63 ± 16.26	122.64 ± 16.01	0.513
DBP, mmHg	74.92 ± 9.48	74.63 ± 8.80	0.738
MAP, mmHg	92.91 ± 11.65	93.17 ± 10.84	0.806

[a]Group E was treated with nalbuphine hydrochloride diluted with saline to 1 mg/L. Group C was administered tramadol hydrochloride diluted with saline to 10 mg/L.

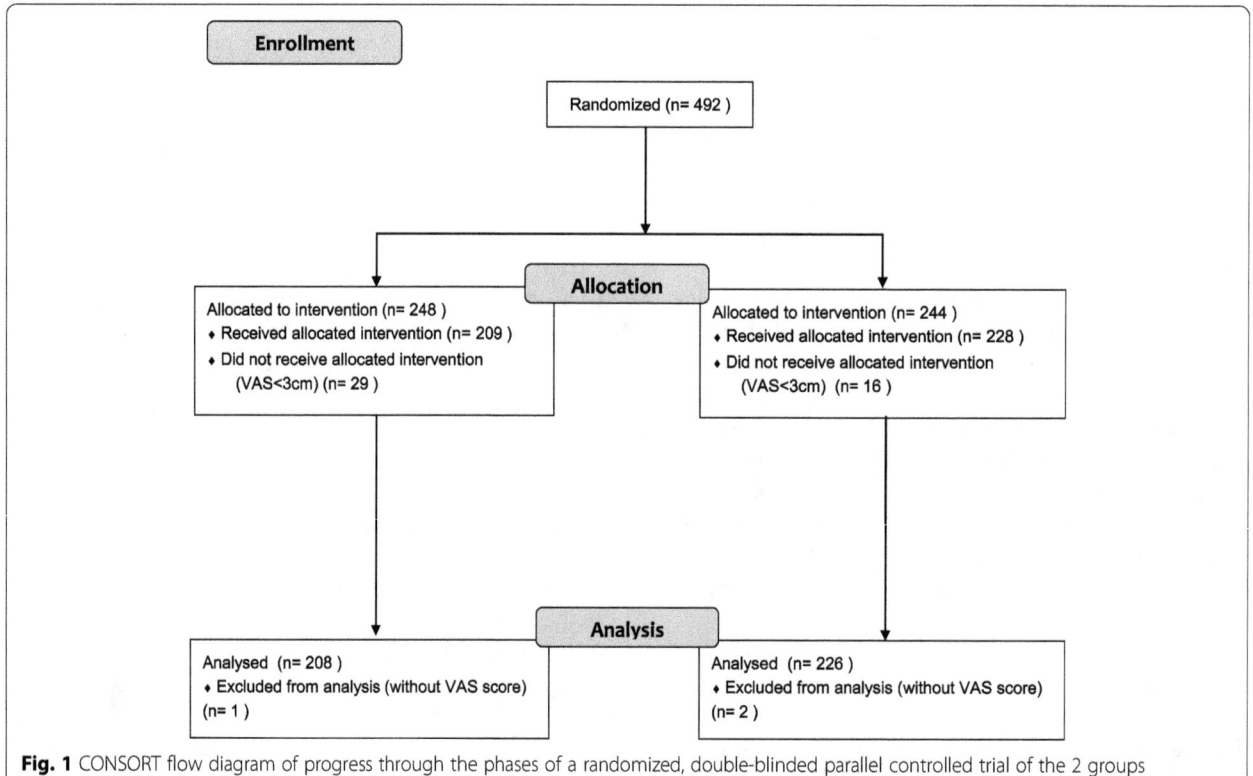

Fig. 1 CONSORT flow diagram of progress through the phases of a randomized, double-blinded parallel controlled trial of the 2 groups

Table 2 Types of surgery, n (%)[a]

	Total, n	Breast	Thyroid	Hysteroscopy	LC	Others
Group E	209	27 (12.9)	41 (19.6)	39 (18.7)	91 (43.5)	11 (5.3)
Group C	228	26 (11.4)	45 (19.7)	44 (19.3)	106 (46.5)	7 (3.1)

[a]Reported as n (%), unless indicated otherwise. Group E was treated with nalbuphine hydrochloride diluted with saline to 1 mg/L. Group C was administered tramadol hydrochloride diluted with saline to 10 mg/L. Other surgeries included: lumbar disc exploration, laparoscopic gastric perforation repair, endoscopic sinus surgery, surgical removal of internal fixation of fractured bones.LC, laparoscopic cholecystectomy

Outcomes

Primary outcome

A pairwise comparison of the VASs determined at rest at different timepoints between groups E and C revealed no difference between the VAS scores at T_1, T_2, T_3, or T_4, respectively. However, at T_5 the VAS at rest of group E was significantly lower than that of group C (Fig. 2). A decrease in pain intensity of more than 25% compared with the baseline (T_1) was used as an indicator of analgesic efficacy (Table 3). The analgesic efficacy experienced by group E at T_2 and T_3 was significantly higher than that of group C.

Adverse events

Adverse events occurred in 6 (2.9%) subjects in group E and 3 (1.3%) subjects in group C, with no serious adverse events or deaths occurring in either group. The number of adverse events was higher in group E compared with group C, but the difference was not statistically significant (Table 4).

Secondary outcome

The vital signs (SBP, DBP, respiratory rate, and heart rate) of groups E and C at all timepoints were statistically similar (Table 5). For both groups, the mean SBP, DBP, and heart rate at each of the timepoints T_2, T_3, T_4, and T_5 were significantly lower than at T_1. However, the blood pressures at T_2 to T_5 were comparable to that at admission (T_0), and there was no significant difference in respiratory rates.

Discussion

In this prospective, multicenter study, 437 patients were randomized to receive either nalbuphine (group E) or tramadol (group C) to treat pain after ambulatory surgery. Group E experienced significantly longer duration of analgesia compared with group C. At each timepoint, the vital signs (SBP, DBP, respiratory rate, and heart rate) of the 2 groups were statistically comparable. However, within each group there were significant differences in SBP, DBP, and heart rate at T_2, T_3, T_4, and T_5, relative to T_1. Overall, the analgesic effect of nalbuphine was comparable to that of tramadol, with nalbuphine having a longer duration of analgesia.

In China, the number of day surgeries is increasing due to improvements in surgery and anesthesia, with shorter recovery time and patients discharged within 24 h after surgery. Therefore, there is a higher demand for

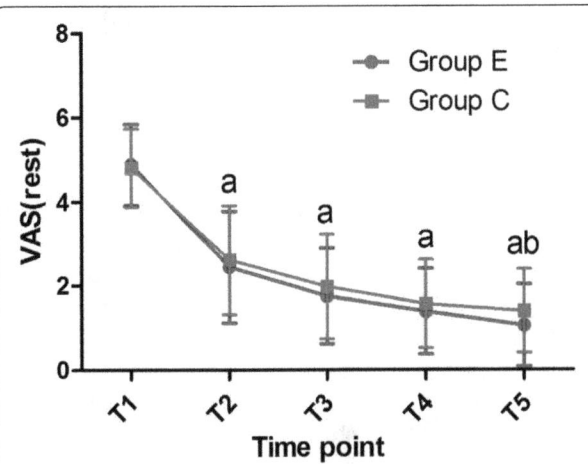

Fig. 2 The VAS at rest in the experimental (Group E) and control group (Group C). Time points: T_1: before administration; T_2: after administration at 30 min; T_3: after administration at 2 h; T_4: after administration at 4 h; T_5: after administration at 6 h. [a]After administration, the VAS of Group E was lower than that of Group C, from T_2-T_5; [b]there was a statistically significant difference in VAS between the 2 groups at T_5. Data are expressed as mean ± standard deviation

Table 3 Pain reduction when compared to baseline (T_1), n (%)[a]

		Group E[b]	Group C[c]	χ^2	P
T_2[d]	Effective	186 (89.0)	178 (78.4)	8.837	0.003
	Noneffective	23 (11.0)	49 (21.6)		
T_3[e]	Effective	192 (97.0)	195 (90.7)	6.874	0.009
	Noneffective	6 (3.0%)	20 (9.3%)		
T_4[f]	Effective	190 (97.4)	203 (97.1)	0.036	0.850
	Noneffective	5 (2.6)	6 (2.9)		
T_5[g]	Effective	189 (97.9)	201 (97.6)	0.000	1.000
	Noneffective	4 (2.1)	5 (2.4)		

[a]Effective pain reduction is defined as a decrease in pain intensity > 25%, compared with the baseline (T_1). Noneffective is defined as a decrease in pain intensity < 25%, compared with the baseline (T_1)
[b]Group E (n = 209) was treated with nalbuphine hydrochloride diluted with saline to 1 mg/L.
[c]Group C (n = 228) was administered tramadol hydrochloride diluted with saline to 10 mg/L.
[d]T_2: after administration at 30 min
[e]T_3: after administration at 2 h
[f]T_4: after administration at 4 h
[g]T_5: after administration at 6 h

Table 4 Patients experiencing adverse events, n

	Group E	Group C
Total subjects experiencing adverse events	6	3
Vasculitis, medication extravasation	1	0
Dizziness, nausea, vomiting	5	2
Hidrosis	0	1

anesthesia and a need to improve the quality of analgesics. While achieving rapid recovery, patients also need to avoid complications related to surgery and anesthesia, such as pain, nausea, and vomiting. Numerous studies [17, 18] have shown that after day surgery nearly 80% of patients experience pain. Postoperative pain not only affects patients' rehabilitation and prolongs hospitalization, it can also result in progression from acute to chronic

Table 5 Vital signs at each timepoint [a]

	Vital signs	Group E[b]	Group C[c]	P
T_0	SBP	121.63 ± 16.26	122.64 ± 16.01	0.513
	DBP	74.92 ± 9.48	74.63 ± 8.80	0.738
	Respiratory rate	17.09 ± 1.81	17.04 ± 2.18	0.808
	Heart rate	74.45 ± 8.43	74.48 ± 9.75	0.978
T_1	SBP	128.96 ± 17.74**	130.18 ± 17.05**	0.465
	DBP	79.04 ± 11.32**	78.85 ± 11.45**	0.864
	Respiratory rate	16.52 ± 2.40	16.89 ± 2.56	0.121
	Heart rate	78.69 ± 16.33	78.89 ± 14.97	0.893
T_2	SBP	123.87 ± 16.07*	126.10 ± 16.68*	0.157
	DBP	76.20 ± 9.88*	77.12 ± 12.16*	0.390
	Respiratory rate	16.74 ± 2.19	17.12 ± 2.46	0.092
	Heart rate	76.82 ± 13.95*	76.54 ± 12.06*	0.822
T_3	SBP	118.37 ± 15.23*	121.18 ± 15.53*	0.065
	DBP	72.82 ± 9.19*	74.00 ± 9.70*	0.209
	Respiratory rate	16.53 ± 1.85	16.72 ± 2.13	0.321
	Heart rate	74.06 ± 10.82*	74.59 ± 9.58*	0.598
T_4	SBP	116.72 ± 15.43*	118.82 ± 15.19*	0.169
	DBP	71.27 ± 9.36*	72.07 ± 9.73*	0.399
	Respiratory rate	16.44 ± 1.78	16.62 ± 2.20	0.366
	Heart rate	72.81 ± 9.44*	73.62 ± 8.99*	0.378
T_5	SBP	116.53 ± 14.86*	117.11 ± 14.46*	0.691
	DBP	70.64 ± 9.39*	70.63 ± 9.45*	0.986
	Respiratory rate	16.46 ± 1.84	16.54 ± 2.07	0.682
	Heart rate	72.65 ± 9.35*	72.76 ± 9.22*	0.905

[a]T_0: at admission, T_1: before administration, T_2: after administration at 30 min, T_3: after administration at 2 h, T_4: after administration at 4 h, T_5: after administration at 6 h
[b]Group E ($n = 209$) was treated with nalbuphine hydrochloride diluted with saline to 1 mg/L.
[c]Group C ($n = 228$) was administered tramadol hydrochloride diluted with saline to 10 mg/L.
*Difference is statistically significant compared with T_1; **difference is statistically significant compared with T_0

pain, which is the main cause of readmission after day surgery [19].

According to the Chinese Society of Anesthesiology [20], systemic opioids given to patients undergoing ambulatory surgery with general anesthesia activate opioid receptors and stimulate various organs. This often results in nausea and vomiting, pruritus, urinary retention, excessive sedation and respiratory inhibition. Thus, in principle, systemic opioids are not used for postoperative pain relief after day surgery. The analgesic and adverse reactions of mixed agonist-antagonist opioids, such as nalbuphine and dezocine, also exhibit a ceiling effect. Implementation of multimodal analgesia using NSAIDs can significantly reduce the dose of opioid and adverse reactions, and can be used postoperatively to manage moderate pain after ambulatory surgery.

Nalbuphine, a mixed agonist-antagonist opioid, is associated with milder μ receptor-related side effects. Its plasma half-life is 5 h, and in clinical studies the duration of analgesic activity ranges from 3 to 6 h [21]. In our study, the VAS at rest of group E was less than 4 points, and the difference was statistically significant compared with the VAS at rest before administration. This indicates that nalbuphine could effectively relieve pain after ambulatory surgery. Similar results were also observed in animal studies that showed amelioration of somatic and visceral pain in mice after treatment with nalbuphine [22].

In the present study, the VAS at rest at timepoints T_1 to T_4 of the nalbuphine group (group E) did not differ from that of the control. At T_5, the VAS at rest of the nalbuphine group was significantly lower than that of the tramadol group. This indicates that the duration of nalbuphine for pain relief after ambulatory surgery was longer than that of tramadol. There were 6 cases (2.8%) of adverse reactions in the nalbuphine group, which was not significantly different from the 3 cases (1.3%) in the tramadol group.

The incidence of adverse reactions associated with nalbuphine is relatively low compared with other opioid medications. A meta-analysis of randomized controlled trials by Zeng et al. [23] showed that nalbuphine has similar analgesic effects compared to morphine, and a better drug safety profile with a low incidence of postoperative pruritus, respiratory inhibition, nausea, and vomiting. In addition, studies have reported that antagonism of the μ receptor by nalbuphine could reduce the adverse reactions of other opioids, as seen in the combination of morphine and nalbuphine in patient-controlled analgesia or patient-controlled epidural analgesia [24, 25]; and the rate of adverse effects such as urinary retention related to morphine, pruritus, and nausea was significantly less. Nalbuphine with sufentanil used in patient-controlled analgesia could reduce the incidence of opioid-related nausea and vomiting and improved patients' satisfaction with analgesia [26, 27].

In the present study, the difference in respiratory rates before and after administration in both the nalbuphine and tramadol groups was not statistically significant, and no respiratory depression was observed. Many studies have reported that respiratory depression caused by nalbuphine is small and has a ceiling effect [28, 29]. In one study, a neonate was wrongly administered a ten-fold higher dose than required of nalbuphine, and it resulted in only prolonged sedation with no respiratory failure [30].

Studies have shown that pre-anesthetic injections of nalbuphine could reduce stress responses and fluctuations in blood pressure and heart rate during intubation [31, 32]. In the present study, the blood pressures and heart rates of both groups after administration were significantly lower than at T_1, although still within normal ranges. The blood pressure at T_0 (Inception of the study) was compared to the blood pressure after surgery (T_1-T_5); the blood pressure at T_1 was significantly higher than at T_0. However, at the later timepoints, T_2 to T_5, there were no statistical differences in the blood pressures compared to T_0. The decrease in blood pressure after administration (T_2-T_5) may have been due to the alleviation of pain. If so, then the lowered blood pressure could also indicate the analgesic efficacy of nalbuphine.

There are several limitations in this study. First, a limited number of parameters (VAS score, adverse events, and change of vital signs) were observed within the half-life of the medication. Secondly, the VAS scores were recorded at rest and not during movement. Finally, due to ethical issues a placebo control group was not possible. Therefore, we were not able to assess the effectiveness of nalbuphine or tramadol at 4 and 6 h after administration. Fortunately, none of the patients dropped out during the 4 or 6 h after administration of medication for pain. However, the present results warrant further experiments to determine comprehensively the effectiveness and safety of nalbuphine for the treatment of pain after ambulatory surgery.

Conclusion

This study indicates that nalbuphine at a recommended dose of 0.2 mg/kg is safe and effective for pain management after ambulatory surgery.

Abbreviations

ALT: alanine aminotransferase; ASA: American Society of Anesthesiologists; AST: Aspartic aminotransferase; BIS: Bispectral index; BMI: Body mass index; BUN: Blood urea nitrogen; C: Control; CONSORT: Consolidated Standards of Reporting Trials; Cr: Creatinine; DBP: Diastolic pressure; E: Experimental; MAP: Mean arterial pressure; SBP: Systolic blood pressure; VAS: Visual analog scale

Acknowledgements
Not applicable.

Authors' contributions
GYJ: This author contributed to the data collection, contributed to the data analysis and wrote the manuscript. WL: This author contributed to the data collection and analysis. LQ: This author contributed to the data collection and analysis. FQW: This author contributed to the data collection and analysis. HN This author contributed to the data collection and analysis. HCF: This author contributed to the data collection and analysis. MCH: This author contributed to the data collection and analysis. LCJ: This author contributed to the data collection and analysis. WHB: This author contributed to the data collection and analysis. CH: This author contributed to the data collection and analysis. GQL: This author designed most of the research plan, contributed to the data collection. CZG: This author designed most of the research plan, contributed to the data collection. All of the authors have read and approved the manuscript.

Author details
[1]Department of Anesthesiology, Xiangya Hospital of Central South University, No. 87 Xiangya Road, Changsha, Hunan, China. [2]Department of Anesthesiology, Hunan Provincial People's Hospital, Changsha, Hunan, China. [3]Department of Anesthesiology, Third Xiangya Hospital of Central South University, Changsha, Hunan, China. [4]Department of Anesthesiology, Pain Medicine & Critical Care Medicine, Aviation General Hospital of China Medical University & Beijing Institute of Translational Medicine, Chinese Academy of Sciences, Beijing, China. [5]Department of Anesthesiology, Peking University Shouguang Hospital, Beijing, China. [6]Department of Anesthesiology, Shanxi Academy of Medical Sciences, Shanxi Dayi Hospital, Shanxi, China. [7]Department of Anesthesiology, Fudan University Shanghai Cancer Center, Shanghai, China. [8]Department of Anesthesiology, Third Affiliated Hospital of Sun Yat-Sen University, Guangzhou, Guangdong, China. [9]Department of Anesthesiology, First People's Hospital of Foshan, Foshan, Guangdong, China. [10]Department of Anesthesiology, Beijing Ditan Hospital Capital Medical University, Beijing, China.

References
1.	Shirakami G, Teratani Y, Namba T, Hirakata H, Tazuke-Nishimura M, Fukuda K. Delayed discharge and acceptability of ambulatory surgery in adult outpatients receiving general anesthesia. J Anesth. 2005;19:93–101. https://doi.org/10.1007/s00540-004-0297-6.
2.	Tong D, Chung F. Postoperative pain control in ambulatory surgery. Surg Clin North Am. 1999;79:401–30.
3.	Rawal N. Postoperative pain treatment for ambulatory surgery. Best Pract Res Clin Anaesthesiol. 2007;21:129–48.
4.	Melnyk M, Casey RG, Black P, Koupparis AJ. Enhanced recovery after surgery (ERAS) protocols: Time to change practice? Can Urol Assoc J. 2011;5:342–8. https://doi.org/10.5489/cuaj.11002.
5.	Lee JH. Anesthesia for ambulatory surgery. Korean J Anesthesiol. 2017;70: 398–406. https://doi.org/10.4097/kjae.2017.70.4.398.
6.	Acalovschi I, Cristea T, Margarit S, Gavrus R. Tramadol added to lidocaine for intravenous regional anesthesia. Anesth Analg. 2001;92:209–14.
7.	Jankovic RJ, Visnjic MM, Milic DJ, Stojanovic MP, Djordjevic DR, Pavlovic MS. Does the addition of ketorolac and dexamethasone to lidocaine intravenous regional anesthesia improve postoperative analgesia and tourniquet tolerance for ambulatory hand surgery? Minerva Anestesiol. 2008;74:521–7.
8.	Kumar A, Sharma D, Datta B. Addition of ketamine or dexmedetomidine to lignocaine in intravenous regional anesthesia: A randomized controlled study. J Anaesthesiol Clin Pharmacol. 2012;28:501–4. https://doi.org/10.4103/0970-9185.101941.
9.	Abdel-Ghaffar HS, Kalefa MA, Imbaby AS. Efficacy of ketamine as an adjunct to lidocaine in intravenous regional anesthesia. Reg Anesth Pain Med. 2014; 39:418–22. https://doi.org/10.1097/AAP.0000000000000128.
10.	Youssef MIEN. Lidocaine-nalbuphine versus lidocaine-tramadol for intravenous regional anesthesia. Ain-Shams J Anesthesiol. 2014;7:198–204.
11.	Bakri MH, Ismail EA, Abd-Elshafy SK. Analgesic effect of Nalbuphine when added to intravenous regional anesthesia: a randomized control trial. Pain Physician. 2016;19:575–81.

12. Vilsbøll T. The effects of glucagon-like peptide-1 on the beta cell. Diabetes Obes Metab. 2009;11 Suppl 3:11–8. https://doi.org/10.1111/j.1463-1326.2009.01073.x.

13. Shin D, Kim S, Kim CS, Kim HS. Postoperative pain management using intravenous patient-controlled analgesia for pediatric patients. J Craniofac Surg. 2001;12:129–33.

14. Mukherjee A, Pal A, Agrawal J, Mehrotra A, Dawar N. Intrathecal nalbuphine as an adjuvant to subarachnoid block: What is the most effective dose? Anesth Essays Res. 2011;5:171–5. https://doi.org/10.4103/0259-1162.94759.

15. Hua X, Chen LM, Zhu Q, Hu W, Lin C, Long ZQ, et al. Efficacy of controlled-release oxycodone for reducing pain due to oral mucositis in nasopharyngeal carcinoma patients treated with concurrent chemoradiotherapy: a prospective clinical trial. Support Care Cancer. 2019;27:3759–67. https://doi.org/10.1007/s00520-019-4643-5.

16. Ali M, Khan FA. Comparison of analgesic effect of tramadol alone and a combination of tramadol and paracetamol in day-care laparoscopic surgery. Eur J Anaesthesiol. 2009;26:475–9. https://doi.org/10.1097/EJA.0b013e328324b747.

17. Chow S-C, Shao J, Wang H. Sample size calculations in clinical research (2nd ed). Boca Raton: Chapman & Hall/CRC; 2008.

18. Apfelbaum JL, Chen C, Mehta SS, Gan TJ. Postoperative pain experience: results from a national survey suggest postoperative pain continues to be undermanaged. Anesth Analg. 2003;97:534–40 table of contents.

19. Aubrun F, Ecoffey C, Benhamou D, Jouffroy L, Diemunsch P, Skaare K, et al. Perioperative pain and post-operative nausea and vomiting (PONV) management after day-case surgery: The SFAR-OPERA national study. Anaesth Crit Care Pain Med. 2018. https://doi.org/10.1016/j.accpm.2018.08.004.

20. Xu J. Expert consensus on analgesia afteradult day surgery. J Clin Anesthesiol. 2017;08:812–5.

21. Web site:LABEL: NALBUPHINE HYDROCHLORIDE- nalbuphine hydrochloride injection, solution. Available at: https://www.dailymed.nlm.nih.gov/dailymed/drugInfo.cfm?setid=6025e8d4-5083-4c3a-58a0-050e7b0b6150. Accessed 26 Feb 2020.

22. Narver HL. Nalbuphine, a non-controlled opioid analgesic, and its potential use in research mice. Lab Anim (NY). 2015;44:106–10. https://doi.org/10.1038/laban.701.

23. Zeng Z, Lu J, Shu C, Chen Y, Guo T, Wu QP, et al. A comparision of nalbuphine with morphine for analgesic effects and safety : meta-analysis of randomized controlled trials. Sci Rep. 2015;5:10927. https://doi.org/10.1038/srep10927.

24. Chen MK, Chau SW, Shen YC, Sun YN, Tseng KY, Long CY, et al. Dose-dependent attenuation of intravenous nalbuphine on epidural morphine-induced pruritus and analgesia after cesarean delivery. Kaohsiung J Med Sci. 2014;30:248–53. https://doi.org/10.1016/j.kjms.2014.01.001.

25. Yeh YC, Lin TF, Chang HC, Chan WS, Wang YP, Lin CJ, et al. Combination of low-dose nalbuphine and morphine in patient-controlled analgesia decreases incidence of opioid-related side effects. J Formos Med Assoc. 2009;108:548–53. https://doi.org/10.1016/S0929-6646(09)60372-7.

26. Zhang S. Clinical observation of low-dose nalbuphine combinedwith sufentanil in PCIA. Acta Acad Med WeiFang. 2016;38:330–2.

27. Niu NYT. nalbuphine combined with sufentanil for clinical observation of analgesia afteradult laparoscopic surgery. World Med Inform Digest. 2017;17:84–6.

28. Gupta M, Gupta P. Nalbuphine pretreatment for prevention of etomidate induced myoclonus: A prospective, randomized and double-blind study. J Anaesthesiol Clin Pharmacol. 2018;34:200–4. https://doi.org/10.4103/joacp.JOACP_210_16.

29. Romagnoli A, Keats AS. Ceiling effect for respiratory depression by nalbuphine. Clin Pharmacol Ther. 1980;27:478–85.

30. Schultz-Machata AM, Becke K, Weiss M. Nalbuphine in pediatric anesthesia. Anaesthesist. 2014;63:135–43. https://doi.org/10.1007/s00101-014-2293-z.

31. Tariq AM, Z. Iqbal and Qadirullah. Efficacy of nalbuphine in preventing haemodynamic response to laryngoscopy and intubation. J Postgrad Med Inst. 2014;28:211–6.

32. Chawda PM, Pareek MK, Mehta KD. Effect of nalbuphine on haemodynamic response to orotracheal intubation. J Anaesthesiol Clin Pharmacol. 2010;26:458–60.

8

Application of preoperative assessment of pain induced by venous cannulation in predicting postoperative pain in patients under laparoscopic nephrectomy

Fei Peng, Yanshuang Li, Yanqiu Ai, Jianjun Yang and Yanping Wang[*]

Abstract

Background: Postoperative pain is the most prominent concern among surgical patients. It has previously been reported that venous cannulation-induced pain (VCP) can be used to predict postoperative pain after laparoscopic cholecystectomy within 90 mins in the recovery room. Its potential in predicting postoperative pain in patients with patient-controlled intravenous analgesia (PCIA) is worth establishing. The purpose of this prospective observational study was to investigate the application of VCP in predicting postoperative pain in patients with PCIA during the first 24 h after laparoscopic nephrectomy.

Methods: One hundred twenty patients scheduled for laparoscopic nephrectomy were included in this study. A superficial vein on the back of the hand was cannulated with a standard-size peripheral venous catheter (1.1×3.2 mm) by a nurse in the preoperative areas. Then the nurse recorded the VAS score associated with this procedure estimated by patients, and dichotomized the patients into low response group (VAS scores < 2.0) or high response group (VAS scores $\geq$2.0). After general anesthesia and surgery, all the patients received the patient-controlled intravenous analgesia (PCIA) with sufentanil. The VAS scores at rest and on coughing at 2 h, 4 h, 8 h, 12 h, 24 h, the effective number of presses and the number of needed rescue analgesia within 24 h after surgery were recorded.

Results: Peripheral venous cannulation-induced pain score was significantly correlated with postoperative pain intensity at rest ($r_s = 0.64$) and during coughing ($r_s = 0.65$), effective times of pressing ($r_s = 0.59$), additional consumption of sufentanil ($r_s = 0.58$). Patients with venous cannulation-induced pain intensity $\geq$2.0 VAS units reported higher levels of postoperative pain intensity at rest ($P < 0.0005$) and during coughing ($P < 0.0005$), needed more effective times of pressing ($P < 0.0005$) and additional consumption of sufentanil ($P < 0.0005$), and also needed more rescue analgesia ($P = 0.01$) during the first 24 h. The odds of risk for moderate or severe postoperative pain (OR 3.5, 95% CI 1.3–9.3) was significantly higher in patients with venous cannulation-induced pain intensity $\geq$2.0 VAS units compared to those <2.0 VAS units.

(Continued on next page)

* Correspondence: 282243756@qq.com

Department of Anesthesiology, Pain and Perioperative Medicine, The First Affiliated Hospital of Zhengzhou University, No.1 Jianshe East Road, Zhengzhou 450052, China

(Continued from previous page)

Conclusions: Preoperative assessment of pain induced by venous cannulation can be used to predict postoperative pain intensity in patients with PCIA during the first 24 h after laparoscopic nephrectomy.

Keywords: Venous cannulation, Pain, Postoperative pain, Pain prediction

Background

Postoperative pain is the most prominent concern among surgical patients. If not adequately controlled, it will affect postoperative rehabilitation, health-related quality of life, and may develop into persistent long-term pain [1–3].

Current postoperative pain management strategies apply a standardized, one-size-fits-all approach to all patients. These standardized protocols are not suitable for the significant difference in patient's pain and may lead to insufficient analgesia in patients with high analgesic needs, or excessive analgesia, which is accompanied by increasing analgesic-related side effects. The ability to preoperative predict who is at risk for developing moderate or severe postoperative pain might allow anaesthetists to optimize pain management by offering personalized, stratified or targeted analgesic treatment protocols. Preoperative pain prediction methods are highly relevant in this regard.

Numerous studies have tried to identify patients who are at risk for postoperative pain in the preoperative period and evaluated the role of psychological factors and experimental pain tests or quantitative sensory tests (QST) [4–8]. However, none of those prediction methods has been used as a routine for prediction of postoperative pain, mainly because expensive equipment, much time and effort are required outside routine preoperative procedures.

Peripheral venous cannulation, a routine procedure of preoperative preparation, induced pain intensity could be assessed easily and rapidly before surgery without specific equipment or training. It was recently shown that peripheral venous cannulation-induced pain (VCP) intensity could be used to predict the risk of postoperative pain. Patients with VCP score at or above 2.0 VAS units reported higher levels of acute postoperative pain intensity and more often have moderate or severe postoperative pain within 90 mins in the recovery room [9]. Its potential in predicting postoperative pain in patients with patient-controlled intravenous analgesia (PCIA) is worth establishing. The purpose of this study was to test if peripheral VCP intensity can be used to predict the risk for pain in patients with PCIA during the first 24 h after laparoscopic nephrectomy.

Methods

Participants

This prospective clinical observational study was approved by the Institutional Scientific Research and Clinical Trials Ethics Committee of the First Affiliated Hospital of Zhengzhou University (ref.: 2019- KY-120) and registered at chictro.org (ref.: ChiCTR1900024352; July 6, 2019).

Patients who were classified as American Society of Anesthesiologists (ASA) physical status I-II, aged between 18 and 65 years, all genders, BMI 18 to 28 kg/m^2, and scheduled to undergo laparoscopic nephrectomy under general anaesthesia, agree to use postoperative analgesia pump for 48 h after surgery, agreed to cooperate and signed the informed consent were recruited.

Patients with the following conditions were excluded: severe heart, lung and metabolic diseases, hepatic or renal dysfunction, a history of neuromuscular system disease, mental illness, and a tendency to malignant hyperthermia, preoperative existing pain, long-term use of sedative and analgesic drugs (> 3 months), drug or alcohol abusers, or severe hypertension, poor understanding or communication difficulty, failed venous cannulation, changed in surgical approach (from laparoscopic to open surgery, the operative time over than 3 h, failed to complete the data collection.

Preoperative pain assessment

An anaesthetist visited the patients the day before surgery, described the visual analogue scale (VAS) for them and instructed on the use of PCIA bump. On the day of surgery, an experienced nurse inserted a peripheral venous catheter (B. Braun Melsungen AG, Germany) with a standard-size (1.1 × 3.2 mm inner diameter) into a superficial vein on the back of the patient's hand in the preoperative preparation room. The patients were asked to estimate, on a horizontal VAS ruler, their maximum pain intensity associated with this procedure, recorded to one decimal point (0.0–10.0). Then the nurse recorded the VAS score estimated (on a horizontal VAS ruler, their maximum pain score associated with this procedure) by the patients, and dichotomized the patients into low response group (VCP score < 2.0 VAS units) or high response group (VCP score ≥ 2.0 VAS units). The nurse was aware of whether the patient was to take part in the study.

Anaesthesia

All patients were anaesthetized by anaesthetists who were blinded to study and did not participate in data collection. Once in the operating room, the standardized monitoring of ECG, SpO_2, noninvasive blood pressure was established. Before the induction of anaesthesia, the patients were given IV Penehyclidine Hydrochloride 0.5 mg, and a loading dose of dexmedetomidine with 0.5 µg kg^{-1} was infused over 10 min. The bispectral index (BIS) was used to monitor the depth of anaesthesia. Then anaesthesia was induced with midazolam 2 mg, sulfentanil 0.5 µg kg^{-1}, etomidate 2–3 mg kg^{-1}. Cisatracurium 0.2 mg kg^{-1} was given to facilitate endotracheal intubation. Anaesthesia was maintained with sevoflurane (1–2%), remifentanil 0.1–0.3 µg kg^{-1} min^{-1}. The cisatracurium was used to provide a satisfactory level of muscle relaxation. The BIS value was maintained between 40 to 60. The pneumoperitoneum pressure with carbon dioxide was set at 13–15 mmHg, and the $EtCO_2$ was maintained at 35 to 45 mmHg. Thirty minutes before the end of the surgery, sulfentanil 10 µg and flurbiprofen axetil 100 mg were given as postoperative analgesia, and tropisetron 5 mg was given to prevent postoperative nausea and vomiting. At the end of the surgery, sevoflurane and remifentanil were stopped. Immediately after surgery, the PCIA pump was attached to the peripheral venous line by the anaesthetist. Then the patients were sent to the post anaesthetic care unit for anaesthetic resuscitation. All patients were sent to the general ward after being fully awake. Upon arrival in the general ward, all the patients were once again instructed on the use of the PCIA pump and VAS.

Postoperative analgesia regimen

The PCIA with sulfentanil regimen was applied to 48 h after surgery. The PCIA regimen consisted of sulfentanil 3.0 µg kg^{-1} and 5 mg tropisetron, mixed with 0.9% normal saline to a total volume of 150 ml. The PCIA was programmed to deliver a 2 ml bolus on demand, with a lock-out interval of 10 min, and a background infusion rate of 2 ml h^{-1}. In the ward, patients pressed PCA when VAS score at rest > 3.0. If patients still reported pain or the VAS scores ≥4.0, supplemental rescue boluses of intravenous flurbiprofen axetil injection of 50 mg were administered. The complete history of continuous infusion, bolus infusion, and bolus demand for the PCIA device was downloaded after surgery.

Outcome variables measures and data collection

The study outcomes variables and the vital parameters were recorded at 2, 4, 8, 12 and 24 h after surgery. During the studied period, pain intensity, sulfentanil consumption, pressing times of the PCIA, and the number of rescue analgesia were recorded at above time points. Overall satisfaction index of the patients was recorded at 24 h. Pain intensity was assessed with VAS at rest and during coughing.

The primary outcome was maximum postoperative pain scores at rest and during coughing within the first 24 h. The secondary outcome was effective times of pressing, additional consumption of sulfentanil and satisfaction index at 24 h. Also, the number of rescue analgesia within the first 24 h was also measured.

Postoperative data collector was blinded to the preoperative peripheral venous cannulation-induced pain score of the patients.

Sample size and statistical analyses

The sample size was based on a pilot experiment of 20 cases resulted in our observation that patients with VCP score ≥ 2.0 VAS units was present in 8 out of 20 patients and that mean maximum postoperative pain score (VAS) at rest within 24 h after surgery was 3.9 (± 1.3). Therefore, in order to show a 20% difference between the patients with VCP score ≥ 2.0 VAS units and the patients with VCP score ≥ 2.0 VAS units, the number of patients in each group was expected to be 41 ($\alpha = 0.05$, $\beta = 0.8$). Since the groups are unequal, assuming a 40% of patients with VCP score ≥ 2.0 VAS units, and allow for up to 15% dropouts, a total of 120 patients (48 patients with VCP score ≥ 2.0 VAS units and 72 patients with VCP score < 2.0 VAS units) would be sufficient to test our hypothesis.

The IBM SPSS version 22.0 software packages were used for statistical analyses. The normality of the continuous data was tested by the Shapiro-Wilk test. Normally distributed continuous variables were expressed as mean ± SD and compared between groups using a two-sample Student t-test. IF the distribution was not normal, the median with inter-quartile range (IQR) were expressed, and a Mann–Whitney U-test was used. Categorical data were expressed as frequency (n) and percentage (%) and were statistically tested using the chi-square or Fisher's exact test. Correlations between variables were assessed with Spearman's rank correlation coefficients. Logistic regression analysis was used to evaluate the predictive abilities of cannulation-induced pain intensity. All P values <0.05 were considered to be statistically significant.

Results

A total of 139 patients undergoing laparoscopic nephrectomy were screened between August and October 2019, of which 19 were excluded because they did not meet the inclusion criteria, refused to participate in the trial, and failed venous cannulation. Among the remaining 120 patients, some were eliminated due to transferred to ICU, converted to open surgery, surgery duration over 3 hours, or incomplete recording, and 106 study patients were available for analysis (Fig. 1).

Patients' demographic characteristics and perioperative data are shown in Table 1. The median (inter-quartile

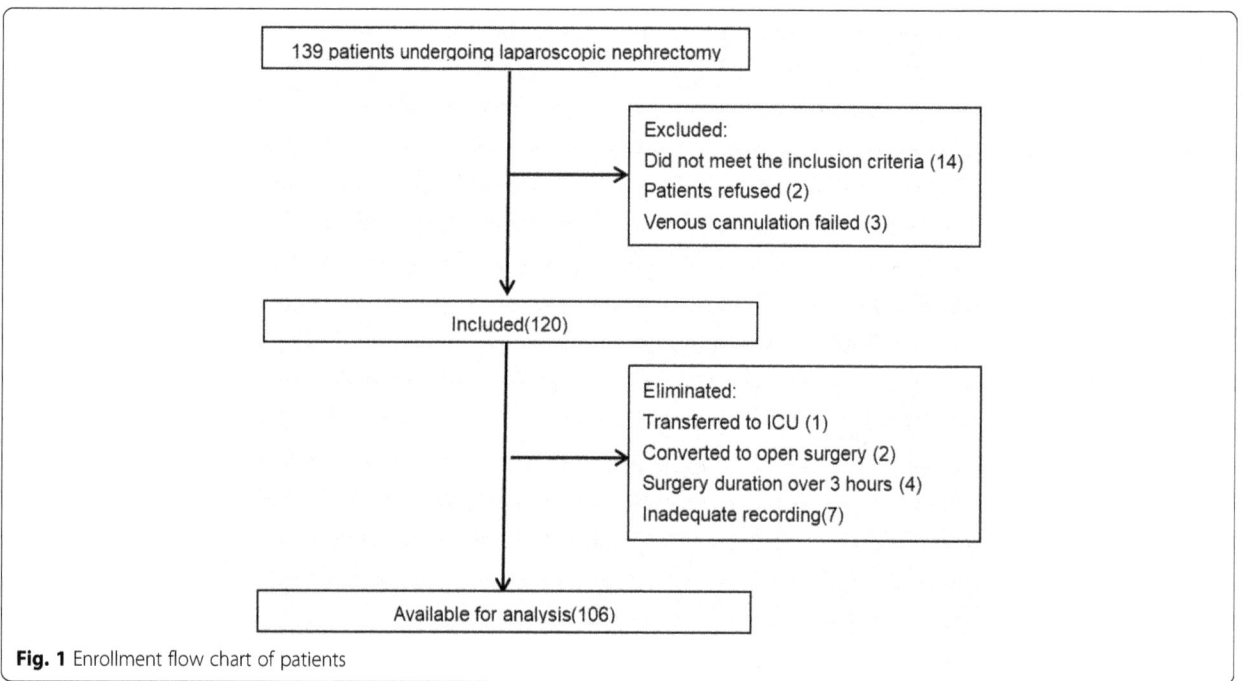

Fig. 1 Enrollment flow chart of patients

range) of peripheral venous cannulation-induced pain score, postoperative maximum pain score at rest, postoperative maximum pain score during coughing, effective times of pressing, additional consumption of sulfentanil were 1.8 (1.4–2.6), 3.4 (3.0–3.9), 5.8 (5.5–6.3), 1 (0–5), 3.18 (0–12.56) μg. The cut-off point of classification according to VCP pain score (2.0 VAS units) was close to the median level of peripheral venous-induced pain score.

Bivariate correlations between peripheral venous cannulation-induced pain score and outcome variables are shown in Fig. 2 and Table 2. Postoperative maximum pain score at rest ($r_s = 0.64$, $P < 0.001$) (Fig. 2a), postoperative maximum pain score during coughing ($r_s = 0.65$, $P < 0.001$) (Fig. 2b), effective times of pressing ($r_s = 0.59$, $P < 0.001$), additional consumption of sulfentanil ($r_s = 0.58$,

Table 1 Patients' demographic characteristics and perioperative data

Variable	
Age (years)	53 (40–59)
Gender (M/F)	57/49
ASA (i/II)	38/68
BMI (kg/m^2)	24.8 (22.1–26.5)
Peripheral venous cannulation-induced pain score	1.8 (1.4–2.6)
Postoperative maximum pain score at rest	3.4 (3.0–3.9)
Postoperative maximum pain score during coughing	5.8 (5.5–6.3)
Effective times of pressing	1 (0–5)
Additional consumption of sulfentanil, μg	3.18 (0–12.56)

Data are presented as median (range) or number

$P < 0.001$) were statistically significantly correlated with peripheral venous cannulation-induced pain score, respectively.

Patients' demographic characteristics and perioperative data between the two groups are shown in Table 3. There were no significant differences in age, gender, BMI, ASA, history of surgery, type of surgery, approaches of surgery, duration of anaesthesia and surgery, consumption of remifentanil between the two groups. Patients with venous cannulation-induced pain intensity ≥2.0 VAS units reported higher levels of postoperative pain intensity at rest (3.7 vs. 3.2 VAS units; $P < 0.0005$) and during coughing (6.2 vs. 5.6 VAS units; $P < 0.0005$), needed more effective times of pressing (3 vs. 1; $P < 0.0005$) and additional consumption of sulfentanil (7.46 vs. 2.56 μg; $P < 0.0005$), and also needed more rescue analgesia (33.3% vs. 12.5%; $P = 0.01$) during the first 24 h. While the satisfaction index was significantly lower (3 vs.5; $P < 0.0005$).

The number of patients experiencing maximum pain (at rest) exceeding 4.0 VAS units during the first 24 h between high response group and low response group were shown in Table 4. In high response group, 33.3% reported moderate or severe postoperative pain. While, in low response group, 12.5% reported moderate or severe pain. There was statistically significant in the risk for moderate or severe pain between two groups ($P = 0.01$).

After controlling for possible factors affecting postoperative pain (gender, age, history of surgery, type of surgery and approaches of surgery), the odds of risk for moderate or severe postoperative pain (OR 3.5, 95% CI 1.3–9.3) was significantly higher in patients with venous

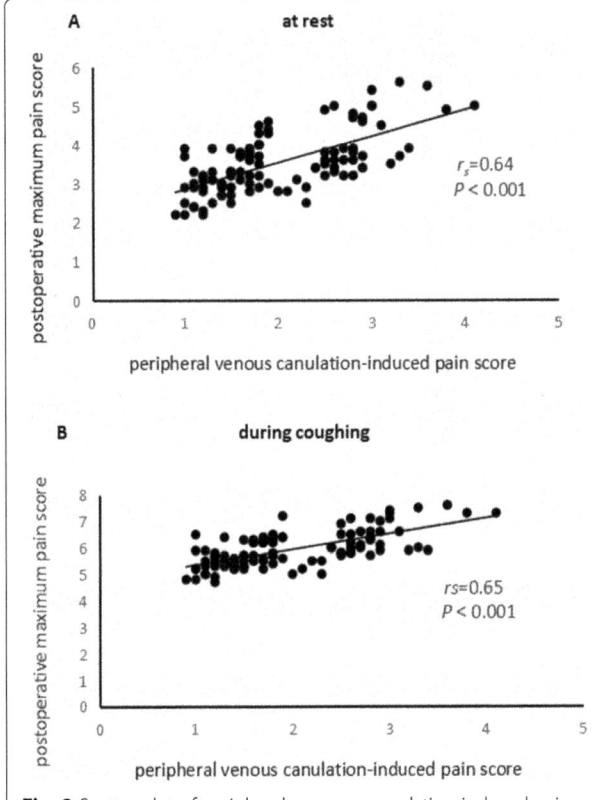

Fig. 2 Scatter plot of peripheral venous cannulation-induced pain score and postoperative maximum pain score (**a**) at rest, (**b**) during coughing

cannulation-induced pain intensity ≥2.0 VAS units compared to those < 2.0 VAS units (Table 5).

Discussion

This study shows that peripheral venous cannulation-induced pain score is positively correlated with postoperative maximum pain and addition consumption of sulfentanil during the first 24 h after laparoscopic nephrectomy. Patients with VCP score ≥ 2.0 VAS units are more likely to report higher postoperative pain scores and additional consumption of sulfentanil. Furthermore, patients with VCP score ≥ 2.0 VAS units have a 3.5 times higher risk for moderate or severe postoperative pain.

Peripheral venous cannulation, is a routine practice before surgery, has been reported by patients to be

Table 2 Bivariate correlations between venous cannulation-induced pain score and outcome variables

	Correlation coefficient (r_s)
Postoperative maximum pain score at rest	0.64[*]
Postoperative maximum pain score during coughing	0.65[*]
Effective times of pressing	0.59[*]
Additional consumption of sulfentanil, μg	0.58[*]

[*]meant $P < 0.05$

painful. The pain intensity is associated with cannula site, cannula size, failed venipuncture attempts and process times [10, 11]. In the present study, we did not include patients with failed venipuncture, and this procedure was performed by the experienced nurse with same diameter puncture needle on the same site. The results showed that the median level of pain intensity associated with venous cannulation on the hand was 1.8 VAS units, which was close to current study proposed the cut-off level of the VCP (2.0 VAS units). Furthermore, the cut-off level of the VCP was found to be 2.0 VAS units in predicting postoperative pain in Persson et al. Study [9]. Another study reported that 2.0 VAS units represented a more reasonable cut-off level of VCP for prediction of postoperative pain [12].

Prior researchers have also reported similar results to ours. Persson et al. [9] study reported that the VCP score was significantly correlated with postoperative maximum pain score at rest within 90 mins after laparoscopic cholecystectomy. Patients with VCP score ≥ 2.0 VAS units had higher postoperative pain and risk for moderate or severe postoperative pain in the recovery room. However, the proportion of moderate or severe postoperative pain in patients with VCP score ≥ 2.0 VAS units and < 2.0 VAS units were higher than the present study reported. In our study, 33.3 and 12.5% of patients reported moderate or severe postoperative pain between patients with VCP score ≥ 2.0 VAS units and < 2.0 VAS units, while in Persson et al. [9] study, the proportions were 77 and 35%. A possible explanation as to the difference is that patients are administered opioid through PCIA with continuous background infusion instead of on-demand. Carvalho et al. [13] study used VCP score to predict labor pain of 50 women and found that pain intensity of intravenous cannulation was correlated with time to epidural request during the course of induction of labour. A recently study [12] evaluated the usefulness of VCP score in 4 categories surgery (presumed to with hardly any postoperative pain, slight, moderate and severe levels of postoperative pain) and reported that the method of VCP score was only statistically significant in the patients subjected to surgery presumed to result in moderate levels of postoperative pain.

Numerous studies have been developed to predict postoperative pain in the last decade. The pain intensity of QST stimuli, including pressure, electric, and thermal stimulus, have been reported to correlate with the intensity of postoperative pain [6–8, 14–17]. Werner et al. [18] reported that QST assessments might predict up to 54% of the variance in the postoperative pain experience. The predictive ability of the tests is much higher than previously reported for single-factor analyses of demographics and psychologic factors. However, these methods may be time-consuming and not necessarily available in a fast-

Table 3 Demographic characteristics and perioperative data in patients dichotomized for peripheral venous cannulation-induced pain score

	venous cannulation-induced pain score (VAS units)		P values
	<2.0	≥ 2.0	
Total number of patients	64	42	
Gender (M/F)	39/25	18/24	0.068
Age (years)	53 (48–62)	52 (38–58)	0.248
BMI (kg/m^2)	24.2 (22.1–25.9)	25.1 (22.1–27.8)	0.076
ASA (I/II)	23/41	15 /27	0.981
History of surgery (No/Yes)	40 /24	22/20	0.301
Type of surgery (Partial/Radical)	24/40	13/29	0.489
Approaches of surgery (Retroperitoneal/Transperitoneal)	15/49	9/33	0.809
Duration of anaesthesia, min	134 (100–157)	133 (113–170)	0.339
Refentanil, mg	1.05 (0.80–1.40)	1.10 (1.00–1.36)	0.361
Postoperative maximum pain score at rest	3.2 (2.9–3.7)	3.7 (3.4–4.7)	< 0.0005
Postoperative maximum pain score on coughing	5.6 (5.3–6.2)	6.2 (5.8–7.0)	< 0.0005
Additional consumption of sulfentanil, μg	2.56 (0–7.86)	7.46 (2.71–22.91)	< 0.0005
Effective times of pressing	1 (0–3)	3 (1–8)	< 0.0005
Needed rescue analgesia	8 (12.5%)	14 (33.3%)	0.01
satisfaction index	5 (4–5)	3 (3–4)	< 0.0005

Variables are presented as median (range) or number

paced clinical environment. The VCP assessment is easy to perform, timely and rapid clinical test and requires no special equipment.

Our finding has important clinical implications since pain management in the postoperative period still present a challenge. There is large individual variability in response to opioids and the potential side effects such as respiratory depression, nausea, vomiting and constipation. The ability to preoperative identification of patients at greater risk for moderate or severe postoperative pain and having higher opioids requirements is very beneficial. Using peripheral VCP intensity as a predictor of postoperative pain may allow anaesthetists more convenient to adjust the dosage of opioids and can potentially improve postoperative pain management.

There are some limitations to the present study. Known risk factors of postoperative pain are female gender, lower age, preoperative pain, intraoperative factors and psychological factors, and so on [8, 19–21]. Furthermore, it was reported that psychological factors were correlated with venous cannulation-induced pain score [22]. This study did not take psychological factors into account. The psychological variables may affect the levels of postoperative pain and venous cannulation-induced pain score. Besides, this method did not be evaluated in other surgical patients.

Conclusions

In conclusion, peripheral venous cannulation-induced pain score was associated with postoperative pain and

Table 4 Cross-tabulation for a prediction model for maximum postoperative pain according to peripheral venous cannulation-induced pain score

	Venous cannulation-induced pain score (VAS units)		Total number of patients
	< 2.0	≥ 2.0	
Patients reporting maximum postoperative pain intensity at rest (VAS units)			
< 4	56 (87.5%)	28 (66.7%)	84
≥ 4	8 (12.5%)	14 (33.3%)	22
Total number of patients	64	42	106

Comparison of the number of patients experiencing pain exceeding VAS 4.0 within 24 h between high response group and low response group (P = 0.01)

Table 5 Logistic regression analysis of the ability of venous cannulation-induced pain score (≥ / < 2.0 VAS units) to predict postoperative pain intensity ≥4.0 VAS units

	multivariate analysis	
	OR(95% CI)	P value
Venous cannulation-induced pain score (VAS units)		
< 2.0	1.0(ref)	0.012
≥ 2.0	3.5 (1.3–9.3)	

Abbreviations = OR (odds ratio), CI (confidence interval)
The model adjusted for gender, age, history of surgery, type of surgery and approaches of surgery

addition consumption of sulfentanil during the first 24 h after laparoscopic nephrectomy. Patients with VCP score ≥ 2.0 VAS units had higher postoperative pain scores, additional consumption of sulfentanil and risk for moderate or severe postoperative pain. Therefore, peripheral venous cannulation-induced pain intensity can be considered as a simple and useful method to predict postoperative pain in patients with PCIA during the first 24 h after laparoscopic nephrectomy.

Abbreviations
VCP: Venous cannulation-induced pain; PCIA: Patient-controlled intravenous analgesia; VAS: Visual analogue scale; QST: Quantitative sensory tests; ASA: American Society of Anesthesiologists; BMI: Body mass index

Acknowledgements
This research was supported by the department of Urinary surgery at the First Affiliated Hospital of Zhengzhou University. The authors thank Jian Li, Lang Yan, and Xuepei Zhang for performing the operation.

Authors' contributions
FP contributions to the study concept and design, acquisition of data, analysis and interpretation of data, drafting and revising the manuscript. YSL contributions to the study design, acquisition of data. YQA contributions to the study concept and design. JJY helped revise the manuscript. YPW contribution to the study concept and design, analysis and interpretation of data, revising the manuscript. All authors read and approved of the final manuscript.

References
1. Glare P, Aubrey KR, Myles PS. Transition from acute to chronic pain after surgery. Lancet. 2019;393(10180):1537–46. https://doi.org/10.1016/S0140-6736(19)30352-6.
2. Gan TJ, Habib AS, Miller TE, White W, Apfelbaum JL. Incidence, patient satisfaction, and perceptions of post-surgical pain: results from a US national survey. Curr Med Res Opin. 2014;30(1):149–60. https://doi.org/10.1185/03007995.2013.860019.
3. Lavand'homme P. Transition from acute to chronic pain after surgery. Pain. 2017;158 Suppl 1:S50–S54;doi:https://doi.org/10.1097/j.pain.0000000000000809.
4. Pan PH, Tonidande AM, Aschenbrenner CA, Houle TT, Harris LC, Eisenach JC. Predicting acute pain after cesarean delivery using three simple questions. Anesthesiology. 2013;118(5):1170–9. https://doi.org/10.1097/ALN.0b013e31828e156f.
5. Rehberg B, Mathivon S, Combescure C, Mercier Y, Savoldelli GL. Prediction of acute postoperative pain following breast cancer surgery using the pain sensitivity questionnaire: a cohort study. Clin J Pain. 2017;33(1):57–66.
6. Buhagiar LM, Cassar OA, Brincat MP, Buttigieg GG, Inglott AS, Adami MZ, et al. Pre-operative pain sensitivity: a prediction of post-operative outcome in the obstetric population. J Anaesthesiol Clin Pharmacol. 2013;29(4):465–71. https://doi.org/10.4103/0970-9185.119135.
7. Werner MU, Jensen EK, Stubhaug A. Preoperative quantitative sensory testing (QST) predicting postoperative pain: image or mirage? Scand J Pain. 2017;15:91–2. https://doi.org/10.1016/j.sjpain.2017.01.012.
8. Gamez BH, Habib AS. Predicting severity of acute pain after cesarean delivery: a narrative review. Anesth Analg. 2018;126(5):1606–14. https://doi.org/10.1213/ANE.0000000000002658.
9. Persson AK, Pettersson FD, Dyrehag LE, Åkeson J. Prediction of postoperative pain from assessment of pain induced by venous cannulation and propofol infusion. Acta Anaesthesiol Scand. 2016;60(2):166–76. https://doi.org/10.1111/aas.12634.
10. Goudra BG, Galvin E, Singh PM, Lions J. Effect of site selection on pain of intravenous cannula insertion: a prospective randomised study. Int J Anesth. 2014;58:732–5. https://doi.org/10.4103/0019-5049.147166.
11. Rüsch D, Koch T, Spies M, Hj Eberhart L. Pain during venous cannulation. Dtsch Arztebl Int. 2017;114(37):605–11. https://doi.org/10.3238/arztebl.2017.0605.
12. Persson AK, Åkeson J. Prediction of acute postoperative pain from assessment of pain associated with venous catheterization. Pain Prac. 2019;19(2):158–67. https://doi.org/10.1111/papr.12729.
13. Carvalho B, Zheng M, Aiono-Le TL. Evaluation of experimental pain tests to predict labour pain and epidural analgesic consumption. Br J Anaesth. 2013;110(4):600–6. https://doi.org/10.1093/bja/aes423.
14. Buhagiar L, Cassar OA, Brincat MP, Azzopardi LM. Predictors of post-caesarean section pain and analgesic consumption. J Anaesthesiol Clin Pharmacol. 2011;27(2):185–91. https://doi.org/10.4103/0970-9185.81822.
15. Wilder-Smith CH, Hill L, Dyer RA, Torr G, Coetzee E. Postoperative sensitization and pain after cesarean delivery and the effects of single im doses of tramadol and diclofenac alone and in combination. Anesth Analg. 2003;97(2):526–33.
16. Granot M, Lowenstein L, Yarnitsky D, Tamir A, Zimmer EZ. Postcesarean section pain prediction by preoperative experimental pain assessment. Anesthesiology. 2003;98(6):1422–6.
17. Strulov L, Zimmer EZ, Granot M, Tamir A, Jakobi P, Lowenstein L. Pain catastrophizing, response to experimental heat stimuli, and post-cesarean section pain. J Pain. 2007;8(3):273–9.
18. Werner MU, Mjöbo HN, Nielsen PR, Rudin A. Prediction of postoperative pain: a systematic review of predictive experimental pain studies. Anesthesiology. 2010;112:1494–502. https://doi.org/10.1097/ALN.0b013e3181dcd5a0.
19. Richebé P, Capdevila X, Rivat C. Persistent postsurgical pain: pathophysiology and preventative pharmacologic considerations. Anesthesiology 2018;129(3):590–607; doi:https://doi.org/10.1097/ALN.0000000000002238.
20. Horn-Hofmann C, Scheel J, Dimova V, Parthum A, Carbon R, Griessinger N, et al. Prediction of persistent post-operative pain: pain-specific psychological variables compared with acute post-operative pain and general psychological variables. Eur J Pain. 2018;22(1):191–202. https://doi.org/10.1002/ejp.1115.
21. Tan CO, Chong YM, Tran P, Weinberg L, Howard W. Surgical predictors of acute postoperative pain after hip arthroscopy. BMC Anesthesiol. 2015;15:96. https://doi.org/10.1186/s12871-015-0077-x.
22. Suren M, Kaya Z, Gokbakan M, Okan I, Arici S, Karaman S, et al. The role of pain catastrophizing score in the prediction of venipuncture pain severity. Pain Pract. 2014;14(3):245–51. https://doi.org/10.1111/papr.12060.

9

Comparison of intrathecal morphine with continuous patient-controlled epidural anesthesia versus intrathecal morphine alone for post-cesarean section analgesia

Izumi Sato[1†], Hajime Iwasaki[1*†] (ID), Sarah Kyuragi Luthe[1,2], Takafumi Iida[1] and Hirotsugu Kanda[1]

Abstract

Background: Several neuraxial techniques have demonstrated effective post-cesarean section analgesia. According to previous reports, it is likely that patient-controlled epidural analgesia (PCEA) without opioids is inferior to intrathecal morphine (IM) alone for post-cesarean section analgesia. However, little is known whether adding PCEA to IM is effective or not. The aim of this study was to compare post-cesarean section analgesia between IM with PCEA and IM alone.

Methods: Fifty patients undergoing elective cesarean section were enrolled in this prospective randomized study. Patients were randomized to one of two groups: IM group and IM + PCEA group. All patients received spinal anesthesia with 12 mg of 0.5% hyperbaric bupivacaine, 10 μg of fentanyl, and 150 μg of morphine. Patients in IM + PCEA group received epidural catheterization through Th11–12 or Th12-L1 before spinal anesthesia and PCEA (basal 0.167% levobupivacaine infusion rate of 6 mL/h, bolus dose of 3 mL in lockout interval of 30 min) was commenced at the end of surgery. A numerical rating scale (NRS) at rest and on movement at 4,8,12,24,48 h after the intrathecal administration of morphine were recorded. In addition, we recorded the incidence of delayed ambulation and the number of patients who requested rescue analgesics. We examined NRS using Bonferroni's multiple comparison test following repeated measures analysis of variance; $p < 0.05$ was considered as statistically significant.

Results: Twenty-three patients in each group were finally analyzed. Mean NRS at rest was significantly higher in IM group than in IM + PCEA group at 4 (2.7 vs 0.6), 8 (2.2 vs 0.6), and 12 h (2.5 vs 0.7), and NRS during mobilization was significantly higher in IM group than in IM + PCEA group at 4 (4.9 vs 1.5), 8 (4.8 vs 1.9), 12 (4.9 vs 2), and 24 h (5.7 vs 3.5). The number of patients who required rescue analgesics during the first 24 h was significantly higher in IM group compared to IM + PCEA group. No significant difference was observed between the groups in incidence of delayed ambulation.

Conclusions: The combined use of PCEA with IM provided better post-cesarean section analgesia compared to IM alone.

(Continued on next page)

* Correspondence: iwasakih@asahikawa-med.ac.jp
†Izumi Sato and Hajime Iwasaki contributed equally to this work.
[1]Department of Anesthesiology and Critical Care Medicine, Asahikawa Medical University, Midorigaoka-higashi 2-1-1-1, Asahikawa, Hokkaido 078-8510, Japan

(Continued from previous page)

Keywords: Cesarean section, Postoperative analgesia, Intrathecal morphine, Patient-controlled epidural analgesia

Background

Several neuraxial techniques have demonstrated effective postoperative analgesia following cesarean section [1–4]. Intrathecal or epidural morphine and patient-controlled epidural anesthesia (PCEA) are generally used for post-cesarean section analgesia. One study reported that intrathecal morphine alone was superior to epidural morphine alone or PCEA without opioids for postoperative analgesia following cesarean section [1]. Both intrathecal and epidural morphine are reported to be effective for post-cesarean section analgesia [5, 6], however, it is unknown if there is a meaningful difference between the route through which a single dose of neuraxial morphine is administered. Another study concluded that the combined use of intrathecal morphine and PCEA improved post-cesarean section analgesia compared to PCEA without opioids [2]. Based on the literature and one retrospective study [7], it is likely that PCEA without opioids is inferior to intrathecal morphine alone for post-cesarean section analgesia. In other words, performing PCEA without opioids may not be a reason to omit intrathecal morphine. However, little is known whether adding epidural anesthesia to intrathecal morphine is effective or not. We hypothesized that the combined use of PCEA and intrathecal morphine may have an advantage in post-cesarean section analgesia compared to intrathecal morphine alone.

Methods

This study was registered in the University Hospital Medical Information Network under registration number UMIN000032475 with approval from the hospital's ethics committee. This study adheres the applicable CONSORT guidelines. Healthy pregnant women scheduled for cesarean section at Kushiro Red Cross Hospital (Hokkaido, Japan) were enrolled in this study. Written informed consent was obtained from all the patients. We included patients of the American Society of Anesthesiologists physical status classification scale I and II. We excluded patients with contraindications for spinal or epidural anesthesia due to hemodynamic, infectious, hemostatic, neurological statuses, and medication use. In addition, we excluded cases of which we were unable to obtain informed consent such as extremely emergent cesarean sections, and cases of which general anesthesia was selected for reasons such as urgency or predicted massive hemorrhage. Using sealed envelopes, patients were randomly divided into two groups: Group IM (intrathecal morphine alone) and Group IM + PCEA (intrathecal morphine combined with PCEA).

Patients in the IM + PCEA group received epidural catheterization prior to spinal anesthesia. A 19-gauge epidural catheter with an 18-gauge epidural Tuohy needle was inserted 5 cm through the Th11–12 or Th12-L1 vertebral interspace. All patients received spinal anesthesia at the L2–3 or L3–4 vertebral interspace with a 25-gauge Quincke spinal needle (TOP Corp., Tokyo, Japan) with 0.5% hyperbaric bupivacaine (12 mg), fentanyl (10 mcg), and morphine (150 mcg) administered. Prior to spinal anesthesia, rapid infusion of 6% hydroxyethyl starch 130/0.4 (Voluven, Fresenius Kabi Japan, Tokyo, Japan) and a total of 1000 ml was administered during surgery. Systolic blood pressure was maintained above 100 mmHg using boluses of phenylephrine 100mcg. A bolus of droperidol 1.25 mg was administered to treat intraoperative nausea and vomiting when necessary. In the IM + PCEA group, continuous epidural infusion of 0.167% levobupivacaine using disposable PCEA infusers (Smiths Medical Japan, Tokyo, Japan) were commenced at the end of surgery and ceased after 24 h. The PCEA settings were basal infusion rate of 6 mL/h, patient-controlled analgesia (PCA) demand dose of 3 mL, and lockout interval of 30 min. To confirm the effect of PCEA, cold sensory blockade was assessed prior to removal of the epidural catheter. We excluded patients with insufficient or unilateral sensory block from the analysis. In the IM + PCEA group, the epidural catheter was removed 24 h after intrathecal administration of morphine but prior to ambulation. All patients began ambulation 24 h after intrathecal administration of morphine. Oxygen saturation was monitored for 24 h after surgery for concerns of respiratory depression potentially related to morphine.

We recorded postoperative pain scores using an 11-point verbal score numerical rating scale (NRS) ranging from 0 as no pain to 10 as worst imaginable pain, at rest and on movement (sitting in an upright position and movement of lower extremities) at 4, 8, 12, 24, 48 h after intrathecal administration of morphine. In addition, we assessed the intensity of motor blockade of lower extremities according to the Bromage score [8] (score 1 = free movement of legs and feet; score 2 = just able to flex knees with free movement of feet; score 3 = unable to flex knees, but with free movement of feet; and score 4 = unable to move legs or feet). Inadequate analgesia was managed with 50 mg diclofenac suppository or a drip infusion of 50 mg flurbiprofen axetil for the first 24 h. Morphine-induced side effects including pruritus and postoperative nausea and vomiting (PONV) were treated with 25 mg of hydroxyzine hydrochloride drip infusion and 10 mg of intravenous metoclopramide infusion, respectively. All data were collected by an investigator who was not involved in providing anesthesia. In addition, patients were asked to rate their satisfaction with analgesia before discharge as follows; 5:completely satisfied, 4:satisfied, 3:fair, 2:unsatisfied, 1:completely unsatisfied.

The primary outcome of this study was postoperative pain as measured by NRS at 12 h after intrathecal administration of morphine during mobilization. Secondary outcomes were NRS at 12 h after intrathecal administration of morphine at rest, NRS and Bromage score at 4, 8, 24, 48 h after intrathecal administration of morphine at rest and during mobilization, the number of patients who requested rescue analgesics, the number of requests for rescue analgesics per patient, the interval time before the first request of rescue analgesics, the incidence of delayed ambulation, the incidence of requested treatment for pruritus and PONV during the first 24 h after intrathecal administration of morphine, and patient satisfaction before discharge.

Statistical analysis

The sample size calculation of 21 patients for each group to provide an α value of 0.05 and a β value of 0.1, was based on NRS of 10 previous post-cesarean section patients who were not included in the final analysis (5 patients who received intrathecal morphine and 5 patients who received both intrathecal morphine and PCEA) during mobilization at 12 h after intrathecal administration of morphine. We adjusted our sample size of 25 patients for each group for anticipated dropouts.

Results are expressed as mean ± standard deviation (SD), unless stated otherwise. We examined NRS and Bromage scores using Bonferroni's multiple comparison test following repeated measures analysis of variance. Differences between groups were compared using unpaired t-test for patient characteristics and analgesic satisfaction, and Mann-Whitney U test for rescue analgesics and morphine-induced side effects. For categorical data, we used Fisher's exact test. All statistical analyses were performed using GraphPad Prism® version 7.03 (GraphPad Software, Inc., La Jolla, CA) and a P-value of < 0.05 was considered statistically significant.

Results

Fifty pregnant women (aged 20–45 years) scheduled for cesarean section were enrolled in this study between January 2017 and April 2018. The CONSORT diagram is showed in Fig. 1. We excluded 2 patients in IM group due to use of rescue analgesic during the surgery and 2 patients in IM + PCEA group due to insufficient effect of PCEA and early removal of epidural catheter. Finally, 23 patients in each group were analyzed. Patient characteristics and intraoperative data were comparable among the groups (Table 1). Twelve patients in the IM group and 11 patients in the IM + PCEA group used antiemetic drugs during surgery.

NRS obtained during the first 48 h are shown in Fig. 2. Mean NRS at rest (Fig. 2a) was significantly higher in IM group than in IM + PCEA group at 4 (2.7 vs 0.6), 8 (2.2 vs 0.6), and 12 h (2.5 vs 0.7), and NRS during mobilization (Fig. 2b) was significantly higher in IM group than in IM + PCEA group at 4 (4.9 vs 1.5), 8 (4.8 vs 1.9), 12 (4.9 vs 2), and 24 h (5.7 vs 3.5). In IM + PCEA group, 6 out of 23 patients (26.1%) used PCA after surgery, and the frequency of use of PCA was 0.78 ± 1.86 (mean ± SD).

With respect to requests for rescue analgesics, significant differences were observed among the two groups (Fig. 3). The number of patients who required rescue analgesics during the first 24 h was 18 (78.3%) in IM group, and 7 (30.4%) in IM + PCEA group (Fig. 3a). The number of requests for rescue analgesics per patient was also significantly higher in IM group (1.22 ± 0.80) than in IM + PCEA group (0.3 ± 0.47) (Fig. 3b). The interval time before the first request for rescue analgesics in IM + PCEA group (1254 ± 120 min) was significantly higher than IM group (521 ± 421 min) (Fig. 3c).

Three patients required treatment for pruritus in IM group and 2 in IM + PCEA group. One patient in IM group requested treatment for PONV. The difference among the groups was not statistically significant for morphine induced side effects.

There were no significant differences in Bromage scores during the first 48 h between two groups (Fig. 4). All patients were evaluated as 1 in Bromage score from 24 h after intrathecal administration of morphine. Ambulation was delayed for approximately 24 h in one patient in IM group due to postoperative pain. Two patients in IM + PCEA group experienced delayed ambulation for approximately 1 and 6 h, respectively, due to weakness of lower extremities. There were no patients who experienced neurological complications or respiratory depression. All patients discharged from the hospital on day 7 after the surgery as scheduled. We obtained patient satisfaction score from 89% of the participants (21/23 in IM group and 20/23 in IM + PCEA group). There was no significant difference in patient satisfaction score between IM group (3.57 ± 1.36) and IM + PCEA group (4.23 ± 0.73) ($p = 0.0651$). Although no patient gave satisfaction score of 1 in IM + PCEA group, three patients in IM group scored 1.

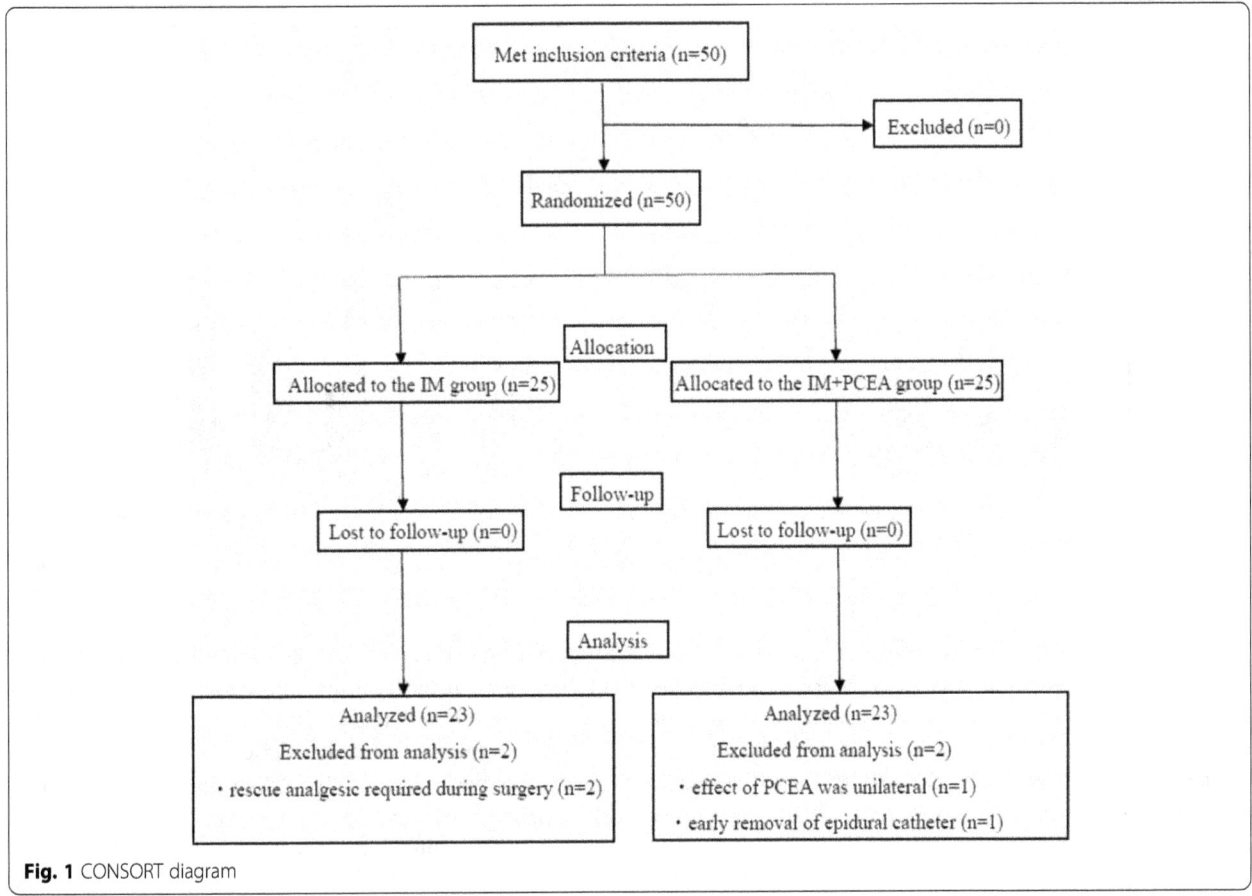

Fig. 1 CONSORT diagram

Discussion

By analyzing 46 patients scheduled for cesarean delivery in this prospective randomized study, we found that the combined use of PCEA and intrathecal morphine provides better post-cesarean section analgesia in the first 12 h at rest and in the first 24 h at movement compared to intrathecal morphine alone. In addition, although no significant difference in patient satisfaction score between IM group and IM + PCEA group was observed, a trend of higher satisfaction was seen in IM + PCEA group. To the best of our knowledge, this is the first study to compare intrathecal morphine with PCEA and intrathecal morphine alone. Similarly to our results,

when focusing on the advantages of PCEA, a previous study concluded that the combined use of intrathecal morphine and PCEA improved post-cesarean section analgesia compared to PCEA without opioids [2]. Another study reported that intrathecal morphine alone was superior to epidural morphine alone or PCEA without opioids [1]. Accordingly, PCEA alone is likely to be inferior to intrathecal morphine alone for post-cesarean section analgesia. While the literature showed that intrathecal morphine provided better post-cesarean section analgesia compared to epidural morphine or PCEA without opioids [1], the pain scores during mobilization in the IM group in our study were similar to the present study.

Table 1 Patient characteristics and intraoperative data

	IM group (n = 23)	IM + PCEA group (n = 23)	P value
Age (years)	33.30 ± 5.46	32.74 ± 4.98	0.7155
Height (cm)	157.87 ± 6.27	158.00 ± 5.89	0.9423
Weight (kg)	65.48 ± 10.20	64.65 ± 7.84	0.7596
Duration of surgery (minutes)	53.48 ± 10.30	51.13 ± 9.60	0.4281
Previous history of caesarean section	13 (56.5)	14 (60.9)	> 0.9999
ASA physical status I/II	12 (52.2)/11 (47.8)	16 (69.6)/7 (30.4)	0.3651

Results are expressed as mean ± SD or as n (%). *IM* Intrathecal morphine, *IM + PCEA* Intrathecal morphine combined with patient-controlled epidural anesthesia, *ASA* American Society of Anesthesiologists

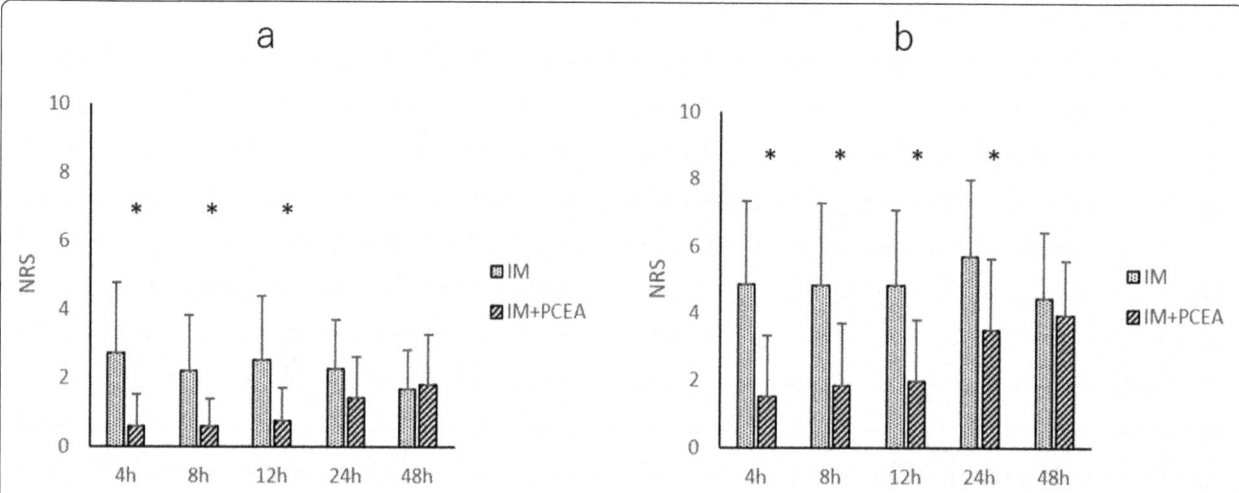

Fig. 2 Numerical rating scale (NRS) during the first 48 h after intrathecal administration of morphine at rest and at movement. **a**. NRS at rest for the first 48 h after intrathecal administration of morphine. **b**. NRS at movement for the first 48 h after intrathecal administration of morphine. *P<0.01. IM = intrathecal morphine. IM + PCEA = intrathecal morphine combined with patient-controlled epidural anesthesia

Therefore, intrathecal morphine alone may not be the best post-cesarean section analgesia. Moreover, previous studies have demonstrated that the suitable target for optimal analgesia is NRS score of below 3–3.3/10 and reductions in pain scores of 30–40% [9–13]. Therefore, despite the statistical differences, postoperative analgesia at rest seems to be sufficient in both IM group and IM + PCEA group. By contrast, postoperative analgesia during mobilization in IM group seems to be insufficient (mean NRS range 4.8–5.7/10) and additional thoracic PCEA (IM + PCEA group) provided clinically meaningful reduction (reduction to mean NRS range 1.5–3.5/10) in pain scores and optimal analgesia.

High quality post-cesarean section analgesia is crucial for postoperative recovery, as patients are recovering from major abdominal surgery while breastfeeding and caring for a newborn [14, 15]. To provide adequate post-cesarean section analgesia, clinical management guidelines for obstetrician-gynecologists recommends a multimodal approach in which systematic opioids can be reduced [16]. In guidelines of Enhanced Recovery After Surgery (ERAS) Society, thoracic epidural analgesia is an alternative to intrathecal morphine for post-open general gynecologic surgery analgesia [17]. Further, despite the benefit in analgesia, several risks of adding thoracic epidural anesthesia should be taken into consideration. First, patients will receive needle puncture twice to perform lumbar spinal and thoracic epidural anesthesia. Second, use of a combined lumbar epidural and spinal technique will save an additional procedure, however, lumbar epidural analgesia may increase motor blockade which can contribute to delay in ambulation. In the present study, all patients in IM + PCEA group were evaluated as 1 on Bromage score, indicating free movement of legs and feet, with two patients (8.7%) experiencing delayed ambulation. The low incidence of delayed ambulation may be linked to the level of placement of the epidural catheter, which in the present study was the lower thoracic vertebral interspace (Th11–12 or Th12-L1). While motor blockade during thoracic epidural analgesia has been reported to be 6.7% at 24 h after cesarean section [2], the incidence of motor blockade

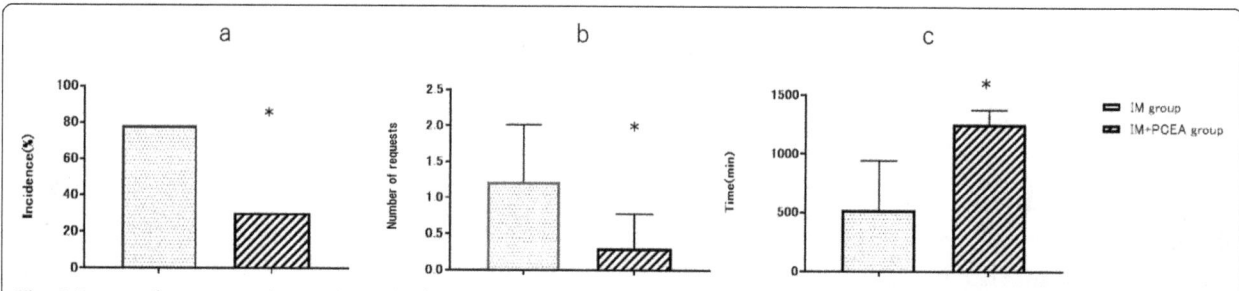

Fig. 3 Requests for rescue analgesics during the first 24 h after intrathecal administration of morphine. **a**. Percentage of patients who requested rescue analgesics. **b**. Number of requests for rescue analgesics per patient. $P<0.0001$. **c**. Interval time (minutes) before the first request for rescue analgesics. $P = 0.0005$. IM = intrathecal morphine. IM + PCEA = intrathecal morphine combined with patient-controlled epidural anesthesia

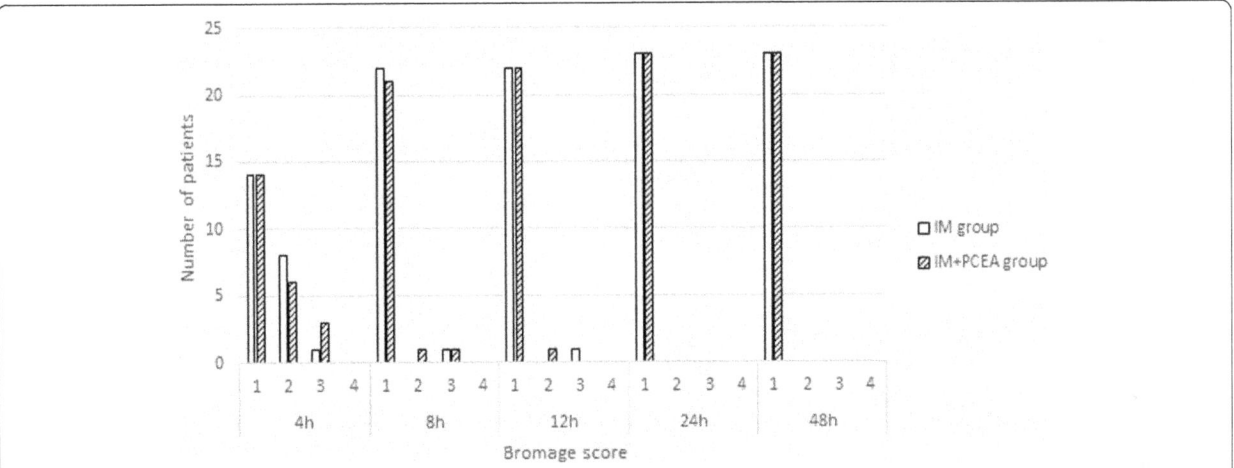

Fig. 4 Bromage score of postoperative pain during the first 48 h after intrathecal administration of morphine. Bromage score: score 1 = free movement of legs and feet; score 2 = just able to flex knees with free movement of feet; score 3 = unable to flex knees, but with free movement of feet; and score 4 = unable to move legs or feet. IM = intrathecal morphine. IM + PCEA = intrathecal morphine combined with patient-controlled epidural anesthesia

was shown to be 26% at 12 h after cesarean section during continuous epidural infusion via L2–3 or L3–4 vertebral interspace in prior studies [18]. Therefore, lumbar epidural analgesia may increase the risk of motor blockade compared to thoracic epidural analgesia. Furthermore, it is known that adequate postoperative analgesia is necessary for early ambulation in addition to recovery of the motor function [19]. Likewise, one patient (4.3%) in the IM group (who did not receive epidural anesthesia) experienced delayed ambulation for approximately 24 h due to postoperative pain. Third, neurological complications are a rare but serious complication associated with epidural anesthesia. Although there were no patients with neurological complications in our study, previous literature has reported the incidence of permanent neurological injury after epidural anesthesia as 0–7.6:1000 [20].

In addition, the choice and concentration of epidural local anesthetic play an important role in post-cesarean section analgesia and early ambulation. The choice of local anesthetic usually depends on the speed of onset required for the particular clinical situation. Epidural local anesthetics commonly used for cesarean section analgesia include lidocaine, bupivacaine, ropivacaine, and chloroprocaine. Previous studies have used 0.1 to 0.2% ropivacaine or levobupivacaine for PCEA following cesarean section [1, 2, 4, 21]. One study comparing 0.15% of plain ropivacaine and levobupivacaine for post-cesarean section PCEA showed no significant differences regarding postoperative analgesic efficacy and motor weakness [4]. Another study which compared low concentration (0.15%) and high concentration (0.5%) levobupivacaine for postoperative epidural analgesia after

major abdominal surgery reported that there were no significant differences in analgesic effect with consistent low motor blockade [22]. Therefore, low concentrated levobupivacaine may be a potential alternative for ropivacaine. In the present study we chose 0.167% levobupivacaine as literature on levobupivacaine for post-cesarean section PCEA was limited. The present study showing low NRS scores without motor weakness in IM + PCEA group supports that low concentrated levobupivacaine may be optimal for post-cesarean section PCEA.

The study has several potential limitations. First, although patients were randomly divided into two groups, PCEA did not allow a full blinding. However, the data was collected by an investigator who was not involved in providing anesthesia. Another method to minimize performance bias is to compare IM + PCEA with levobupivacaine versus IM + PCEA with saline alone as control group, however, we were unable to conduct this for ethical concerns. Second, only elective cesarean sections were included in our study as we were unable to obtain informed consent in extremely emergent cesarean sections. This may limit the generalizability of our inferences to more severe cases. However, our findings remain highly relevant to the majority of the population who receive cesarean sections. Third, scheduled acetaminophen and/or non-steroidal anti-inflammatory drugs (NSAIDs) were not used in our study. Scheduled acetaminophen and/or NSAIDs is a less invasive form of multimodal pain control compared to epidural anesthesia and previously reported to improve post-cesarean section analgesia [23, 24]. If the scheduled acetaminophen and/or NSAIDs were used in this study, it might decrease the impact of PCEA. Forth, patients were not allowed to ambulate with the epidural in place and the thoracic epidural catheter was removed in 24 h after intrathecal administration of morphine. We speculate that a thoracic PCEA might be beneficial in the setting of a longer period of infusion and patients being permitted to ambulate with the epidural catheter in place.

Conclusions

A combined use of PCEA and spinal anesthesia with intrathecal morphine provided better postoperative analgesia following cesarean section without delay in ambulation compared to single shot spinal anesthesia with intrathecal morphine alone. Although there are several risks that require consideration, thoracic epidural catheterization and 24 h of PCEA in addition to intrathecal morphine may be a reasonable option to improve post-cesarean section analgesia especially during mobilization.

Abbreviations

PCEA: Patient-controlled epidural anesthesia; PCA: Patient-controlled anesthesia; NRS: Numerical rating scale; PONV: Postoperative nausea and vomiting; SD: Standard deviation; ERAS: Enhanced Recovery After Surgery; NSAIDs: Non-steroidal anti-inflammatory drugs

Acknowledgments

Izumi Sato and Hajime Iwasaki are equally contributing first authors of this article. Part of the data in this article was presented at the 7th Annual Meeting of the Japanese Society of Anesthesiologists Hokkaido-Tohoku Region site (Akita, 2017). We express our gratitude to Professor Yasuaki Saijo for suggestions on statistical analysis. We also thank Obstetrics and Gynecology physicians (Dr. Tatsumi Yamaguchi, Dr. Masaki Azuma, Dr. Toshie Yonehara, Dr. Yukiko Aoyagi, Dr. Rieko Tanaka, Dr. Hiroki Higashi, Dr. Hiroki Hashimoto, Dr. Goro Maeda, Dr. Keiko Tanaka, Dr. Shotaro Fujino, Dr. Tetsuya Nakajin, and Dr. Tomono Shimabukuro), 4A ward medical staff, and operating room medical staff of Kushiro Red Cross Hospital for compliance with study protocol.

Authors' contributions

Study design: IS and HI. Advisor for study protocol and management of the study: TI and HK. Study conduction: IS and HI. Data analysis: IS, HI and SKL. Manuscript preparation: IS, HI and SKL. Editing and approval of the manuscript: TI and HK. All authors have read and approved the manuscript.

Author details

[1]Department of Anesthesiology and Critical Care Medicine, Asahikawa Medical University, Midorigaoka-higashi 2-1-1-1, Asahikawa, Hokkaido 078-8510, Japan. [2]Department of Anesthesiology, Indiana University School of Medicine, 1130 W. Michigan Street, Fesler Hall 204, Indianapolis, IN 46202, USA.

References

1. Kaufner L, Heimann S, Zander D, Weizsacker K, Correns I, Sander M, Spies C, Schuster M, Feldheiser A, Henkelmann A, Wernecke KD, Heymann CVON. Neuraxial anesthesia for pain control after cesarean section: a prospective randomized trial comparing three different neuraxial techniques in clinical practice. Minerva Anestesiol. 2016;82:514–24.
2. Mikuni I, Hirai H, Toyama Y, Takahata O, Iwasaki H. Efficacy of intrathecal morphine with epidural ropivacaine infusion for postcesarean analgesia. J Clin Anesth. 2010;22:268–73.
3. Vercauteren M, Vereecken K, La Malfa M, Coppejans H, Adriaensen H. Cost-effectiveness of analgesia after caesarean section. A comparison of intrathecal morphine and epidural PCA. Acta Anaesthesiol Scand. 2002;46: 85–9.
4. Matsota P, Batistaki C, Apostolaki S, Kostopanagiotou G. Patient-controlled epidural analgesia after Caesarean section: levobupivacaine 0.15% versus

5. ropivacaine 0.15% alone or combined with fentanyl 2 microg/ml: a comparative study. Arch Med Sci. 2011;7:685–93.
5. Duale C, Frey C, Bolandard F, Barriere A, Schoeffler P. Epidural versus intrathecal morphine for postoperative analgesia after caesarean section. Br J Anaesth. 2003;91:690–4.
6. Sarvela J, Halonen P, Soikkeli A, Korttila K. A double-blinded, randomized comparison of intrathecal and epidural morphine for elective cesarean delivery. Anesth Analg. 2002;95:436–40 table of contents.
7. Suzuki H, Kamiya Y, Fujiwara T, Yoshida T, Takamatsu M, Sato K. Intrathecal morphine versus epidural ropivacaine infusion for analgesia after cesarean section: a retrospective study. JA Clin Rep. 2015;1:3.
8. Bromage PR. A comparison of the hydrochloride and carbon dioxide salts of lidocaine and prilocaine in epidural analgesia. Acta Anaesthesiol Scand Suppl. 1965;16:55–69.
9. Myles PS, Myles DB, Galagher W, Boyd D, Chew C, MacDonald N, Dennis A. Measuring acute postoperative pain using the visual analog scale: the minimal clinically important difference and patient acceptable symptom state. Br J Anaesth. 2017;118:424–9.
10. Hartrick CT, Kovan JP, Shapiro S. The numeric rating scale for clinical pain measurement: a ratio measure? Pain Pract. 2003;3:310–6.
11. Campbell WI, Patterson CC. Quantifying meaningful changes in pain. Anaesthesia. 1998;53:121–5.
12. Bodian CA, Freedman G, Hossain S, Eisenkraft JB, Beilin Y. The visual analog scale for pain: clinical significance in postoperative patients. Anesthesiology. 2001;95:1356–61.
13. Farrar JT, Portenoy RK, Berlin JA, Kinman JL, Strom BL. Defining the clinically important difference in pain outcome measures. Pain. 2000;88:287–94.
14. McDonnell NJ, Keating ML, Muchatuta NA, Pavy TJ, Paech MJ. Analgesia after caesarean delivery. Anaesth Intensive Care. 2009;37:539–51.
15. Kerai S, Saxena KN, Taneja B. Post-caesarean analgesia: what is new? Indian J Anaesth. 2017;61:200–14.
16. Practice Bulletin No ACOG. 209: obstetric analgesia and anesthesia. Obstet Gynecol. 2019;133:e208–e25.
17. Nelson G, Altman AD, Nick A, Meyer LA, Ramirez PT, Achtari C, Antrobus J, Huang J, Scott M, Wijk L, Acheson N, Ljungqvist O, Dowdy SC. Guidelines for postoperative care in gynecologic/oncology surgery: enhanced recovery after surgery (ERAS(R)) society recommendations--part II. Gynecol Oncol. 2016;140:323–32.
18. Buggy DJ, Hall NA, Shah J, Brown J, Williams J. Motor block during patient-controlled epidural analgesia with ropivacaine or ropivacaine/fentanyl after intrathecal bupivacaine for caesarean section. Br J Anaesth. 2000;85:468–70.
19. Gandhi KA, Jain K. Management of anaesthesia for elective, low-risk (category 4) caesarean section. Indian J Anaesth. 2018;62:667–74.
20. Brull R, McCartney CJ, Chan VW, El-Beheiry H. Neurological complications after regional anesthesia: contemporary estimates of risk. Anesth Analg. 2007;104:965–74.
21. Chen LK, Lin PL, Lin CJ, Huang CH, Liu WC, Fan SZ, Wang MH. Patient-controlled epidural ropivacaine as a post-cesarean analgesia: a comparison with epidural morphine. Taiwan J Obstet Gynecol. 2011;50:441–6.
22. Dernedde M, Stadler M, Bardiau F, Boogaerts JG. Comparison of 2 concentrations of levobupivacaine in postoperative patient-controlled epidural analgesia. J Clin Anesth. 2005;17:531–6.
23. Valentine AR, Carvalho B, Lazo TA, Riley ET. Scheduled acetaminophen with as-needed opioids compared to as-needed acetaminophen plus opioids for post-cesarean pain management. Int J Obstet Anesth. 2015;24:210–6.
24. Akhavanakbari G, Entezariasl M, Isazadehfar K, Kahnamoyiagdam F. The effects of indomethacin, diclofenac, and acetaminophen suppository on pain and opioids consumption after cesarean section. Perspect Clin Res. 2013;4:136–41.

10

Ultrasound-guided ilioinguinal-iliohypogastric block (ILIHB) or perifocal wound infiltration (PWI) in children: A prospective randomized comparison of analgesia quality

Bjoern Grosse[1]*[iD], Stefan Eberbach[1], Hans O. Pinnschmidt[2], Deirdre Vincent[3], Martin Schmidt-Niemann[1] and Konrad Reinshagen[1,3]

Abstract

Background: Ilioinguinal-iliohypogastric block (ILIHB) is a well-established procedure for postoperative analgesia after open inguinal surgery in children. This procedure is effective and safe, especially when ultrasound is used. Data availability for comparing ultrasound-guided blocks versus wound infiltration is still weak. The study was designed to determine the efficacy of ultrasound-guided ILIHB (US-ILIHB) on postoperative pain control in pediatric patients following a inguinal daycase surgery, compared with perifocal wound infiltration (PWI) by the surgeon.

Methods: This randomized, double-blinded trail was conducted in pediatric patients aged from 6 months to 4 years. The total number of children included in the study was 103. Patients were allocated at random in two groups by sealed envelopes. The ILIHB group recieved 0,2% ropivacain for US-ILIHB after anesthesia induction. The PWI group recieved 0,2% ropivacain for PWI performed by a surgeon before wound closure. Parameters recorded included the postoperative pain score, pain frequency, time to first analgesics and consumption of analgesics. *Results:* US-ILIHB significantly reduced the occurrence of pain within the first 24 h after surgery (7.7%, $p = 0.01$). Moreover, the pain-free interval until administration of the first dose of opioids was 21 min longer, on average ($p = 0.003$), following US-ILIHB compared to perifocal wound infiltration. 72% of children who received US-ILIHB did not require additional opioids, as compared to 56% of those who received PWI.

Conclusion: Thus our study demonstrates that US-ILIHB ensures better postoperative analgesia in children and should be prioritized over postoperative PWI.

Keywords: Regional, Ultrasound, opioids, Pain, outpatient, Ambulatory, local, Anesthetics, Drugs, infant, Age

* Correspondence: Bjoern.Grosse@kinderkrankenhaus.net
[1]Department of Pediatric Anesthesiology, Altona Children's Hospital, Bleickenallee 38, 22763 Hamburg, Germany

Background

The ratio of surgeries performed in an outpatient setting has been increasing rapidly for years and this trend is extend to continue in the future. Open inguinal surgery in children is an outpatient procedure that requires efficient and long-acting analgesia to facilitate early discharge. However, the prevalence of compromising and persistent post-surgery pain in children remains high [1]. Once a child has left the hospital, their parents are tasked with administering medication. Unfortunately, parents often encounter difficulties handling the dosing of painkillers, which results in inadequate or inefficient pain management [2]. Due to the lack of experience and insufficient knowledge of the parents, with respect to pain management, children consequently experience high levels of emotional stress associated with pain. In fact, their understanding of pain has been shown to depend on their psycho-social development stage. Thus, inadequate medical care may result in lasting psychological damage [3]. We must, therefore, focus on the best possible pain treatment. Various randomized studies have demonstrated that local anaesthetic procedures are more effective in children than systemic ones [4, 5]. Local anaesthetic procedures allow for a reduction of the opioid dose which in turn reduces the rate of systemic side effects caused by opioids [6, 7]. A multicentre study by the "Pediatric Regional Anesthesia Network" based on 15,000 cases has demonstrated that the risk of side effects from local anaesthesia in children is low with no observable long-term damage [8]. Hence, the "S3 Guideline on Treatment of Acute Perioperative and Posttraumatic Pain" from 2007, which is currently being revised, recommends using regional anaesthetic procedures, whenever possible, rather than systemic oral painkillers (recommendation grade A) [9]. In fact, the latest Cochrane Review demonstrate that ultrasound-guided regional anaesthetic procedures allow for more targeted blocks using lower doses of local anaesthetics in children, which further reduces the incidence of side effects [10]. Coming to the conclusion that optimal analgesia in surgical interventions can be achieved by means of regional nerve blocks, and the resulting implementation of ultrasound to increase the effectiveness of these nerve blocks, makes the use of ultrasound-assisted nerve blocks virtually indispensable for the prevention of pain in children [11, 12]. The ILIHB to be investigated in this study was first introduced in the 1980's as an anaesthetic procedure for inguinal surgery in children and did not include ultrasound support. Even though ILIHB is an established regional anaesthesia procedure, data availability for comparing ultrasound-guided blocks versus wound infiltration is still weak due to the lack of evidence [13–18]. Unequivocal data demonstrating that either method provides a high quality of analgesia, in

children or in adults, is not yet available making the choice of the right anaesthetic procedure to ensure optimal analgesia difficult.

Our study tested the primary hypothesis that US-ILIHB provides a more adequate analgesia in pediatric inguinal surgery with correspondingly lower pain levels on the pediatric scale of discomfort and pain (KUSS) within 24 h, as compared to surgical perifocal wound infiltration (PWI). Secondarily, we tested the hypothesis that the demand for analgesics after pediatric inguinal surgery is much later in patients of the US-ILIHB group while the amount of painkillers as well as the frequency of their administration is correspondingly lower than in patients of the PWI group.

Methods

Approval

The study was reviewed by the ethics committee of the Hamburg Medical Council and approved by the doctoral committee of the University of Hamburg. Parents were informed about the purposes of the study and how their children would be involved at each visit, and their consent was provided in writing. All children were recruited from the pediatric and urological clinic of the Altona Children's Hospital of the University of Hamburg.

Power and sample size calculation

The number of cases was calculated using G * Power 3.1. An effect size of 0.6 was derived from previous studies [13, 15]. The alpha was set at 5%. Experience has shown that the drop-out rate is around 10%. Therefore, with a power set to 0.9, the number of 102 cases was calculated, 120 cases are targeted.

Study population

One hundred sixteen children aged from 6 months to 4 years with a minimum weight of 6 kg; with an American Society of Anesthesiologists Classification (ASA) of I or II and scheduled for a unilateral outpatient inguinal surgery were enrolled in equal randomized (1:1), double-blind, parallel group study conducted in Germany. The initial maximum age of 3 years was extended to 4 years during the study due to the little recruitment number. The following exclusion criteria were applied: mental illness, allergies to relevant drugs, renal insufficiency, coagulation disorders, local infections, emergency procedures, and additional interventions. Demographic data such as gender, age, and weight were collected. Subjects were randomized and allocated to two groups using sealed envelopes including the respective technique (US-ILIHB group, $n = 53$, and PWI group, $n = 50$). After 120 envelopes were numbered 1 to 120, they were filled 1:1 with the technique protocol of the corresponding group. An computer generated simple randomisation allocated the envelops to patients. Only the anaesthesiologist was notified the group and which block technique to use immediately before the induction of anaesthesia when the envelope was opened. After performing the procedure and in accordance with a specified "standardized operation procedure" (SOP), he put the completed technique protocol back into the envelope and sealed it, so that group and corresponding procedure remained hidden from the patient and the personnel performing pain measurements.

Anatomy

The ilioinguinal and iliohypogastric nerves originate from the spinal cord at the level of L1 and Th12. They cross the inside of the quadratus lumborum muscle to the aponeurosis of the transverse abdominal muscle, which they pierce at the lumbar triangle. Thereafter, they pass between the internal oblique muscle and the transverse abdominal muscle, until entering the internal oblique muscle 1–3 cm medially to the anterior superior iliac spine. In children, on a line between the anterior superior iliac spine and the navel, the ilioinguinal nerve is 9–11 mm away and the iliohypogastric nerve is 13–18 mm away from the anterior superior iliac spine. The ilioinguinal nerve provides sensory innervation to part of the groin: mons pubis and labia or scrotum, with a great range of anatomical variability, especially with respect to the innervation of the labia and scrotum. In 40% of cases, innervation is supplied by the genitofemoral nerve. Iliohypogastric nerve provides sensory innervation to the groin and the skin above mons pubis [19].

Standardized introduction

Thirty minutes before the induction of anaesthesia, all children were premedicated with midazolam 0.5 mg/kg per os. All patients were intubated and anesthetized according to the SOP as follows: Anaesthesia was induced with sevoflurane via a face mask, 0.3 µg/kg IV sufentanil, and 0.05 mg/kg IV vecuronium. All patients were intubated. Anaesthesia was maintained with 10 mg/kg/h of propofol 1%. IV fluid maintenance therapy was achieved using 1% glucose solution (< 12 months) or 0.9% acetate Ringer's solution at an infusion rate of 10 ml/kg/h. Children also received 10 mg/kg ibuprofen as at rectal suppository. Lastly 0.1–0.2 µg/kg of sufentanil was administered as a "rescue analgesia" if there were signs of intraoperative pain were detected.

Block technique

As local anaesthetics 0.2 ml/kg of naropin 0,2% was used. This bloc was administered to all patients using sterile conditions and in general anaesthesia. Target structures of the nerve block were the ilioinguinal and iliohypogastric nerves, which run within the fasciae between the oblique abdominal muscles, the internal oblique muscle, and the transverse abdominal muscle (Fig. 1).

All patients in the US-ILIHB group were treated by well experienced paediatric anaesthesiologists from the paediatric anaesthesia department of the Altona Children's Hospital. Immediately after anaesthesia was induced, the main anatomical structures: the external oblique muscle, the internal oblique muscle, and the transverse abdominal muscle were visualized using the ultrasound SonoSite S-Nerv, linear probe (Fig. 1b). A weight-adapted amount of naropin was applied between the internal oblique muscle and the transverse abdominal muscle layers, using a needle guided ultrasound-assisted "in-plane" technique. Prior to injection with naropin a negative aspiration test, via a 25 gauge cannula with 0.5 mm outer diameter, had to be performed (Fig. 2a).

All patients in the *PWI group* were treated by paediatric surgeons from the Department of Paediatric Surgery of the Altona Children's Hospital. At the end of the surgery, immediately after closing the aponeurosis of external oblique muscle, a negativ aspiration test using a 20 gauge cannula with 0.9 mm outside diameter was administered followed by weight-adapted administration of naropin in macroscopic view through a suture gap (Fig. 2b).

Pain measurement and postoperative management

Since preverbal children (< 4 years) are not yet able to adequately assess or communicate their level of pain, pain intensity was measured using third-party assessments based on an approved multidimensional pain scale [20, 21], namely the "pediatric scale of discomfort and pain" (KUSS) was used [22]. As primary outcome measure pain measurement datapoints were collected in three instalments within the first 24 h post-surgery. For this purpose, children were transferred to the recovery room, known as the "post-anesthesia care unit (PACU)", immediately at the end of anaesthesia at which point the first assessment took place. Trained nurses performed four measurements in 15 minute intervals. Measurements based on KUSS, signs of pain in the categories: crying, facial expression, trunk stance, posture, motor restlessness are each rated with 1-3 points and finally result in a pain score between 0-10, which is intended to reflect pain intensity. Thus a score of 0 means "no pain" while a score of 10 reflects "maximum pain". In general, analgesia (0.05 mg/kg piritramide) was provided to children who scored 3 or higher on the KUSS scale until their pain subsided or was at a level of less than 3. Following the stay at PACU patients were transferred from PACU to the discharge station, konwn as the "outpatient surgery ward" (OSW). During the stay at the OSW,

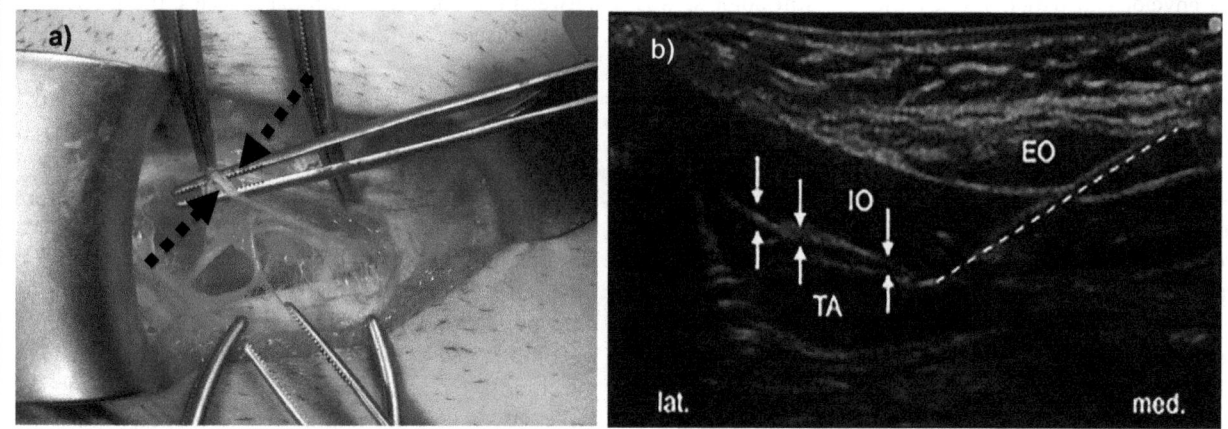

Fig. 1 Anatomy: **a** macroscopic: Black arrows = ilioinguinal-iliohypogastric nerves; **b** Ultrasound image: EO = abdominal external oblique muscle, IO = abdominal internal oblique muscle, TA = transverse abdominal muscle; White arrows = Ilioinguinal and iliohypogastric nerves between fasciae, Dotted line = needle in situ; lat.=lateral, med.=medial

the second assessment episode took place, in which nurses performed four measurements at 30 min intervals. After the final examination of the patients and their full recovery, all parents were briefed in detail on the administration of the KUSS scale before the children were discharged. Therefore, the fourth and last assessment episode was performed at home, during which parents performed four measurements at four-hour intervals. In addition to the KUSS scores, complaining of nausea or occurrence of vomiting events, and other abnormalities were queried on the phone the following morning. Secondary outcome measures that were recorded was the time until the first pain medication was administered after surgery (piritramide, ibuprofen, or paracetamol) and lastly, the duration of surgery, and the frequency and total dose of piritramide were also assessed.

Data analysis
The Statistical data processing was carried out in cooperation with the Institute for Medical Biometry & Epidemiology of the Hamburg Eppendorf University

Hospital. The descriptive statistics for continuous variables were based on the mean value and standard deviation per group. Absolute and percentage frequencies per group were determined and presented as categorical variables. Group differences with respect to continuous variables were tested using the Mann–Whitney U test, while group differences with respect to categorical variables were tested with χ^2– and Fisher's exact test. The effects of group, time interval, and their interaction with the dichotomous dependent variable were tested using a mixed logistic regression model. A linear mixed model was fit to the continuous dependent variable with the fixed effects of group and point in time, and with the points in time within patients as repeated measures representing repeated measurements. The group-specific course of analgesia administration was analysed and visualized using the Kaplan-Meier method and a comparison of the groups was conducted using logrank tests. The significance level for all tests was set to 0.05 and all statistical tests were set to be bilateral. All analyses were performed using SPSS version 25.0 (IBM, NY, US).

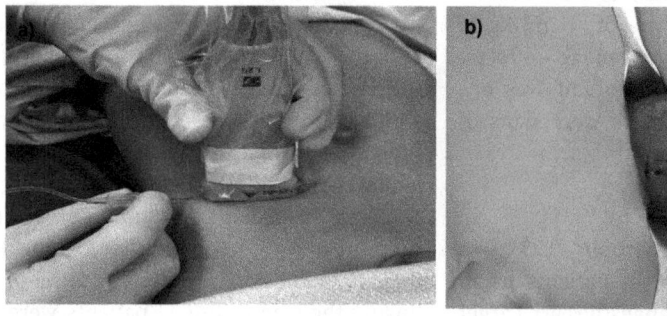

Fig. 2 Technique: **a** Ultrasound-guided ilioinguinal-iliohypogastric block; **b** Perifocal wound infiltration after fascial suture, injection through suture gap (arrow)

Since the mean values of the collected pain scores of both groups (US-ILIHB and PWI) demonstrated extreme differences among the four measurement episodes, the statistical evaluation was not adequate as planned initially. Pain scores assessed in PACU and OSW were very low in both groups, while pain scores measured at home were relatively high. One reason for this difference was the particularly high occurrence of reports of absolute freedom from pain in the PACU and OSW measurement episodes. In order to be able to present the difference in analgesia between both methods, we planned to analyse the pain scores within the three individual measurement episodes (PACU, OSW, at home), and not on the entire time frame. Thus, in a second step, the data was dichotomized, i.e. divided into values = 0 and > 0. As such, all pain scores > 0 represent pain that occurred at the time of measurement, while pain scores = 0 indicate that there was no occurrence of pain. This allowed us to represent the "relative frequency of occurrence of pain" (rel.freq.), with the resulting differences in rel.freq. Within the episodes ($p = 0.000$) and measurement times ($p = 0.001$), and between groups ($p = 0.009$) being highly significant.

Results

A total of 116 patients were selected for the study, of which, 115 were randomized. Twelve patients were excluded. 53 patients were enrolled and analysed in the US-ILIHB group and 50 patients in the PWI group (see Fig. 3). In the follow up phase we lost contact with four patients, and the study was discontinued for three cases, due to additional interventions having been required. One patient with bronchospasm, during reversal of anaesthesia, and one patient with a known ibuprofen allergy were excluded from the study. Other reasons for exclusion were e.g. gaps in the documentation, or imprecise implementation of the technique due to anatomical challenges. As stated previously, demographics and characteristics of all subjects were recorded (gender, age, weight, ASA, duration of surgery) and shown to have negligible difference on the two groups. The average age in both groups was 2 years, while 83–92% of patient population were boys. The average surgery time was calculated to be 36 min in both groups (Tab. 1). None of the patients treated in the course of this study experienced any complications that could be related to the block technique being investigated. As seen below, Fig. 4 shows a clear trend: Most pain events occurred in the measurement episode at home, with more frequent occurrences of pain in the PWI group than in the US-ILIHB group. Following, results with regards to the respective group (US-ILIHB and PWI) (Fig. 5a) are discussed. The relative frequency of all pain events in the US-ILIHB group was 12.6% (SD = 1.9), whereas in the PWI group it was 20.3% (SD = 2.5), resulting in a difference of 7.7% in favour of the US-ILIHB group ($p =$

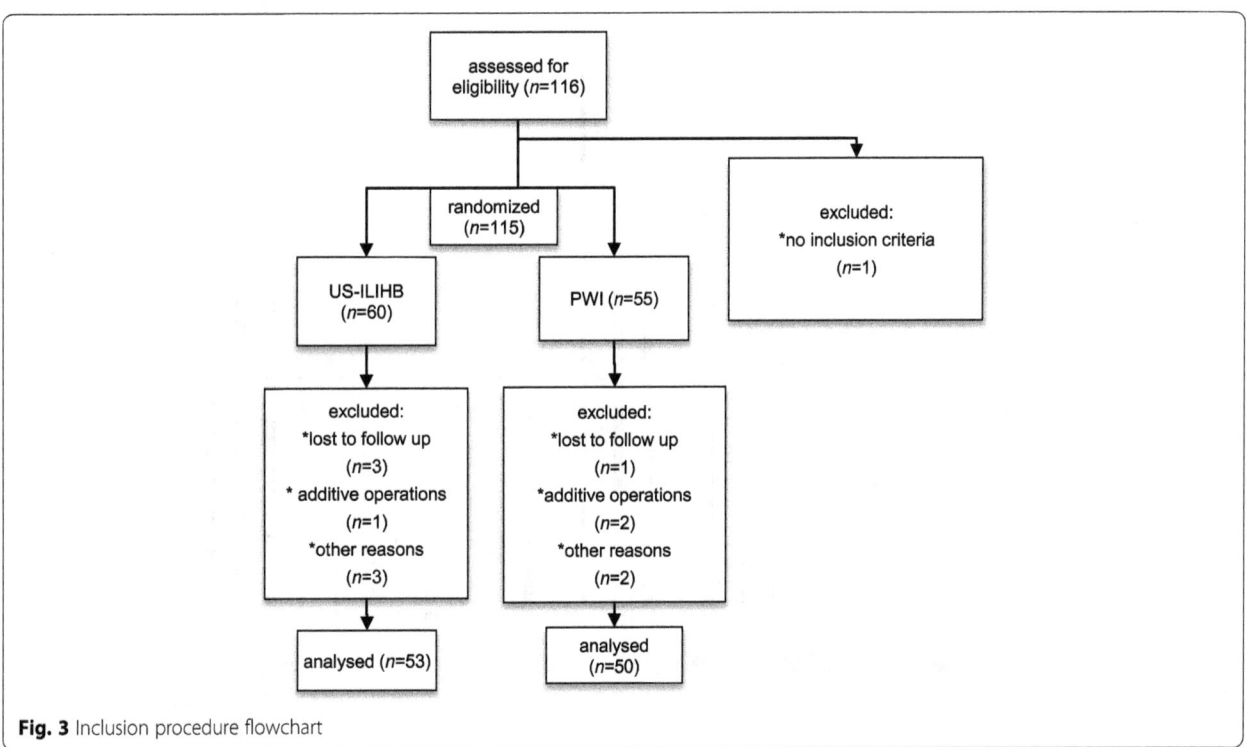

Fig. 3 Inclusion procedure flowchart

Table 1 Descriptive statistics (upper part), MV = mean value, SD = standard deviation, n = number. Consumption of analgesicis (lower part) for US-ILIHB and PWI group, p = significance

		US-ILIHB (n = 53)				PWI (n = 50)			
		MW	SD	n	(%)	MW	SD	n	(%)
Sex	F (n/ %)			9	17.0			4	8.0
	M (n/ %)			44	83.0			46	92.0
ASA	I			50	94.3			41	82.0
	II			3	5.7			9	18.0
Age (months)		27.8	14.0	53		26.0	12.9	50	
Body weight (kg)		13.0	3.1	53		12.5	2.8	50	
Duration of surgery (min.)		36.3	14.4	53		36.7	13.4	50	
		MW	SD	n		MW	SD	n	
(n)Piritramide p = 0.082		0.4	0.6	53		0.6	0.8	50	
Σ Piritramide (mg) p = 0.059		0.2	0.4	53		0.4	0.5	50	
(n)Clonidine p = 0.048		0.2	0.6	53		0.4	0.6	50	
Σ Clonidine (µg) p = 0.049		3.0	6.5	53		5.9	8.4	50	

0.01). That is, the relative frequency of all pain events in the PWI group is about 50% greater than in the US-ILIHB group. Figure 5b demonstrates the following results obtained with regards to the respective measurement episode (PACU, OSW, at home) and all subjects of both groups, with the frequency of pain being 9.2%

(SD = 3.2) in PACU, and 10.0% in OSW (SD = 1.9). Overall, pain was detected most frequently at home with 38.4% (SD = 3.2) ($p = <0.001$). The time until the administration of piritramide, within the first 2 h after surgery, yielded following results (Fig. 6a): The US-ILIHB group averaged 1.97 h (95% CI 1.93–2.00) until the first piritramide application in comparison to the PWI group, which averaged 1.62 h until the first piritramide application (95% CI 1.48–1.77). This results in a difference of 0.35 h or 21 min of earlier pain treatment in the PWI group ($p = 0.003$). With respect to caregivers' first administration of either ibuprofen or paracetamol, within the first 15 h of arrival at home, the following results were obtained (Fig. 6b): In the US-ILIHB group, parents administered the first peripheral analgesic after 11.94 h (95% CI 6.07–11.09), whereas in the PWI group required analgesia after 8.58 h (95% CI 9.24–14.64). However, even though the difference is quite large, the findings were not statistically significant ($p = 0.078$) due to large variances in both groups. There were no significant differences regarding the frequency of postoperative nausea and vomiting in both groups within 24 h measurement period: 5 out of 53 versus 5 out of 50 patients reported nausea and vomiting in the US-ILHIB and in the PWI group, respectively. The absolute amounts of administered analgesics and the frequency of analgesia applications did not differ significantly (see Table 1). However, in absolute terms, only 15 children in the US-ILIHB

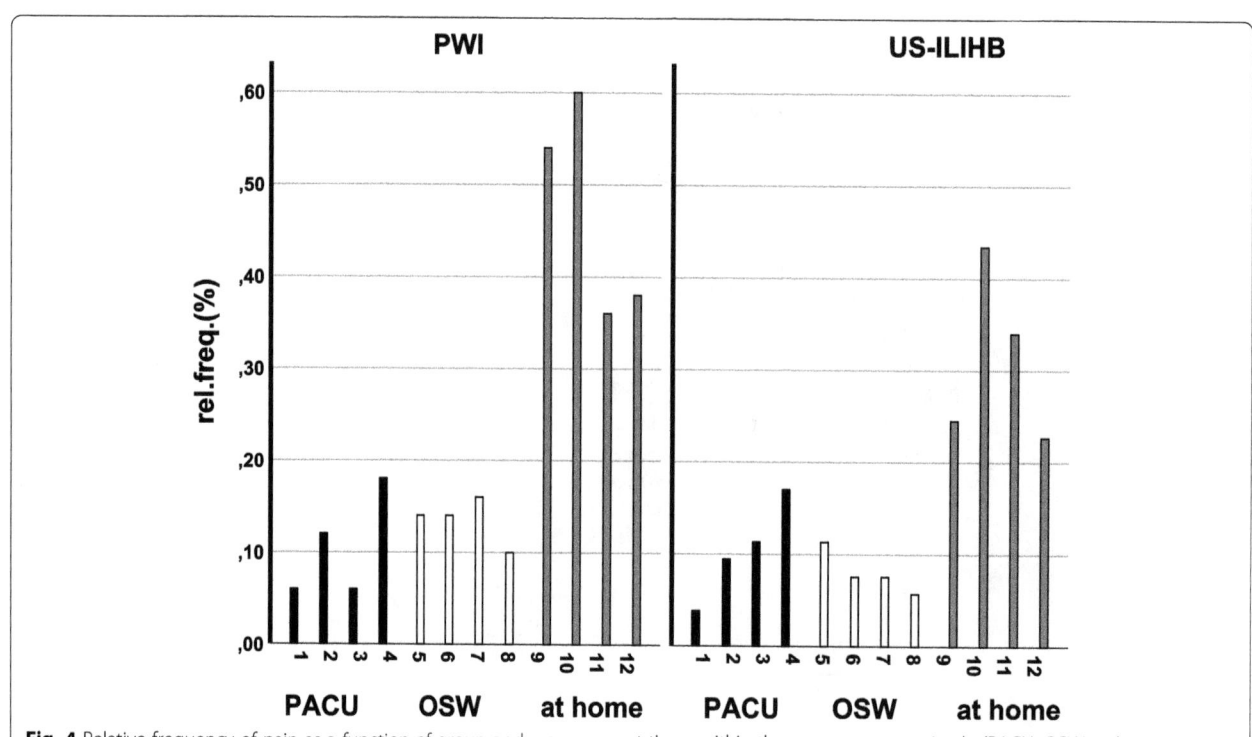

Fig. 4 Relative frequency of pain as a function of group and measurement times within the measurement episode (PACU, OSW, at home), 1–12 = measurement times within 24 h

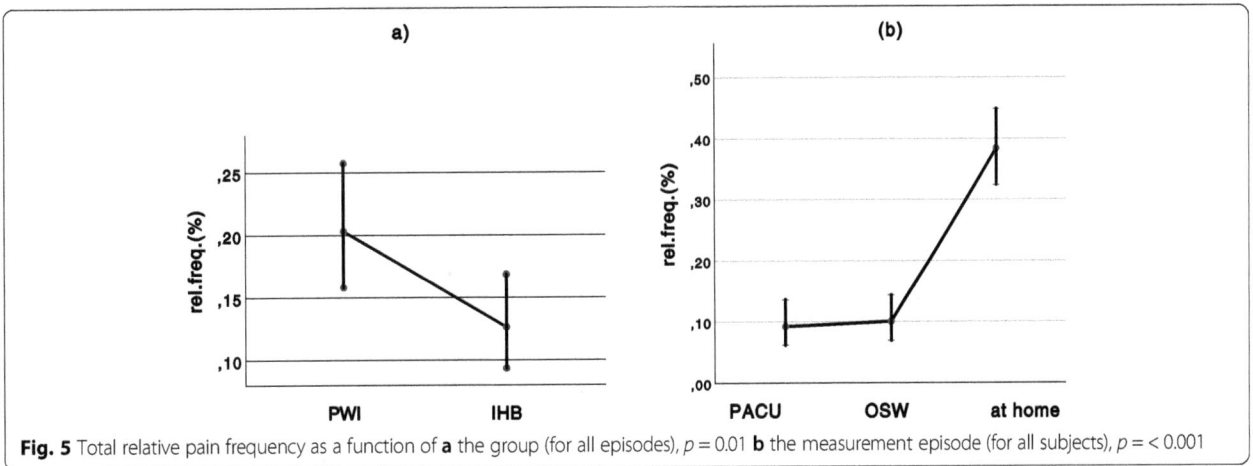

Fig. 5 Total relative pain frequency as a function of **a** the group (for all episodes), $p = 0.01$ **b** the measurement episode (for all subjects), $p = < 0.001$

group (28.3%) versus 22 children in the PWI group (44%) received an opioid in PACU. Overall, no analgesics were given to 7 children in the PWI group (14%) versus 15 children (28.3%) in the US-ILIHB group during the 24-h monitoring (Fig. 7).

Discussion

The primary objective of our research was to demonstrate that targeted ultrasound-guided ILIHB in young children after conventional inguinal surgery, provides better analgesia than surgical infiltration, as this research question has not been answered as to date. In fact, Reid et al. were amongst the first to conducted a study on 49 children in 1987, comparing (1) ILIHB performed using the landmark technique with (2) surgical infiltration, resulting in no significant difference in analgesic effects between both groups [18]. As the block technique was less efficient, since it used anatomical landmarks, it has now been largely replaced by more effective ultrasound technology. Moreover, the number of subjects enrolled in Reid at al.' s study may have been too low to detect

unambiguous differences. Thus, in 1992, Spittal et al. carried out another investigation comparing ILIHB, performed in landmark technique, to surgical infiltration, with a sample of 50 participants. However, this study did not demonstrate any difference either. In 2013, Sahin et al. examined the effectiveness of another abdominal wall block, namely the transverse abdominis plane (TAP) block, that ultimately, achieved a better outcome than the surgical block technique with regards to demonstrate that targeted and ultrasound-guided nerve block achieves better outcomes than a surgical block with regards to (1) time until the first pain medication administration and (2) amount of analgesia used [15]. As Sahin et al.'s results are promising, we decided to investigate the commonly performed ultrasound-guided ilioinguinal-iliohypogastric block. As the ILIHB better targets the anatomical area for inguinal surgical interventions, it has been shown to be more precise, allows for better analgesia, and lower doses of local anaesthetics than the ultrasound-guided TAP method [23, 24]. Our study design enabled us to demonstrate, for the first

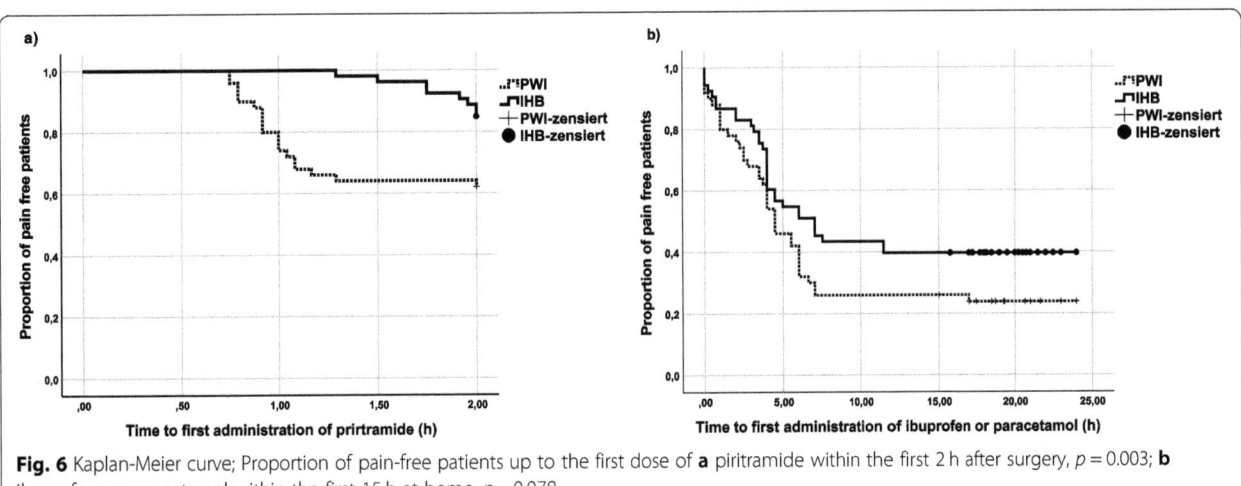

Fig. 6 Kaplan-Meier curve; Proportion of pain-free patients up to the first dose of **a** piritramide within the first 2 h after surgery, $p = 0.003$; **b** ibuprofen or paracetamol within the first 15 h at home, $p = 0.078$

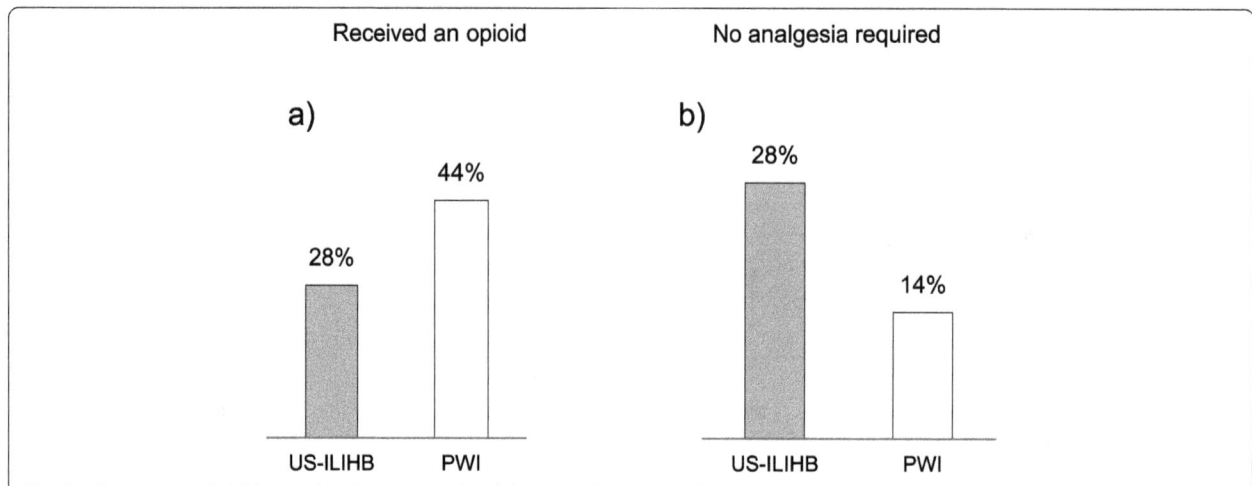

Fig. 7 a Percentage of children within their group who did not need analgesics; **b** Percentage of children within their group who received an opioid (piritramide). Grey: children in the US-ILIHB group, white: Children in the PWI group

time, this effect of ultrasound-guided TAP using the example of ultrasound-guided ILIHB. Contrary to the study by Sahin et al., we used a low, uniform dose of 0.2 ml/kg instead of 0.2 and 0.5 ml/kg for both groups in order to more accurately demonstrate the difference in effect between both groups, as overdoses or different dosages between groups can result in possible cofounders.

After many contradictory study findings, the present study provides significant evidence that the relative frequency of pain events is approximately 50% lower in the first 24 h after surgery (12.6% versus 20.4%) when applying US-ILIHB block prior to inguinal interventions in children. In the US-ILIHB group, only every eighth child (6.7 out of 53 children) showed signs of pain, however when surgical infiltration was used, it was every fifth child (10.2 out of 50 children).

We also were able to demonstrate that the frequency of pain events increased the longer the period after block. (Fig. 5b). Thus, as the occurrence of pain in the hospital setting during the first 3 hours was assessed to have been 10%, this was most likely caused by a still intact block. In line with findings, pain increased three times over the next 16 h, as the effect of the block was decreasing.

We also demonstrated that children who received US-ILIHB were longer pain-free, 21 min on average, than children with surgical infiltration, as measured by the time spent until the first opioid administration. Although not statistically significant, the same trend was seen in the time to first administration of peripheral analgesics administered by parents (ibuprofen, paracetamol): In fact, children having received ultrasound block intervention requested an analgesic on average of 3 h later in comparison to their PWI counterparts.

With regards to the consumption of analgesics, the overall volume of consumed opioid analgesics (piritramide) was lower, and they were consumed less frequently following ultrasound block. While these were only minor differences without significance, in context this effect can be interpreted as a trend due to the fact it is also reflected significantly for co-analgesics like clonidine (frequency of clonidine: $p = 0.048$, total clonidine in µg: $p = 0.049$) (Tab. 1, lower part). In general, nearly 50% more children in the PWI group (22/44%) received an opioid in PACU than in the US-ILIHB group (15/28%) (Fig. 7b). However, during 24-h monitoring, no analgesics was given to 7 children (14%) in the PWI group, about half as many as in the US-ILIHB group (15 children, or 30%) (Fig. 7a). Even though differences between the analgesia usage were observed, our study was not set up statistically to answer the question regarding which analgesia was better in terms of quality or intensity, as measured in postoperative pain scores. One reason for this is the high number of pain-free children and this insufficient differentiation of pain scores between the groups. For example, 80% of pain measurements yielded zero in both groups. However, in terms of the quantity and application of analgesics, the cumulation of our results, clearly indicate that the use of US-ILIHB prior to inguinal surgery in young children reduces pain and, consequently, ensures prolonged postoperative freedom from pain with fewer analgesia usages than the surgical PWI at the end of the surgery. Thus, in accordance with almost all investigational criteria, US-ILIHB appears to be significantly superior to PWI, or appears to show a clear trend in that direction.

One reason for our findings is the slow release of anaesthetics, as the preoperative ultrasound-guided application of local anaesthetic in-between fascia of the oblique abdominal wall muscles results in the formation of a deposit. This deposit is then slowly absorbed, thus generating a long-lasting effect (Fig. 1b). Another explanation for US-ILIHB's superiority over PWI in analgesia properties, is the fact that a surgical injection of analgesia performed before wound closure may be absorbed faster, or may seep through gaps in the fascial suture, resulting in a decreased effectiveness (Fig. 2b). This would also explain the shortened interval until the first administration of analgesics, and the more frequent need for analgesics.

Even though the study's findings are promising, there are several limitations to address. Firstly, the investigated techniques were not performed by a single person but by several people. However, despite the fact that the group of investigators consisted of a fixed number of specialists within each of departments, all of which have high levels of experience with regional anaesthesia in children, the methods employed were implemented according to a well-established SOP. Therefore, this bias presumably has little effect, given the large number of patients included. Secondly, pain assessments were carried out by nursing staff in the hospital, and by parents at home. Both groups were provided with precise instructions on how to use the same pain scale prior to data collection. The KUSS pain scale is a commonly used and approved scale for the assessment of pain in neonates and small children, however it might still permits a degree of objectivity. Lastly, the temporal offset between applications of local anaesthetics (preoperativ US-ILIHB; postoperativ PWI) could influence pain assessment due to the different residence times of local anaesthetics. However, a clear difference between preoperative or postoperative block in terms of the reduction of pain has not been demonstrated so far [25, 26]. This probably means that this effect is negligible.

Conclusions

Both methods, ILIHB and PWI, have proven to be effective, with the evidence for better analgesia by one or the other method being thin and ambiguous. Taking into consideration all results presented here, this study demonstrates that the use of pre-operative ultrasound-guided ILIHB could be an improved analgesia method in children (< 4 years old) subjects undergoing open inguinal surgery.

Abbreviations
ASA: American society of anesthesiologists classification; ILIHB: Ilioinguinal-iliohypogastric block; KUSS: Pediatric scale of discomfort and pain; OSW: Outpatient surgery ward; PACU: Post anesthesia care unit; PWI: Surgical perifocal wound infiltration; rel.freq.: Relative frequency of occurence of pain; SOP: Standardized operation procedure; TAP: Transverse abdominis plane block; US-ILIHB: Ultrasound guided ilioinguinal-iliohypogastric block

Acknowledgements
Not applicable in this section.

Authors' contributions
B.G. and S.E. conceived of the presented idea, they designed the study and planned the experiments. H.P. performed the computations and verified the analytical methods. S.E. and K.R. aided in interpreting the results. B.G. wrote the manuscript with support from D.V. and with input from all authors. M.S-N. contributed to the final version of the manuscript. K.R. supervised the project. All authors discussed the results and contributed to the final manuscript. The authors read and approved the final manuscript.

Author details
[1]Department of Pediatric Anesthesiology, Altona Children's Hospital, Bleickenallee 38, 22763 Hamburg, Germany. [2]Center of Experimental Medicine, Institute of Medical Biometry and Epidemiology, University Hospital Hamburg-Eppendorf, Hamburg, Germany. [3]Department of Pediatric Surgery, University Hospital Hamburg-Eppendorf, Hamburg, Germany.

References
1. Groenewald CB, Rabbitts JA, Schroeder DR, Harrison TE. Prevalence of moderate-severe pain in hospitalized children. Paediatr Anaesth. 2012;22(7): 661–8.
2. Rony RY, Fortier MA, Chorney JM, Perret D, Kain ZN. Parental postoperative pain management: attitudes, assessment, and management. Pediatrics. 2010;125(6):e1372–8.
3. Zernikow B, Hechler T. Pain therapy in children and adolescents. Dtsch Arztebl Int. 2008;105(28–29):511–21 quiz 521-512.
4. Gunes Y, Gunduz M, Unlugenc H, Ozalevli M, Ozcengiz D. Comparison of caudal vs intravenous tramadol administered either preoperatively or postoperatively for pain relief in boys. Paediatr Anaesth. 2004;14(4):324–8.
5. Khalil SN, Hanna E, Farag A, Govindaraj R, Vije H, Kee S, Chuang AZ. Presurgical caudal block attenuates stress response in children. Middle East J Anaesthesiol. 2005;18(2):391–400.
6. Michaloliakou C, Chung F, Sharma S. Preoperative multimodal analgesia facilitates recovery after ambulatory laparoscopic cholecystectomy. Anesth Analg. 1996;82(1):44–51.
7. Eriksson H, Tenhunen A, Korttila K. Balanced analgesia improves recovery and outcome after outpatient tubal ligation. Acta Anaesthesiol Scand. 1996; 40(2):151–5.
8. Polaner DM, Taenzer AH, Walker BJ, Bosenberg A, Krane EJ, Suresh S, Wolf C, Martin LD. Pediatric regional anesthesia network (PRAN): a multi-institutional study of the use and incidence of complications of pediatric regional anesthesia. Anesth Analg. 2012;115(6):1353–64.
9. Hea L. S3-Leitlinie "Behandlung akuter perioperativer und posttraumatischer Schmerzen". In: Deutsche Interdisziplinäre Vereinigung für Schmerztherapie; 2007.
10. Guay J, Suresh S, Kopp S. The use of ultrasound guidance for perioperative neuraxial and peripheral nerve blocks in children. Cochrane Database Syst Rev. 2019;2:CD011436.
11. Lam DK, Corry GN, Tsui BC. Evidence for the Use of Ultrasound Imaging in Pediatric Regional Anesthesia: a systematic review. Reg Anesth Pain Med. 2016;41(2):229–41. https://doi.org/10.1097/AAP.0000000000000208. PMID: 25675289.
12. Willschke H, Marhofer P, Bosenberg A, Johnston S, Wanzel O, Cox SG, Sitzwohl C, Kapral S. Ultrasonography for ilioinguinal/iliohypogastric nerve blocks in children. Br J Anaesth. 2005;95(2):226–30.
13. Aveline C, Le Hetet H, Le Roux A, Vautier P, Cognet F, Vinet E, Tison C, Bonnet F. Comparison between ultrasound-guided transversus abdominis plane and conventional ilioinguinal/iliohypogastric nerve blocks for day-case open inguinal hernia repair. Br J Anaesth. 2011;106(3):380–6.
14. Lorenzo AJ, Lynch J, Matava C, El-Beheiry H, Hayes J. Ultrasound guided transversus abdominis plane vs surgeon administered intraoperative regional field infiltration with bupivacaine for early postoperative pain control in children undergoing open pyeloplasty. J Urol. 2014;192(1):207–13.
15. Sahin L, Sahin M, Gul R, Saricicek V, Isikay N. Ultrasound-guided transversus abdominis plane block in children: a randomised comparison with wound infiltration. Eur J Anaesthesiol. 2013;30(7):409–14.
16. Trainor D, Moeschler S, Pingree M, Hoelzer B, Wang Z, Mauck W, Qu W. Landmark-based versus ultrasound-guided ilioinguinal/iliohypogastric nerve blocks in the treatment of chronic postherniorrhaphy groin pain: a retrospective study. J Pain Res. 2015;8:767–70.

17. Spittal MJ, Hunter SJ. A comparison of bupivacaine instillation and inguinal field block for control of pain after herniorrhaphy. Ann R Coll Surg Engl. 1992;74(2):85–8.

18. Reid MF, Harris R, Phillips PD, Barker I, Pereira NH, Bennett NR. Day-case herniotomy in children. A comparison of Ilio-inguinal nerve block and wound infiltration for postoperative analgesia. Anaesthesia. 1987;42(6):658–61.

19. Benz-Worner J, Johr M. Regional anaesthesia in children--caudal anaesthesia and trunk blocks. Anasthesiol Intensivmed Notfallmed Schmerzther. 2013; 48(4):272–7.

20. DNQP DNfQidP. Expertenstandard Schmerzmanagement in der Pflege. Schriftenreihe des Deutschen Netzwerks für Qualitätsentwicklung in der Pflege. 2004.

21. Johnston CC, Stevens BJ, Yang F, Horton L. Differential response to pain by very premature neonates. Pain. 1995;61(3):471–9.

22. Buttner W, Finke W, Hilleke M, Reckert S, Vsianska L, Brambrink A. Development of an observational scale for assessment of postoperative pain in infants. Anasthesiol Intensivmed Notfallmed Schmerzther. 1998;33(6): 353–61.

23. Fredrickson MJ, Paine C, Hamill J. Improved analgesia with the ilioinguinal block compared to the transversus abdominis plane block after pediatric inguinal surgery: a prospective randomized trial. Paediatr Anaesth. 2010; 20(11):1022–7.

24. Faiz SHR, Nader ND, Niknejadi S, Davari-Farid S, Hobika GG, Rahimzadeh P. A clinical trial comparing ultrasound-guided ilioinguinal/iliohypogastric nerve block to transversus abdominis plane block for analgesia following open inguinal hernia repair. J Pain Res. 2019;12:201–7.

25. Dahl V, Raeder JC, Erno PE, Kovdal A. Pre-emptive effect of pre-incisional versus post-incisional infiltration of local anaesthesia on children undergoing hernioplasty. Acta Anaesthesiol Scand. 1996;40(7):847–51.

26. Bourget JL, Clark J, Joy N. Comparing preincisional with postincisional bupivacaine infiltration in the management of postoperative pain. Arch Surg. 1997;132(7):766–9.

11

Regional versus systemic analgesia in video-assisted thoracoscopic lobectomy

Benedikt Haager[1], Daniel Schmid[1,2], Joerg Eschbach[2], Bernward Passlick[1] and Torsten Loop[2]* (ID)

Abstract

Background: The optimal perioperative analgesic strategy in video-assisted thoracic surgery (VATS) for anatomic lung resections remains an open issue. Regional analgesic concepts as thoracic paravertebral or epidural analgesia were used as systemic opioid application. We hypothesized that regional anesthesia would provide improved analgesia compared to systemic analgesia with parenteral opioids in VATS lobectomy and would be associated with a lower incidence of pulmonary complications.

Methods: The study was approved by the local ethics committee (AZ 99/15) and registered (germanctr.de; DRKS00007529, 10th June 2015). A retrospective analysis of anesthetic and surgical records between July 2014 und February 2016 in a single university hospital with 103 who underwent VATS lobectomy. Comparison of regional anesthesia (i.e. thoracic paravertebral blockade (group TPVB) or thoracic epidural anesthesia (group TEA)) with a systemic opioid application (i.e. patient controlled analgesia (group PCA)). The primary endpoint was the postoperative pain level measured by Visual Analog Scale (VAS) at rest and during coughing during 120 h. Secondary endpoints were postoperative pulmonary complications (i.e. atelectasis, pneumonia), hemodynamic variables and postoperative nausea and vomiting (PONV).

Results: Mean VAS values in rest or during coughing were measured below 3.5 in all groups showing effective analgesic therapy throughout the observation period. The VAS values at rest were comparable between all groups, VAS level during coughing in patients with PCA was higher but comparable except after 8–16 h postoperatively (PCA vs. TEA; $p < 0.004$). There were no significant differences on secondary endpoints. Intraoperative Sufentanil consumption was significantly higher for patients without regional anesthesia ($p < 0.0001$ vs. TPVB and vs. TEA). The morphine equivalence postoperatively applicated until POD 5 was comparable in all groups (mean ± SD in mg: 32 ± 29 (TPVB), 30 ± 27 (TEA), 36 ± 30 (PCA); $p = 0.6046$).

Conclusions: Analgesia with TEA, TPVB and PCA provided a comparable and effective pain relief after VATS anatomic resection without side effects. Our results indicate that PCA for VATS lobectomy may be a sufficient alternative compared to regional analgesia.

Keywords: Minimal-invasive lung surgery, Thoracic paravertebral blockade, Thoracic epidural anesthesia, Patient controlled anesthesia

* Correspondence: torsten.loop@uniklinik-freiburg.de
[2]Department of Anesthesiology and Intensive Care Medicine, Medical Center, University of Freiburg, Hugstetter Straße 55, 79106 Freiburg, Germany

Background

Video-assisted thoracic surgery (VATS) is considered as the standard minimal invasive surgical procedure for anatomic lung resections [1]. The advantages of VATS compared with open thoracotomy include faster recovery, reduced perioperative pain intensity, and decreased postoperative morbidity [2–4]. Nevertheless, persistent pain after VATS affects the ability to cough, impairs deep breathing and lung function, resulting in cardiorespiratory complications (> 15%), delayed recovery and increased costs [2].

The optimal perioperative analgesic strategy after VATS lobectomy remains contradictory. Thoracic epidural analgesia (TEA) is commonly considered as the gold standard for pain relief after open thoracotomy and is preferred by the majority of clinicians. In times of enhanced recovery and fast track concepts after surgery thoracic paravertebral block (TPVB) is an upcoming regional anesthesia technique in thoracic anesthesia. It can be used as single injection or continuous technique. However, there are also anesthesiologists in the field of thoracic anesthesia preferring patient-controlled analgesia (PCA) instead of the regional anesthesia techniques [5–7]. Regional analgesia techniques such as TEA may be not suitable for all patients for technical reasons or anticoagulative drug therapy and may be associated with numerous risks (e.g. dural perforation, spinal cord damage by formation of hematoma, infection and abscess; hypotension; urinary retention) [8, 9]. The role of TPVB in this context has not been as clear but shown to be effective for pain relief with less hemodynamic side effects than TEA [5, 10–15]. As there is no evidence for one superior regional technique for pain relief after VATS, single-shot or continuous TPVB may be a suitable alternative to TEA or systemic opioid application. Intravenous patient-controlled analgesia with morphine analogue (PCA) is a widely used, simple, and convenient method [16].

After implementation of VATS as a standard for anatomic lung resection in our department the procedure-specific pain protocol was based on multimodal systemic analgesia with non-opioid and opioid drugs. Although less invasive, the thoracoscopic approach, resulted in unexpectedly high intensity of postoperative pain [17]. In this respect, regional analgesia (i.e. TEA or TPVB) was considered to be the crucial component of multimodal postoperative pain management in our department.

Accordingly, we wanted to analyze and undertook a retrospective analysis to establish whether thoracic regional analgesia (TPVB with ropivacaine alone or TEA) would provide improved analgesia compared with systemic analgesia with parenteral opioids and non-steroidal analgesics leading to a reduction postoperative pulmonary complications such as atelectasis, pneumonia, hypoxia or pulmonary dysfunctions.

Methods

The study was approved by the local ethics committee (AZ 99/15) and registered (germanctr.de; DRKS00007529). Inclusion criteria were age older than 18 years and anatomic lung resection via VATS approach. Exclusion criteria were conversion to open thoracotomy, non-anatomic ("wedge") lung resections and additional chest wall resections. Data were retrospectively collected between July 2014 und February 2016. Patients signed a written informed consent approving their data could be used for scientific purposes. From July 2014 until January 2015 all patients received either a TPVB or a TEA. From January 2015 the perioperative analgesia was changed by interdisciplinary institutional decision and included systemic opioid application with piritramide as patient controlled analgesia (PCA; Graseby 3300; PCA Syringe Pump; SMITHS MEDICAL INTERNATIONAL LIMITED, Watford, Hertfordshire, United Kingdom).

Anesthetic management

The perioperative anesthetic regimen is standardized. Pre-medication before arrival in the operating room was performed with midazolam (3.75–7.5 mg p.o.). The responsible consultant preoperatively decided indication and choice for TPVB or TEA. Three experienced anesthesiologists performed all TEA and TPVB following the same protocol. Patients in the group TEA received an epidural catheter, using an 18G Tuohy needle, the epidural catheter (20G) will be placed at T4/5, T5/6, or T6/7 interspace (depending on the site of surgery) using the midline approach and hanging drop technique [18]. Epidural block analgesia was induced with 10 ml of ropivacaine 0.2% and sufentanil (0.2–0.3 µg/kg, maximally 25 µg) administered as three separate injections, followed by a continuous infusion of ropivacaine 0.2% and sufentanil 0.5 µg/ml with a fixed infusion rate at 8 ml/h until 24 h after operation. The paravertebral space is located by using the technique described as previously described [13, 19]. After introduction of the catheter (3 cm into the paravertebral space), gentle aspiration, and test dose application (3 ml of ropivacaine 0.5% with adrenalin (5 µg/ml)), thoracic paravertebral blockade (TPVB) was induced with 30 ml ropivacaine 0.5% with adrenaline (5 µg/ml) followed by continuous paravertebral application of ropivacaine 0.2% (fixed infusion rate 8 ml/h). The patients with systemic analgesia received an intravenous PCA, which was started immediately postoperative with a PCA device programmed to deliver piritramide i.v. (bolus dose of 1.5 mg, with a lockout time of 5 min and restricted total dose of 40 mg/4 h). After an initial dose of 0.4–0.6 µg/kg of sufentanil, additional bolus doses of 0.1–0.2 µg/kg of sufentanil are administered as needed. Induction of anesthesia was performed by a target-controlled infusion (TCI) of with propofol (Propofol 1%

MCT & Injectomat® TIVA Agilia, Fresenius-Kabi GmbH, Bad Homburg, Germany) at plasma concentrations of 2–4 µg*ml^{-1}. The Bispectral Index of the encephalogram (BIS) was monitored (BIS® A-2000 monitor, Aspect Medical Systems, Newton, MA, USA) and the propofol concentration was decreased to 2.2 µg/ml at the lowest, if the BIS value decreases to below 30. Propofol concentration was increased to 4 µg*ml^{-1} to avoid arterial blood pressure values above 20% of baseline and BIS values above 60. Core temperature was kept above 36.0 °C using a forced-air warming system. All patients were endotracheally intubated with a double-lumen endobronchial tube for one-lung ventilation.

Surgical management

VATS lobectomy was performed using a utility incision of 5 cm length entering the 4th intercostal space regardless which lobe was resected. Two further incisions of 1–2 cm were placed in posterior and anterior axillary line at level of the diaphragm in the 7th or 8th intercostal space. At the end of the procedure a 24 Fr chest tube was placed exiting the anterior lower incision in the 7th or 8th intercostal space. Following the same protocol two thoracic surgeons performed all procedures (B.P., B.H.). Chest tubes were removed when there was no air leakage for 6 h and the pleural fluid amount for 24 h did not exceed 200 ml.

Postoperative pain management

In the author's institution surgical patients were preoperatively instructed in the use of the visual analog scale (VAS). The VAS Score consisted of an unmarked 10 cm line, with 0 cm representing no pain and 10 cm the worst imaginable pain. Postoperatively all patients received a basic analgesic therapy containing either metamizole 4 × 1 g per day or acetaminophen 3 × 1 g depending on comorbidities (i.e. renal/liver dysfunction, allergies) and oxycodone 2 × 20 mg per day directly in the intermediate care unit. When the pain intensity exceeded 3 cm a bolus of piritramide 1.5 mg was applicated and repeated until the pain level decreased below 3 (VAS) again. Patients of the PCA group were directly connected to an i.v. PCA device, delivering piritramide bolus doses of 1.5 mg with a lockout time of 5 min and a total dose of 40 mg in 4 h. Nursing staff assessed pain intensity on the intermediate care unit in intervals of 4 h until 24 h after surgery, following once a day until 5th postoperative day. Morphine equianalgesic conversion was calculated using the calculator based on the American Pain Society guideline (http://americanpainsociety.org/uploads/education/PAMI_Pain_Mangement_and_Dosing_Guide_02282017.pdf).

Postoperative non-pain management

Heart rate and arterial blood pressure were monitored continuously for the first 24 h postoperatively on the intermediate care unit and every 8 h after discharge to the ward. Hypotension was defined by mean arterial pressure below 60 mmHg. A chest x-ray was routinely performed immediately after the operation and on the day following the removal of the chest tube. Radiologic infiltrates were defined by the written result from a consultant of the department of radiology. Pneumonia was defined by either radiologic proven infiltrate with necessity of antibiotic treatment or microbiological proof of bacteria making an antibiotic treatment necessary. A blood cell count was routinely performed on POD 1, leukocytosis was observed when leucocyte count exceeded 9.800/ml. Pruritus, postoperative nausea and vomiting (PONV) and paresthesia were checked twice daily during the morning and afternoon round of the medical staff on the intensive care unit.

Outcome measures

Primary endpoint was the postoperative pain intensity assessed by the VAS in cm at different times after the procedure. VAS scores (0–10) were assessed by the nursing staff at the beginning of the shift routinely at rest and during coughing on ICU. When transferred to the ward after 24 h, pain scores were documented once daily during the morning round of the nursing staff. Secondary outcome parameters were pulmonary (i.e. atelectasis, pneumonia, pulmonary embolism and respiratory failure) and surgical complications (i.e. leukocytosis, time to chest tube removal, pleural effusion) as well as side effects of the analgesic therapy (hypotension, pruritus, paresthesia, PONV). Atelectasis was defined by radiological criteria, pneumonia as fever, radiologic infiltration, positive microbiology or leukocytosis requiring antibiotic treatment.

Statistical analyses

Data were presented as mean and standard deviation (± SD) or median and IQR if not indicated otherwise. Patient characteristic data were compared by analysis of variance (ANOVA) for multiple comparisons with Tukey post-hoc test. Comparisons of serial measurements (VAS for pain) were performed with repeated-measures ANOVA. Ranked data were analyzed with the Kruskal–Wallis and Mann–Whitney U-tests when appropriate. Categorical data were examined by Fisher's exact or Chi-square test. Probability values under 0.05 were considered significant.

Results

From July 2014 to February 2016, 103 patients who underwent VATS lobectomy for oncologic reasons were examined retrospectively and initially included. In 62 patients analgesia was performed by regional anesthesia (28 patients with TPVB and 34 with TEA). From May 2015 patients were scheduled without regional anesthesia due to change in local procedures and 41 patients underwent VATS lobectomy with systemic opioid-based analgesia (PCA). Four patients were excluded due to conversion to systemic analgesia because of postoperative catheter dislocation, inadequate data sheet or open thoracotomy. The patient's demographic data are described in Table 1.

Mean VAS score was measured below 3.5 in all groups showing effective perioperative analgesia (Figs. 1 and 2). The VAS values at rest were comparable between all groups, VAS values during coughing were also effective and comparable with except higher in patients with PCA compared to TEA after 16 h postoperatively (Fig. 2). The intraoperative dose of sufentanil was significantly higher in the PCA group (Fig. 3; $p < 0.0001$; mean dose 67 ± 4 µg for the PCA group vs. 47 ± 3 µg vs. patients with TPVB and 34 ± 2 vs. patients with TEA). The postoperative morphine equivalence dose applicated postoperatively until postoperative day 5 was comparable in all groups (Fig. 3: median (25–75%) in mg: 25 (15–51) (TPVB), 20 (11–52) (TEA), 24 (16–51) (PCA); $p = 0.60$).

Secondary endpoints showed no difference between the three groups (Table 2). Hemodynamic complications like hypotension demanding a vasopressor therapy were observed in 4 patients each with TPVB and PCA compared to 7 patients with TEA (Table 2). There was no pulmonary complication such as pulmonary embolism or respiratory failure. Pneumonia was diagnosed in 3 patients with TPVB, two patients with TEA, and 6 patients in the PCA group (Table 2). Pruritus was observed in one patient with TPVB and in 3 with TEA. No patient with PCA had pruritus (Table 2).

Discussion

This retrospective study analyzed two regional analgesic concepts (TPVB and TEA) and one systemic concept via opioid application using a PCA for postoperative analgesia in patients undergoing VATS lobectomy or VATS anatomic resections. The main findings can be summarized as follows: (i) TPVB, TEA and systemic analgesia provided effective analgesia (VAS < 4) during the perioperative period; (ii) the postoperative pain relief was comparable with similar opioid doses in all groups with the exception of 16 h postoperative while coughing favoring regional anesthesia; (iii) secondary outcome measures as respiratory or surgical complications did not differ among the three groups.

There are two major issues influencing the postoperative fast track concept in thoracic surgery demanding an optimal pain relief. First, early effective pain relief augments early mobilization with possible reduction of pulmonary complications (e.g. atelectasis, pneumonia) leading to early discharge and reduced health costs [20]. Secondly, thoracic surgery (especially thoracotomy) is associated with one of the highest incidences of chronic pain syndrome (up to 50%) [21]. There was a significantly lower incidence for VATS procedures, though still a number of patients (34%) emerge from VATS thoracic surgery suffering from chronic pain [22]. Placement of trocars and utility incision can cause intercostal nerve injury and pleural irritation as thoracotomy does, promoting pain transmission to the central nervous system leading to pain memory. Effective block of neural afferents can reduce acute postoperative pain and avoid the development of a pain consciousness [18].

For VATS resections the reports on different analgesic strategies are still very heterogeneous [7, 23, 24]. TEA is established as gold standard for thoracotomy and is

Table 1 Patient and surgical characteristics

	TPVB ($n = 25$)	TEA ($n = 31$)	PCA ($n = 41$)	Total ($n = 97$)	P value
Sex					$P < 0.04$
female	7	9	22*	38	
male	18	22	19	59	
Age (median/range) (yr)	69 (45–81)	72 (46–88)	68 (43–81)	70 (43–88)	0.865
ASA Score (n)					0.520
I	0	0	0	0	
II	4	1	9	14	
III	20	29	31	80	
IV	1	1	1	3	
Type of surgery					0.225
Lobectomy	20	24	29	73	
Segment resection	3	6	12	21	
Pneumonectomy	2	1	0	3	

TPVB Thoracic paravertebral blockade, TEA Thoracic epidural analgesia, PCA Patient controlled analgesia, ASA American Society of Anesthesiology; *p-value < 0.05

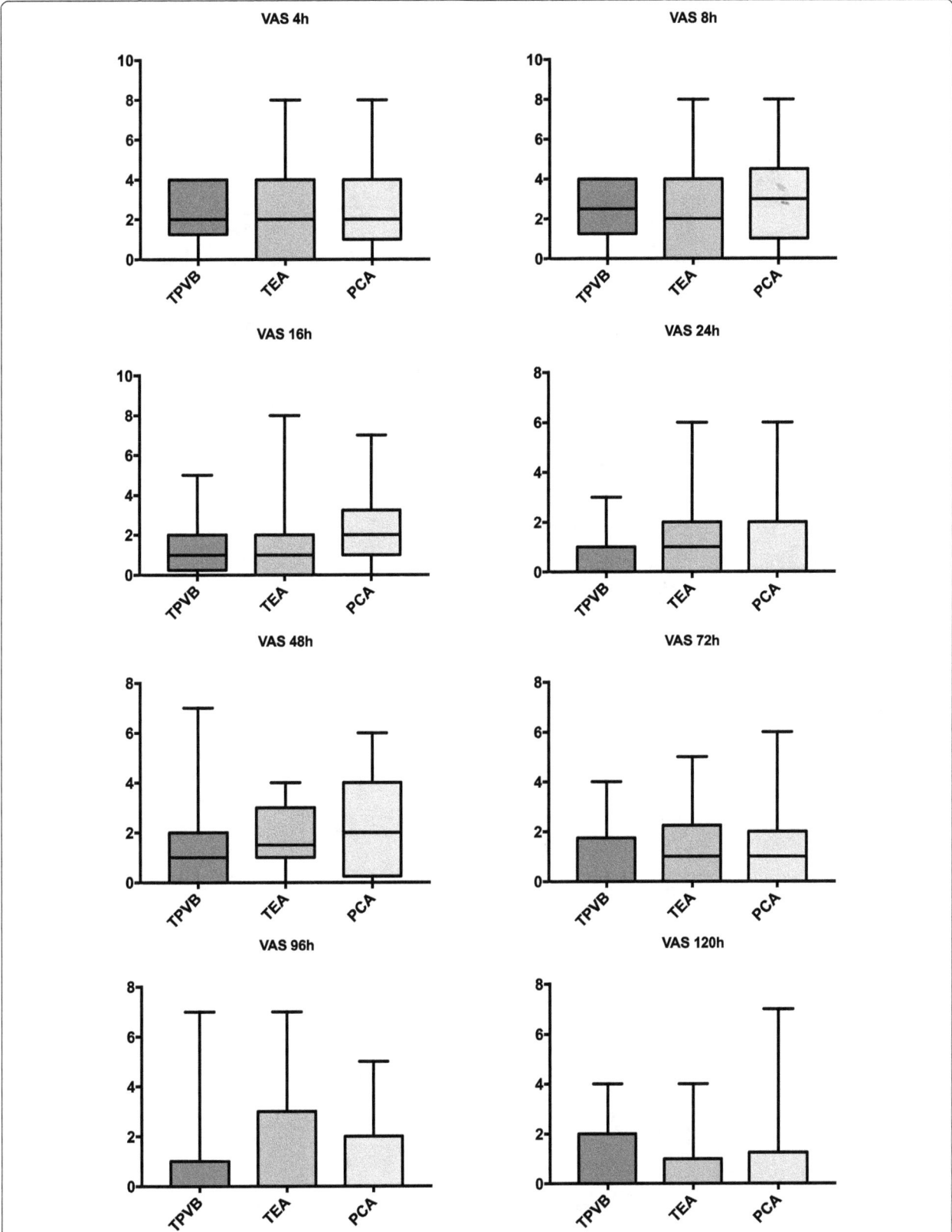

Fig. 1 VAS at rest. TEA. thoracic epidural analgesia; TPVB, thoracic paravertebral blockade; PCA, patient controlled analgesia. Boxplots show median, 25/75th, and 5/95th percentiles

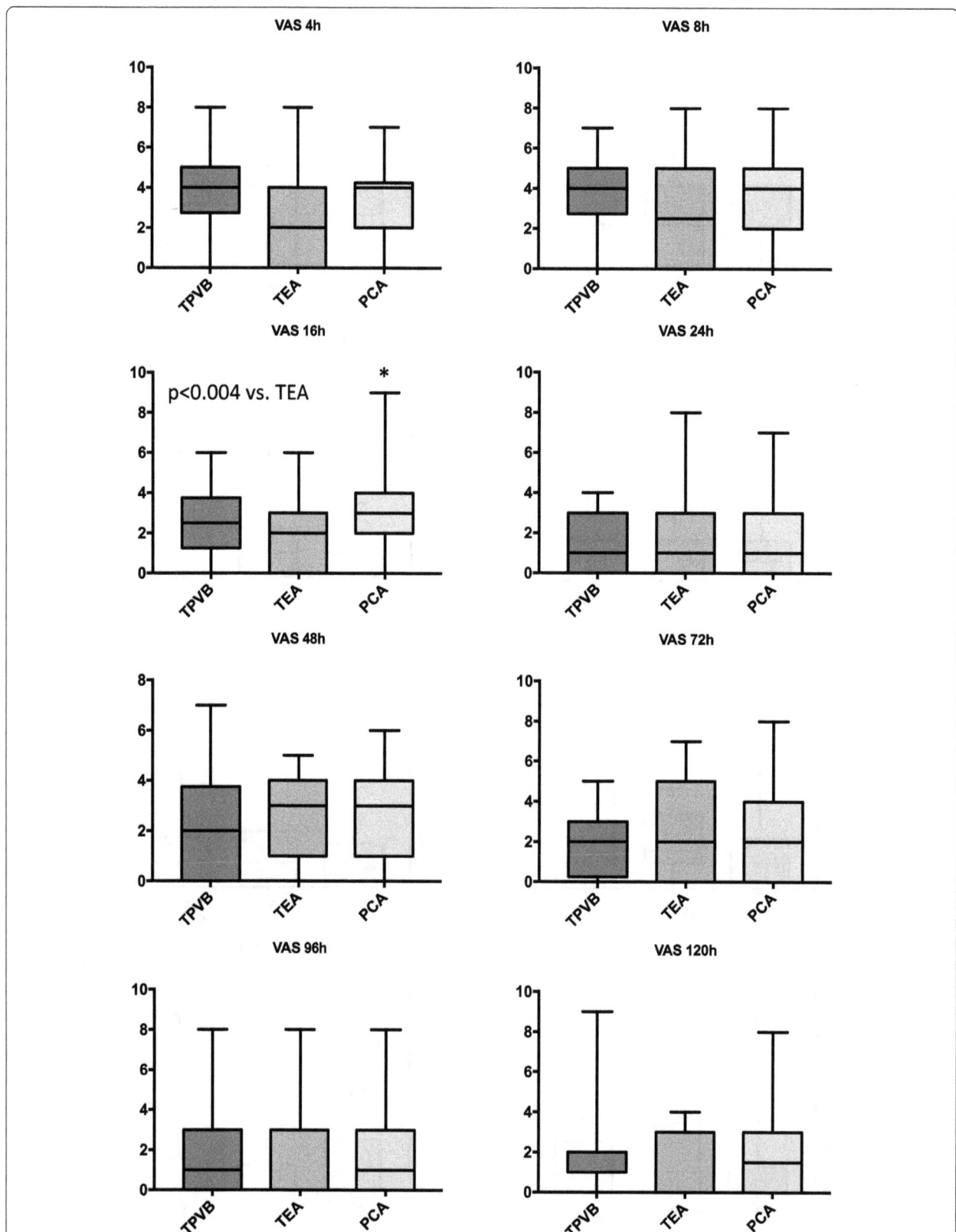

Fig. 2 VAS during coughing. TEA, thoracic epidural analgesia; TPVB, thoracic paravertebral blockade; PCA, patient controlled analgesia. Boxplots show median, 25/75th, and 5/95th percentiles. (*$p < 0.004$ vs. TEA)

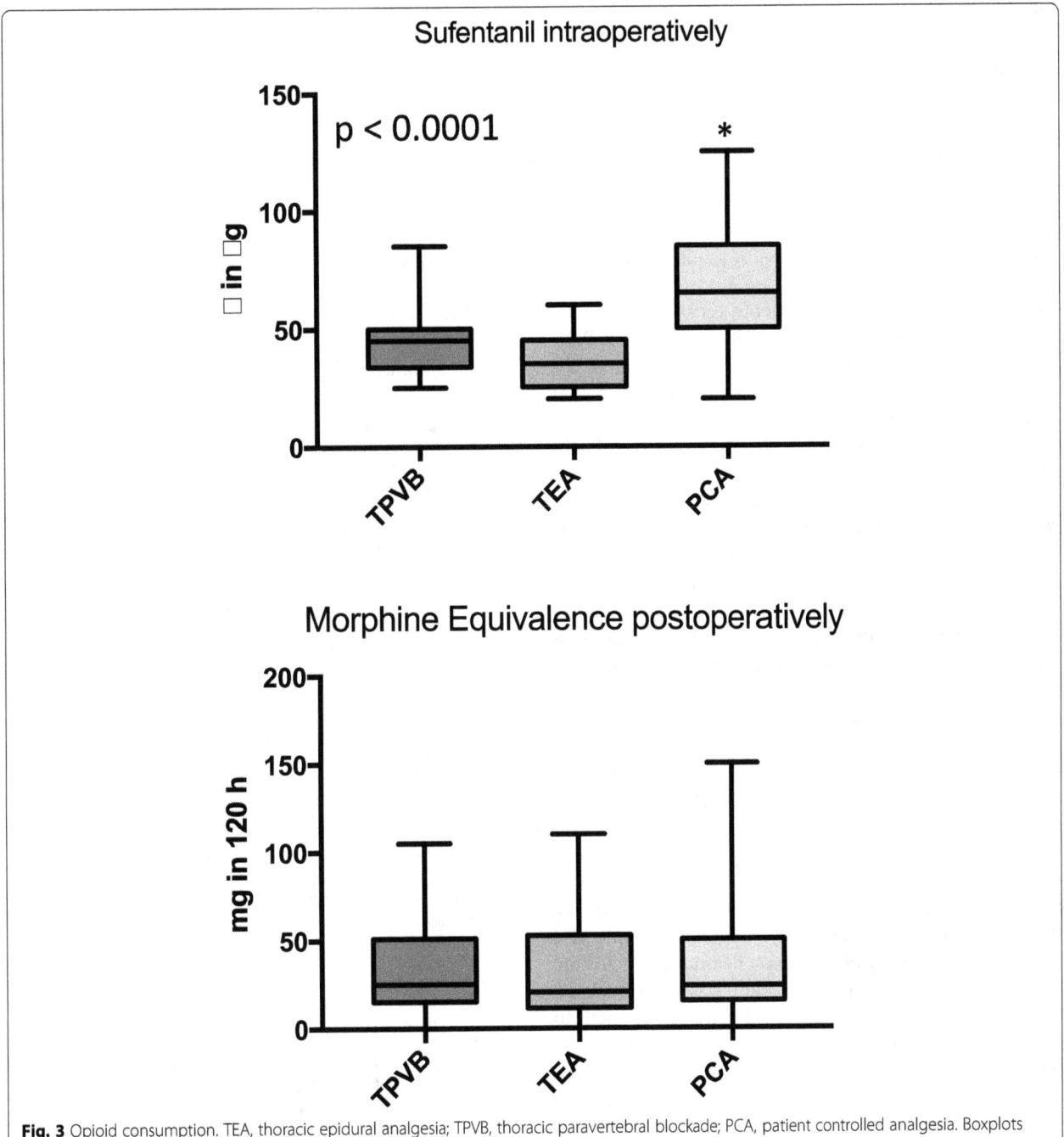

Fig. 3 Opioid consumption. TEA, thoracic epidural analgesia; TPVB, thoracic paravertebral blockade; PCA, patient controlled analgesia. Boxplots show median, 25/75th, and 5/95th percentiles. (*p < 0.0001 vs. TEA and TPVB)

widely used for anatomic VATS resections as well as intravenous delivery of opioids via PCA [25–27]. The results of meta-analyses and reviews demonstrated that TPVB with local anesthetics has a comparable efficacy and a higher safety profile [14, 28, 29]. Kosinski et al. compared continuous epidural with paravertebral analgesia in a prospective randomized study and demonstrated a favorable effect for the paravertebral block on pain scores on the POD 1 and 2. The consumption of opioids was comparable and the authors found a higher

rate of side effects for example urinary retention and hypotension in the TEA group. Beyond that the use of paravertebral block was recommended due to the better safety profile and comparable analgesic effect [30].

In this study, TEA, TPVB, and PCA provided a comparable pain relief. Two studies compared TEA with systemic opioid analgesia for thoracoscopic lobectomy. Kim et al. demonstrated in a non-blinded RCT of 37 patients that there were no differences in pain scores, supplementary analgesic requirements or adverse events [25].

Table 2 Secondary Endpoints

	TPVB (n = 25)	TEA (n = 31)	PCA (n = 41)	Total (n = 97)	P value
Hemodynamics (n)					
Hypotension	4	7	4	15	0.445
Hypertension	23	28	35	86	0.976
Pneumonia (n)	3	2	6	11	0.617
Pruritus (n)	1	3	0	4	0.149
Leucocytosis (n)	16	13	21	50	0.653

TPVB Thoracic paravertebral blockade, *TEA* Thoracic epidural analgesia, *PCA* Patient controlled analgesia

Yie et al. investigated 105 patients retrospectively and found a lower VAS in the TEA group, but only on POD 2. Incidence of dizziness was shown to be higher in the morphine group on POD 1, whereas pruritus was higher in the TEA group on POD 2 and 3 [26].

There were no differences with respect to the pain intensity between opioid PCA and TEA or TPVB. The cost implications of a regional analgesia concept, TEA or TPVB, compared with i.v. analgesia is well documented. The cost difference is mainly caused by the professional manpower costs and the treatment of complications [31].

In addition to the comparable pain relief we found no difference between the secondary outcomes (e.g. pulmonary complications, surgical complications, PONV) not supporting our hypothesis that there would be less pulmonary complications using a regional anesthetic procedure.

This study had some limitations. The trial was not a prospective, randomized, and double-blinded clinical study, but technique and expertise in TEA or TPVB was very homogeneous and performed exclusively by three consultants and reflects clinical practice. In addition, pain assessment was routinely evaluated only at the described time points. Secondly, the small sample size limited the possibility of drawing a definitive conclusion. Thirdly, the sample size of the study was not calculated due to the retrospective design and therefore to small to evaluate the secondary outcomes of respiratory function, pulmonary complications, nausea and vomiting, degree of sedation, hypotension, and pruritus. Finally, assessment of the level of analgesic effect or sensory block of the TEA and TPVB were not routinely performed.

Conclusions

In conclusion, our findings indicated that application of systemic opioids via PCA device was an effective and acceptable alternative to regional anesthesia with TEA or TPVB for postoperative pain relief for patients undergoing VATS lobectomy.

Abbreviations
ANOVA: Analysis of variance; PCA: Patient-controlled analgesia; POD: Postoperative day; PONV: Postoperative nausea and vomiting; TCI: Target-controlled infusion; TEA: Thoracic epidural analgesia; TPVB: Thoracic paravertebral block; VAS: Visual analog scale; VATS: Video-assisted thoracic surgery

Acknowledgements
Not applicable.

Authors' contributions
BH initiated and designed the study, DS designed the study database and collected the case reports, JE is responsible for the acute pain service and the corresponding documentation. BP proofread the manuscript and contributed to the study design. TL performed statistical processing, writing and drafting of the manuscript. All authors read and approved the manuscript in its final version.

Author details
¹Department of Thoracic Surgery, Medical Center, University of Freiburg, Hugstetter Straße 55, 79106 Freiburg, Germany. ²Department of Anesthesiology and Intensive Care Medicine, Medical Center, University of Freiburg, Hugstetter Straße 55, 79106 Freiburg, Germany.

References
1. Steinthorsdottir KJ, Wildgaard L, Hansen HJ, et al. Regional analgesia for video-assisted thoracic surgery: a systematic review. Eur J Cardiothorac Surg. 2014;45:959–66.
2. Falcoz PE, Puyraveau M, Thomas PA, et al. Video-assisted thoracoscopic surgery versus open lobectomy for primary non-small-cell lung cancer: a propensity-matched analysis of outcome from the European Society of Thoracic Surgeon database. Eur J Cardiothorac Surg. 2016;49:602–9.
3. Bendixen M, Jorgensen OD, Kronborg C, et al. Postoperative pain and quality of life after lobectomy via video-assisted thoracoscopic surgery or anterolateral thoracotomy for early stage lung cancer: a randomised controlled trial. Lancet Oncol. 2016;17:836–44.
4. McKenna RJ Jr, Houck W, Fuller CB. Video-assisted thoracic surgery lobectomy: experience with 1,100 cases. Ann Thorac Surg. 2006;81:421–5.
5. Joshi GP, Bonnet F, Shah R, et al. A systematic review of randomized trials evaluating regional techniques for postthoracotomy analgesia. Anesth Analg. 2008;107:1026–40.
6. Wenk M, Schug SA. Perioperative pain management after thoracotomy. Curr Opin Anaesthesiol. 2011;24:8–12.
7. Shanthanna H, Moisuik P, O'Hare T, et al. Survey of postoperative regional analgesia for thoracoscopic surgeries in Canada. J Cardiothorac Vasc Anesth. 2018;32:1750–5.
8. Popping DM, Wenk M, Van Aken HK. Neurologic complications after epidural analgesia. AINS. 2012;47:336–43.
9. Horlocker TT. Regional anaesthesia in the patient receiving antithrombotic and antiplatelet therapy. Br J Anaesth. 2011;107(Suppl 1):i96–106.
10. Messina M, Boroli F, Landoni G, et al. A comparison of epidural vs. paravertebral blockade in thoracic surgery. Minerva Anestesiol. 2009;75:616–21.
11. Thavaneswaran P, Rudkin GE, Cooter RD, et al. Brief reports: paravertebral block for anesthesia: a systematic review. Anesth Analg. 2010;110:1740–4.
12. Marret E, Bazelly B, Taylor G, et al. Paravertebral block with ropivacaine 0.5% versus systemic analgesia for pain relief after thoracotomy. Ann Thorac Surg. 2005;79:2109–13.
13. Karmakar MK. Thoracic paravertebral block. Anesthesiology. 2001;95:771–80.
14. Davies RG, Myles PS, Graham JM. A comparison of the analgesic efficacy and side-effects of paravertebral vs epidural blockade for thoracotomy--a systematic review and meta-analysis of randomized trials. Br J Anaesth. 2006;96:418–26.

15. Powell ES, Cook D, Pearce AC, et al. A prospective, multicentre, observational cohort study of analgesia and outcome after pneumonectomy. Br J Anaesth. 2011;106:364–70.

16. Hudcova J, McNicol E, Quah C, et al. Patient controlled opioid analgesia versus conventional opioid analgesia for postoperative pain. Cochrane Database Syst Rev. 2006;4:CD003348.

17. Dango S, Harris S, Offner K, et al. Combined paravertebral and intrathecal vs thoracic epidural analgesia for post-thoracotomy pain relief. Br J Anaesth. 2013;110:443–9.

18. Richardson J, Lonnqvist PA. Thoracic paravertebral block. Br J Anaesth. 1998; 81:230–8.

19. Kehlet H, Dahl JB. Anaesthesia, surgery, and challenges in postoperative recovery. Lancet. 2003;362:1921–8.

20. Gottschalk A, Ochroch EA. Clinical and demographic characteristics of patients with chronic pain after major thoracotomy. Clin J Pain. 2008;24: 708–16.

21. Shanthanna H, Aboutouk D, Poon E, et al. A retrospective study of open thoracotomies versus thoracoscopic surgeries for persistent postthoracotomy pain. J Clin Anesth. 2016;35:215–20.

22. Hutchins J, Sanchez J, Andrade R, et al. Ultrasound-guided paravertebral catheter versus intercostal blocks for postoperative pain control in video-assisted thoracoscopic surgery: a prospective randomized trial. J Cardiothorac Vasc Anesth. 2017;31:458–63.

23. Duale C, Gayraud G, Taheri H, et al. A French Nationwide survey on anesthesiologist-perceived barriers to the use of epidural and paravertebral block in thoracic surgery. J Cardiothorac Vasc Anesth. 2015;29:942–9.

24. Kim JA, Kim TH, Yang M, et al. Is intravenous patient controlled analgesia enough for pain control in patients who underwent thoracoscopy? J Korean Med Sci. 2009;24:930–5.

25. Yie JC, Yang JT, Wu CY, et al. Patient-controlled analgesia (PCA) following video-assisted thoracoscopic lobectomy: comparison of epidural PCA and intravenous PCA. Acta Anaesthesiol Taiwanica. 2012;50:92–5.

26. Yoshioka M, Mori T, Kobayashi H, et al. The efficacy of epidural analgesia after video-assisted thoracoscopic surgery: a randomized control study. Ann Thorac Cardiovasc Surg. 2006;12:313–8.

27. Baidya DK, Khanna P, Maitra S. Analgesic efficacy and safety of thoracic paravertebral and epidural analgesia for thoracic surgery: a systematic review and meta-analysis. Interact Cardiovasc Thorac Surg. 2014;18:626–35.

28. Demmy TL, Nwogu C, Solan P, et al. Chest tube-delivered bupivacaine improves pain and decreases opioid use after thoracoscopy. Ann Thoracic Surg. 2009;87:1040–6.

29. Kosinski S, Fryzlewicz E, Wilkojc M, et al. Comparison of continuous epidural block and continuous paravertebral block in postoperative analgaesia after video-assisted thoracoscopic surgery lobectomy: a randomised, non-inferiority trial. Anaesthesiol Intens Ther. 2016;48:280–7.

30. Macario A, Scibetta WC, Navarro J, et al. Analgesia for labor pain: a cost model. Anesthesiology. 2000;92:841–50.

31. Bartha E, Carlsson P, Kalman S. Evaluation of costs and effects of epidural analgesia and patient-controlled intravenous analgesia after major abdominal surgery. Br J Anaesth. 2006;96:111–7.

12

Differential rates of intravascular uptake and pain perception during lumbosacral epidural injection among adults using a 22-gauge needle versus 25-gauge needle

Robin Raju[1*] [ID], Michael Mehnert[2], David Stolzenberg[2], Jeremy Simon[2], Theodore Conliffe[2] and Jeffrey Gehret[2]

Abstract

Background: Inadvertent intravascular injection has been suggested as the most probable mechanism behind serious neurological complications during transforaminal epidural steroid injections. Authors believe a smaller gauge needle may lead to less intravascular uptake and less pain. Theoretically, there is less chance for a smaller gauge needle to encounter a blood vessel during an injection compared to a larger gauge needle. Studies have also shown smaller gauge needle to cause less pain. The aim of the study was to quantify the difference between a 22-gauge needle and 25-gauge needle during lumbosacral transforaminal epidural steroid injection in regards to intravascular uptake and pain perception.

Methods: This was a prospective single blind randomized clinical trial performed at outpatient spine practice locations of two academic institutions. One hundred sixty-two consecutive patients undergoing lumbosacral transforaminal epidural injections from February 2018 to June 2019 were recruited and randomized to each arm of the study – 84 patients were randomized to the 22-gauge needle arm and 78 patients to 25-gauge arm. Each transforaminal injection level was considered a separate incidence, hence total number of incidence was 249 (136 in 22-gauge arm and 113 in 25-gauge arm). The primary outcome measure was intravascular uptake during live fluoroscopy and/or blood aspiration. The secondary outcome measure was patient reported pain during the procedure on the numerical rating scale.

Results: Fisher exact test was used to detect differences between 2 groups in regards to intravascular uptake and paired t-tests were used to detect differences in pain scores. The incidence of intravascular uptake for a 22-gauge needle was 5.9% (95% confidence interval: 1.9 to 9.8%) and for a 25-gauge needle, 7.1% (95% confidence interval: 2.4 to 11.8%) [$p = 0.701$]. Average numerical rating scale scores during the initial needle entry for 22-gauge and 25-gauge needle was 3.46 (95% confidence interval: 2.94 to 3.98) and 3.13 (95% confidence interval: 2.57 to 3.69) respectively [$p = 0.375$].

Conclusions: The study showed no statistically significant difference in intravascular uptake or pain perception between a 22-gauge needle and 25-gauge needle during lumbosacral transforaminal epidural steroid injections.

Keywords: Intravascular uptake, Epidural, Transforaminal, Needle gauge, Fluoroscopy, Pain perception

* Correspondence: robin.raju@yale.edu
[1]Department of Orthopedics and Rehabilitation, Yale New Haven Hospital/
Yale University, 1 Long Wharf Drive, New Haven, CT 06511, USA

Background

Over 40 million epidural injections are administered every year in the United States as per data obtained from Centers for Medicare & Medicaid Services [1]. Although generally considered a safe procedure, epidural steroid injections are not exempt from serious complications. There are three approaches to performing epidural injections – interlaminar approach, transforaminal approach and caudal approach. Transforaminal epidural steroid injections (TFESI) offer the advantage of placing steroids into ventral epidural space directly over the painful spinal nerve in patients with low back pain and/or leg pain. Hence many practitioners prefer this technique over interlaminar or caudal approach, although there is no definitive evidence to suggest one is superior to the other. Serious but rare complications have been reported with TFESI including spinal cord infarction, epidural hematoma, paralysis, and even death. Proposed mechanisms of action behind these devastating outcomes are arterial dissections/vasospasms, inadvertent intravascular injections or embolization of particulate corticosteroids [2–5].

Inadvertent intravascular injection has been suggested as the most probable mechanism behind serious neurological complications during TFESI [4–6]. The incidence of inadvertent intravascular injection during TFESI has been estimated to be 6–26% depending on the level of the injection [7–12]. A review of current literature reveals several studies evaluating factors involved in intravascular uptake during TFESI such as needle type, level of injection, injection approach, underlying comorbidities and so on. Among all these factors, needle type has been studied the most. Different bevel types do not appear to be a substantial factor in intravascular uptake during TFESI [13–17]. Although not conclusive, blunt type needles have shown a trend towards decreased intravascular uptake in few studies [14, 16]. In regards to level of injection, increased vascularity has been reported at the sacral foramen and at other spinal foramen (especially cervical, thoracic and higher lumbar levels) which can lead to increased intravascular uptake [11, 18, 19]. The artery of Adamkewicz, a major radicular artery often implicated in spinal cord infarction during TFESI, has been reported in anatomical studies to be found not only at higher lumbar levels but also at lower lumbar levels [20–22]. Several lumbosacral transforaminal epidural approaches targeting different parts of neuroforamen have been studied and no single approach has shown to be superior to the others in reducing intravascular uptake [17, 23, 24].

Although several needle types have been studied in the past, needle gauge has never been assessed with respect to intravascular uptake. It can be beneficial to know whether needle size plays a factor in intravascular uptake during TFESI. This study aims to look at two needle sizes – 22-gauge and 25-gauge needle. It can be hypothesized that 25-gauge needle due to its smaller diameter can potentially lead to less intravascular uptake. Theoretically, when taken into account the surface area covered by a needle while it traverses through tissue planes, there is less chance for a smaller diameter needle to encounter/puncture a blood vessel during an injection compared to a larger diameter needle. Studies have also shown smaller diameter needle to cause less pain [25]. Authors hypothesize that the smaller 25-gauge needle can be less painful for patients, hence making the procedure more tolerable. On the other hand, most practitioners tend to prefer 22-gauge needle for TFESI as it is easier to steer through tissue planes.

There are multiple ways to assess intravascular uptake during TFESI. Traditionally, blood aspiration, local anesthetic test dose and/or live fluoroscopy have been used to detect intravascular uptake during spinal procedures, but none of these methods have shown to be particularly sensitive. Digital subtraction angiography (DSA) has gained traction over the last decade and it has shown to be much more sensitive than other methods in detecting intravascular uptake [7, 26–28]. Although very sensitive, DSA has not been routinely used on lumbosacral TFESI due to the cost and increased radiation exposure to providers (and to patients) associated with its use.

Methods

Institutional Review Board approval was obtained prior to the initiation of this study. There was no funding source involved in this study. Data is presented in accordance with the Consolidated Standards of Reporting Trials (CONSORT) statement and is available as Supplement. All patients provided written informed consent before participation in the study. Consecutive patients at two academic institutions from February 2018 to June 2019 were enrolled in the study. Injections were performed by five fellowship-trained interventional pain physicians. All injections were administered with Quincke needles (sharp bevel) and performed in outpatient fluoroscopy suites. Authors chose sharp bevel needle as it is the most commonly used needle in transforaminal epidural injections. 25-gauge blunt or short bevel needle is hard to steer through tissue planes lending itself limited clinical utility in transforaminal epidural injections.

Inclusion criteria included 1) patients with low back pain and/or radicular pain, 2) patients scheduled for lumbosacral TFESI. Exclusion criteria included 1) patients with contrast/local anesthetic allergy, 2) patients with pregnancy, coagulopathy, systemic infection, and inability to provide informed consent, 3) vulnerable patient population including prisoners, 4) patients with severe anxiety, 5) patients with prior lumbar surgery, 6) age < 18 years old, and 7) Body Mass Index (BMI) > 40.

One hundred sixty-two consecutive patients were recruited and randomized to each arm of the study – 22-gauge vs 25-gauge (randomization was done separately for each provider based on a computer generated algorithm). Eighty-four patients were randomized to 22-gauge arm and 78 patients to 25-gauge arm (Fig. 1). Initial goal was to recruit around 250 patients, but due to logistical reasons and difficulty in recruitment, study was terminated early after enrolling 162 patients.

All injections were administered by Physical Medicine and Rehabilitation (physiatry) specialists who had completed a fellowship in interventional spine procedures and had at least 1 year of experience in interventional spine care. All practitioners used a similar approach for lumbosacral TFESI – subpedicular/supraneural approach. The target for L1-L5 TFESI was at the superior and posterior aspect (six o'clock position of the pedicle in the AP projection) of the lumbar neuroforamen. The target for S1 TFESI was at the supero-lateral aspect of dorsal S1 foramen. Providers were allowed to switch the TFESI approach to infraneural 'Kambin's' triangle or interlaminar/caudal approach if the planned injection could not be administered with the initial approach.

The primary outcome measure was intravascular uptake during live fluoroscopy and/or blood aspiration. DSA was not available at all study locations and was therefore not utilized. The secondary outcome measure was patient reported pain during the procedure from 1 to 10 on the numerical rating scale (NRS).

After obtaining informed consent, patients were asked to record pre-procedure pain level on the NRS. Study coordinator explained the study design to the patients and specifically asked patients to pay attention to pain scores during 2 occasions – first one, during the initial needle entry after they feel the burn of the numbing agent and the second, during the administration of the steroids towards the end of the procedure. Interventionalists would also remind the patients to assess their pain during these 2 phases of the procedure. Patients were then brought to the fluoroscopy suite and placed in prone position on the fluoroscopy table. A procedural time-out was then conducted as per facility guidelines. The patients were prepped and draped in a standard sterile fashion in the prone position and the C-arm was positioned so that an oblique view of the neuroforamen was visualized and target marked. The soft tissues overlying this structure were infiltrated with 1–5 mL of 1% lidocaine (10 mg/mL) without epinephrine using a 27-gauge 1.5 in. needle. Lidocaine was injected at the skin (without creating a significant skin wheel) and through the subcutaneous tissue to 1 to 1.5 in. depth (maximum of 2 passes through the subcutaneous tissue). Then, a 22-gauge or 25-gauge (as per randomization) Quincke needle was inserted toward the target using an ipsilateral oblique trajectory view. Patients were blinded to the gauge of the needle. The needle was advanced under an oblique, AP and lateral visualization, to confirm correct needle tip placement. Aspiration was confirmed to be negative for cerebrospinal fluid and/or blood. Then a 1–2 mL volume of contrast dye (Omnipaque-240/Iohexol 240 mg/mL) was injected under live fluoroscopy to look

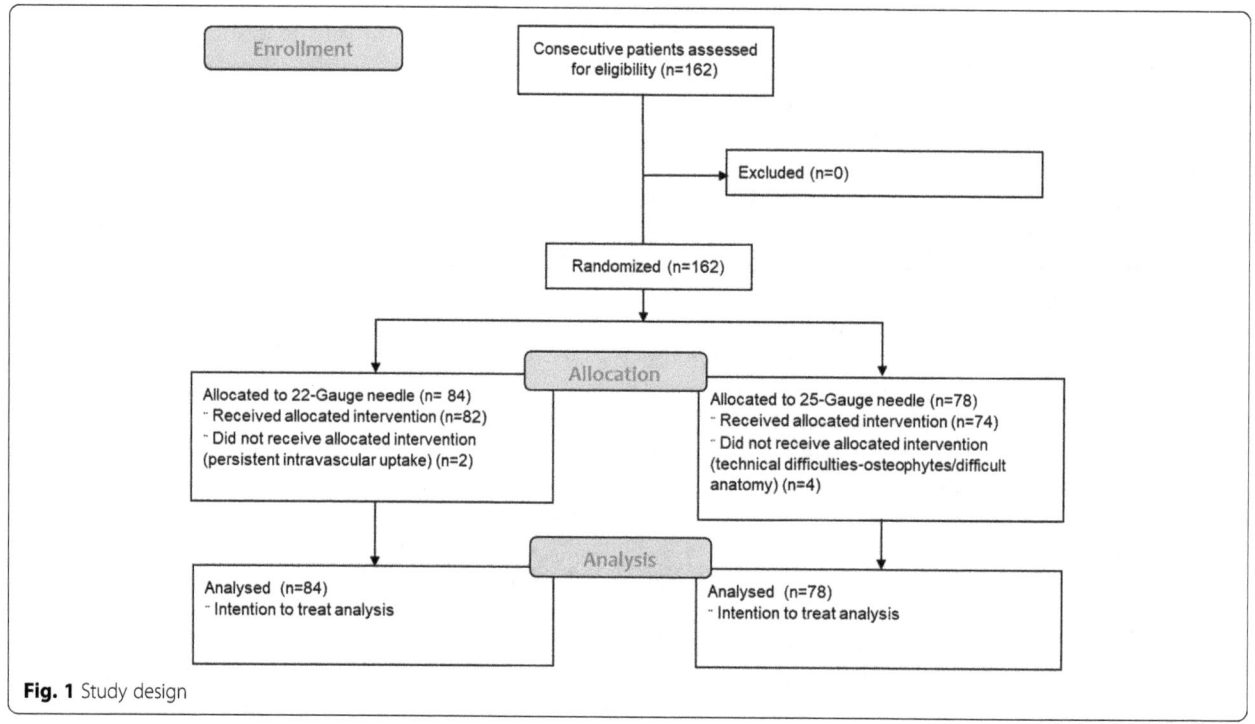

Fig. 1 Study design

for intravascular uptake. Needle tip was repositioned until an epidural only contrast pattern was observed prior to injecting the steroid. After obtaining satisfactory contrast flow pattern and negative blood aspiration, the injectate (3 mL of injectate per level - mixture of 1–2 mL of dexamethasone 10 mg/mL, 1-2 mL of 1% lidocaine and/or 1-2 mL of normal saline) was administered at each level along the nerve root and into the epidural space very slowly based on patient tolerance. Patients were reminded by interventionalists to assess their pain during this time. For the purposes of this study, only the initial contrast pattern was utilized. If an epidural only contrast flow was not obtained or persistent intravascular uptake was noted despite multiple needle redirections, the procedure was either abandoned or another approach was utilized (infraneural vs caudal vs interlaminar approach) as per patient and provider discretion. Live fluoroscopy and blood aspiration were utilized to confirm intravascular uptake at every injection level. Intravascular injection noted by either method was reported as 'present' for each level. Digital subtraction angiography or lidocaine test dose method was not used to confirm intravascular spread. At the conclusion of the procedure, all needle(s) were re-styletted, withdrawn and sterile dressings were placed. Patients were then brought to the recovery area and study coordinator or nurse (who had no knowledge of needle allocation) presented patients with written post-procedural questionnaire (paper form). Patients were specifically asked to rate the pain during the initial needle entry and also during the administration of injectate (steroid mixture). Overall tolerability of the procedure was also measured on an ordinal scale ('well tolerated' at 1 and 'poorly tolerated' at 4).

Statistical analysis
Each needle entry at any given lumbosacral level was considered a separate incidence. For instance, a bilateral L5 TFESI was considered 2 separate incidences. Fisher exact test was used to detect differences between 2 groups in regards to intravascular uptake and paired t-tests were used to detect differences in pain scores. Both primary and secondary outcome measures were analyzed based on intent-to-treat principle.

Results
A total of 249 TFESI injections were completed on 162 subjects. No serious complications were reported in any patients. Baseline demographics for both study groups are listed in Table 1.

Eighty-seven patients received 2 level injections and the remaining 75 patients received 1 level injections. Each level was considered a separate incidence, hence total number of incidence was 249. Patients enrolled had TFESI at L2 to S1 levels. The most common level of injection was L5 neuroforamen for both groups. In four

patients, the target could not be obtained (all in 25-gauge arm) due to technical difficulties (osteophytes/difficult anatomy) hence reassigned to 22-gauge needle arm and was completed successfully. Two other patients in 22-gauge group (both at S1 neuroforamen) were reassigned to interlaminar or caudal approach due to persistent intravascular uptake. All other patients had successful completion of the injection according to their assignments.

The overall incidence of intravascular uptake for both the 22-gauge and 25-gauge group was 6.4% (16 out of 249) in this study. The incidence of intravascular uptake for 22-gauge group was 5.9% (8 out of 136, 95% confidence interval: 1.9 to 9.8%). The incidence of intravascular uptake for 25-gauge group was 7.1% (8 out of 113, 95% confidence interval: 2.4 to 11.8%). There was no statistically significant difference between both groups in regards to intravascular uptake ($p = 0.701$, Fig. 2).

Further analysis of intravascular uptake between different levels yielded no statistically significant differences (Table 2). There was a trend towards increased intravascular uptake incidence at S1 level among both groups, but was not statistically significant (p value = 0.767, Table 2).

Pain scores (NRS) for 22-gauge and 25-gauge groups are listed in Table 3. There was no statistically significant difference in pain scores (during initial needle entry and administration of injectate) between both groups (Table 3). Injection tolerability was also measured (well tolerated =1, poorly tolerated = 4) and average score for 22-gauge group and 25-gauge group was 1.24 and 1.23 respectively ($p = 1.000$). Again, both groups showed no statistically significant difference in overall tolerability.

Discussion
The results of this study showed no statistically significant difference between the use of a 22-gauge and 25-gauge needle in regards to intravascular uptake or pain scores. One would expect the smaller gauge needle to reduce incidence of intravascular uptake but this study did not demonstrate any benefit in using a smaller bore 25-gauge needle as opposed to a larger bore 22-gauge needle. On the contrary, there seemed to be some disadvantage in using the 25-gauge needle as it can be hard to

Table 1 Patient baseline demographic data

	22-gauge (n = 84)	25-gauge (n = 78)	p-value
Age (years)	60.0	57.7	0.322
Sex (M:F)	M-45%; F-55%	M-52%; F-48%	0.543
Diagnosis			
-Radiculopathy	73.8%	80.7%	
-Spinal Stenosis	22.6%	14.1%	
-Other	3.6%	5.2%	

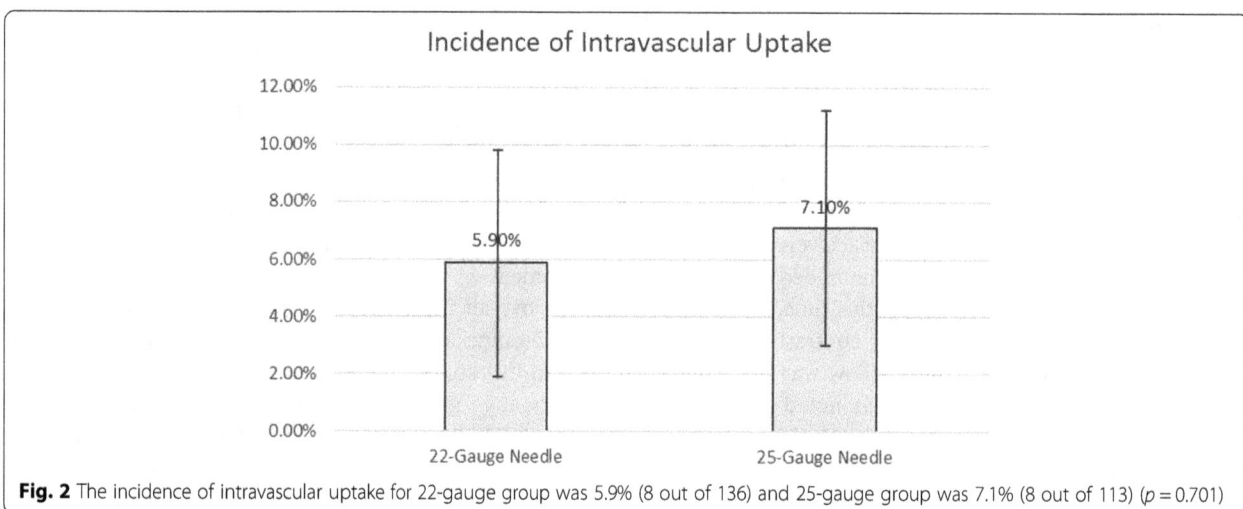

Fig. 2 The incidence of intravascular uptake for 22-gauge group was 5.9% (8 out of 136) and 25-gauge group was 7.1% (8 out of 113) ($p = 0.701$)

penetrate firm ligaments/skin and navigate around osteophytes, hence harder to steer and reach the target. Even though this study excluded patients with BMI > 40, all interventionalists found it less desirable to use 25-gauge needle as it took longer and required more fluoroscopic images to complete the procedure. In addition, it is to be noted that there were 6 cases in this study which switched assignment after randomization, and 4 of them were in 25-gauge arm (all of them due to technical challenge in obtaining the target at L4 and/or L5 levels). The other 2 assignment changes were due to persistent intravascular uptake, hence reassigned to interlaminar approach. Although not quantified in this study, 25-gauge needle can be difficult to steer through deeper tissue planes limiting its potential use in clinical practice. In this study, there was no outcome measure to gauge the difficulty level associated with completing a lumbosacral TFESI using 25-gauge needle. Authors recommend future studies looking at procedure time/exposure to further quantify this phenomenon in a more objective manner.

Although patients with lumbar surgery were excluded from the study, low thoracic and sacral surgeries can also result in increased vascularity in lumbar region due to post-surgical changes. On post-hoc analysis, none of the patients had documented low thoracic or sacral surgeries prior to enrolling in the study.

Table 2 Intravascular uptake incidence per level

Levels	22-gauge ($n = 136$)	25-gauge ($n = 113$)	p-value
L2	1/4	0/7	
L3	0/17	3/19	
L4	0/33	0/32	
L5	2/66	0/32	
S1	5/16	5/23	0.767
Overall incidence	8/136 (5.9%)	8/113 (7.1%)	0.701

The study may also suggest that a smaller gauge needle may not lead to less pain. Although the study was not well designed to detect the differences in pain perception, the results suggest no difference in pain scores or tolerability between the 2 groups. Patients were specifically asked to rate the pain during the initial needle entry and also during the administration of injectate (steroid mixture) hoping to differentiate pain experienced at various stages of the procedure, but no statistically significant differences were observed.

Limitations

Similar to prior studies on intravascular uptake, one of the limitations of this study was also the relatively small sample size. A sample size of 249 was not enough to detect small changes that may exist between the 2 groups especially given the low overall incidence of intravascular uptake during TFESI. Also true randomization at injection event level was not possible as one patient could have had multiple events. Although initial goal was to recruit around 250 patients, study was terminated early at 162 patients, hence an 'event' was changed from patients to level of injections for statistical analysis possibly implying cluster randomization.

Authors did not use digital subtraction angiography to detect intravascular uptake as it was not available at all study locations. Instead, standard live fluoroscopy and/ or vascular aspiration were used. Studies have shown DSA to increase the sensitivity of detecting intravascular uptake [7, 26–28].

Pain scores were obtained after the procedure when patients were in the recovery room which could have led to recall bias. When patients were asked to rate pain during the initial needle entry, they could in fact be assessing the needle used for local anesthetic infiltration. More accurate pain scores could have been obtained if asked during the procedure immediately after placement

Table 3 Pain scores (NRS 1–10) between 22-gauge and 25-gauge groups

Pain scores	22-gauge (95% CI[a]) n = 84	25-gauge (95% CI[a]) n = 78	p-value
Average NRS before the procedure	5.88 (5.42 to 6.34)	6.21 (5.73 to 6.69)	0.330
Average NRS during the initial needle entry	3.46 (2.94 to 3.98)	3.13 (2.57 to 3.69)	0.375
Average NRS during the administration of steroid	4.01 (3.44 to 4.58)	3.77 (3.20 to 4.34)	0.554

There was no statistically significant difference in pain scores between 22-gauge and 25-gauge needle at various stages of the procedure
[a]CI confidence interval

of the needle and administration of steroids. Although the procedure was standardized in the research protocol, there may still be differences in how the injection was performed between various interventionalists (five in this study) which can affect patients' pain perception. Sensitivity analysis (taking into consideration individual provider variability) appeared to affect pain scores but had limited impact on the rate of intravascular uptake.

Conclusions

One would expect the smaller 25-gauge needle to reduce incidence of intravascular uptake and be less painful during TFESI, but the study finds no conclusive evidence. In conclusion, the study showed no statistically significant difference in intravascular uptake or pain perception between a 22-gauge needle and 25-gauge needle during lumbosacral TFESI.

Abbreviations
TFESI: Transforaminal epidural steroid injection; BMI: Body Mass Index (BMI); DSA: Digital subtraction angiography (DSA); NRS: Numerical rating scale

Acknowledgements
The authors would like to thank Dr. Mitchell Freedman and Dr. Matthew Sherman for their help with analysis and development of the article.

Authors' contributions
RR, JS, JG, TC, MM, and DS were instrumental in design of the study, interpretation of data along with recruitment of the subjects. RR was a major contributor in writing the manuscript. All authors read, revised and approved the final manuscript.

Author details
[1]Department of Orthopedics and Rehabilitation, Yale New Haven Hospital/Yale University, 1 Long Wharf Drive, New Haven, CT 06511, USA.
[2]Department of Physical Medicine and Rehabilitation, Rothman Orthopaedic Institute/Thomas Jefferson University Hospital, 925 Chestnut Street, Philadelphia, PA 19107, USA.

References
1. Manchikanti L, Pampati V, Hirsch JA. Retrospective cohort study of usage patterns of epidural injections for spinal pain in the US fee-for-service Medicare population from 2000 to 2014. BMJ. 2016;6(12):e013042.
2. Muro K, O'Shaughnessy B, Ganju A. Infarction of the cervical spinal cord following multilevel transforaminal epidural steroid injection: case report and review of the literature. J Spinal Cord Med. 2007;30:385–8.
3. Rozin L, Rozin R, Koehler SA, et al. Death during transforaminal epidural steroid nerve root block (C7) due to perforation of the left vertebral artery. Am J Forensic Med Pathol. 2003;24:351–5.
4. Tiso RL, Cutler T, Catania JA, Whalen K. Adverse central nervous system sequelae after selective transforaminal block: the role of corticosteroids. Spine J. 2004;4:468–74.
5. Lyders EM, Morris PP. A case of spinal cord infarction following lumbar transforaminal epidural steroid injection: MR imaging and angiographic findings. AJNR Am J Neuroradiol. 2009;30:1691–3.
6. Baker R, Dreyfuss P, Mercer S, Bogduk N. Cervical transforaminal injection of corticosteroids into a radicular artery: a possible mechanism for spinal cord injury. Pain. 2003;103:211–5.
7. Lee MH, Yang KS, Kim YH, Jung HD, Lim SJ, Moon DE. Accuracy of live fluoroscopy to detect intravascular injection during lumbar transforaminal epidural injections. Korean J Pain. 2010;23(1):18–23.
8. Kranz PG, Amrhein TJ, Gray L. Incidence of inadvertent intravascular injection during CT fluoroscopy-guided epidural steroid injections. AJNR Am J Neuroradiol. 2015;36(5):1000–7.
9. Smuck M, Fuller BJ, Yoder B, Huerta J. Incidence of simultaneous epidural and vascular injection during lumbosacral transforaminal epidural injections. Spine J. 2007;7(1):79–82.
10. Furman MB, O'Brien EM, Zgleszewski TM. Incidence of intravascular penetration in transforaminal lumbosacral epidural steroid injections. Spine (Phila Pa 1976). 2000;25(20):2628–32.
11. Nahm FS, Lee CJ, Lee SH, Kim TH, Sim WS, Cho HS, Park SY, Kim YC, Lee SC. Risk of intravascular injection in transforaminal epidural injections. Anaesthesia. 2010;65(9):917–21.
12. Hong JH, Lee YH. Comparison of incidence of intravascular injections during transforaminal epidural steroid injection using different needle types. Korean J Anesthesiol. 2014;67(3):193–7.
13. Smuck M, Yu AJ, Tang CT, Zemper E. Influence of needle type on the incidence of intravascular injection during transforaminal epidural injections: a comparison of short-bevel and long-bevel needles. Spine J. 2010;10(5):367–71.
14. Ozcan U, Sahin S, Gurbet A, Turker G, Ozgur M, Celebi S. Comparison of blunt and sharp needles for transforaminal epidural steroid injections. Agri. 2012;24(2):85–9.
15. Smuck M, Paulus S, Patel A, Demirjian R, Ith MA, Kennedy DJ. Differential rates of inadvertent intravascular injection during lumbar transforaminal epidural injections using blunt-tip, pencil-point, and catheter-extension needles. Pain Med. 2015;16(11):2084–9.
16. Hong J, Jung S, Chang H. Whitacre needle reduces the incidence of intravascular uptake in lumbar transforaminal epidural steroid injections. Pain Physician. 2015;18(4):325–31.
17. Shin J, Kim YC, Lee SC, Kim JH. A comparison of Quincke and Whitacre needles with respect to risk of intravascular uptake in S1 transforaminal epidural steroid injections: a randomized trial of 1376 cases. Anesth Analg. 2013;117(5):1241–7.
18. Park SJ, Kim SH, Kim SJ, Yoon DM, Yoon KB. Comparison of incidences of intravascular injection between medial and lateral side approaches during traditional S1 transforaminal epidural steroid injection. Pain Res Manag. 2017;2017:6426802.
19. Simon J, McAuliffe M, Smoger D. Location of radicular spinal arteries in the lumbar spine from analysis of CT angiograms of the abdomen and pelvis. Pain Med. 2016;17(1):46–51.
20. Taterra D, Skinningsrud B, Pekala PA, Hsieh WC, Cirocchi R, Walocha JA, Tubbs RS, Tomaszewski KA, Henry BM. Artery of Adamkiewicz: a meta-analysis of anatomical characteristics. Neuroradiology. 2019;61(8):869–80.
21. Houten JK, Errico TJ. Paraplegia after lumbosacral nerve root block: report of three cases. Spine J. 2002;2(1):70–5.
22. Tvetea L. Spinal cord vascularity. V. The venous drainage of the spinal cord in the rat. Acta Radiol Diagn (Stockh). 1976;17(5B):653.
23. Park JW, Nam HS, Cho SK, Jung HJ, Lee BJ, Park Y. Kambin's triangle approach of lumbar transforaminal epidural injection with spinal stenosis. Ann Rehabil Med. 2011;35(6):833–43.
24. Levi D, Horn S, Corcoran S. The incidence of intradiscal, intrathecal, and

intravascular flow during the performance of retrodiscal (infraneural) approach for lumbar transforaminal epidural steroid injections. Pain Med. 2016;17(8):1416–22.

25. Arendt-Nielsen L, Egekvist H, Bjerring P. Pain following controlled cutaneous insertion of needles with different diameters. Somatosens Mot Res. 2006; 23(1–2):37–43.

26. McLean JP, Sigler JD, Plastaras CT, Garvan CW, Rittenberg JD. The rate of detection of intravascular injection in cervical transforaminal epidural steroid injections with and without digital subtraction angiography. PMR. 2009;1(7): 636–42.

27. Kim YH, Park HJ, Moon DE. Rates of lumbosacral transforaminal injections interpreted as intravascular: fluoroscopy alone or with digital subtraction. Anaesthesia. 2013;68(11):1120–3.

28. Hong JH, Huh B, Shin HH. Comparison between digital subtraction angiography and real-time fluoroscopy to detect intravascular injection during lumbar transforaminal epidural injections. Reg Anesth Pain Med. 2014;39(4):329–32.

13

Intraoperative dexmedetomidine attenuates norepinephrine levels in patients undergoing transsphenoidal surgery

RyungA Kang[1], Ji Seon Jeong[1]*⊙, Justin Sangwook Ko[1], Soo-Youn Lee[2], Jong Hwan Lee[1], Soo Joo Choi[1], Sungrok Cha[1] and Jeong Jin Lee[1]

Abstract

Background: Dexmedetomidine has sympatholytic effects. We investigated whether dexmedetomidine could attenuate stress responses in patients undergoing endoscopic transnasal transseptal transsphenoidal surgery.

Methods: Forty-six patients were randomized to receive a continuous infusion of 0.9% saline ($n = 23$) or dexmedetomidine (n = 23). Immediately after general anesthesia induction, the dexmedetomidine group received a loading dose of 1 mcg/kg dexmedetomidine over 10 min, followed by a maintenance dose of 0.2–0.7 mcg/kg/h and the control group received 0.9% saline at the same volume until 30 min before the end of surgery. Serum levels of epinephrine, norepinephrine, and glucose were assessed before surgery (T1) and the end of drug infusion (T2). The primary outcome was the change in norepinephrine levels between the two time points.

Results: Changes (T2-T1 values) in perioperative serum norepinephrine levels were significantly greater in the dexmedetomidine group than in the control group (median difference, 56.9 pg/dL; 95% confidence interval, 20.7 to 83.8 pg/dL; $P = 0.002$). However, epinephrine level changes did not show significant intergroup differences ($P = 0.208$). Significantly fewer patients in the dexmedetomidine group than in the control group required rescue analgesics at the recovery area (4.3% vs. 30.4%, $P = 0.047$).

Conclusions: Intraoperative dexmedetomidine administration reduced norepinephrine release and rescue analgesic requirement. Dexmedetomidine might be used as an anesthetic adjuvant in patients undergoing transnasal transseptal transsphenoidal surgery.

Keywords: Dexmedetomidine, Norepinephrine, Stress response, Pituitary

* Correspondence: jiseon78.jeong@samsung.com
[1]Department of Anesthesiology and Pain Medicine, Samsung Medical Center, Sungkyunkwan University School of Medicine, 81 Irwon ro, Gangnam gu, Seoul 06351, South Korea

Background

The endoscopic transnasal transseptal transsphenoidal approach (TSA) is commonly used for the excision of pituitary tumors [1]. This surgical approach enables improved visualization of the sellar and parasellar areas, but is associated with an increase in intraoperative stress responses due to intense noxious stimuli at various stages of the surgery, including the insertion of epinephrine-soaked nasal packing, nasal speculum insertion, sphenoidal drilling, and sellar dissection, induce a variety of stress responses [2]. These surgical stimuli induce stress hormone release and sympathetic hyperactivation, resulting in hypertension and tachycardia [3]. To attenuate stress responses during surgery, dexmedetomidine as an anesthetic adjuvant has been used [4, 5].

Dexmedetomidine is a highly selective α2-adrenoceptor agonist, and it has been widely used in the perioperative setting to provide sedation, analgesia, and sympatholysis [6–8]. Recently, dexmedetomidine has become an appealing adjunct during neurosurgical anesthesia because of several properties, including its potential for neuroprotection, minimal impact on neuronal function, stable hemodynamics, opioid- and anesthesia-sparing effects, and minimal respiratory depression [4, 6, 9]. In addition, unlike other sedatives such as propofol, remifentanil, and etomidate, dexmedetomidine has the characteristics of natural sleep-like sedation, in which the patient can still cooperate for a neurologic exam [6]. However, dexmedetomidine may result in hemodynamic compromise including severe bradycardia and hypotension, and thus should be used very cautiously in patients with compromised brain perfusion [6].

In this randomized, placebo-controlled trial, we hypothesized that intraoperative dexmedetomidine administration would reduce intraoperative stress hormone release during TSA surgery. Accordingly, we investigated epinephrine and norepinephrine levels with and without dexmedetomidine administration during TSA surgery.

Methods
Study participants
This prospective, randomized, double-blinded, placebo-controlled trial was approved by the Samsung Medical Center Research Ethics Board, Seoul, Korea (SMC 2018–08–022-002), and was prospectively registered with an extension of the Clinical Trial Registry of Korea (http://cris.nih.go.kr; identifier, KCT0003636; principal investigator, Ji Seon Jeong) on November 21, 2018. This study was adhered to CONSORT guideline. One investigator identified eligible patients from the surgeon's operating list and contacted them the day before surgery to inform them of the study protocol. Written informed consent was obtained from all participants. We enrolled 46 adult patients with American Society of Anesthesiologists Physical Status

classification I to III scheduled for elective endoscopic transnasal transseptal TSA surgery for the excision of nonfunctioning pituitary adenoma between January 2019 and April 2019, at Samsung Medical Center, Seoul, Korea. We included only the patients with nonfunctioning pituitary adenoma that were not associated with clinical evidence of hormonal hypersecretion approved by preoperative hormonal tests. We excluded patients with adrenal disorder or pheochromocytoma, as well as those who refused to participate in this study, those with a history of cardiac, renal, or hepatic disease; preexisting atrioventricular block, conduction disorder, or arrhythmia; or allergy to study drugs. We further excluded patients scheduled to undergo planned biopsy of the tumor and revision surgery.

Randomization and blinding
A member of the Samsung Medical Center who was not otherwise involved in the study performed computer-generated block randomization (www.randomizer.org) at a 1:1 ratio: dexmedetomidine group ($n = 23$) and control group (n = 23). Allocation of patients to each study group was concealed in an opaque envelope that was opened only by the hospital pharmacist who was not involved in either perioperative management or outcome assessment. The hospital pharmacist prepared visually identical study solutions in 50-mL syringes and labeled them using deidentified study code names for double-blinding. The 50-mL syringes contained 2 mL of 200 mcg dexmedetomidine (Dexmedine Inj, Hana Pharmacy, Seoul, Korea) in 48 mL of 0.9% saline to make a total volume of 50 mL (4 mcg/mL) for the dexmedetomidine group, or 50 mL of 0.9% saline for the control group. All enrolled patients, the anesthesiologist performing perioperative management, care givers, every other observer assessing the patient outcomes, and one surgeon who performed all the surgeries were blinded to group allocation until the end of study.

Interventions and intraoperative management
After applying standard monitoring including electrocardiogram, non-invasive arterial blood pressure measurement, and pulse oximetry, all patients received standardized general anesthesia comprising propofol and remifentanil using syringe pump in target-controlled infusion (TCI) mode (Injectomat TIVA Agilia, Fresinius KABI, France) as a standard of our center. The pharmacokinetic sets used to calculate target effect-site concentrations (Ce) for propofol and remifentanil were Marsh and Minto models, respectively. Ce was set to 3–5 mcg/mL for propofol and 1–3 mcg/mL for remifentanil. During the maintenance of anesthesia, the propofol dose was adjusted to achieve a target bispectral index of 40–60, and the remifentanil dose was adjusted to maintain

the mean arterial blood pressure and heart rate within 20% of the preinduction values. Immediately after the induction of general anesthesia, the patients underwent an arterial line cannulation for invasive continuous arterial pressure monitoring and blood sampling, and the study drugs were administered using a syringe pump until 30 min before the end of surgery. The dexmedetomidine group received intravenous dexmedetomidine at a loading dose of 1 mcg/kg over 10 min, followed by a maintenance dose of 0.2–0.7 mcg/kg/h. The maintenance dose of dexmedetomidine was started at a dose of 0.7 mcg/kg/h and was reduced by 0.1 intervals if there was no effect after treatment of hypotension or bradycardia. The control group received intravenous 0.9% saline at the same volume. To treat bradycardia (heart rate < 50 beats per minutes) or hypotension (decreases in mean blood pressure > 20%), the doses of propofol and remifentanil were adjusted first. If it was ineffective, intravenous atropine (0.25–0.5 mg) or ephedrine (2.5–5 mg) was administered for the treatment of bradycardia or hypotension, respectively. After that, we reduced the dose of dexmedetomidine lastly. All patients received 0.1 mg/kg of intravenous hydromorphone before the end of surgery for postoperative analgesia. TCI infusion was maintained until the end of surgery even though the study drug was stopped 30 min before the end of surgery. All patients were extubated after the end of surgery and prior to being transferred to the post-anesthesia care unit (PACU). All surgeries were performed by a single neurosurgeon [1].

Postoperative management

After the end of surgery, the patients were transferred to the PACU, and stayed there until they met the PACU discharge criteria. Postoperative supplemental analgesia was standardized. Pain severity was measured at rest by using a numerical rating scale (NRS; 11-point scale where 0 = no pain and 10 = worst pain). Patients with NRS scores > 4 were treated using rescue analgesics comprising intravenous ketorolac 30 mg. If this was ineffective after 15 min, intravenous pethidine 25 mg was administered. Postoperative nausea or vomiting was treated using intravenous metoclopramide 10 mg. The level of sedation was assessed during the PACU stay by using the Richmond Agitation-Sedation Scale (RASS) [10], and the duration of sedation was defined as the time from the end of surgery to the time of reaching the score of 0 on the RASS at the PACU. The Glasgow Coma Scale (GCS) was measured at alert and calm state to assess the overall level of consciousness after surgery in PACU. Blinded PACU nurses recorded all PACU data, including opioid consumption, presence or absence of nausea or vomiting, pain scores, and GCS scores.

Data collection

Blood samples (7 mL) for the measurement of plasma epinephrine and norepinephrine levels were collected through radial arterial cannulation at two predetermined time points: 10 min before surgery (T1), which corresponded to the time immediately after radial arterial cannulation, and the end of drug infusion (i.e., 30 min before the end of surgery) (T2). The collected blood samples were centrifuged, and the plasma and serum were separated and frozen at − 80 °C until analysis. Plasma concentrations of epinephrine and norepinephrine were analyzed by using high-performance liquid chromatography (HPLC) (Agilent 1200 HPLC system, Agilent Technologies, CA, USA) with electrochemical detection by a blinded laboratory investigator. An HPLC kit (Plasma Catecholamines by HPLC, Bio-Rad Laboratories, Hercules, CA, USA) including all reagents, calibrators, controls and column was used. The linear assay range was 10–2000 pg/mL for both epinephrine and norepinephrine. The intra- and inter-day assay precisions were coefficient of variation ≤10% at two concentrations for each analyte. We participated in the proficiency testing provided by the Korean Association of External Quality Assessments Service twice a year. Glucose level was measured using a blood gas/chemistry analysis device (RAPIDLAB1265, Siemens Healthcare Diagnostics Inc., Berlin, Germany) at the same predetermined time intervals (T1 and T2).

Intraoperative hemodynamic variables (mean blood pressure and heart rate) were automatically recorded in the electronic medical records. Intraoperative propofol and remifentanil consumption was also recorded.

Outcomes

The primary outcome was the change in perioperative serum norepinephrine level. The secondary outcomes included perioperative serum epinephrine and glucose levels, dexmedetomidine-related side effects (hypotension, bradycardia, and sedation), the incidence of postoperative nausea or vomiting, and postoperative pain score measured at discharge from PACU.

Statistical analysis

The sample size was calculated on the basis of the findings of a previous study by Aho et al. [11] The mean difference (standard deviation [SD]) in serum norepinephrine levels between the baseline and the highest level during surgery between patients who received intramuscular dexmedetomidine and those who received 0.9% saline was 2.2 (1.5) mcg/dL. We expected that, compared to the controls, patients receiving intravenous dexmedetomidine would show a reduction in serum norepinephrine level by at least 50% [12]. We calculated that 21 patients per group were required to detect this degree of difference with a power of 80% and an α = 0.05. Considering a 10% dropout rate, we decided to enroll 46 patients in total.

After determining the normality of data distribution by using the Shapiro-Wilk test, continuous variables were analyzed using the *t* test or Mann-Whitney U test as appropriate. Parametric and non-parametric data were reported as mean ± SDs and median [interquartile ranges], respectively. Categorical variables were analyzed using the chi-square test or Fisher's exact test. Bonferroni correction was used for multiple comparisons. Data analysis was conducted using IBM SPSS Statistics for Windows/Macintosh, Version 25.0 (IBM Corp., Armonk, NY, USA). For all analyses, a *P*-value < 0.05 was considered significant, and two-sided tests were used.

Availability of data and materials
The datasets generated and/or analysed during the current study are available from the corresponding author on reasonable request.

Results
Study participants
Between January 2019 and April 2019, 48 patients scheduled for TSA surgery for the excision of nonfunctioning pituitary adenoma were assessed for eligibility, and 2 patients were excluded. All enrolled patients were randomly assigned to one of the two study groups (*n* = 23 each) and completed the study (Fig. 1).

All patients underwent their planned surgical procedure and completed the protocol for measurement of the primary outcome. The baseline patient and surgical characteristics were similar between the two groups (Table 1).

Outcomes
Changes (T2-T1 values) in perioperative serum norepinephrine levels were significantly greater in the dexmedetomidine group than in the control group (median difference, 56.9 pg/dL; 95% confidence interval [CI], 20.7 to 83.8 pg/dL; *P* = 0.002). However, changes in perioperative serum epinephrine levels were not significantly affected by the administration of dexmedetomidine (median difference, −12.4 pg/dL; 95% CI, −40.1 to 9.2 pg/dL; *P* = 0.208). Baseline (T1) epinephrine and norepinephrine levels (median [interquartile range]) were not significantly different between the two groups (control vs. dexmedetomidine: epinephrine, 10 [10–22] vs. 11 [10–26] pg/dL, *P* = 0.395; norepinephrine, 153 [125–184] vs. 172 [143–195] pg/dL; *P* = 0.249) (Table 2).

At T2, norepinephrine level was significantly lower in the dexmedetomidine group than in the control group (52 [41–72] vs. 103 [79–144] pg/dL; *P* < 0.001), but epinephrine level was not significantly different between the two groups (control vs. dexmedetomidine: 36 [25–43] vs. 44 [36–83] pg/dL; *P* = 0.066). Glucose level was similar in both groups at T1 (*P* = 0.124), but it was significantly higher in the dexmedetomidine group than in

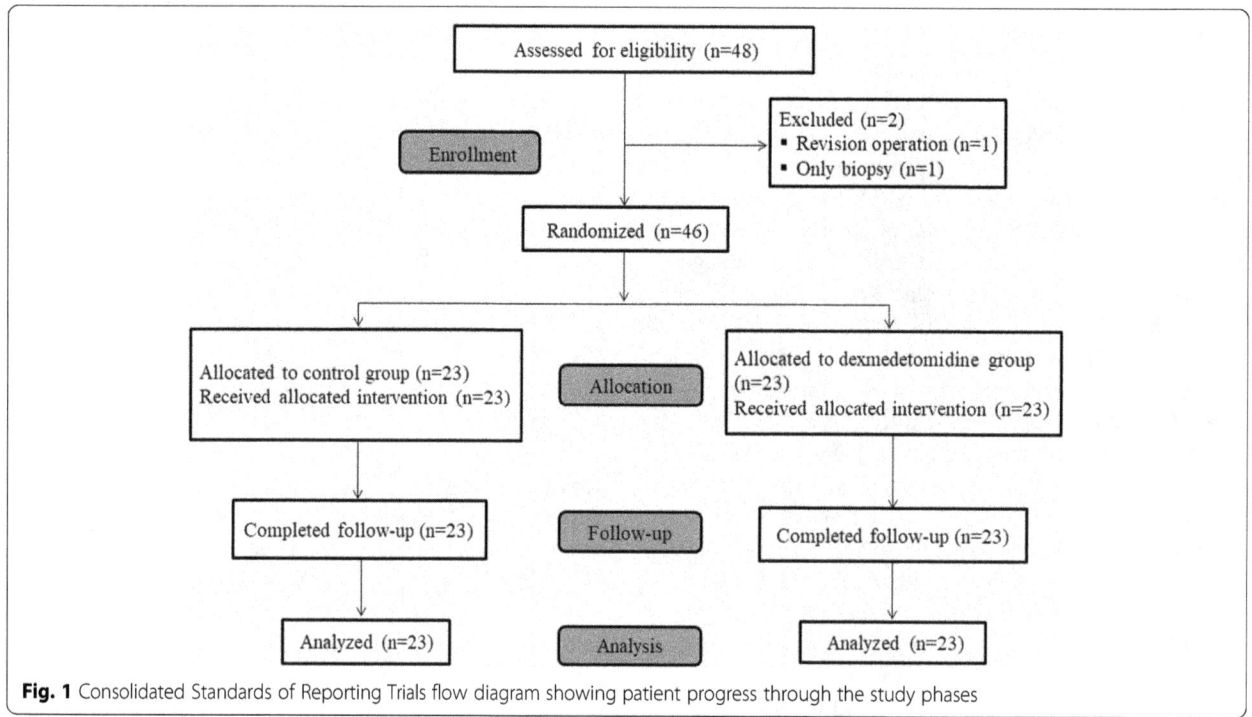

Fig. 1 Consolidated Standards of Reporting Trials flow diagram showing patient progress through the study phases

Table 1 Patients' characteristics

Parameter	Control (**n** = 23)	Dexmedetomidine (**n** = 23)	**P** value
Age (years)	48 [39–56]	55 [43–62]	0.111
Sex (male/female)	11/12	8/15	0.550
Body mass index (kg/m^2)	26.0 ± 4.6	25.2 ± 2.8	0.491
ASA physical status (I/II)	18/5	17/6	0.665
Duration of surgery (hours)	2.8 ± 1.6	2.3 ± 1.0	0.262

Values are mean ± standard deviations, median [interquartile ranges], or number. *ASA* American Society of Anesthesiologist

the control group at T2 (control vs. dexmedetomidine: 128 [112–140] vs. 147 [125–161] mg/dL; P = 0.03).

Intraoperative mean blood pressure and heart rate are shown in Fig. 2.

Significant hemodynamic instability was not observed in either group. The incidence of intraoperative hypotension was similar between the two groups, but the incidence of intraoperative bradycardia was significantly higher in the dexmedetomidine group than in the control group (Table 2). Postoperative pain score at the recovery area was similar between the two groups (control vs. dexmedetomidine: 2 [1–3] vs. 2 [1–2]; P = 0.188). The number of patients requiring rescue analgesics at the PACU was significantly lower in the dexmedetomidine group than in the control group (7 [30.4%] vs. 1 [4.3%] patients; P = 0.047). Nevertheless, no significant

difference was observed in the length of PACU stay (P = 0.308).

Discussion

In this randomized, placebo-controlled trial, we demonstrated that intraoperative intravenous dexmedetomidine administration attenuates the increase in plasma norepinephrine level during TSA surgery. Patients administered dexmedetomidine showed frequent intraoperative bradycardia but did not show impaired hemodynamic instability and had less requirements for rescue analgesics in the immediate postoperative period.

Surgical stimulus initiates a cascade of stress responses through direct activation of the sympathetic nervous system and increased secretion of pituitary hormones [3, 13]. Attenuation of these stress responses to intense

Table 2 Perioperative clinical outcomes

Parameters	Control (**n** = 23)	Dexmedetomidine (**n** = 23)	**P**^{a} value
Stress hormone level at baseline (T1)			
Norepinephrine (pg/mL)	153.3 [125–183.6]	172.3 [142.8–195.2]	0.249
Epinephrine (pg/mL)	10 [10–21.7]	10.6 [10–25.6]	0.395
Glucose (mg/dL)	102 [93–119]	97 [84–108]	0.124
Stress hormone level at the end of infusion (T2)			
Norepinephrine (pg/mL)	102.5 [78.9–143.8]	52.2 [41.2–71.6]	< 0.001
Epinephrine (pg/mL)	35.9 [24.9–43.3]	43.9 [36.1–83.1]	0.066
Glucose (mg/dL)	128 [112–140]	147 [125–161]	0.030
Propofol dose (mg/kg/h)	7.0 [6.3–7.7]	6.8 [6.3–7.2]	0.668
Remifentanil dose (mcg/kg/h)	4.4 [3.4–5.4]	4.5 [3.6–6.3]	0.267
Lowest BIS value during maintenance	40 [40–41]	40 [36–40]	0.088
Highest BIS value during maintenance	50 [47–53]	48 [44–52]	0.136
Intraoperative hypotension, n	6 (26.1%)	9 (39.1%)	0.530
Intraoperative bradycardia, n	1 (4.3%)	9 (39.1%)	0.010
Postoperative nausea or vomiting at PACU, n	4 (17.4%)	1 (4.3%)	0.346
Pain score at PACU (NRS, 0–10)	2 [1–3]	2 [1–2]	0.188
Number of patients requiring rescue analgesics at PACU, n	7 (30.4%)	1 (4.3%)	0.047
GCS score at PACU	15 [15–15]	15 [15–15]	> 0.999
Duration of recovery at PACU (minutes)	60 ± 10	64 ± 9	0.308

Values are mean ± standard deviation, median [interquartile ranges] or number (percentages). ^{a}The P value for the t-test, Mann-Whitney U test, and the Fisher's exact test is set at 0.05. *BIS* Bispectral index, *GCS* Glasgow Coma Scale, *PACU* Post-anesthesia care unit

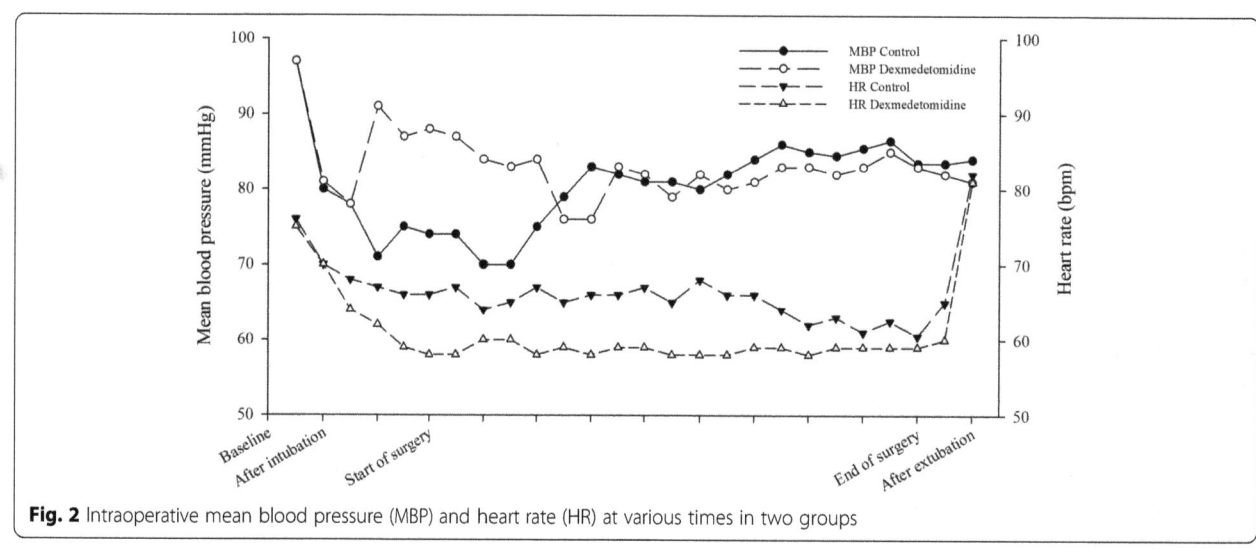

Fig. 2 Intraoperative mean blood pressure (MBP) and heart rate (HR) at various times in two groups

noxious stimuli during surgery improved outcomes by exerting beneficial effects on the postoperative outcomes [14]. Our findings indicated that propofol-remifentanil anesthesia supplemented with dexmedetomidine attenuated surgical stress by inhibiting the secretion of norepinephrine. Dexmedetomidine exerts its sympatholytic effects by activating inhibitory α2-receptors, both in the central nervous system and on peripheral sympathetic nerve endings [3, 11, 12, 14, 15]. However, because plasma norepinephrine passes the blood-brain barrier poorly, attenuated plasma norepinephrine levels do not simultaneously reflect both the central and peripheral sympatholytic effects of dexmedetomidine [16]. Based in this, it can be inferred that plasma norepinephrine was released into the blood from the adrenal medulla in response to sympathetic stimulation separately from the central nervous system. Therefore, attenuated plasma norepinephrine in our study might be due to the peripheral sympatholytic effects of dexmedetomidine. In our study, norepinephrine level was more significantly attenuated in the dexmedetomidine group than in the control group, which showed that dexmedetomidine effectively blunted the stress responses. These findings are consistent with those of a previous study, which showed that dexmedetomidine attenuated catecholamine increase after major spine surgery [12]. However, epinephrine level was unaffected by the administration of dexmedetomidine in our study. The possible reason for this is that dexmedetomidine mainly inhibits release of norepinephrine from presynaptic sympathetic nerve terminals [17]. Another possible reason is that epinephrine-soaked nasal packing may have affected plasma epinephrine levels. Therefore, the true effect of dexmedetomidine on plasma epinephrine level might be masked by epinephrine-soaked nasal packing.

Previous studies have shown that perioperative administration of dexmedetomidine reduced glucose levels that surgical stress produces [14, 18]. However, recent meta-analysis demonstrated that reduced blood glucose levels in dexmedetomidine group were shown in only in abdominal surgery, not in cardiac surgery or other surgery subgroups [3]. In our study, glucose levels were significantly higher in the dexmedetomidine group than in the control group (147 mg/dL vs. 128 mg/dL). The possible reason might be ascribed to the pharmacological properties of the α2-adrenoceptor agonists itself, which can cause hyperglycemia by a mechanism that involves the postsynaptic α2-adrenoceptor stimulation of pancreatic beta cells, which inhibits insulin secretion [19]. Another possible reason might be due to attenuated surgical stress response caused by a dose-related sympatholytic effect of dexmedetomidine based on a study evaluating the effects of dexmedetomidine on glucose levels in children undergoing general anesthesia [20]. Moreover, exogenous epinephrine infusion can cause a transient increase in glucose production and a sustained inhibition of glucose clearance, resulting in hyperglycemia, but is unlikely [21].

The use of intravenous dexmedetomidine during the intraoperative period reduces postoperative opioid consumption [22]. This analgesic-sparing effect was also found in our study. Patients in the dexmedetomidine group had significantly lower requirements of rescue analgesics. Dexmedetomidine has side effects such as hypotension, bradycardia, and oversedation [17]. In our study, typical biphasic hemodynamic effects of dexmedetomidine, including transient hypertension, bradycardia, and hypotension, were explained by the results from the peripheral vasoconstrictive and sympatholytic properties of dexmedetomidine [23]. However, the use of remifentanil with propofol might have obscured the true incidence of hypotension. In addition, a concern regarding the use of dexmedetomidine infusion during surgery is delayed recovery due to the sedative effect of dexmedetomidine. However, in our study, dexmedetomidine administration was discontinued 30 min before the end of surgery, and thus it did not affect the patients' recovery time [12].

Our study has several limitations. First, we evaluated the effect of dexmedetomidine as an adjuvant under the standard anesthetic regimen of our center (propofol-remifentanil). Therefore, it may be difficult to interpret the true effect of dexmedetomidine owing to study design. In addition, we planned to adjust the maintenance dose of dexmedetomidine, which may impact on the stress response to surgery. However, the loading dose of dexmedetomidine accounts for over 50% of the total dose during surgery. Therefore, we considered the effect of adjustable maintenance dose would be minimal. Second, baseline stress hormone levels were measured immediately after tracheal intubation, which was one of the most important noxious stimuli during surgery. Therefore, these measured values may not reflect the actual reference value. However, since stress hormone levels were measured at the same time point between the two groups, the differences between the two time points could be interpreted as demonstrating the effect of dexmedetomidine. Nevertheless, it would have been better to measure stress hormone levels before the induction of general anesthesia. Third, we measured two types of hormones (epinephrine and norepinephrine) at two time points. The selection of the time points was based on judgment and our experience, but they may not be optimal. The overall effect of dexmedetomidine on surgery could be measured, but the effects of stress intensity, dose, and time of administration could not be measured. Moreover, it would have been better to measure cortisol, a more suitable marker for stress response to evaluate stress response [3]. Further study is needed for the serial measurement of the effects of dexmedetomidine at various stages of surgery, as is the incorporation of other stress responses markers, such as cortisol, glucagon, plasma interleukin-6 [19], to establish more accurate responses to the administration of dexmedetomidine.

Conclusions

In conclusion, intraoperative dexmedetomidine administration reduced norepinephrine release and reduced rescue analgesic requirements. Dexmedetomidine can be used as an anesthetic adjuvant in patients undergoing TSA surgery.

Abbreviations

GCS: Glasgow Coma Scale; PACU: Post-anesthesia care unit; TSA: Transsphenoidal approach; NRS: Numerical rating scale; RASS: Richmond Agitation-Sedation Scale

Acknowledgments

Not applicable.

Authors' contributions

RAK contributed to study design, interpretation of data, and drafted the manuscript. JSJ contributed to study design, analysis, and interpretation of the data, revised the manuscript, and approved the final version. JSK contributed to study design, critically revised the manuscript, and approved the final version. SYL was primarily responsible for the processing and analysis of blood samples. JHL and SJC contributed to critically revised the manuscript, and approved the final version. SC and JJL contributed to study design, acquisition of data, and approved the final version.

Author details

[1]Department of Anesthesiology and Pain Medicine, Samsung Medical Center, Sungkyunkwan University School of Medicine, 81 Irwon ro, Gangnam gu, Seoul 06351, South Korea. [2]Department of Laboratory Medicine and Genetics, Samsung Medical Center, Sungkyunkwan University School of Medicine, Seoul, South Korea.

References

1. Hong SD, Nam DH, Kong DS, Kim HY, Chung SK, Dhong HJ. Endoscopic modified transseptal transsphenoidal approach for maximal preservation of sinonasal quality of life and olfaction. World Neurosurg. 2016;87:162–9.
2. Jan S, Ali Z, Nisar Y, Naqash IA, Zahoor SA, Langoo SA, Azhar K. A comparison of dexmedetomidine and clonidine in attenuating the hemodynamic responses at various surgical stages in patients undergoing elective transnasal transsphenoidal resection of pituitary tumors. Anesth Essays Res. 2017;11(4):1079–83.
3. Wang K, Wu M, Xu J, Wu C, Zhang B, Wang G, Ma D. Effects of dexmedetomidine on perioperative stress, inflammation, and immune function: systematic review and meta-analysis. Br J Anaesth. 2019;123(6): 777–94.
4. Kadarapura N, Gopalakrishna PKD, Chatterjee N, Hariharan V. Easwer, and Arimanickam Ganesamoorthi: Dexmedetomidine as an anesthetic adjuvant in patients undergoing transsphenoidal resection of pituitary tumor. J Neurosurg Anesthesiol. 2015;27:209–15.
5. Gupta D, Srivastava S, Dubey RK, Prakash PS, Singh PK, Singh U. Comparative evaluation of atenolol and clonidine premedication on cardiovascular response to nasal speculum insertion during trans-sphenoid surgery for resection of pituitary adenoma: a prospective, randomised, double-blind, controlled study. Indian J Anaesth. 2011;55(2):135–40.
6. Lin N, Vutskits L, Bebawy JF, Gelb AW. Perspectives on dexmedetomidine use for neurosurgical patients. J Neurosurg Anesthesiol. 2019;31(4):366–77.
7. Hall JE, Uhrich TD, Barney JA, Arain SR, Ebert TJ. Sedative, amnestic, and analgesic properties of small-dose dexmedetomidine infusions. Anesth Analg. 2000;90(3):699–705.
8. Lee S. Dexmedetomidine: present and future directions. Korean J Anesthesiol. 2019;72(4):323–30.
9. Darmawikarta D, Sourour M, Couban R, Kamath S, Reddy KK, Shanthanna H. Opioid-free analgesia for supratentorial craniotomies: a systematic review. Can J Neurol Sci. 2019;46(4):415–22.
10. Sessler CN, Gosnell MS, Grap MJ, Brophy GM, O'Neal PV, Keane KA, Tesoro EP, Elswick RK. The Richmond agitation-sedation scale: validity and reliability in adult intensive care unit patients. Am J Respir Crit Care Med. 2002; 166(10):1338–44.
11. Aho M, Scheinin M, Lehtinen AM, Erkola O, Vuorinen J, Korttila K. Intramuscularly administered dexmedetomidine attenuates hemodynamic and stress hormone responses to gynecologic laparoscopy. Anesth Analg. 1992;75(6):932–9.
12. Kim MH, Lee KY, Bae SJ, Jo M, Cho JS. Intraoperative dexmedetomidine attenuates stress responses in patients undergoing major spine surgery. Minerva Anestesiol. 2019;85(5):468–77.
13. Desborough JP. The stress response to trauma and surgery. Br J Anaesth. 2000;85(1):109–17.
14. Uyar AS, Yagmurdur H, Fidan Y, Topkaya C, Basar H. Dexmedetomidine attenuates the hemodynamic and neuroendocrinal responses to skull-pin head-holder application during craniotomy. J Neurosurg Anesthesiol. 2008; 20(3):174–9.

15. Keniya VM, Ladi S, Naphade R. Dexmedetomidine attenuates sympathoadrenal response to tracheal intubation and reduces perioperative anaesthetic requirement. Indian J Anaesth. 2011;55(4):352–7.

16. Patrick A, Vdq S, Foti A, Curzon G. Effects of clonidine on central and peripheral nerve tone in primary hypertension. Hypertension. 1986;8:611–7.

17. Ralph Gertler HCB, Mitchell DH, Silvius EN. Dexmedetomidine: a novel sedative-analgesic agent. BUMC Proc. 2001;14:13–21.

18. Harsoor SS, Rani DD, Lathashree S, Nethra SS, Sudheesh K. Effect of intraoperative dexmedetomidine infusion on sevoflurane requirement and blood glucose levels during entropy-guided general anesthesia. J Anaesthesiol Clin Pharmacol. 2014;30(1):25–30.

19. AB RMV, Hall GM, Grounds RM. Effects of dexmedetomidine on adrenocortical function, and the cardiovascular, endocrine and inflammatory responses in postoperative patients needing sedation in the intensive care unit. Br J Anaesth. 2001;86(5):650–6.

20. Gorges M, Poznikoff AK, West NC, Brodie SM, Brant RF, Whyte SD. Effects of dexmedetomidine on blood glucose and serum potassium levels in children undergoing general anesthesia: a secondary analysis of safety endpoints during a randomized controlled trial. Anesth Analg. 2019;129(4): 1093–9.

21. Vranic M, Gauthier C, Bilinski D, Wasserman D, El Tayeb K, Hetenyi G Jr, Lickley HL. Catecholamine responses and their interactions with other glucoregulatory hormones. Am J Phys. 1984;247(2 Pt 1):E145–56.

22. Kang R, Jeong JS, Yoo JC, Lee JH, Choi SJ, Gwak MS, Hahm TS, Huh J, Ko JS. Effective dose of intravenous Dexmedetomidine to prolong the analgesic duration of Interscalene brachial plexus block: a single-center, prospective, double-blind, randomized controlled trial. Reg Anesth Pain Med. 2018;43(5): 488–95.

23. Weerink MA, Struys MM, Hannivoort LN, Barends CR, Absalom AR, Colin P. Clinical pharmacokinetics and pharmacodynamics of dexmedetomidine. Clin Pharmacokinet. 2017;56(8):893–913.

14

Efficacy of programmed intermittent bolus epidural analgesia in thoracic surgery

M. Higashi[1], K. Shigematsu[2], E. Nakamori[1], S. Sakurai[1] and K. Yamaura[1]* ⓘD

Abstract

Background: Continuous epidural infusion (CEI) has some disadvantages, such as increased local anesthetic consumption and limited area of anesthetic distribution. Programmed intermittent bolus (PIB) is a technique of epidural anesthesia in which boluses of local anesthetic are automatically injected into the epidural space. The usefulness of PIB in thoracic surgery remains unclear. In this study, we aimed to compare the efficacies of PIB epidural analgesia and CEI in patients undergoing thoracic surgery.

Methods: This randomized prospective study was approved by the Institutional Review Board. The study included 42 patients, who were divided into CEI ($n = 21$) and PIB groups ($n = 21$). In the CEI group, patients received continuous infusion of the local anesthetic at a rate of 5.1 mL/90 min. In the PIB group, a pump delivered the local anesthetic at a dose of 5.1 mL every 90 min. The primary endpoints were the frequency of patient-controlled analgesia (PCA) and the total dose of local anesthetic until 36 h following surgery. Student's t-test, the chi-square test, and the Mann–Whitney U test were used for statistical analyses.

Results: The mean number of PCA administrations and total amount of local anesthetic were not significantly different between the two groups up to 24 h following surgery. However, the mean number of PCA administrations and total amount of local anesthetic at 24–36 h after surgery were significantly lower in the PIB group than in the CEI group (median [lower–upper quartiles]: 0 [0–2.5] vs. 2 [0.5–5], $P = 0.018$ and 41 [41–48.5] vs. 47 [43–56], $P = 0.035$, respectively). Hypotension was significantly more frequent in the PIB group than in the CEI group at 0–12 h and 12–24 h (3.3% vs. 0.5%, $P = 0.018$ and 7.9% vs. 0%, $P = 0.017$, respectively).

Conclusion: PIB can reduce local anesthetic consumption in thoracic surgery. However, it might result in adverse events, such as hypotension.

Keywords: Anesthesia, Epidural anesthesia, Programmed intermittent bolus, Thoracic surgery

* Correspondence: keny@kuaccm.med.kyushu-u.ac.jp
[1]Department of Anesthesiology, Fukuoka University School of Medicine,

7-45-1, Nanakuma, Jonan-ku, Fukuoka 814-0180, Japan

Background

Continuous epidural infusion (CEI) of a local anesthetic combined with patient-controlled analgesia (PCA) is an effective postoperative analgesic approach for thoracic surgery [1]. However, CEI has some disadvantages, such as increased local anesthetic consumption and a limited area of anesthetic distribution [2].

Programmed intermittent bolus (PIB) is a technique of epidural anesthesia in which boluses of local anesthetic are automatically injected into the epidural space. This technique increases the analgesic area [3]. Reports have indicated that intermittent epidural bolus administration reduces local anesthetic usage and improves maternal satisfaction in labor analgesia [4–6]. However, the usefulness of PIB in thoracic surgery is unclear.

The purpose of this study was to compare the efficacies of PIB epidural analgesia and CEI in patients undergoing thoracic surgery.

Methods

This randomized prospective study was approved by the Institutional Review Board (IRB No. 15-9-06) of Fukuoka University Hospital, Fukuoka, Japan, and was registered in the clinical trials database UMIN (ID 000019904) on 24 November 2015. Written informed consent was obtained from all patients.

Patients

Patients undergoing open lung lobectomy or partial lobectomy at the Fukuoka University Hospital, Fukuoka, Japan between March 2016 and March 2017 were recruited. The exclusion criteria were age < 20 years and contraindication for epidural anesthesia. Patients were randomly divided into a CEI or PIB group by computer generated randomization using Excel 2013 (Microsoft Inc., Redmond, WA) by KY (Fig. 1).

The study was discontinued when epidural analgesia was ineffective, when the patient's hypotension continued even after the administration of vasopressor, or when motor paralysis appeared owing to epidural analgesia.

Anesthesia

Under standard monitoring, thoracic epidural anesthesia was performed at Th4–6 in the lateral position. An 18G epidural Tuohy needle (Uniever®, Unisis Corp., Saitama, Japan) was used, and the epidural space was identified using the loss-of-resistance technique. A 20G epidural catheter (Uniever®, Unisis Corp.) was inserted 5 cm to the head side. Following a 3-mL test dose of 1% mepivacaine, the epidural catheter was fixed.

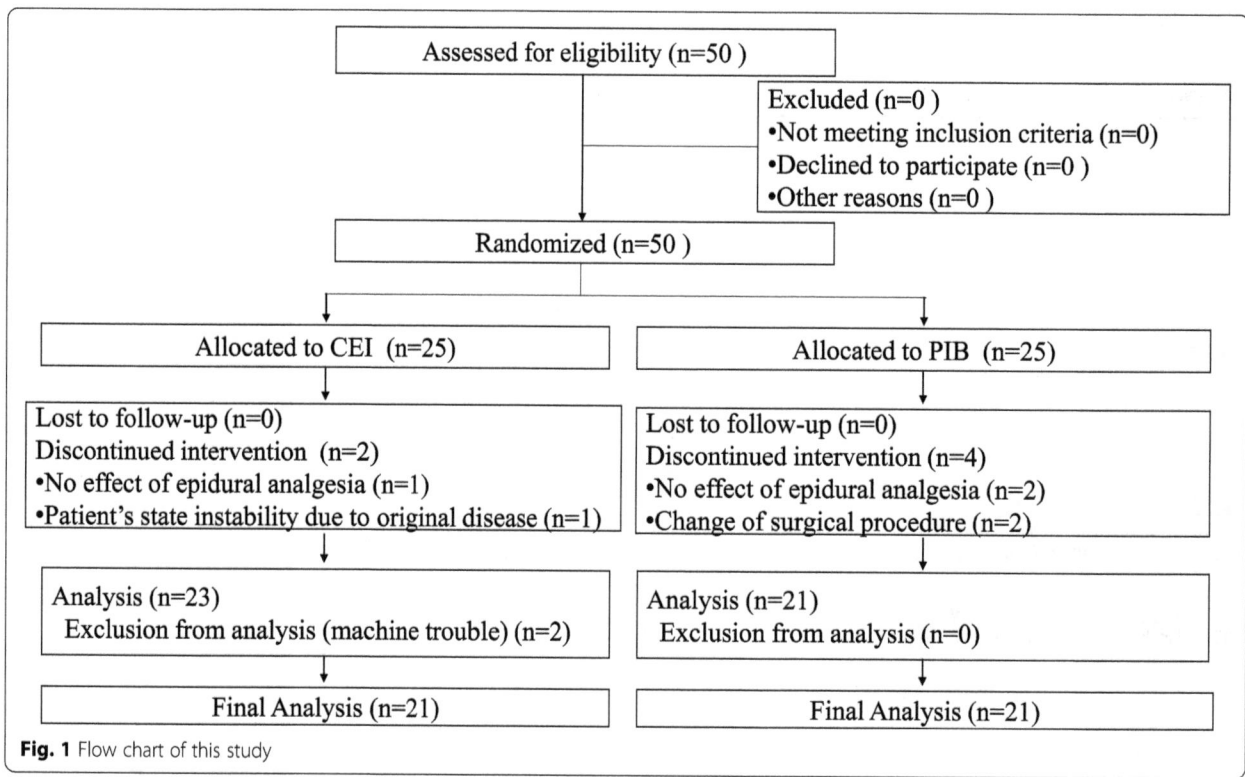

Fig. 1 Flow chart of this study

General anesthesia was induced with intravenous fentanyl (2 μg/kg), propofol (1 mg/kg), and rocuronium (0.9 mg/kg) and was maintained with sevoflurane (1.5–2%) and remifentanil (0.1–0.2 μg/kg/min). Fentanyl was used intravenously up to 5 μg/kg. A local anesthetic via the epidural catheter was not used during the operation.

After surgery, all patients were extubated in the operating room, observed in the post-anesthesia care unit for 30 min to 1 h, and then transferred to the ward.

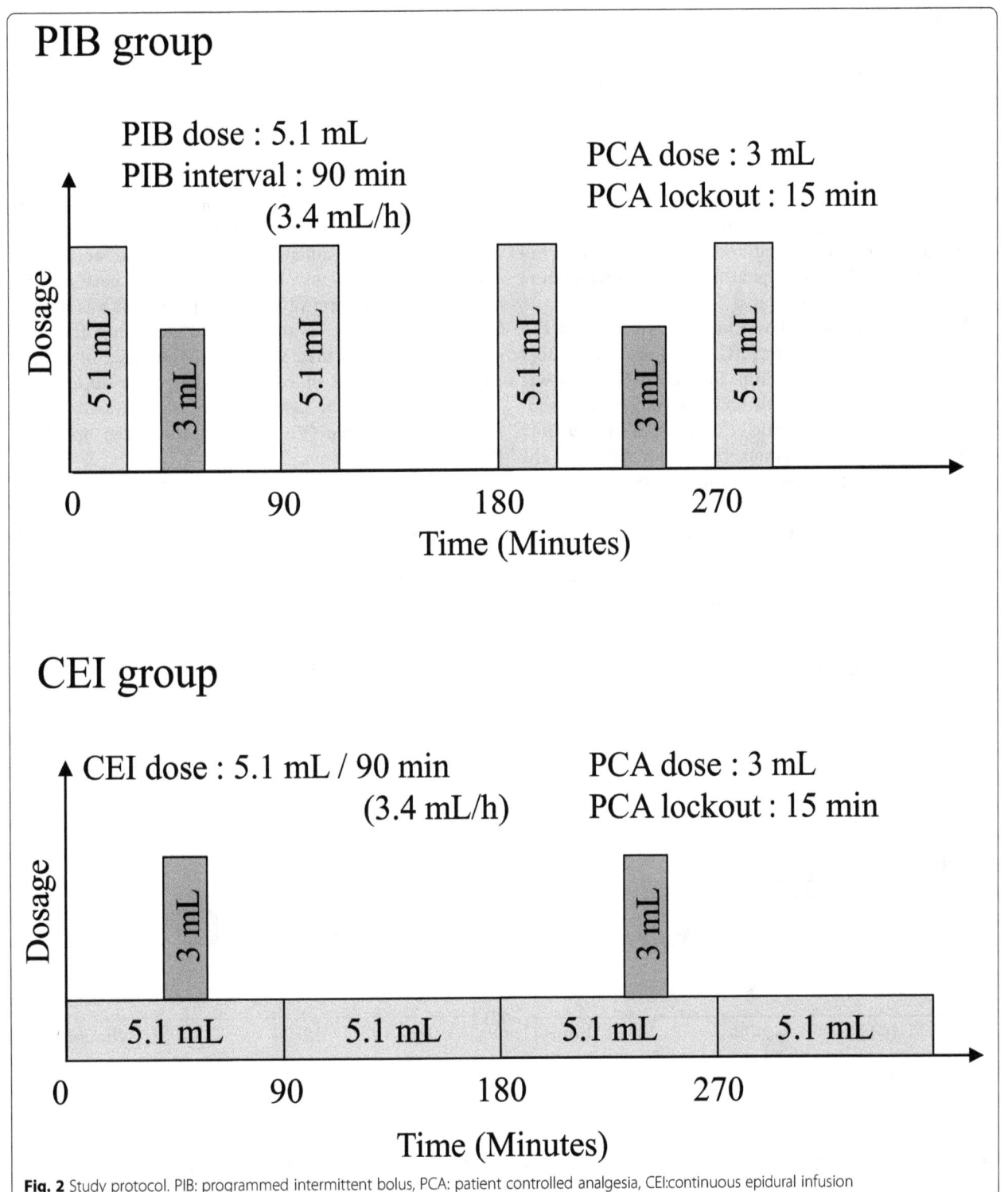

Fig. 2 Study protocol. PIB: programmed intermittent bolus, PCA: patient controlled analgesia, CEI:continuous epidural infusion

Table 1 Patient characteristics

	PIB (n = 21) mean ± SD	CEI (n = 21) mean ± SD	P-value
Age (years)	63 ± 2.8	67 ± 2.6	0.34
BMI (kg/m²)	24.5 ± 1.1	22.4 ± 0.5	0.08
SBP (mmHg)	122 ± 2	121 ± 2	0.72
Use of analgesics during the operation			
Fentanyl (μg)	171 ± 35	193 ± 35	0.67
Remifentanil (mg)	1.5 ± 0.2	1.8 ± 0.2	0.32
Operation time (min)	249 ± 20	263 ± 18	0.61
Anesthesia time (min)	334 ± 22	351 ± 18	0.56

Intervention

At the end of surgery, a 5-mL initial dose of local anesthetic (ropivacaine 2 mg and fentanyl 2 μg in 1 ml) was administered via the epidural catheter after closure of thoracotomy in both groups.

The study protocol is shown in Fig. 2. In both the PIB and CEI groups, a pump (CADD-Solis ambulatory infusion pump, Smith Medical, St Paul, MN, USA) was used. In the CEI group, patients received continuous infusion of the local anesthetic at a rate of 5.1 mL/90 min (3.4 mL/h). In the PIB group, the pump delivered the local anesthetic at a dose of 5.1 mL every 90 min. The PCA system was programmed to deliver a 3-mL bolus of the local anesthetic with a lockout interval of 15 min in both groups.

The primary endpoints were the frequency of PCA and total dose of local anesthetic during 36 h of

postoperative period. The secondary endpoints were pain intensity, frequency of rescue analgesics, including nonsteroidal anti-inflammatory drugs and acetaminophen, adverse events, hypotension, and postoperative nausea and vomiting (PONV). Hypotension was defined as systolic blood pressure (SBP) 20% less than the baseline value or less than 90 mmHg. The onset of adverse reactions and use of rescue analgesics postoperatively were examined. The pain intensity was assessed using a visual analog scale (VAS) during rest, deep breathing, cough, and movement.

Statistical analysis

Continuous variables are expressed as mean ± standard deviation or median [lower–upper quartiles]. From the results of preliminary study, total dose of local anesthetics in CEI was 24 ml more than in PIB,

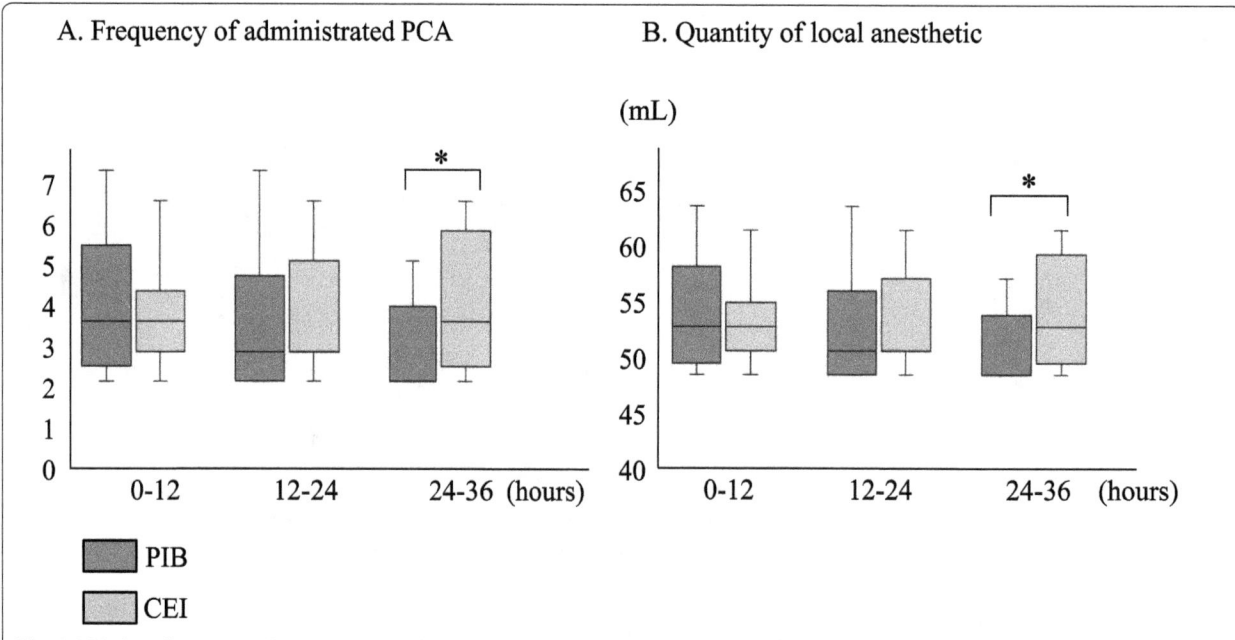

Fig. 3 PCA data after surgery. Data are presented as median [lower–upper quartiles]. The Mann–Whitney U test was used for comparison of categorical variables. *P < 0.05. PCA: patient-controlled analgesia, PIB: programmed intermittent bolus, CEI: continuous epidural infusion

Table 2 Use of rescue analgesics postoperatively

	PIB (n = 21)	CEI (n = 21)	P-value
	n (%)	n (%)	
Use of analgesics			
Loxoprofen	20(95.2)	19(85.6)	0.55
Acetaminophen	1(4.7)	3(14.3)	0.61
Celecoxib	1(4.7)	2(9.5)	0.55
Tramadol	2(9.5)	1 (4.7)	0.55

and SD of CEI was 32. Based on these results, we estimated that the following: SD = 32, Δ = 0.78, α = 0.05, and beta = 0.2. The required number of cases was estimated to be 21 for each group. We considered a 10–20% dropout rate; therefore, 50 patients were enrolled. Differences between groups were examined for statistical significance by using student's t-test after logarithmic transformation. Student's t-test, the chi-square test, and the Mann–Whitney U test were used for statistical analyses. A P-value < 0.05 was considered statistically significant.

Results

Fifty patients who underwent open lung lobectomy or partial lobectomy were randomly divided into the CEI group (n = 25) and PIB group (n = 25). In the CEI group, 2 patients were excluded because of ineffectiveness of epidural analgesia and instability in the patient's state due to the original disease. In the remaining 23 patients of the CEI group, additional 2 patients were excluded from the analysis because of machine trouble; finally, 21 patients were included in the analysis. In PIB group, 4 patients were excluded (2 patients owing to ineffectiveness of epidural analgesia and 2 patients owing to change in surgical procedure), and 21 patients were finally included in the analysis (Fig. 1). Patient characteristics are shown in Table 1.

The mean number of PCA administrations and total amount of local anesthetic were not significantly different between the two study groups up to 24 h after surgery. However, the mean number of PCA administrations was significantly lower in the PIB group than in the CEI group at 24–36 h after surgery (median [lower–upper quartiles]: 0 [0–2.5] vs. 2 [0.5–5], P = 0.018) and total amount of local anesthetic was also significantly lower in the PIB group than in the CEI group at 24–36 h after surgery (median [lower–upper quartiles]: 41 [41–48.5] vs. 47 [43–56] mL, P = 0.035) (Fig. 3). The use of rescue analgesics was not significantly different between the two study groups (Table 2). The VAS scores during

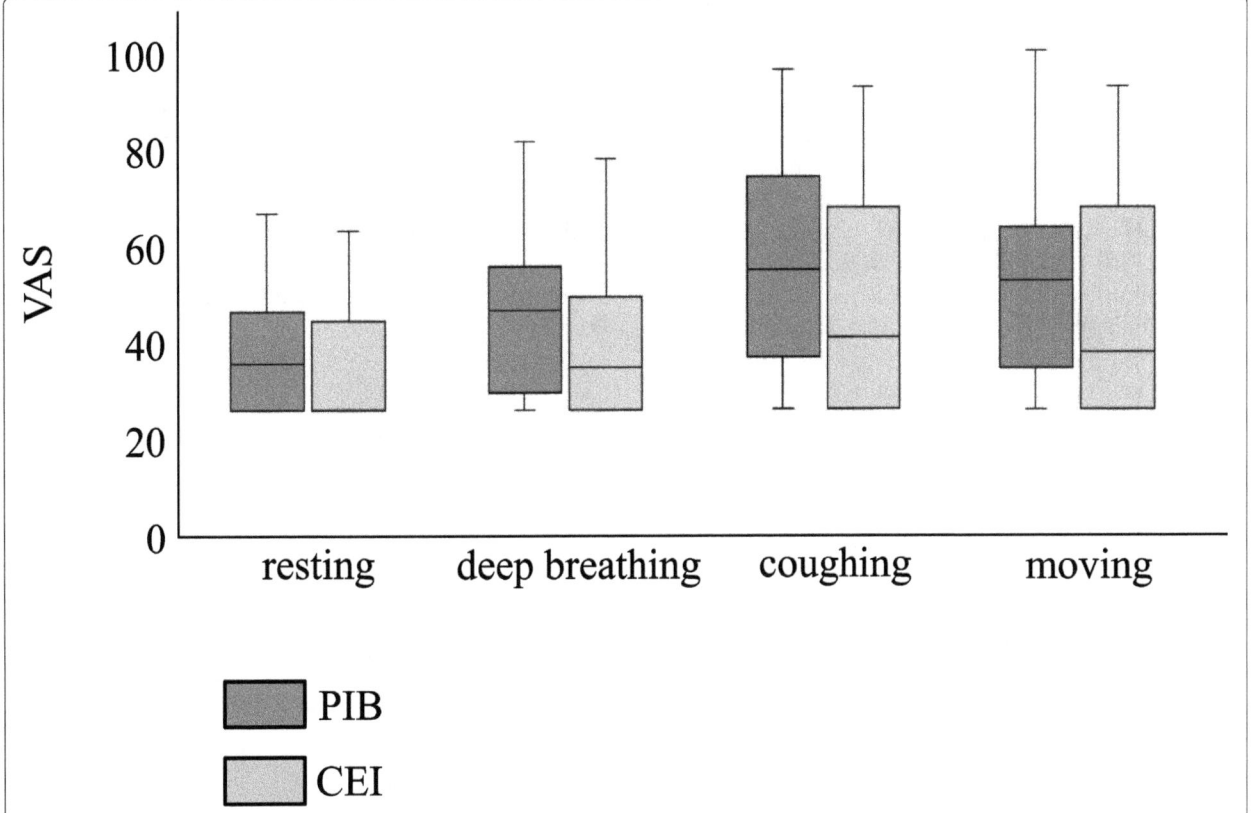

Fig. 4 VAS scores at POD 1. Data are presented as median [lower–upper quartiles]. The Mann–Whitney U test was used for comparison of categorical variables. VAS: visual analog scale, PIB: programmed intermittent bolus, CEI: continuous epidural infusion, POD: postoperative day

Table 3 Adverse events

	PIB ($n = 21$)	CEI ($n = 21$)	P-value
	n (%)	n (%)	
Adverse effects			
Nausea, vomiting	8(38.1)	5(23.8)	0.32
Urinary retention	2(9.5)	3(14.3)	0.63
Feeling dizzy on standing up	4(19.0)	1(4.7)	0.15

resting, deep breathing, coughing, and moving after the surgery were also not significantly different between the two study groups (Fig. 4).

The frequencies of adverse events, such as nausea, vomiting, and dizziness on standing up, were not significantly different between the two study groups (Table 3). The frequency of hypotension was greater in the PIB group than in the CEI group at 0–12 h and 12–24 h postoperatively (3.3% vs. 0.5%, $P = 0.018$ and 7.9% vs. 0%, $P = 0.017$, respectively) (Table 4).

Discussion

Our results showed that PIB has an analgesic effect comparable with that of CEI and reduces the required amount of local anesthetic on the first day after thoracotomy. However, adverse events, such as hypotension, need attention.

To compensate for the limitations of CEI, such as a restricted area of analgesic effect, the technique of intermittent bolus infusion of epidural analgesics has been developed. The advantage of PIB is mainly in the maintenance of labor analgesia [5, 7]. Its use has been recently demonstrated in total knee arthroplasty and major abdominal and gynecological surgery, and its utility has been shown [8–10]. However, to our knowledge, this is the first randomized study to show the advantage of PIB in thoracotomy.

The reduction in the total amount of local anesthetic with intermittent bolus infusion compared with continuous infusion is consistent with the findings in labor analgesia reports and postoperative reports. In major

abdominal and gynecological surgery, the beneficial effect of PIB is noted on the first postoperative day and not on the day of the operation [9]. Sequential epidural bolus infusion provides superior epidural block compared with CEI [2].

Compared with bolus infusion, hemodynamic stability with CEI without bolus administration is superior; the incidence of hypotension reduced by 67% without using bolus infusion compared with that using bolus infusion [11]. However, PIB studies for postsurgical analgesia indicated no adverse effects [8–10]. With regard to the incidence of hypotension, the difference between our results and those of previous reports might be associated with differences in the site of epidural anesthesia and dose of local anesthetic. Hypotension occurred but was not significant in both groups, and there was a need for noradrenalin when epidural anesthesia involved puncture at Th8–10 [9]. On the other hand, when epidural anesthesia involved puncture at Th10–12 in open gynecological surgery [8] or L3–5 in total knee arthroplasty, [8] there was no hypotension requiring intervention. The bolus dose was 6 mL every hour in the major surgical study that reported hypotension, [9] and among studies that did not report hypotension, the doses were 4 mL every hour for open gynecological surgery [10] and 3 mL every hour for total knee arthroplasty [8]. We used a bolus of 5.1 mL every 90 min (3.4 mL every hour). Therefore, when PIB and CEI are used for a higher level of thoracic epidural anesthesia, attention should be paid to the bolus dose to avoid hypotension.

The present study has limitations. First, this is not double blinded study. Second, in this study, the dose and concentration of local anesthetic was single, and the total dose of local anesthetic and counts of PCA were less than that of preliminary studies. We need to re-examine the small dose and concentration of local anesthetics in future studies.

Conclusions

PIB can reduce local anesthetic consumption in thoracic surgery. However, it might result in adverse events, such as hypotension.

Abbreviations

BMI: Body mass index; CEI: Continuous epidural infusion; PCA: Patient-controlled analgesia; PIB: Programmed intermittent bolus; PONV: Postoperative nausea and vomiting; SBP: Systolic blood pressure; UMIN: University hospital medical information network; VAS: Visual analog scale

Acknowledgements

The authors would like to thank Enago (https://www.enago.jp/) for the English language review.

Authors' contributions

MH, KY: conceptualized and designed the study and wrote the manuscript; KS: analyzed data; and EN, SS: collected the data. All authors read and approved the manuscript.

Table 4 Frequency of hypotension events after surgery

	PIB ($n = 21$)	CEI ($n = 21$)	P-value
	n (%)	n (%)	
20% less than baseline SBP			
0-12 h	7(3.3)	1(0.5)	0.018
12-24 h	6(9.5)	3(4.7)	0.26
24-36 h	6(9.5)	4(6.3)	0.47
SBP less than 90 mmHg			
0-12 h	10(4.8)	4(1.9)	0.0495
12-24 h	5(7.9)	0(0.0)	0.017
24-36 h	4(6.3)	1(1.6)	0.15

Author details
[1]Department of Anesthesiology, Fukuoka University School of Medicine, 7-45-1, Nanakuma, Jonan-ku, Fukuoka 814-0180, Japan. [2]Operation rooms, Fukuoka University Hospital, Fukuoka, Japan.

References
1. Saeki H, Ishimura H, Higashi H, Kitagawa D, Tanaka J, Maruyama R, et al. Postoperative management using intensive patient-controlled epidural analgesia and early rehabilitation after an esophagectomy. Surg Today. 2009;39:476–80.
2. Ueda K, Ueda W, Manabe M. A comparative study of sequential epidural bolus technique and continuous epidural infusion. Anesthesiology. 2005; 103:126–9.
3. Patkar CS, Vora K, Patel H, Shah V, Modi MP, Parikh G. A comparison of continuous and intermittent bolus administration of 0.1% ropivacaine with 0.0002% fentanyl for epidural labor analgesia. J Anaesthesiol Clin Pharmacol. 2015;31:234–8.
4. George RB, Allen TK, Habib AS. Intermittent epidural bolus compared with continuous epidural infusions for labor analgesia: a systematic review and meta-analysis. Anesth Analg. 2013;116:133–44.
5. Carvalho B, George RB, Cobb B, McKenzie C, Riley ET. Implementation of programmed intermittent epidural bolus for the maintenance of labor analgesia. Anesth Analg. 2016;123:965–71.
6. Sng BL, Zeng Y, de Souza NNA, Leong WL, Oh TT, Siddiqui FJ, et al. Automated mandatory bolus versus basal infusion for maintenance of epidural analgesia in labour. Cochrane Database Syst Rev. 2018;5:CD011344.
7. Onuoha OC. Epidural analgesia for labor: continuous infusion versus programmed intermittent bolus. Anesthesiol Clin. 2017;35:1–14.
8. Kang S, Jeon S, Choe JH, Bang SR, Lee KH. Comparison of analgesic effects of programmed intermittent epidural bolus and continuous epidural infusion after total knee arthroplasty. Korean J Anesthesiol. 2013;65:S130–1.
9. Wiesmann T, Hoff L, Prien L, Torossian A, Eberhart L, Wulf H, et al. Programmed intermittent epidural bolus versus continuous epidural infusion for postoperative analgesia after major abdominal and gynecological cancer surgery: a randomized, triple-blinded clinical trial. BMC Anesthesiol. 2018;18:154.
10. Satomi S, Kakuta N, Murakami C, Sakai Y, Tanaka K, Tsutsumi YM. The efficacy of programmed intermittent epidural bolus for postoperative analgesia after open gynecological surgery: a randomized double-blinded study. Biomed Res Int. 2018. https://doi.org/10.1155/2018/6297247.
11. Gerhardt MA, Gunka VB, Miller RJ. Hemodynamic stability during labor and delivery with continuous epidural infusion. J Am Osteopath Assoc. 2006;106: 692–8.

15

Modified technique for thermal radiofrequency ablation of thoracic dorsal root ganglia under combined fluoroscopy and CT guidance

Raafat M. Reyad[1], Hossam Z. Ghobrial[1], Ehab H. Shaker[1]*[iD], Ehab M. Reyad[2], Mohammed H. Shaaban[3], Rania H. Hashem[3] and Wael M. Darwish[4]

Abstract

Background: This study is comparing thermal radiofrequency ablation (TRFA) of the thoracic dorsal root ganglia (TDRG) guided by Xper CT and fluoroscopy with the standard fluoroscopy.

Methods: This randomized clinical trial included 78 patients suffering from chronic refractory pain due to chest malignancies randomly allocated into one of two groups according to guidance of TRFA of TDRG. In CT guided group ($n = 40$) TRFA was done under integrated Xper CT-scan and fluoroscopy guidance, while it was done under fluoroscopy guidance only in standard group ($n = 38$). The primary outcome was pain intensity measured by visual analog scale (VAS) score, functional improvement and consumption of analgesics. The secondary outcome measures were patient global impression of changes (PGIC) and adverse effects.

Results: VAS scores decreased in the two groups compared to baseline values ($p < 0.001$) and were lower in CT guided group up to 12 weeks. Pregabalin and oxycodone consumption was higher in the standard group at 1, 4 and 12 weeks ($p < 0.001$). Functional improvement showed near significant difference between the two groups ($P = 0.06$ at week 1, 0.07 at week 4 respectively) while the difference was statistically significant at week 12 ($P = 0.04$). PGIC showed near significant difference only at week 1 ($P = 0.07$) while the per-patient adverse events were lower in CT guided group ($p = 0.027$).

Conclusions: Integrated modality guidance with Xper CT-scan and fluoroscopy together with suprapedicular inferior transforaminal approach may improve efficacy and safety of TRFA of TDRG for the treatment of intractable chest pain in cancer patients.

Keywords: Thermal radiofrequency ablation, Intractable pain, Chest malignancies, Transforaminal approach, Dorsal root ganglia, Suprapedicular approach

* Correspondence: ehabhanafy2006@yahoo.com
[1]Department of Anesthesia & Pain Management, National Cancer Institute, Cairo University, Cairo, Egypt

Background

Thoracic pain represents approximately 3–5% of patient visits to pain clinic worldwide [1]. Lung cancer is one of the three most common malignancies that are highly associated with pain,together with head and neck, breast cancers, and advanced or metastatic diseases increase the prevalence of pain from 51 to 66% in cancer patients [2]. Lung cancer is the most common cancer worldwide; 1.8 million cases are diagnosed annually (13% of all cancers diagnoses) [3]. Post-thoracotomy pain occurs in 30–50% of patients undergoing thoracotomy [4].

Pain is the presenting symptom in 20% of cases of lung cancer and it may be more distressing to patients with lung cancer than to patients with other cancers [5]. Pain affects the patient's psyche, sleep, behavior and ultimately quality of life. The management of such pain is challenging and it may be either medical or interventional. Interventional treatment of such refractory pain due to lung cancer could be attributed to multiplicity of pain generators (visceral-somatic-neuropathic) such as chest wall pain, costo-pleural syndrome, pancoast tumor, rib metastasis, post-thoracotomy pain syndrome, post-herpetic neuralgia and pain related to diagnostic or therapeutic procedures e.g. chemotherapy or radiotherapy-induced pain. Interventional therapies include epidural or intrathecal drug injection, intercostal nerve block, sympathectomy, rhizotomy, and percutaneous cervical cordotomy (PCC) [6]. Rhizotomy refers to the selective, segmental destruction of the dorsal sensory rootlets to interrupt pain perception by the spinal cord. This could be accomplished using neurosurgical or chemical means or using selective percutaneous procedures, such as cryoanalgesia and radiofrequency (RF) ablation [6].

There are many technical difficulties in approaching the deep-seated thoracic dorsal root ganglia (DRG) through the transforaminal route. The spine is kyphotic, with the tip at T6, and slightly scoliotic to the right side even in normal subjects [7]. Spinous processes are acute, especially at the T5-T8 level. In addition, broad and wide laminae together with narrow intervertebral foramina are also obstacles [8]. The intervertebral foramina are further masked by the facet joints and the crowded nature of the costovertebral and the costotransverse joints [9].

The extra guidance of Xper CT than conventional fluoroscopy may improve the success of the transforaminal approach to thoracic DRG considering all these factors of technical difficulties due to natural anatomical barriers lowering the efficacy of dorsal rhizotomy (which is still the standard interventional therapy for treating lung cancer pain worldwide). The authors hypothesize that combining the Xper CT scan with fluoroscopy to guide RF ablation through the transforaminal route can enhance its efficacy and safety in relieving the intractable pain of chest malignancies. The current study aimed to compare the results of thermal radiofrequency ablation (TRFA) of the thoracic DRG under combined Xper CT - fluoroscopy guidance with the standard fluoroscopy technique.

Methods

This single-blinded, parallel group, randomized clinical trial was conducted in the National Cancer Institute, Cairo University during the period from April 2017 to March 2018 after obtaining the approval of the Institutional Review Board (approval No.: 201617013. 2P). The study was retrospectively registered at clinicaltrials.gov on 04/22/2018 (Registration No.: NCT03533413). The study fulfilled the principles of the Helsinki Declaration and followed the Medical Research Involving Human Subjects Act (WMO). This study adheres to CONSORT guidelines for reporting clinical trials. The purpose, benefits, possible risks and expectations were explained to all patients before their enrollment in the study and a written informed consent was obtained from each patient. Patients were recruited from the pain clinic. Eligible patients were 18 years or older and suffering from chronic moderate-to-severe pain (VAS score ≥ 40 mm), due to chest malignancies and pain was refractory to the maximally tolerated dose of opioids for at least four weeks [10]. The malignancies included lung cancer, pleural mesothelioma, chest wall tumors and metastatic deposits of the chest. The exclusion criteria were sepsis, coagulopathy, malignant epidural invasion, distorted local anatomy, severe cardiorespiratory compromise, neuropsychiatric illness, history of drug dependence and known allergy to contrast media or the medications used.

Randomization, allocation, and concealment

Eighty patients were randomly allocated into one of two equal groups. In CT group ($n = 40$) TRFA of the thoracic DRG was conducted under Xper Guided CT fluoroscopy guidance, while the procedure was conducted under fluoroscopy guidance only in the standard group ($n = 40$). The random number list was concealed and checked just before a patient's allocation by personnel blinded to the study.

Technique for the fluoroscopy-guided procedure

The procedure was conducted in the fluoroscopy room where all anesthetic and resuscitation facilities were available. ASA-standard monitors (NIBP, pulse-oximetry, and EKG) were connected to the patient. A G20 intravenous (IV) line was fixed and O_2 via nasal prongs and a 1 g ceftriaxone (Longacef GSK, Cairo, Egypt) IV infusion was initiated. The procedure was conducted under the ASA recommendation of conscious alert sedation with a 0.5–1.0 µg/kg fentanyl IV (fentanyl citrate 50 µg/mL; Janssen Pharmaceutica, Beerse, Belgium) and a 0.5–1.0 µg/kg dexmedetomidine (Precedex 200 mcg/2 mL, Pfizer, USA) IV in addition to propofol (Diprivan 1%, Fresenius Kabi, USA) IV boluses during TRFA application. The patient was placed prone on a small pillow located under the chest, and the back of the patient was sterilized using 8% povidone iodide and draped. The needle was a Baylis RF needle (100 mm length, 10 mm active tip, curved, G20, sharp needle) (Baylis Medical Company Inc. Montreal, QC Canada). The selected level was checked by history, local examination for rib tenderness and possible neuropathic characters, e.g., allodynia. The fluoroscopic postero/anterior (PA) view was taken and squaring (alignment) of the targeted vertebra was attained by cephalocaudal orientation of the C-arm. An ipsilateral oblique view of 15° was completed and then the port of needle entry was located at the lower 1/3 to 1/4 of the lateral vertebral edge, under the articular pillar and the halo of the transverse process. As a rule, the port of needle entry must be within 4 cm of the midline (Rule of 4) to avoid injuring the parietal pleura [8]. Lidocaine 1% (Debocaine 2%,

Sigma-Tec, Egypt) was used for local infiltration of the skin and subcutaneous tissues. The RF cannula was advanced using the trajectory (tunnel) technique with a 15° oblique view and then with a dead-lateral view until the needle tip stopped at the lower- or mid-foraminal zone and behind the central line to avoid segmental blood supply and nerve root injury (Fig. 1). After a negative aspiration for blood, air or CSF, 0.5–1.0 ml of iohexol contrast medium (Omnipaque TM, Nycomed, Ireland) was injected to delineate the dorsal root ganglia, nerve roots, epidural space and the intercostal nerve path (Fig. 1). A thermocouple electrode was inserted and sensory stimulation at 50 Hz and up to 0.5 v and motor stimulation at 2 Hz and up to 1–1.5 v was conducted to verify the needle tip position (tingling paresthesia and/or intercostal muscle contraction inside the needle). Neural mapping of the affected dermatomal (intercostal) levels to be blocked was additionally performed by asking the patient if their original pain was at, above or below the level of sensory/motor stimulation and if paresthesia is concordant with his original pain. Additionally, the impendence was checked (normal range is 150–250 Ω inside the neural foramen). The pain level was checked again after

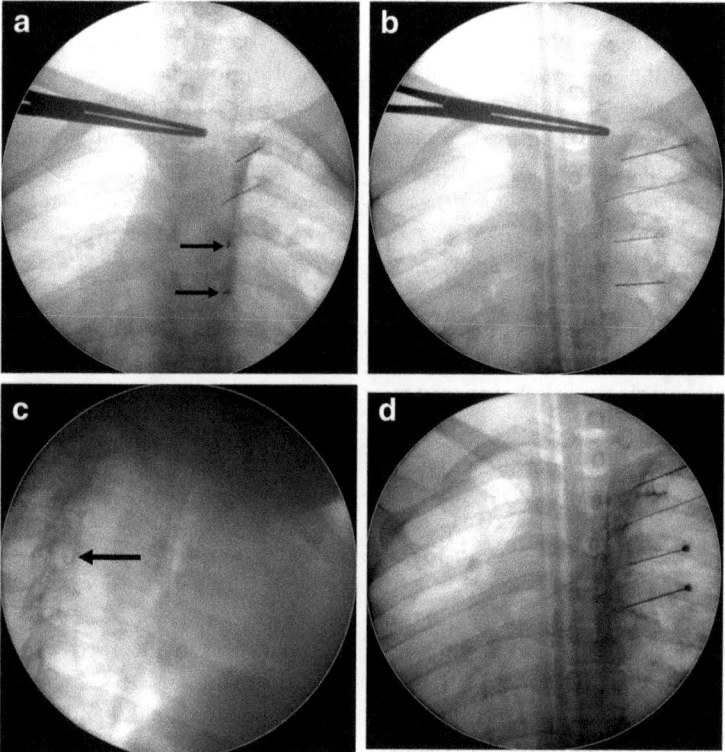

Fig. 1 Fluoroscopic pictures showing the technique of thoracic DRG transforaminal approach: **a)** ipsilateral 15° oblique view with 4 RF needles at T3, 4, 5, 6 levels (black arrows point at trajectory-end-on-needles orientation), **b)** P-A view showing the 4 needles tips nearly at the neural foramina, **c)** lateral view showing the RF needles tips in the transforaminal positions after contrast injection (black arrow points at the characteristic signet ring appearance of DRG), **d)** P-A view showing transforaminal, epidural and intercostal spread of the contrast at the targeted levels

injecting a lidocaine-betamethasone mixture (2 ml of 2% lidocaine/segment and 2 mg/ml betamethasone sodium phosphate plus 5 mg/ml betamethasone dipropionate) (Diprofos 2 mg + 5 mg/ml,MSD/Schering-Plough,NJ, USA). After 2 min, thermal lesioning was conducted using Baylis generator at 80 °C for 120 s twice (up and medial then down and medial to enlarge the lesion size of the DRG), and both sensory and motor stimulation were repeated upon rotation of the needle tip. The patient's back was dressed and the patient was transferred to the recovery unit where vital signs and pain and neurological findings were checked for 1–2 h before discharge. The patient was instructed clearly to consult the pain team if adverse effects happened, namely, chest pain or dyspnea (pneumothorax) and neurological insults (motor deficits).

Technique for the combined CT-fluoroscopy guided procedure

The patient is placed prone on the angio table (Allura Xper FD 20 Flat detector Fluoroscopy with Xper CT, Philips, Netherlands) (Fig. 2) and Xper CT scan of the desired chest levels is performed without contrast to localize the targeted neural foramina with the help of Xper Guide defining the entry point, the needle path and the needle target; thus optimizing the final position of the needle tip. RF stimulation and lesioning are carried out as before, and finally, chest scanogram is performed to rule out pneumothorax (Fig. 3).

In both groups all patients were converted to as needed immediate release oxycodone (Oxynorm® 5- 10 mg Mundipharm) capsules and the average daily required dose to achieve adequate analgesia was calculated then given as sustained release formula (Oxycontin® 10–20-40 mg Mundipharm) in the first visit of the patient after 1 week. Regarding Pregabalin (Lyrica®50–75-150 mg

Pfizer), the dose decreased by 25% each week according to patient response with maximum dose 600 mg per day.

A junior clinician of the pain clinic team that was blinded to the study groups was assigned to collect the data. The demographic data included age, gender, chest pathology, body mass index (BMI), duration of the procedure, the side of lesioning, the number of levels/patient, the estimated dose of irradiation exposure (ED), baseline VAS, and medication use. The patient evaluation was conducted 1, 4, and 12 weeks after the procedure. The patients were not allowed to review their previous scores.

The primary outcome measure was pain intensity measured by the visual analog scale (VAS). A 100 mm VAS was presented to the patient as a horizontal line with two ends; the left end represented no pain experienced and the right end represented experiencing the worst pain imaginable. The functional improvement was assessed as a self-reported score after pain procedures representing the percentage of pain reduction; 0–25% means no or minimal improvement, 25–50% means mild improvement, 50–75% means moderate improvement and 75–100% means marked relief [11]. The consumption of analgesics (mg/day) including oxycodone and pregabalin was recorded. The secondary outcome measure was assessed using patient satisfaction with the patient global impression of changes (PGIC) found in Table 1 [12].

The adverse effects were categorized into minor and major groups. The minor events included back pain, soreness, infection, hematoma, and bruises. The major events included pneumothorax, neuritis, motor deficits, and sensory changes, such as discomforting numbness and hypoesthesia, dysesthesia or anesthesia dolorosa.

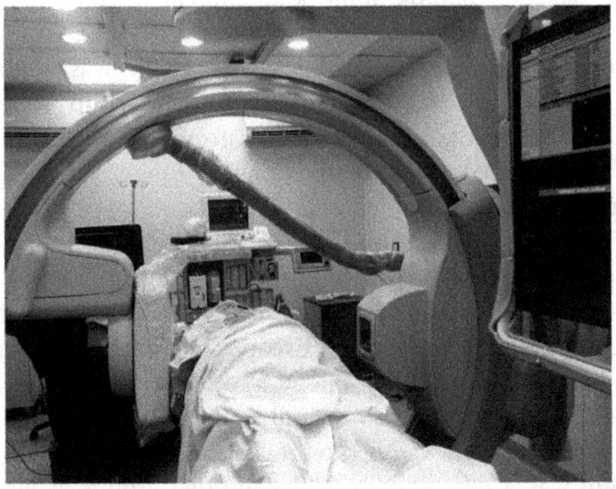

Fig. 2 Allura Xper FD 20 Flat detector Fluoroscopy with Xper CT, Philips, Netherlands

Calculation of the sample size

The required sample size was calculated using G*Power Software version 3.1.9 (Universität Düsseldorf, Germany). There were no previous trials comparing the two studied groups of the current trial. The hypothesis was one of "superiority" (that adding the CT to fluoroscopy- guidance would improve the outcome not just matching the traditional approach). We hypothesized that a difference of 3 in the VAS at 12 weeks after treatment would be clinically meaningful. With this difference and a pooled standard deviation of 4, a total of 29 subjects were needed to detect the difference between the two groups at an alpha level of 0.05 and a power of 0.8. Owing to the repeated measures and possible drop outs, the sample was increased by 20% for each condition. Therefore, a sample of 40 patients in each group was recruited in the study.

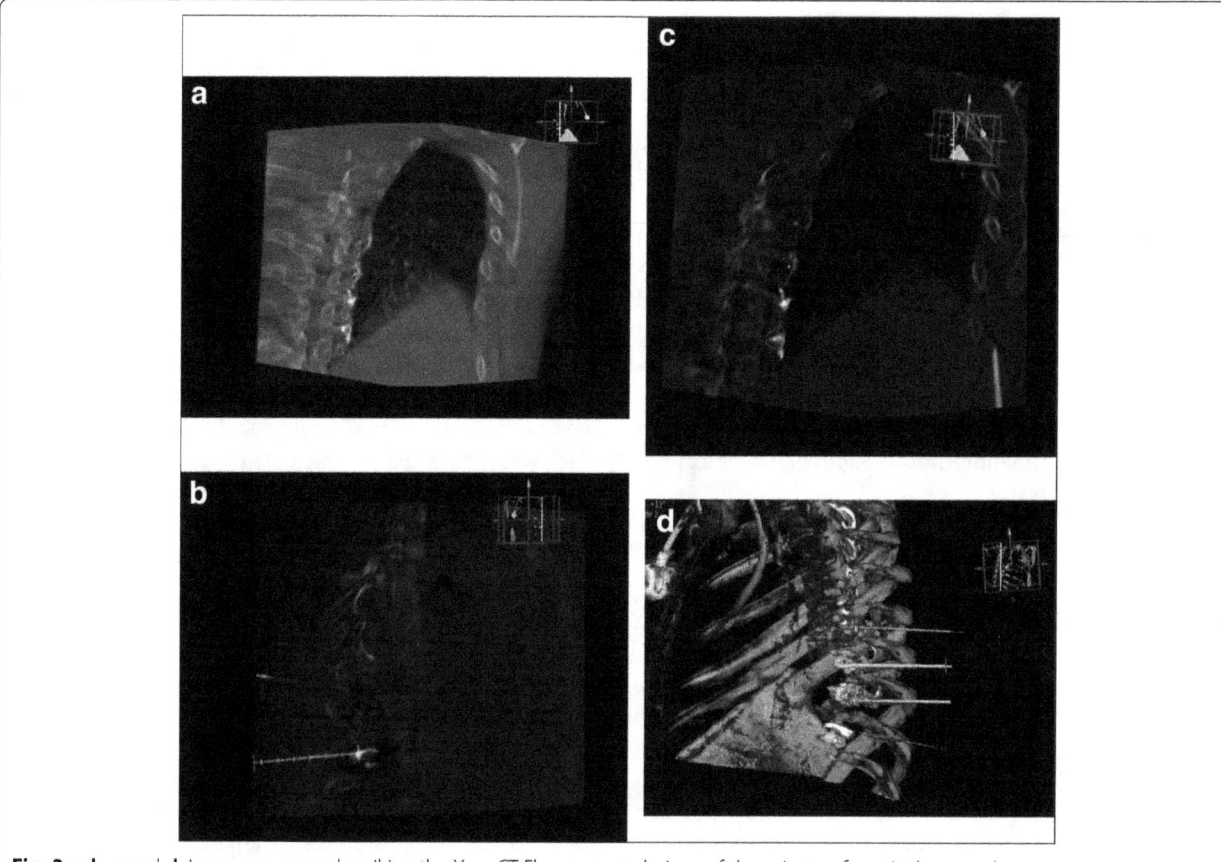

Fig. 3 a, b, c and **d:** image sequence describing the Xper CT-Fluroscopy technique of thoracic transforaminal approach.

Statistical analysis

Data were analyzed using IBM© SPSS© Statistics version 23 (IBM© Corp., Armonk, NY, USA). Data were summarized as a mean and standard deviation or median and range for quantitative data and frequency and percentage for categorical data. The comparisons between quantitative variables were made using the unpaired t-test or the Mann-Whitney test. For comparison of the serial measurements within each group, a mixed linear model was applied. Comparisons of categorical data were made using the Chi-square test or Fisher's exact

test as appropriate. All tests were two-tailed. A p value < 0.05 was considered significant.

Results

Two patients in standard group were lost during the follow-up (Fig. 4). There were no statistically significant differences between the two groups regarding the baseline demographic and clinical characteristics (Table 2) apart from the estimated dose (ED) of irradiation for each injected level, which was highly significant ($p < 0.001$): the CT-guided group was 2 folds higher than the Standard group. The duration of the procedure was significantly longer in the C Group ($p = 0.037$) (Table 3).

The VAS scores decreased significantly in the two groups at all of the follow-up points compared to baseline values ($p < 0.001$ for all comparisons). There was no significant difference in VAS score between both groups at baseline ($p = 0.380$). The VAS scores were lower in the CT-guided group compared to the standard group at 1, 4, and 12 weeks after the procedure (Fig. 5). However, there was a difference between the two groups at week 4, week 8 and week 12 (Fig. 5). Using a linear mixed model, we determined that there was a clear difference

Table 1 Patient Global Impression of Changes (PGIC)

PGIC	Score
Very much improved	1
Much improved	2
Minimally improved	3
No change	4
Worse	5
Much worse	6
Very much worse	7

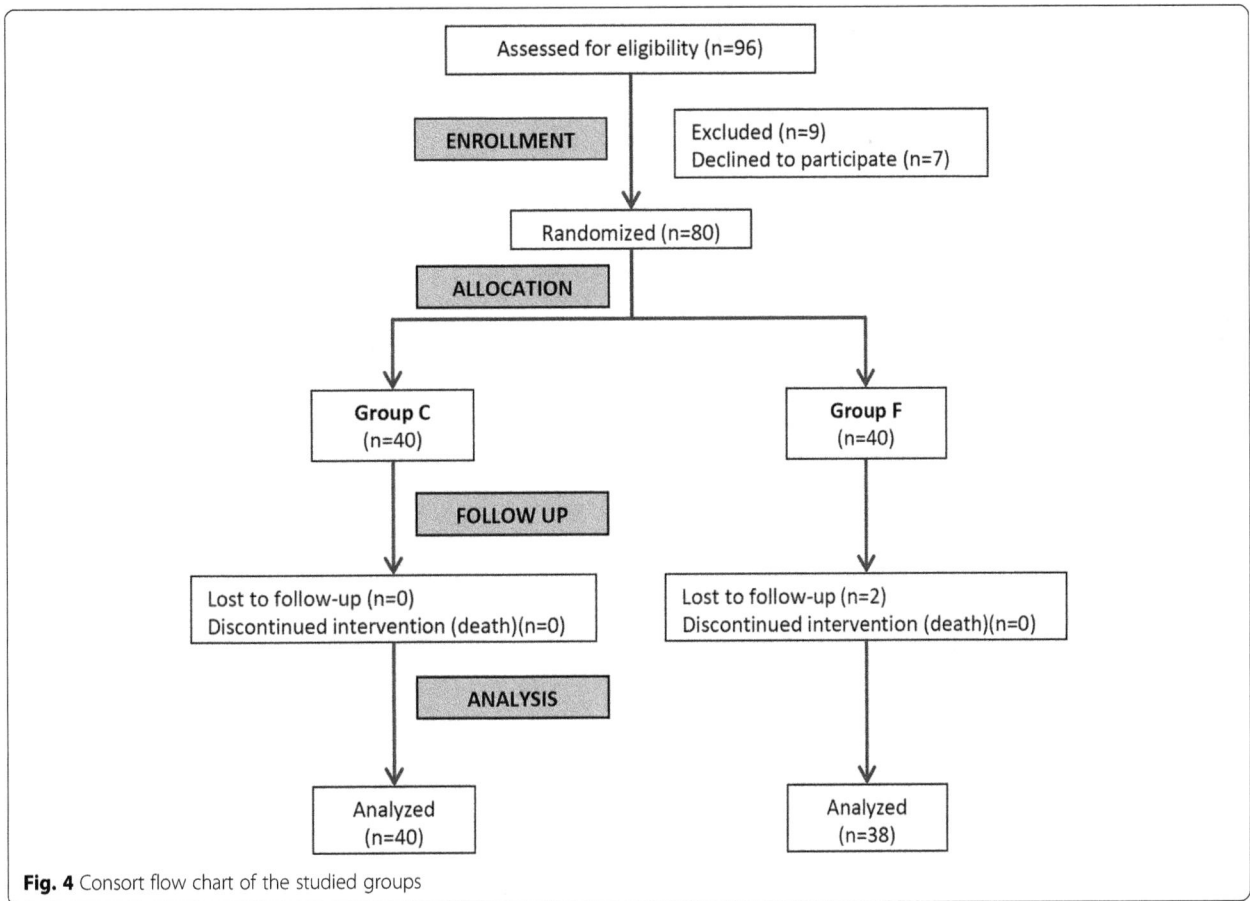

Fig. 4 Consort flow chart of the studied groups

in the average change of VAS score over time between the two groups ($P < 0.001$), as shown in Fig. 5. As a result of comparing between the two groups at each time point, we found that there was a significant difference at week 4 ($P < 0.001$), week 8 ($P < 0.001$), and week 12 ($P = 0.001$).

Table 2 Baseline demographic and clinical characteristics of the two studied groups

	CT-guided group $n = 40$	Standard group $n = 38$	p value
Age (years)	57.0 ± 11.7	59.2 ± 13.2	0.438
Gender (male/female)	29/11	25/13	0.521
Chest pathology			
Lung cancer	19 (47.5%)	20 (52.6%)	1.000
Pleural mesothelioma	14 (35.0%)	13 (34.2)	
Chest secondaries	5 (12.5%)	4 (10.5%)	
Chest wall masses	2 (5.0%)	1 (2.6%)	
Body mass index (kg/m2)	29.2 ± 5.2	28.3 ± 4.3	0.409
Side of treatment (Rt/Lt)	21/19	21/17	0.807

Data are supplied as mean ± SD, numbers (%).

Table 3 Procedural details in the two studied groups

	CT-guided group $n = 40$	Standard group $n = 38$	p value
Duration of procedure (minutes)	26.2 ± 10.7	21.3 ± 9.6	0.037
Number of levels treated/patient			
2 levels	15 (37.5%)	14 (36.8%)	0.862
3 levels	12 (30.0%)	11 (28.9%)	
4 levels	13 (32.5%)	13 (34.3%)	
VAS score before the procedure	72.4 ± 5.2	73.4 ± 4.9	0.385
Oxycodone consumption/day (mg/day)	78 ± 12	80 ± 10	0.428
Pregabalin (mg/day)	311 ± 35	304 ± 23	0.303
Exposure time per level (sec)	21.7 ± 8.1	19.05 ± 6.3	0.112
Estimated dose per level (mGy)	0.28 ± 0.083	0.57 ± 0.23	< 0.001

Data are supplied as mean ± SD, numbers (%).
VAS visual analogue scale, mGy = milligray.

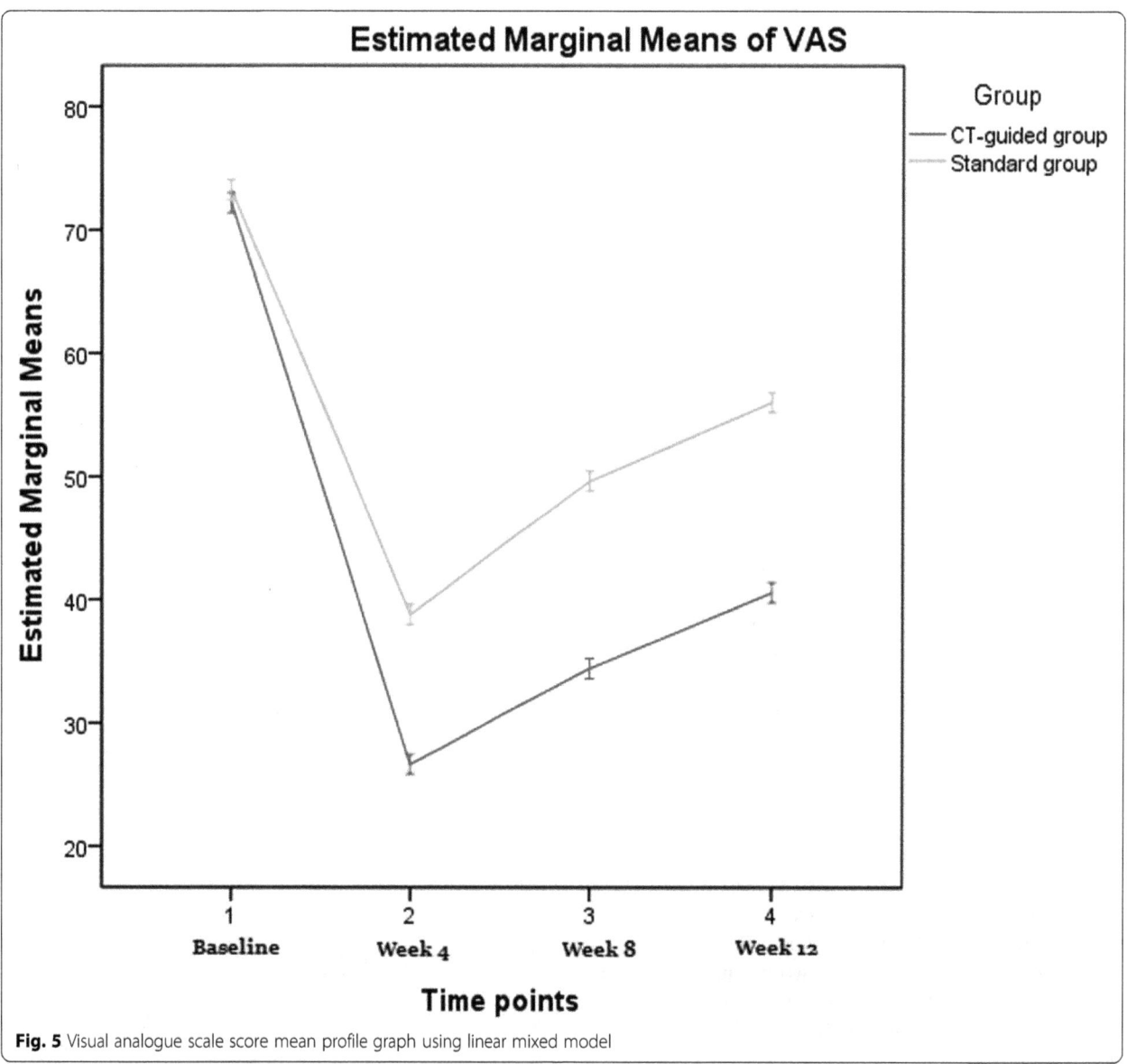

Fig. 5 Visual analogue scale score mean profile graph using linear mixed model

Oxycodone and pregabalin consumption decreased in the two groups at all of the follow-up points compared with the baseline values. There was a significant difference between the two groups in oxycodone and pregabalin consumption (Figs. 6 and 7).

Functional improvement (FI) was better (nearly significant) in the CT-guided group at weeks 1 and 4, while it was significant at week 12 (Fig. 8).

Patient satisfaction (PGIC) showed a higher indication of improvement at weeks 1, 4, and 12, but these were not statistically significant apart from week 1 which was nearly significant (Fig. 9).

The per-patient adverse events occurrence was significantly lower in the CT-guided group (p = 0.027) (Table 4). No infection, motor deficits, or pneumothorax were recorded.

Discussion

The current study demonstrated that selective TRF rhizotomy of thoracic DRG through the inferior transforaminal approach in intractable chest pain cases associated with cancer seems to be of better efficacy if performed under the combined guidance of a CT scan and fluoroscopy (Given the improvement in VAS and FI, and the higher percentages of "very much improvement" in Group C in Weeks 1, 4, and 12, that it is quite likely that the lack of statistical significance for the PGIC was due to insufficient power stemming from the small sample size).

Interventional pain procedures are indicated for refractory pain when analgesic drugs are ineffective or associated with intolerable side effects [13]. In this study, we performed TRFA at the transforaminal station adjacent

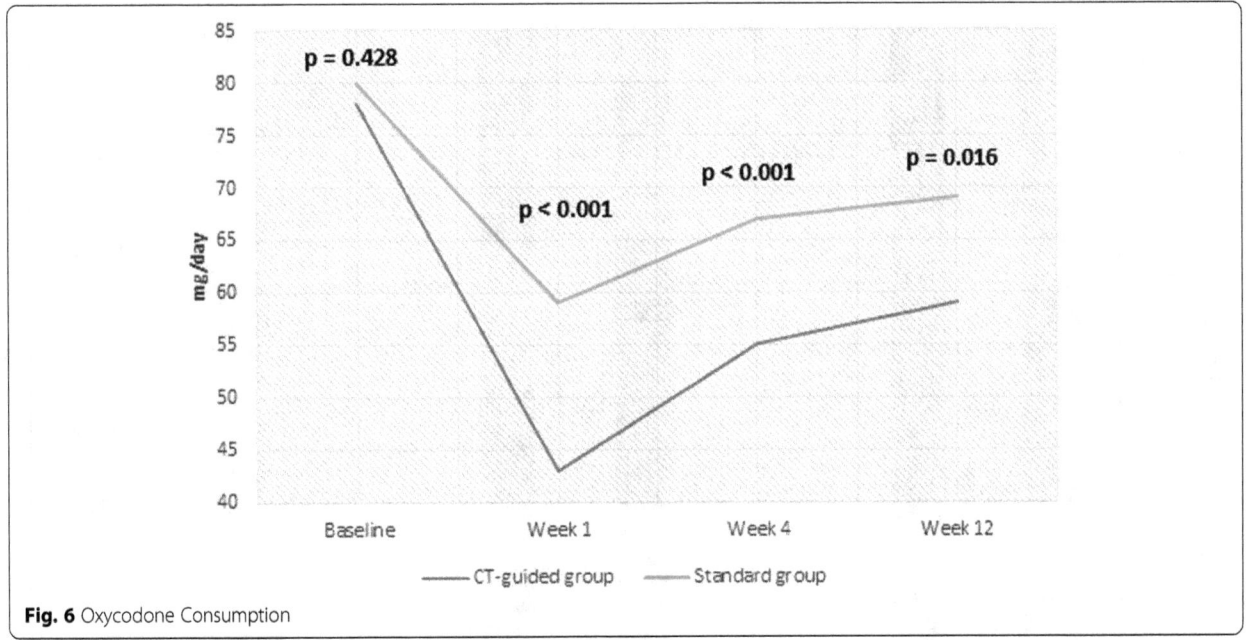

Fig. 6 Oxycodone Consumption

to the DRG assuming its superiority to many interventions. The transforaminal approach may be considered target-specific (i.e. adjacent to DRG), which allows a lower risk of inadvertent dural puncture [14]. It also demonstrated therapeutic values in managing radicular pain in many clinical trials [15]. Lastly, the selected dermatomal segment is only addressed in cases of TRF-DRG without the need to cover the segments above and below as performed in intercostal nerve blocks (the overlap phenomenon).

Paravertebral and intercostal nerve lesioning are efficient and simple procedures that can be performed at the bedside without guidance [16]. They have many drawbacks, such as short-lived, should be repeated [17], lower analgesic efficacy [18], and pneumothorax [13, 16]. Unlike the relative constant position of DRG in the neural foramen, peripheral nerve lesioning may be misplaced in cases of tumor infiltration. Moreover, it may induce deafferentation pain and miss a proximal pain generator [19].

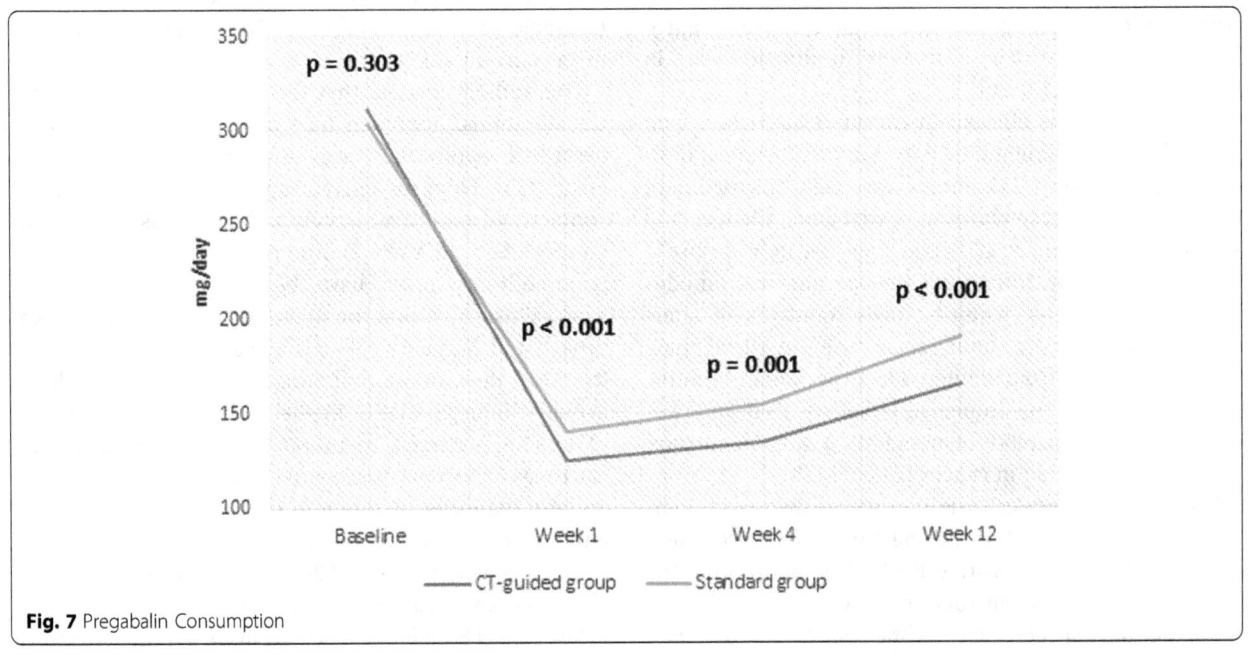

Fig. 7 Pregabalin Consumption

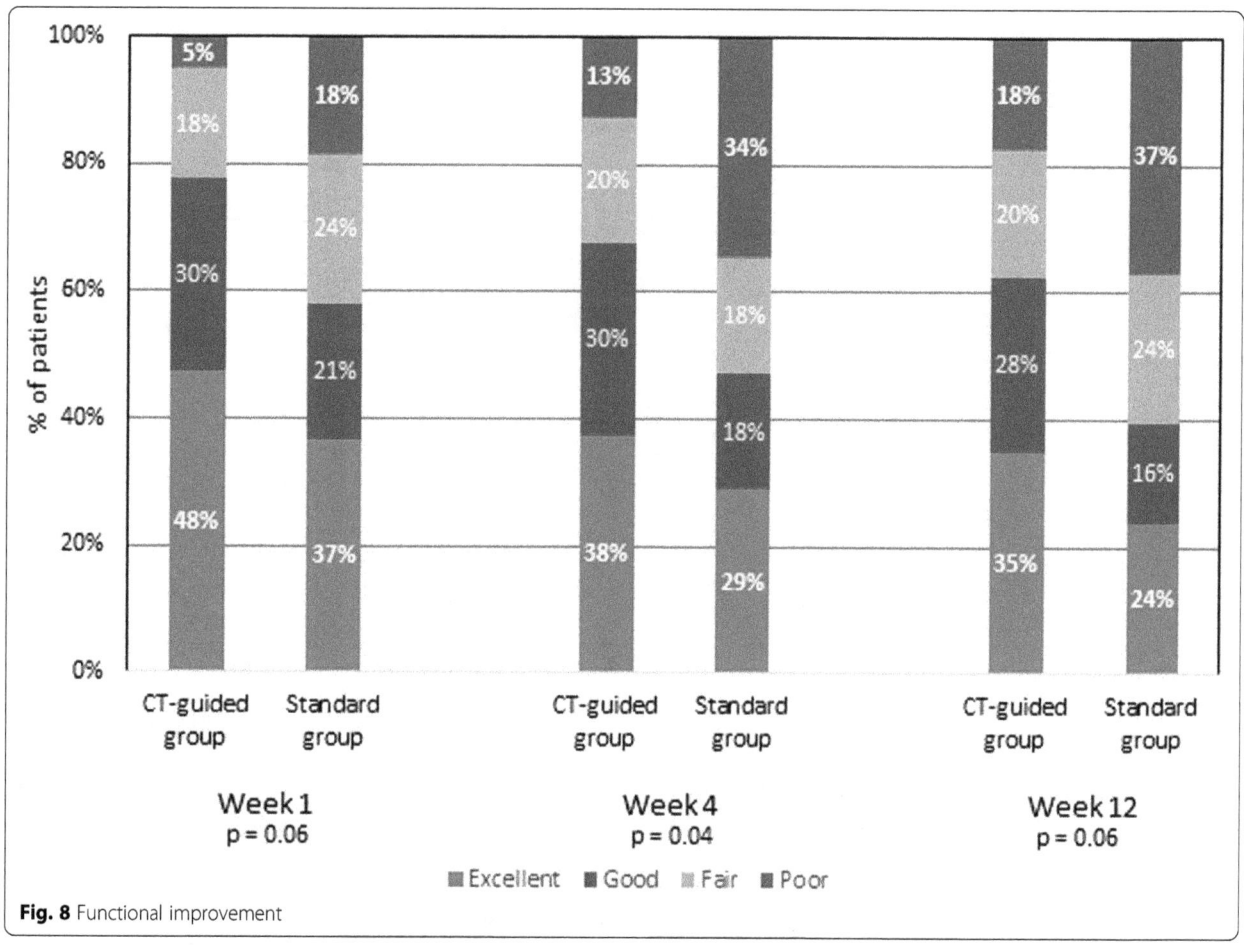

Fig. 8 Functional improvement

Dorsal chemical rhizotomy (epidural or intrathecal) may provide satisfactory analgesia for patients with lung cancer pain. However, it is associated by uncontrolled intraspinal spread and high risk for neurological deficits which ultimately limits its use in clinical practice [13, 20].

Although PCC is efficient in cancer-related chest pain [21] it has many limitations. For example; technical difficulty, 3% mortality, 11% motor weakness, mirror-image dysesthesia, and respiratory, hemodynamic, bladder and sexual dysfunction are all barriers against its widespread use [22]. Similarly, intrathecal therapy and neuromodulation are expensive requiring high standards of aftercare, which greatly limit their use in developing countries. Aside from limited life expectancy, immune compromise and neutropenia, radiation field interference and the possibility of neoplastic epidural invasion are special limitation in cancer patients [23].

Numerous anatomical barriers against the transforaminal approach in the thoracic spine have been previously described [7, 9]. For accurate RF-DRG application at the T7 level and above, van Kleef et al. created small holes in the laminae of thoracic vertebrae using 14G Kirschner

wires to get into the vicinity of the thoracic intervertebral foramina [24]. A CT-scan might provide more precision in locating the thoracic DRG. This can explain the favorable results of combined CT/fluoroscopy guidance in the current study.

The authors assume that the technique of an inferior transforaminal approach may be superior to previously described approaches, e.g. the approach by Charles Gauci [25]. First, the current approach entails less bony contact and periosteal irritation, hence, less patient discomfort. Second, there is little risk of pneumothorax (no pneumothorax cases have been documented in our work).Third, the concept of inferior suprapedicular approach and Kambin's safe triangle achieves greater validity [26] due to several proposed benefits such as avoiding injury to DRG in the superior neural foramen [27]. The peridural membrane of the suprapedicular canal has an evident nociceptive role in a manner similar to what happens in the inflamed synovium or periosteum in the case of joint or bone pain [28].

In the current study, T2-T8 levels were selected to avoid the catastrophic vascular events that may occur below the T8 due to vascular insult of the artery of

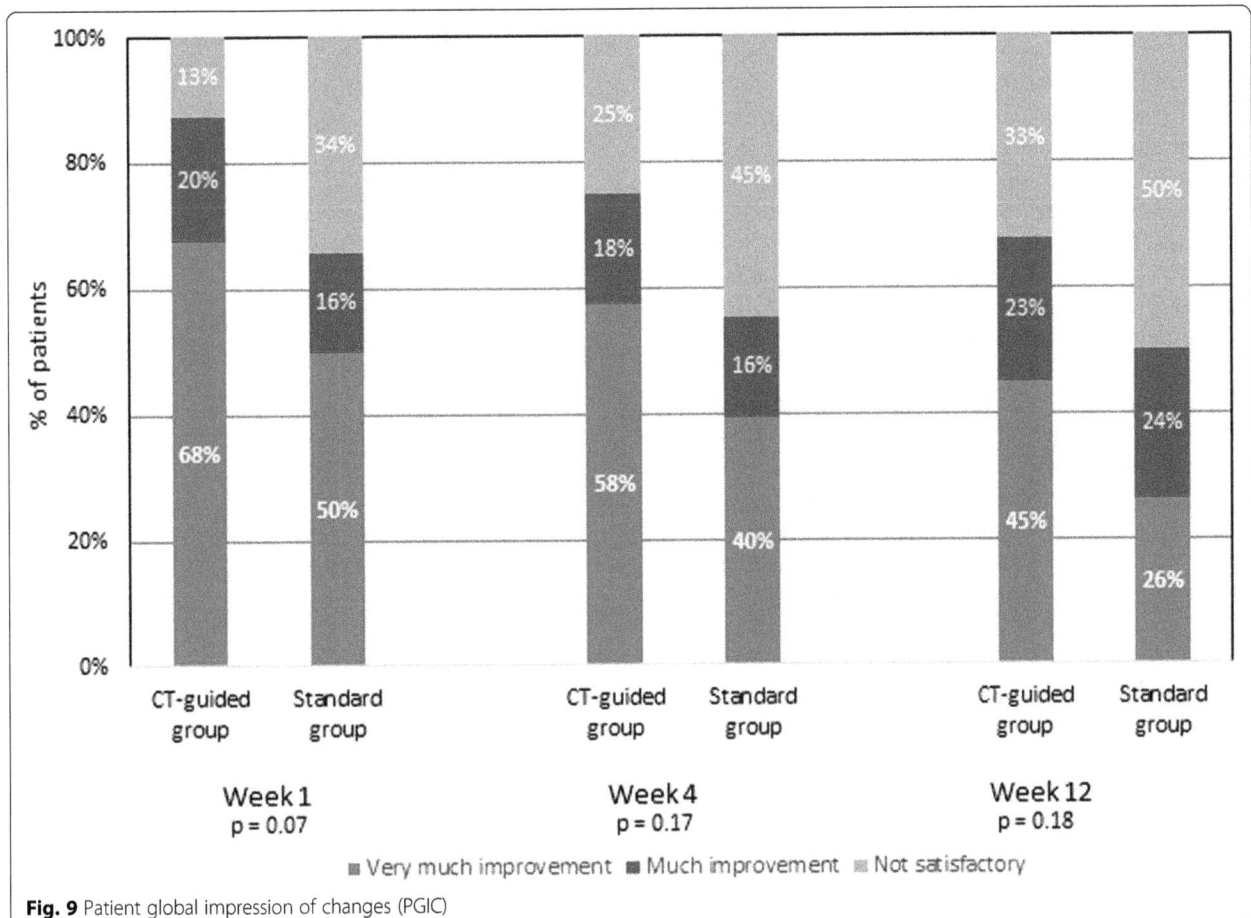

Fig. 9 Patient global impression of changes (PGIC)

Adamkiewicz, "which is the main blood supply of the anterior spinal cord below T8 [29]. Murthy et al. have identified the position of the artery of Adamkiewicz using digital subtraction angiography in the upper half of the neural foramen in 97% of patients and absent in the lower 10% of the foramen [30]. Moreover, the T2 to T8 levels - in general - are the segmental dermatomes commonly affected by chest pain pathologies.

Table 4 adverse effects in both groups

Adverse effects	CT-guided group n = 40	Standard group n = 38	p value
Minor complications			
Back pain	4 (10.0)	5 (13.2)	0.734
Soreness	7 (17.5)	8 (21.1)	0.691
Hematoma	1 (2.5)	2 (5.3)	0.610
Major complications			
Neuritis	3 (7.5)	8 (21.1)	0.086
Sensory deficits	3 (7.5)	5 (13.2)	0.476
Anesthesia dolorosa	1 (2.5)	1 (2.6)	1.000
*Per-patient adverse effects	6 (15)	14 (36.8)	0.027

Data are supplied as number and frequencies.

The neuroablative RF was applied to the DRG and not the pulsed (neuromodulatory) RF for many reasons. Pulsed RF is for short-term pain relief [31], and its neuromodulatory mechanisms take 3–4 weeks to work, which is too long for cancer patients with intractable pain [32]. In addition, TRF has been postulated to be more efficient for different types of pain, e.g., idiopathic trigeminal neuralgia [33], glossopharyngeal therapy for oropharyngeal cancer [34], and facetal medial branch block [11]. Nonparticulate steroids (betamethasone) were used in conjunction with lidocaine before TRF to reduce the occurrence of neuritis (its incidence was 7.5% in the C group versus 32.5% in van Kleef's work). Steroids have potential analgesic effects [35] while lidocaine was used for its analgesic, vasodilator and neuroprotective properties.

In the current work, the extra-guidance technique using the Xper CT reflected a better efficacy with a moderate increase of irradiation hazards (2 folds increase in ED). The implication of CT as a guidance tool has been used for interventional pain procedures, such as celiac plexus and lumbar sympathetic blocks [36, 37]. It allows better visualization of the whole needle path, surrounding soft tissues, and vascular and bony structures [38]. However, CT-associated exposure to excessive irradiation may induce carcinogenesis, genetic mutation and several other hazards [37, 38]. In previous studies conducted by Hoang et al. [39] and Schmid et al. [40] comparing irradiation dose during pain interventions guided by fluoroscopy versus CT, Hoang et al. reported 4 times more radiation exposure during CT than fluoroscopy [39]. In recent work published by Maino et al. [37] in 2018, the ED for lumbar facetal and transforaminal injections was calculated to be 8 to 10 times higher under CT versus fluoroscopy. The lower ED in the current study (2 folds) could be attributed to Xper CT guide technique for fast and accurate RF needle positioning. CT guidance is absolutely contraindicated in pregnant and pediatrics populations; however it improves anatomic localization, technical precision, post-procedures outcome and lessens the complications rate, hence it is widely practiced in many interventional procedures such as CT guided PCC, thoracic DRG-RF and many other techniques according to the clinical situation and physician judgment.

In conclusion, the integrated guidance of Xper CT-scan and fluoroscopy may improve the efficacy of TRF of thoracic DRG for the treatment of intractable chest pain in cancer patients. According to the authors' knowledge, this is the first RCT studying the efficacy and safety of this technique for thoracic DRG-TRF in intractable chest cancer pain. Moreover, we stressed on the inferior transforaminal suprapedicular technique in the thoracic spine region.

Limitations and recommendations, this study is a single center work and single blinded hence multicentric meta-analysis is recommended with a larger sample size of patients for verification of the data of the current work. Furthermore, a longer duration of follow up might be helpful for better evaluation and stratification of guidelines in treating lung cancer pain. Surgical confidence was not considered in the current work and should be respected in further upcoming researches.

Abbreviations
ANOVA: Analysis of variants; ASA: American society of Anesthesiologists; CT: Computerized Tomography; DRG: Dorsal root ganglia; ED: Estimated dose of irradiation exposure; EKG: Electrocardiogram; FI: Functional improvement; IV: Intravenous; mGy: Milligray; NIBP: Non-invasive blood pressure; PA: Postero-anterior; PCC: Pecutaneous cervical cordotomy; PGIC: Patient global impression of changes; PRF: Pulsed radiofrequency; RF: Radiofrequency; TDRG: Thoracic dorsal root ganglia; TRFA: Thermal radiofrequency ablation; VAS: Visual analog scale

Acknowledgements
Not applicable.

Authors' contributions
R M put the research hypothesis, explained to the patients and did the clinical work. H Z carried out statistical analysis of the data and shared the clinical work. E H(corresponding author) wrote the manuscript, analyzed, interpreted the patient data and shared the clinical work. E M collected the data and helped in the statistical analysis. M S and R H shared the radiological part of the study and reviewed the manuscript while W D helped in radiological interpretation of the study and reviewed the manuscript. All authors read and approved the final manuscript.

Author details
[1]Department of Anesthesia & Pain Management, National Cancer Institute, Cairo University, Cairo, Egypt. [2]Department of Clinical Pathology, National Hepatology and Tropical Medicine Research Institute, Cairo, Egypt. [3]Department of Diagnostic & Interventional Radiology, Faculty of Medicine, Cairo University, Cairo, Egypt. [4]Department of Diagnostic & Interventional Radiology, National Cancer Institute, Cairo University, Cairo, Egypt.

References
1. Lou L, Gauci CA. Radiofrequency treatment in thoracic pain. Pain Pract. 2002;2:224–5.
2. Van den Beuken-van Everdingen MHJ, Hochstenbach LMJ, Joosten EAJ, Tjan-Heijnen VC, Janssen DJ. Update on prevalence of pain in patients with Cancer: systematic review and meta-analysis. J Pain Symptom Manag. 2016; 51:1070–90.
3. Ferlay J, Steliarova-Foucher E, Lortet-Tieulent J, Rosso S, Coebergh JW, Comber H, et al. Cancer incidence and mortality patterns in Europe: estimates for 40 countries in 2012. Eur J Cancer. 2013;49(6):1374–403.
4. Humble SR, Dalton AJ, Li L. A systematic review of therapeutic interventions to reduce acute and chronic post-surgical pain after amputation, thoracotomy or mastectomy. Eur J Pain. 2015;19:451–65.
5. Simmons CPL, Macleod N, Laird BJA. Clinical Management of Pain in advanced lung Cancer. Clin Med Insights Oncol. 2012;6:331–46.
6. Zuurmond WWA, Perez RSGM, Loer SA. Role of cervical cordotomy and other neurolytic procedures in thoracic cancer pain. Curr Opin Support Palliat Care. 2010;4:6–10.
7. Ruiz-Lopez R, Pichot C, Raj PP. Spinal neuroaxial blocks. In: Raj PP, Lou L, Erdine S, et al., eds. Interventional Pain Management: Image-Guided Procedures. 2nd ed. Saunders Elsevier; 2008:267.
8. Erdine S, Talu G. Spinal neuroaxial blocks. In: Raj PP, Lou L, Erdine S, et al., eds. Interventional Pain Management: Image-Guided Procedures. 2nd ed. Saunders Elsevier; 2008:255–266.
9. Zhou L, Schneck CD, Shao Z. The anatomy of dorsal ramus nerves and its implications in lower Back pain. Neurosci Med. 2012;03:192.
10. Rad AE, Kallmes DF. Correlation between preoperative pain duration and percutaneous Vertebroplasty outcome. Am J Neuroradiol. 2011;32:1842–5.
11. Costandi S, Garcia-Jacques M, Dews T, Kot M, Wong K, Azer G, et al. Optimal temperature for radiofrequency ablation of lumbar medial branches for treatment of facet-mediated Back pain. Pain Pract. 2016;16(8):961–8.
12. Dworkin RH, Turk DC, Wyrwich KW, Beaton D, Cleeland CS, Farrar JT, et al. Interpreting the clinical importance of treatment outcomes in chronic pain clinical trials: IMMPACT recommendations. J Pain. 2008;9:105–21.
13. Hochberg U, Elgueta MF, Perez J. Interventional analgesic Management of Lung Cancer Pain. Front Oncol. 2017;7:17.
14. Manchikanti L, Singh V, Pampati V, Boswell MV, Benyamin RM, Hirsch JA, ASIPP. Description of documentation in the management of chronic spinal pain. Pain Physician. 2009;12:E199–224.
15. Son K-M, Lee S-M, Lee GW, Ahn MH, Son JH. The impact of lumbosacral transitional vertebrae on therapeutic outcomes of Transforaminal epidural injection in patients with lumbar disc herniation. Pain Pract. 2016;16:688–95.
16. Wong FCS, Lee TW, Yuen KK, Lo SH, Sze WK, Tung SY. Intercostal nerve blockade for cancer pain: effectiveness and selection of patients. Hong Kong Med J. 2007;13:266–70.
17. Axelsson K, Gupta A. Local anaesthetic adjuvants: neuraxial versus peripheral nerve block. Curr Opin Anaesthesiol. 2009;22:649–54.
18. Cohen SP, Sireci A, Wu CL, Larkin TM, Williams KA, Hurley RW. Pulsed radiofrequency of the dorsal root ganglia is superior to pharmacotherapy or pulsed radiofrequency of the intercostal nerves in the treatment of chronic postsurgical thoracic pain. Pain Physician. 2006;9:227–35.
19. Gulati A, Shah R, Puttanniah V, Hung JC, Malhotra V. A retrospective review and treatment paradigm of interventional therapies for patients suffering from intractable thoracic chest wall pain in the oncologic population. Pain Med. 2015;16:802–10.
20. El-Sayed GG. A new catheter technique for thoracic subarachnoid neurolysis in advanced lung cancer patients. Pain Pract. 2007;7:27–30.
21. France BD, Lewis RA, Sharma ML, Poolman M. Cordotomy in mesothelioma-related pain: a systematic review. BMJ Support Palliat Care. 2014;4:19–29.

22. Raslan AM. Percutaneous computed tomography-guided radiofrequency ablation of upper spinal cord pain pathways for cancer-related pain. Neurosurgery. 2008;62:226–34.

23. Pope JE, Deer TR, Bruel BM, Falowski S. Clinical uses of Intrathecal therapy and its placement in the pain care algorithm. Pain Pract. 2016;16:1092–106.

24. van Kleef M, Barendse GA, Dingemans WA. Effects of producing a radiofrequency lesion adjacent to the dorsal root ganglion in patients with thoracic segmental pain. Clin J Pain. 1995;11:325–32.

25. Gauci CA. Thoracic DRG RF/PRF. In: Gauci CA, ed. Manual of RF Techniques: A Practical Manual of Radiofrequency Procedures in Chronic Pain Management, 3rd ed. CoMedical; 2011:128.

26. Bosscher HA, Heavner JE. Treatment of common low Back pain: a new approach to an old problem. Pain Pract. 2015;15:509–17.

27. Civelek E, Solmaz I, Cansever T. Radiological analysis of the triangular working zone during Transforaminal endoscopic lumbar discectomy. Asian Spine J. 2012;6:98–104.

28. Van Dun PLS, Girardin MRG. Embryological study of the spinal dura and its attachment into the vertebral canal. Int J Osteopath Med. 2006;9:85–93.

29. White ML, El-Khoury GY. Neurovascular injuries of the spinal cord. Eur J Radiol. 2002;42:117–26.

30. Murthy NS, Maus TP, Behrns CL. Intraforaminal location of the great anterior radiculomedullary artery (artery of Adamkiewicz): a retrospective review. Pain Med. 2010;11:1756–64.

31. Ke M, Fan Yinghui, Jin Yi, Huang Xuehua , Liu Xiaoming, , Cheng Zhijun, et al. Efficacy of pulsed radiofrequency in the treatment of thoracic postherpetic neuralgia from the angulus costae: a randomized, double-blinded, controlled trial. Pain Physician 2013; 16:15–25.

32. Sluijter M. The physics of radiofrequency and pulsed radiofrequency. In: Gauci CA, ed. Manual of RF Techniques: A Practical Manual of Radiofrequency Procedures in Chronic Pain Management, 3rd ed. CoMedical; 2011:39.

33. Erdine S, Ozyalcin NS, Cimen A, Celik M, Talu GK, Disci R. Comparison of pulsed radiofrequency with conventional radiofrequency in the treatment of idiopathic trigeminal neuralgia. Eur J Pain. 2007;11:309–13.

34. Khan KM, Iqbal M, Ashfaq A. Management of refractory secondary glossobpharyngeal neuralgia with percutaneous radiofrequency thermocoagulation. Anaesth Pain Intensive Care. 2010;14:38–41.

35. Uchida K. Radiofrequency treatment of the thoracic paravertebral nerve combined with glucocorticoid for refractory neuropathic pain following breast cancer surgery. Pain Physician. 2009;12:E277–83.

36. Kambadakone A, Thabet A, Gervais DA, Mueller PR, Arellano RS. CT guided celiac plexus neurolysis: a review of anatomy ,indications , technique , and tips for successful treatment. Radio Graphics. 2011;31:1599–621.

37. Maino P, Presilla S, Franzone PA, Van Kuijk SMJ, Perez R, Koetsier E. Radiation dose exposure for lumabar transforaminal epidural steroid injections and facet joint blocks under CT vs. fluoroscopic guidance. Pain Pract. 2018;18(6):798–804.

38. Wrixon AD. New recommendations from the international commission on radiological protection – a review. Phys Med Biol. 2008;53:R41–60.

39. Hoang JK, Yoshizumi TT, Toncheva G. Radiation dose exposure for lumbar spine epidural steroid injections :a comparison of conventional fluoroscopy data and CT fluoroscopy techniques. Am J Roentgenol. 2011;197:778–82.

40. Schmid G, Schmitz A, Borchardt D. Effective .Dose of CT and fluoroscopic guided perineural/epidural injections of the lumbar spine: a comparative study. Cardio Vasc Intervent Radiol. 2006;29:84–91.

16

Effect of sedation with dexmedetomidine or propofol on gastrointestinal motility in lipopolysaccharide-induced endotoxemic mice

Haiqing Chang[1†], Shuang Li[1†], Yansong Li[1], Hao Hu[2], Bo Cheng[1], Jiwen Miao[1], Hui Gao[1], Hongli Ma[1], Yanfeng Gao[1*] and Qiang Wang[1*]

Abstract

Background: Sepsis often accompanies gastrointestinal motility disorder that contributes to the development of sepsis in turn. Propofol and dexmedetomidine, as widely used sedatives in patients with sepsis, are likely to depress gastrointestinal peristalsis. We queried whether propofol or dexmedetomidine, at sedative doses, aggravated sepsis-induced ileus.

Methods: Sedative/Anesthetic Scores and vital signs of lipopolysaccharide (LPS)-induced endotoxemic mice were measured during sedation with propofol or dexmedetomidine. Endotoxemic mice were divided into 10% fat emulsion, propofol, saline, and dexmedetomidine group. The gastric emptying, small intestinal transit, tests of colonic motility, gastrointestinal transit and whole gut transit were evaluated at 15 mins and 24 h after intraperitoneal injection of sedatives/vehicles respectively.

Results: 40 mg·kg^{-1} propofol and 80 μg·kg^{-1} dexmedetomidine induced a similar depth of sedation with comparable vital signs except that dexmedetomidine strikingly decreased heart rate in endotoxemic mice. Dexmedetomidine markedly inhibited gastric emptying ($P = 0.006$), small intestinal transit ($P = 0.006$), colonic transit ($P = 0.0006$), gastrointestinal transit ($P = 0.0001$) and the whole gut transit ($P = 0.034$) compared with the vehicle, whereas propofol showed no depression on all parts of gastrointestinal motility 15 mins after administration. The inhibitive effects of dexmedetomidine in these tests vanished 24 h after the administration.

Conclusions: Deep sedation with dexmedetomidine, but not propofol, significantly inhibited gastrointestinal peristalsis in endotoxemic mice while the inhibitory effect disappeared 24 h after sedation. These data suggested that both propofol and dexmedetomidine could be applied in septic patients while dexmedetomidine should be used cautiously in patients with cardiac disease or ileus.

Keywords: Endotoxemia, Dexmedetomidine, Gastrointestinal motility, ICU, Propofol, Sedation, Sepsis

* Correspondence: gaoyf2009@126.com; dr.wangqiang@139.com
†Haiqing Chang and Shuang Li contributed equally to this work.
[1]Department of Anesthesiology & Center for Brain Science, The First Affiliated Hospital of Xi'an Jiaotong University, Xi'an 710061, Shaanxi, China

Background

Sepsis has become a life-threatening organ dysfunction with up to 26% mortality in the last decade. It is estimated that there are 19.4 million cases of severe sepsis worldwide, with potentially 5.3 million deaths annually [1]. Impairment of intestinal motility is an inevitable complication of sepsis and sepsis has been identified as one of the risk factors for developing the gastrointestinal (GI) motility problems [2]. In turn, inhibition of propulsive intestinal motility predisposes to gut-derived microbial translocation, which plays a pivotal role in the development of sepsis [3]. It is suggested that a vicious circle might be created by sepsis and GI motility. Thus, in sepsis, GI motility disorder demands our ongoing attention and research.

Severe septic patients who need mechanical ventilation account for 10–20% of all admissions to the intensive care unit (ICU) [4, 5]. Propofol and dexmedetomidine are recommended sedatives for septic patients [6]. Impairment of intestinal peristalsis by sedatives is a major side effect, however, scant attention has been given to it so far [7]. Previous studies demonstrated that symptoms of impaired GI transit such as constipation and feed intolerance occurred in up to 50% of mechanically ventilated patients in ICU and these patients had a longer ICU stay [8, 9]. Thus, we need to devote more attention to the effect of sedatives on GI motility in sepsis.

Propofol as an intravenous anesthetic agent gained US FDA approval for sedation in ICU in 1993 [10]. Some studies showed propofol inhibited gut peristalsis and others showed no alteration on the amplitude of CMMCs in the distal colon and GI transit with propofol [11, 12]. However, extensive researches suggested dexmedetomidine as a popular sedative inhibited GI peristalsis [13, 14]. It is preferable to use a sedative that has fewer inhibitory effects on GI transit, but there is a paucity of data describing this topic in sepsis and there are limited methods that could comprehensively evaluate the motility of all parts of the GI tract in humans. Thus, we sought to examine whether propofol and dexmedetomidine, at sedative doses, can inhibit on GI motility in endotoxemic mice and to compare their differences?

Methods

Animals

Eight–ten weeks old C57BL/6 J male mice were supplied by the Laboratory Animal Center of Xi'an Jiaotong University. A standard laboratory diet was given to the mice in a controlled environment (light: dark: 1:1, the cycle starts at 8 Am every day. All animal protocols followed Animal Research: Reporting of In Vivo Experiments (ARRIVE) Guidelines and were approved by the Institutional Animal Care and Use Committee of Xi'an Jiaotong University. There were no adverse events related to the animals throughout the experiment.

Drugs

Lipopolysaccharide (LPS), Evans blue, methylcellulose, 70 kDa fluorescein isothiocyanate conjugated dextran were bought from Sigma-Aldrich (St Louis, MO, USA). Propofol (Diprivan®, AstraZeneca, London, British), dexmedetomidine (Yangtze River Pharmaceutical Group, Taizhou, Jiangsu, China), isoflurane (RWD Life Science, Shenzhen, Guangdong, China) and 10% fat emulsion (Intralipid®, Fresenius Kabi, Wuxi, Jiangsu, China) were used in present study.

Experimental protocol

First of all, 5 mg·kg^{-1} LPS was applied to build the endotoxemic model. For confirming doses of propofol and dexmedetomidine that could induce similar depth of sedative level, sedative/anesthetic scores of endotoxemic mice was evaluated after those mice were injected i.p. using different doses of propofol and dexmedetomidine.

Then, the pulse oxygen saturation, respiratory rate, heart rate and systolic blood pressure were compared between the mice receiving 40 mg·kg^{-1} propofol and those receiving 80 µg·kg^{-1} dexmedetomidine.

Finally, as described in Fig. 1a, motility tests of different gastrointestinal section were conducted 15 mins and 24 h after the injection of sedatives/vehicles again respectively.

Endotoxemia model

To set up the endotoxemia model, mice would receive a single intraperitoneal injection of 5 mg·kg^{-1} LPS in 0.5 mL 48 h before injection of the sedatives/solvents [15].

Measurement of serum IL-6, TNF-α, and IL-1β levels

A total of 500 µl of blood was collected 48 h after intraperitoneal administration of 5 mg·kg-1 LPS or equal volume saline. Following incubation for 1 h, the blood was centrifuged at 2000 g for 10 mins to obtain the serum. Serum IL-6, TNF-α, and IL-1β levels were measured using enzyme-linked immunosorbent assay (ELISA) kits kit from Assay Designs. ELISA kits of IL-6, TNF-α, and IL-1β were purchased from Beyotime Biotechnology (Shanghai, China).

Euthanasia

In some of the following tests of gastrointestinal motility, the mice were sacrificed to examine the gastrointestinal motor function. According to the 2013 AVMA (American Veterinary Medical Association) Guidelines for the Euthanasia of Animals, animals were euthanized via a continuous 5% isoflurane exposure until 1 min

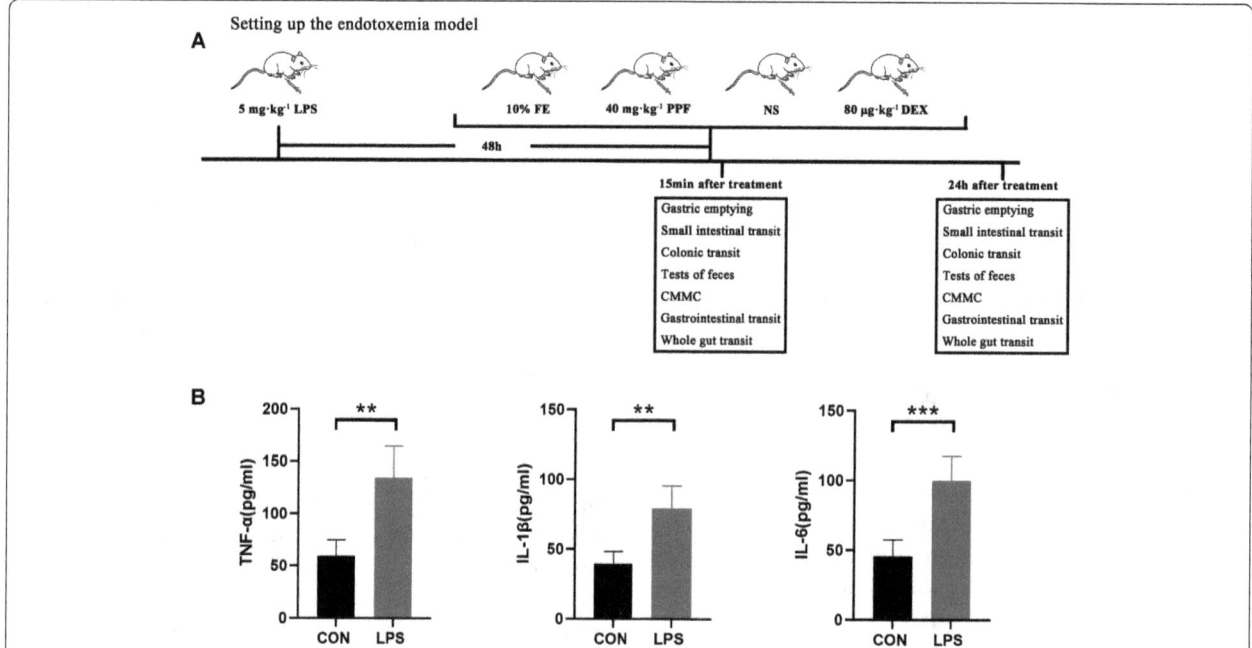

Fig. 1 Protocol of assessing gastrointestinal motility and detection of IL-6, TNF-α, and IL-1β serum levels. *n* = 5 per group. **a**. Firstly, lipopolysaccharide (LPS, 5 mg·kg⁻¹) was used to set up the endotoxemia model. Then the endotoxemic mice were randomized to four groups 48 h after model establishment, and the following drugs were injected intraperitoneally: 10% fat emulsion, 40 mg·kg⁻¹ propofol, normal saline, 80 µg·kg⁻¹ dexmedetomidine. Next, gastric emptying, small intestinal transit, colonic transit, tests of feces, colonic migrating motor complexes, gastrointestinal transit, and whole gut transit were performed 15 mins after injection of sedatives/vehicles. Finally, the same tests were conducted 24 h after the injection of sedatives/vehicles. **b**. The mice in the endotoxemia group have much higher IL-6, TNF-α, and IL-1β serum levels than those mice in the control group. Data were expressed as mean ± SD and analysed by unpaired t test. **P < 0.01, **P < 0.001. CON, control. LPS, lipopolysaccharide. FE, fat emulsion. PPF, propofol. NS, normal saline. DEX, dexmedetomidine

after the breath stop. Then gastrointestinal tissue was obtained in these tests.

Sedative/anesthetic scores

Mice were scored every 5 mins after sedatives/vehicles application: wakefulness (score 0): spontaneous locomotor activity in 1 min observation; light sedation (0.2): no spontaneous locomotion in 1 min observation; deep sedation (0.4): no motor response when placed on a grid inclined (45°) with the head down during 30s observation; light anesthesia (0.6): no righting reflex during 30s observation; moderate anesthesia (0.8): no paw withdrawal reflex and deep anesthesia (1.0): no eye blink reflex [16].

Monitoring of vital signs

Vital signs were measured in 5-min intervals during a 35 mins period. Heart rate and breaths were measured by the BL-420F Data Acquisition & Analysis System (Techman Software Co. LTD, Chengdu, China). Systolic pressure was measured by the tail-cuff system (BP-2000 Blood Pressure Analysis System, Visitech Systems, Apex, NC). Oxygen saturation was measured by Radical 7 (Masimo Corporation, Irvine, USA). Vital signs were recorded at 5 mins after sedation since stable parameters

can be gained only when mice were relatively calm and stationary.

Measurement of gastric emptying (GE) and small intestinal transit (SIT)

Overnight fasting mice were given intragastrically 0.1 ml solution containing 5% Evans blue and 1.5% methylcellulose and were sacrificed 15 mins later. The migrating distance of Evans blue and the total length of the small intestine were measured and transit was expressed in %. The stomach was minced and diluted. And the absorbance of each sample was read at a wavelength of 565 nm (A565). The stomach obtained from a mouse sacrificed immediately after orogastric administration of Evans blue served as a standard (reference stomach). The percentage of GE was calculated by the formula %GE = [(A565reference - A565sample)/A565 reference] × 100% [17].

Colonic transit

Briefly, mice were fasted overnight. A 2 mm glass bead was inserted 2 cm deep into the distal colon after mice were anesthetized using 2% isoflurane. The bead expulsion latency was measured after the recovery of righting reflex [18].

Tests of feces

Mice were housed individually without food for an hour. Fecal pellet output was collected during this period, and numbers and wet weight of feces were recorded. Pellets were dried at 60 °C in the oven overnight, then the dried pellets were weighed right after [19].

Video imaging of colonic migrating motor complexes (CMMCs)

Mice were sacrificed 15 mins after injection of sedatives/solvents. The entire colon was removed and put into Kerbs solution (NaCl 120, KCl 4.7, CaCl$_2$ 2.4, MgSO$_4$ 1.2, NaHCO$_3$ 24.5, KH$_2$PO$_4$ 1.0 and glucose 5.6 in mM, pH 7.4). Then, the colon was mounted to allow spontaneous motor patterns to be imaged for the construction of spatiotemporal maps. The contractile activity was recorded with a Logitech Pro camera and video data were processed with MATLAB® (R2018a, version 9.4). Spatiotemporal maps of the diameter at each point along the proximo-distal length of the colon were constructed and used to quantify the frequency of CMMCs as well as the velocity and length of propagation of CMMCs [20].

Gastrointestinal transit (GIT)

GI transit was examined by calculating the Geometric Center (GC) from the average distribution of a non-absorbable fluorescent marker along the GI tract. FITC-dextran was dissolved at a concentration of 5 mg·ml^{-1} with 0.5% methylcellulose and was given into the stomach (0.1 ml). GI tract of sacrificed mice was harvested 45 mins later and cut averagely into stomach, small bowel (10 segments of equal length), cecum and colon (3 segments of equal length). Tissues were minced, vortexed and centrifuged with 1 ml saline. Supernatants were loaded into a 96 well plate, and the fluorescent signal was read (CytofluorTM plate reader; excitation 492 nm, emission 518 nm). Geometric Center (GC) was calculated as: Σ(S1 x 1 + S2 x 2 + ...S15 x 15), where S was the fraction of the total signal detected in each of the 15 segments [21].

Whole gut transit time (WGTT)

After overnight fasting, mice received intragastrically 0.1 ml of a solution containing Evans blue. Time was recorded from the administration of oral maker to the first appearance of a blue pellet [22].

Statistical analysis

Statistical analyses were performed with Prism 8.0 (GraphPad, San Diego, CA, USA). All of the mice were randomly grouped and tagged, and the statistician was blind to the experimental performer. Shorter migration of maker, longer transit time, less defecation and smaller GC were considered as worse motility. Results are presented as mean ± SD (standard deviation). Data were evaluated for normal distribution and homogeneity of variance, then analysed by one-way ANOVA (between-group differences were detected with Tukey post hoc tests) or Kruskal–Wallis test (followed by Dunn's multiple comparisons test with Bonferroni correction). Two-way repeated-measures ANOVA was used to analyse vital signs (followed by Sidak's post hoc test for multiple comparisons where applicable). An unpaired t test was used to analyse serum IL-6, TNF-α, and IL-1β levels.. Statistical significance was assigned at $P < 0.05$.

Results

Propofol and dexmedetomidine induced dose-dependent sedation in endotoxemic mice

Firstly, we measured the serum levels of IL-6, TNF-α, and IL-1β to confirm the successful establishment of the endotoxemia model (Fig. 1b). Then the depth of sedation of mice with different doses of propofol and dexmedetomidine was evaluated. We found both propofol and dexmedetomidine could induce dose-dependent sedative levels. 40 mg·kg^{-1} propofol and 80 μg·kg^{-1} dexmedetomidine produced a comparable deep sedative level 15 mins after injection and we used these doses to perform the following tests (Fig. 2a, b).

Vital signs of endotoxemic mice during sedation with propofol and dexmedetomidine

Vital signs of sedative endotoxemic mice were measured for 35 mins. It revealed that there was no statistical difference between endotoxemic mice with administration of 40 mg·kg^{-1} propofol and 80 μg·kg^{-1} dexmedetomidine for breaths $(P = 0.920)$, oxygen saturation $(P = 0.925)$, and systolic pressure $(P = 0.608)$, while heart rate decreased strikingly from 10 mins after the dexmedetomidine treatment $(P < 0.0001)$ (Fig. 2c-f).

Dexmedetomidine, but not propofol delayed GE and SIT in endotoxemic mice

Motility of the stomach and small intestine was examined (Fig. 3a, c). We found that GE and SIT were similar in 10% fat emulsion-treated and saline-treated mice. Dexmedetomidine inhibited GE of endotoxemic mice 15 mins after application compared with saline (16.4 ± 7.2% vs 34.7 ± 7.9%, $P = 0.006$) and propofol (16.4 ± 7.2% vs 36.9 ± 11.0%, $P = 0.002$) (Fig. 3b). Similarly, SIT was decreased by dexmedetomidine 15 mins after injection (see images in Fig. 3e), and statistically significant reduction was found as against mice with saline (12.3 ± 5.0% vs 42.5 ± 11.3%, $P = 0.006$) and with propofol (12.3 ± 5.0% vs 42.0 ± 9.4%, $P = 0.008$) (Fig. 3d). However, comparison of GE and SIT among mice with 10% fat emulsion to propofol revealed no significant difference. And

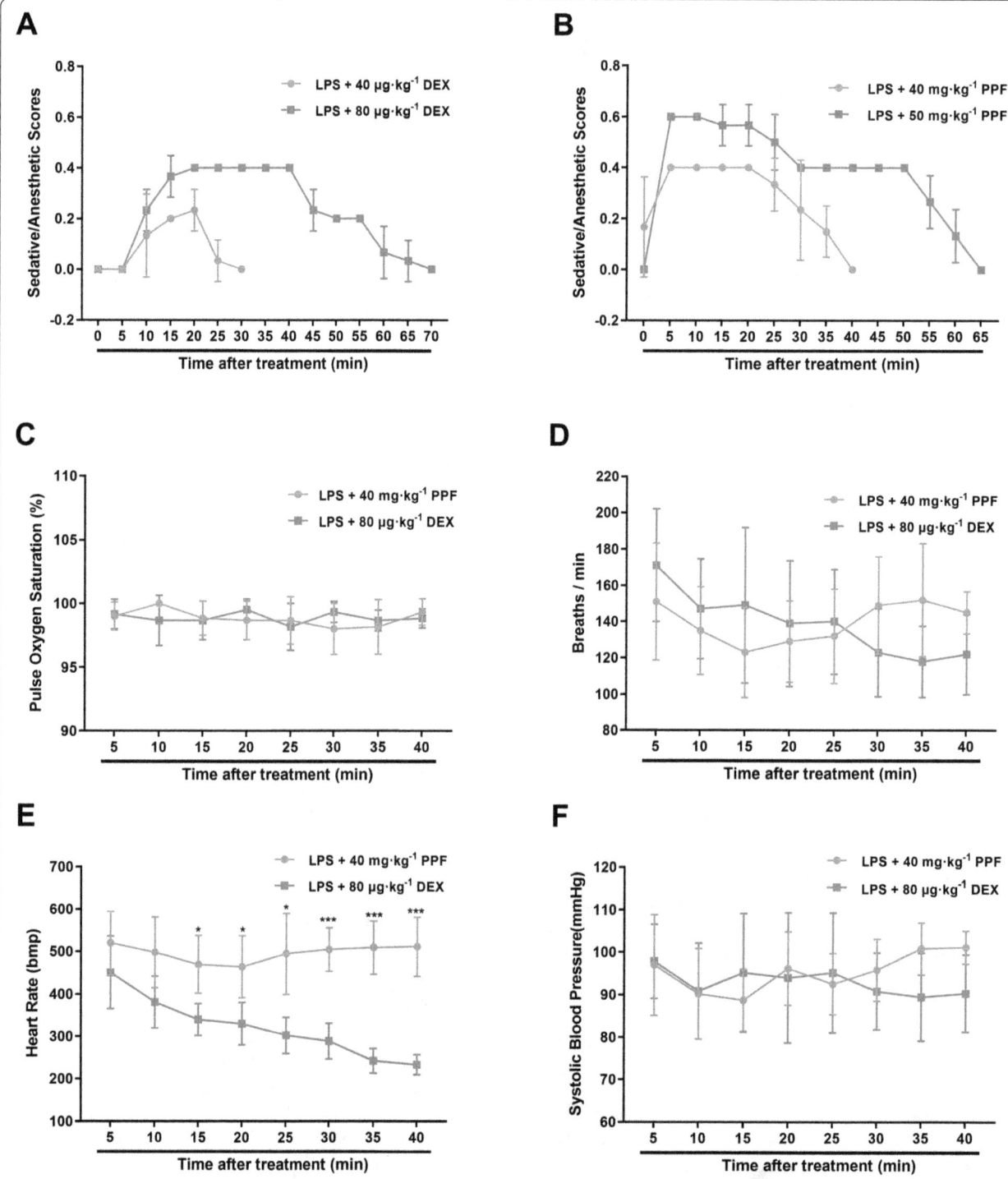

Fig. 2 Depth of sedation and vital signs of endotoxemic mice after administration of propofol or dexmedetomidine. $n = 6$ per group. **a**. Does-dependent sedative depth of endotoxemic mice accepting 40 μg·kg^{-1} and 80 μg·kg^{-1} dexmedetomidine. **b**. Does-dependent sedative depth of endotoxemic mice accepting 40 mg.kg^{-1} and 50 mg.kg^{-1} propofol. **c-f**. The mice with administration of 40 mg·kg^{-1} propofol and 80 μg·kg^{-1} dexmedetomidine had similar pulse oxygen saturation percentage, respiratory rate, and systolic blood pressure over time while dexmedetomidine strikingly decreased heart rate. Vital signs were recorded from 5 mins to 40 mins after sedation. Data were expressed as mean ± SD and analysed by two-way repeated-measures ANOVA. $^{*}P < 0.05$, $^{***}P < 0.001$, LPS + 80 μg·kg^{-1} DEX vs LPS + 40 mg·kg^{-1}PPF. LPS, lipopolysaccharide. PPF, propofol. DEX, dexmedetomidine

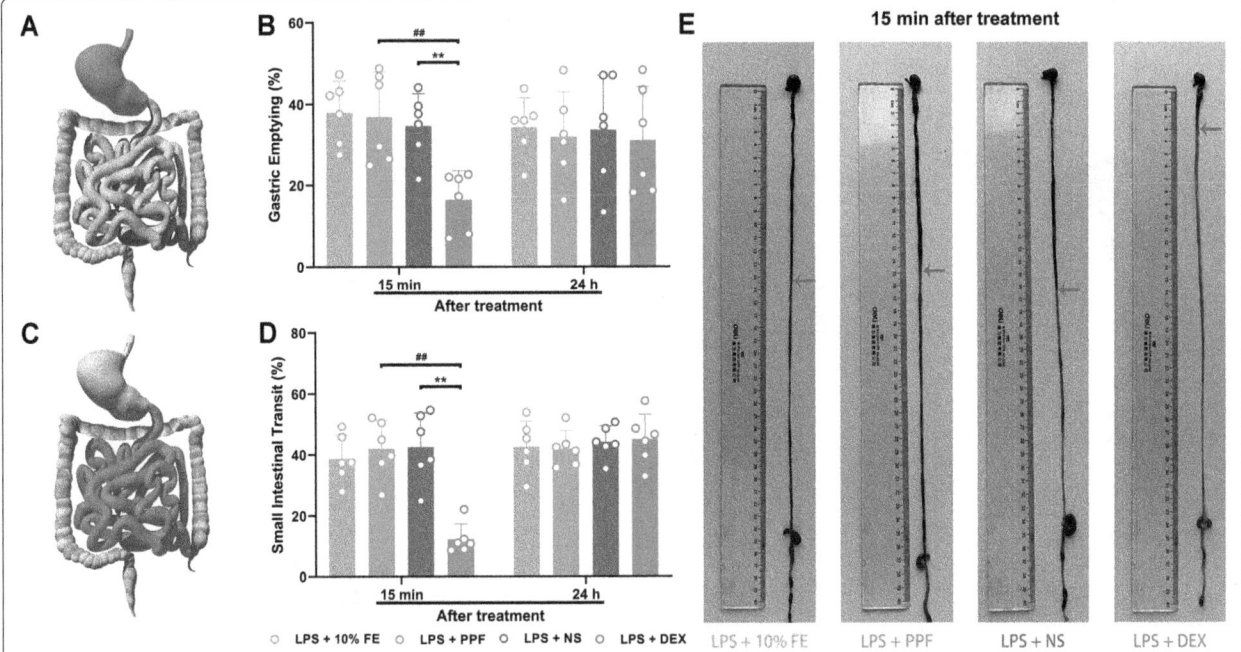

Fig. 3 Effect of dexmedetomidine and propofol on upper gastrointestinal motility in endotoxemic mice. $n = 6$ per group. **a**. A schematic diagram of the stomach that examined in B. **b**. Dexmedetomidine inhibited gastric emptying of endotoxemic mice 15 mins after application compared with saline and propofol, and this depression disappeared 24 h after injection. **c**. A schematic diagram of the small intestine that examined in D. **d**. Dexmedetomidine but not propofol decreased small intestinal transit 15 mins after administration and this inhibition reversed 24 h after injection. **e**. Representative photographs showing small intestinal transit was measured by recording the migration of Evans blue (red arrows) 15 mins after application. Data were expressed as mean ± SD and analysed by one-way ANOVA or Kruskal–Wallis tests. $^{**}P < 0.01$, LPS + DEX vs LPS + NS; $^{##}P < 0.01$, LPS + DEX vs LPS + PPF. LPS, lipopolysaccharide. FE, fat emulsion. PPF, propofol. NS, normal saline. DEX, dexmedetomidine

dexmedetomidine had no inhibitory effect in GE and SIT 24 h after the application.

Not propofol, but dexmedetomidine inhibited colonic transit and defecation in endotoxemic mice

Colonic motility was traced (Fig. 4a). There was no statistical difference between propofol group and 10% fat emulsion group, saline group and 10% fat emulsion group in colonic transit and defecation. Nevertheless, more time was required to expel glass beads in endotoxemic mice with dexmedetomidine ($19,130 \pm 5157$ s) than those with saline (202 ± 49.6 s), $P = 0.0006$ (Fig. 4b). Fewer feces was excreted in an hour in the dexmedetomidine group, and statistic difference exited between dexmedetomidine-treated and saline-treated mice in the wet weight of feces ($P = 0.001$), dry weight of feces ($P = 0.003$) as well as the number of feces ($P = 0.003$) (Fig. 4c-e). This inhibition of dexmedetomidine on colonic transit and defecation reversed 24 h after implement.

Dexmedetomidine, but not propofol suppressed CMMCs in endotoxemic mice

Spontaneous motility of isolated colon was recorded to check the suppressive effect of dexmedetomidine on colon could still be established in vitro. Spatiotemporal

maps of contractile activity patterns were constructed 15 mins (Fig. 5a-d) and 24 h (Fig. 5e-h) after the treatment of sedatives/vehicles. CMMCs frequency was increased (Fig. 5i; $P = 0.033$), while length of propagation was shortened (Fig. 5j; $P = 0.044$) and velocity was reduced (Fig. 5k; $P = 0.012$) by dexmedetomidine 15 mins after injection as against saline. However, CMMCs did not differ significantly in endotoxemic mice receiving 10% fat emulsion and those receiving propofol. This suppression of dexmedetomidine on CMMCs disappeared 24 h after administration.

Dexmedetomidine, not propofol, depressed whole gastrointestinal motility in endotoxemic mice

GIT and WGTT as sensitive methods to assess the motility of the whole GI tract (Fig. 6i). We checked the distribution of FITC-dextran in endotoxemic mice 15 mins (Fig. 6a-d) and 24 h (Fig. 6e-h) after administration of 10% fat emulsion, propofol, saline, and dexmedetomidine respectively. The dexmedetomidine group had smaller GC than the saline group ($P = 0.0001$) or propofol group ($P = 0.0003$) 15 mins after application (Fig. 6j). In respect of the WGTT, dexmedetomidine (554.5 ± 172.6 mins) significantly prolonged latency of the first blue feces expulsion 15 mins after administration compared with saline (224.7 ± 35.3 mins, $P = 0.034$) and

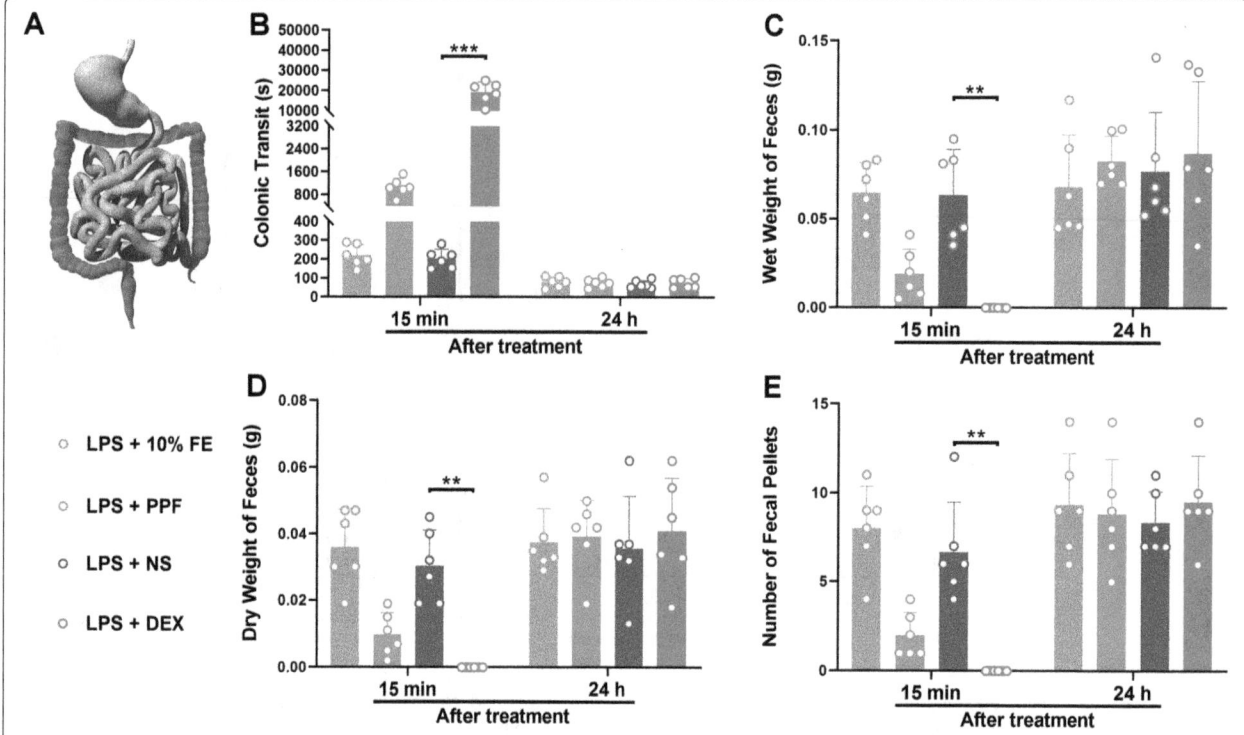

Fig. 4 Effect of dexmedetomidine and propofol on colonic motility in vivo in endotoxemic mice. $n = 6$ per group. **a.** A schematic diagram of the colon. **b.** Dexmedetomidine had inhibitory effect on colonic transit time 15 mins after implement, and 24 h later, this inhibition didn't exist anymore. **c-e.** Dexmedetomidine prevented excretion of feces. There was statistic difference between dexmedetomidine and saline in weight of feces, dry weight of feces and numbers of fecal pellets 15 mins after injection and there was no difference occurred 24 h after application between groups. Data were expressed as mean ± SD and analysed by one-way ANOVA or Kruskal–Wallis test. $^{**}P < 0.01$, $^{***}P < 0.001$, LPS + DEX vs LPS + NS. LPS, lipopolysaccharide. FE, fat emulsion. PPF, propofol. NS, normal saline. DEX, dexmedetomidine

propofol (210.3 ± 46.9 mins, $P = 0.017$) (Fig. 6k). However, propofol had suppression on neither GIT nor WGTT. What's more, this inhibition of dexmedetomidine on the whole gastrointestinal motility had considerable abatement 24 h after injection.

Discussion

Our results showed that deep sedation with dexmedetomidine, but not propofol suppressed motility of various parts of the GI tract including the stomach, small intestine, and colon in endotoxemic mice, whereas such inhibitory effects of dexmedetomidine recovered at 24 h after sedation. Additionally, dexmedetomidine led to heart rate reduction in endotoxemic mice.

Animal models of sepsis are generally divided into 3 categories: bacterial infection models, endotoxin models, and peritonitis models. Cecal ligation and puncture (CLP), a peritonitis model, has been considered a golden standard of sepsis research. However, this model requires an abdominal surgical procedure that may strikingly interfere with GI motility cause the induction of postoperative ileus [23]. Postoperative ileus is possible to obscure the effect of sedatives on GI motility in sepsis. Additionally, the LPS-induced endotoxin model was

more stable compared to usage of bacteria, hence we injected 5 mg·kg^{-1} LPS in mice to build a septic model.

Before comparing the effect of sedatives on GI motility in endotoxemic mice, the sedative depth of different doses of propofol and dexmedetomidine was assessed. Previous study demonstrated that the ED50 and ED95 of propofol for smooth insertion of the laryngeal mask airway were 2.9 mg·kg^{-1} and 3.9 mg·kg^{-1} respectively [24], which equaled to 35.67 and 47.97 mg·kg^{-1} in mice based on human equivalent dose calculation scale [25]. And 50 mg·kg^{-1} and 100 mg·kg^{-1} propofol were used to evaluate the effect on GI motility [12]. Thus, we injected 40 mg·kg^{-1} and 50 mg·kg^{-1} propofol to examine the sedative effect in endotoxemic mice. In addition, 0.5 to 1 mg·kg^{-1} dexmedetomidine had been reported for mice anesthesia [26]. ED50 of dexmedetomidine inhibited gastrointestinal transit was 40 μg·kg^{-1} in rats, it may equal to 80 μg·kg^{-1} for mice [25]. As a consequence, 40 μg·kg^{-1} and 80 μg·kg^{-1} dexmedetomidine was selected to assess sedative depth of mice in present study. Since 40 mg·kg^{-1} propofol and 80 μg·kg^{-1} dexmedetomidine induced comparable deep sedative in endotoxemic mice and the comfort and safety of patients who were undergoing mechanical ventilation ICU entailed deep

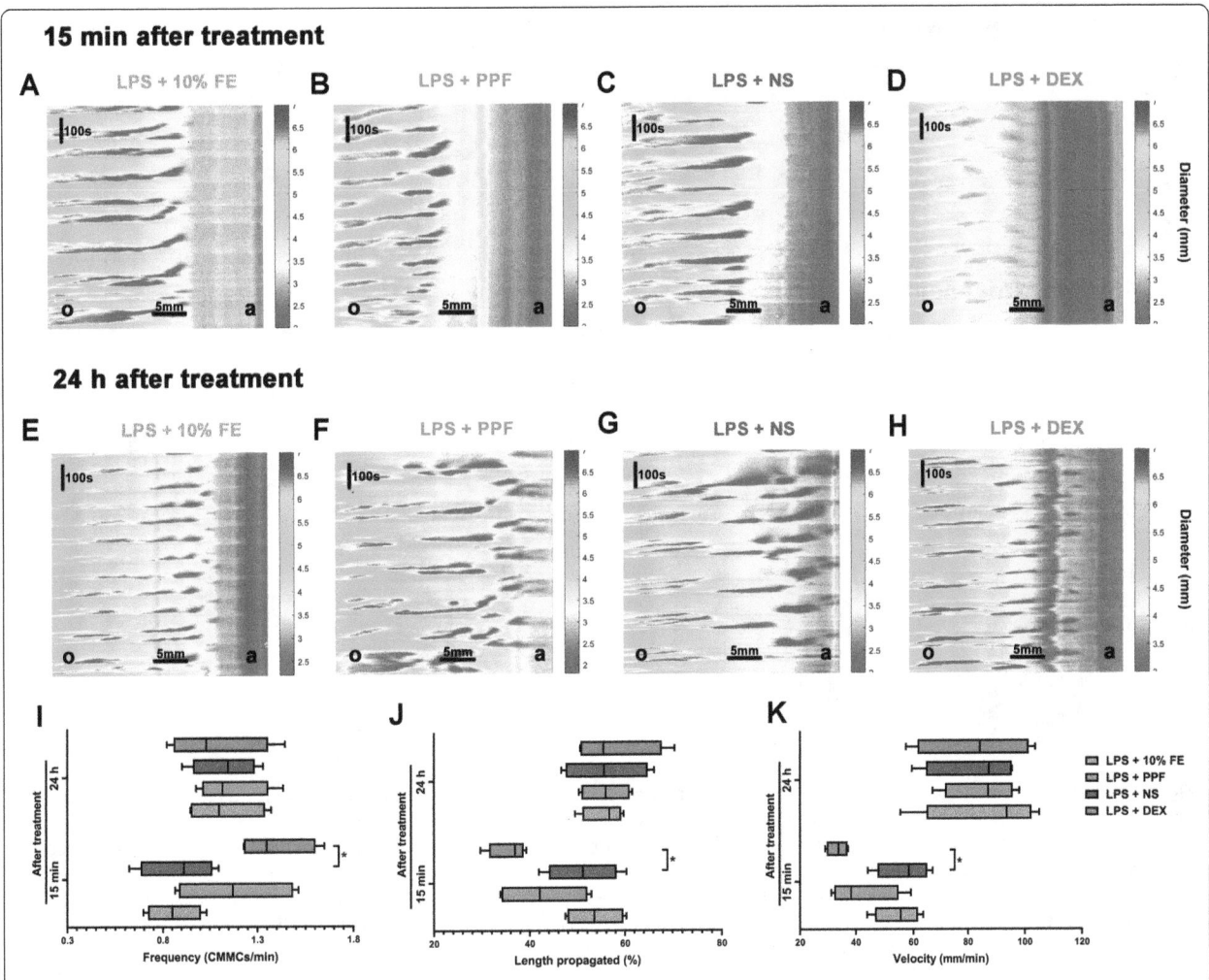

Fig. 5 Effect of dexmedetomidine and propofol on CMMCs in endotoxemic mice. *n* = 4 per group. Typical spatiotemporal maps showed CMMCs in endotoxemic mice receiving 10% fat emulsion, propofol, saline, and dexmedetomidine 15 mins and 24 h after treatment in **a-d** and **e-h** respectively. The ordinate represents time, and the abscissa is indicative of spatial location from the oral end (O) to the anal end (A). The width of the gut (mm), representative of contractions, was pseudocolored. **i-k.** dexmedetomidine not propofol increased CMMCs frequency, shortened percentage of the length of propagation and slowed down velocity of propagation 15 mins after injection. Dexmedetomidine had no effect on CMMCs 24 h after injection. Data were expressed as median and interquartile ranges and analysed by one-way ANOVA. *$P < 0.05$, LPS + DEX vs LPS + NS. LPS, lipopolysaccharide. FE, fat emulsion. PPF, propofol. NS, normal saline. DEX, dexmedetomidine. CMMCs, colonic migrating motor complexes

sedation [27], we employed these doses in the present study. In line with the previous study, dexmedetomidine strongly decreased heart rate [28].

As for administration route, we used a single intraperitoneal injection in present study. Though intravenous injection is more in line with clinical practice, there are practical limitations associated with the technical difficulties of intravenous administration in mice due to their small size, especially in conscious mice [29]. It was not excluded that sedative drugs had directly implication on the gut, but we believed that even intravascular administration of drugs could also act on the gut as drugs would reach gut through blood circulation soon.

We tested GI motility 15 mins and 24 h after drug administration respectively. The maximum sedation depth was reached 15 min after drug administration, therefore we thought it was the right time to access the effect of sedatives on GI motor function. And the terminal half-life of single administration of 100 mg·kg^{-1} propofol in the mouse blood is 140.8 ± 53.55 mins [30] and the elimination half-life of DEX is 2 ~ 3 h. To figure out whether the inhibition of sedatives on GI motor function was sustained after metabolism of these sedatives, we conducted these GI motility tests 24 h after drug implement and found no sustained inhibition existed.

Although some human studies showed that GE [31] and GI motility [32] were uninfluenced by light or sub

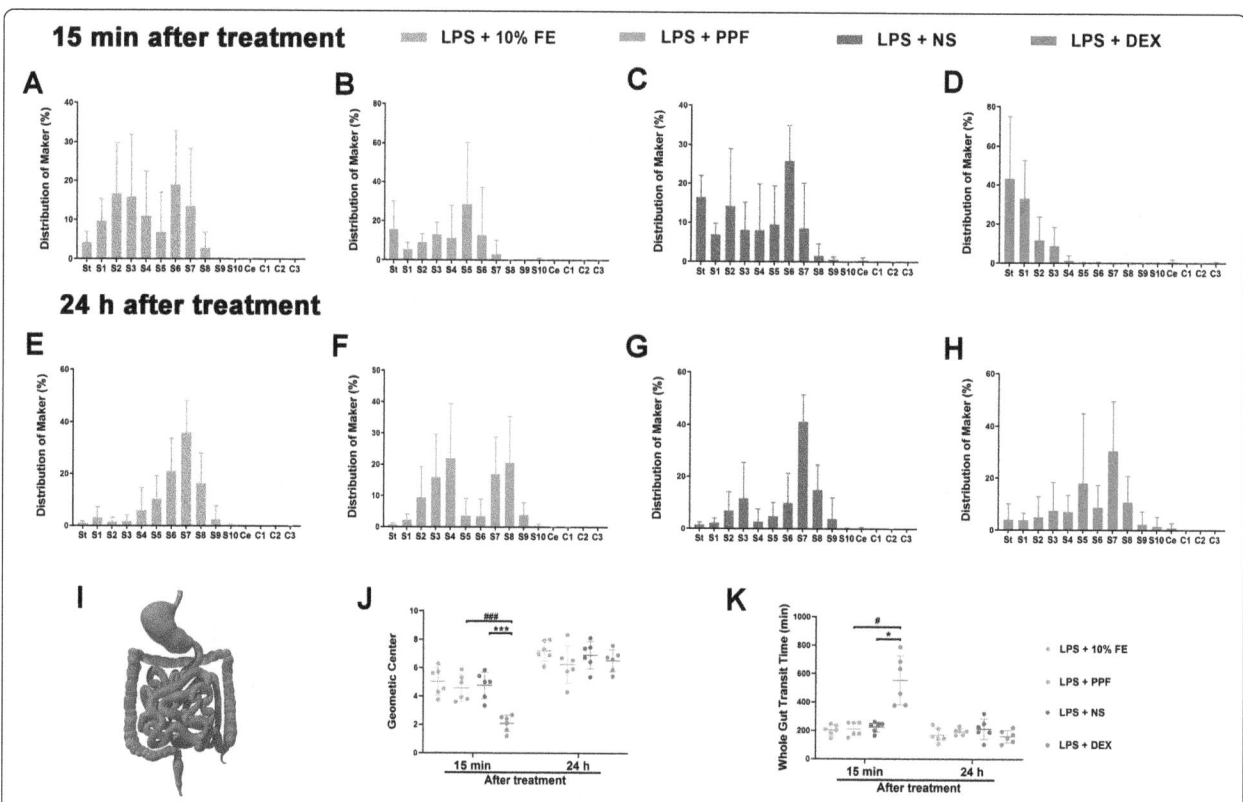

Fig. 6 Effect of dexmedetomidine or propofol on the whole part of gastrointestinal motility in endotoxemic mice. n = 6 per group. Transit histogram for the distribution of non-absorbable fluorescein isothiocyanate through the intestinal segments 15 mins (**a-d**) and 24 h (**e-h**) after administration sedatives/vehicles (St, stomach; S, small intestine; Ce, cecum; C, colon). **i**. A schematic diagram of the whole gastrointestinal tract. 15 mins after treatment, dexmedetomidine depressed the whole gastrointestinal motility that showed smaller geometic center (**j**.) and longer latency of the first blue feces expulsion(**k**.). Results of these two tests were similar between groups 24 h after administration. Data were expressed as mean ± SD and analysed by one-way ANOVA or Kruskal–Wallis test. $^{*}P < 0.05$, $^{***}P < 0.001$, LPS + DEX vs LPS + NS. $^{#}P < 0.05$, $^{###}P < 0.001$, LPS + DEX vs LPS + PPF. LPS, lipopolysaccharide. FE, fat emulsion. PPF, propofol. NS, normal saline. DEX, dexmedetomidine

hypnotic propofol sedation, a human study in vitro founded a dose-dependent depression of propofol on gastric and colonic muscle [33]. Inada et al showed that 50 mg·kg^{-1} propofol weakly repressed GE while 100 mg·kg^{-1} propofol exhibited a marked inhibitory effect on GE and GIT in mice [12]. Thus, it indicated that propofol had a dose-dependent depression on GI motility. Our study explored that, in endotoxemic mice, 40 mg·kg^{-1} propofol was enough to reach deep sedation while had little effect on GI motility. The mechanism of propofol effect on GI motility is complicated and is still a matter of debate. There are three types of GABA receptors (GABA$_A$, GABA$_B$, GABA$_C$) expressed in different regions of GI tract [34]. It was verified that GABA$_A$ involved in the effect of propofol on GI motility [35]. Few studies explored the effect of propofol on GABA$_B$ and GABA$_C$ receptors in respect of GI motility. In a word, the mechanism of propofol on GI motility still needs to be investigated.

The antiperistatical effects in the current study that 80 μg·kg^{-1} dexmedetomidine inhibited all segments of GI tract motor function of endotoxemic mice were consistent with studies in human [13] and animals [7]. Dexmedetomidine increased the frequency of CMMCs while decreased the propagation and velocity of CMMCs in our study. It was in line with the previous study that dexmedetomidine inhibited the guinea pig ileum peristalsis whereas increased the frequency of peristalsis waves in vitro. It might due to the incomplete peristalsis from mouth to anal that triggered an increased peristalsis frequency. Dexmedetomidine is a highly selective α2-adrenoceptor agonist, its inhibitory effect on ileum peristalsis could be prevented only by α2-adrenoceptor antagonist yohimbine instead of α1-adrenoceptor antagonist prazosin [7], which further indicated that the antiperistatical effect of dexmedetomidine may due to α2-adrenoceptor–mediated interruption of excitatory cholinergic pathways in the enteric nervous system [36] or activated inhibitory neural pathways [37]. The α2A subtype in the enteric nervous system was responsible for the suppression of medetomidine on GI motility [38, 39], it might have a potential role in the inhibition of dexmedetomidine on GI peristalsis. Besides, dexmedetomidine inhibited colon motility through a peripheral mechanism in present study, whether the central mechanism involved in this inhibition was speculative.

Conclusion

In conclusion, at a comparable deep sedative level in endotoxemic mice, dexmedetomidine, but not propofol inhibited motilities of all parts of the GI tract, however, such inhibitory effects of dexmedetomidine disappeared after 24 h. So we could speculate that this side effect is short-term, while the prognosis of patients requiring long-term sedation with sedatives remains unknown. Additionally, dexmedetomidine produced obvious heart rate reduction in endotoxemic mice. These data indicated that both propofol and dexmedetomidine can be used in patients with sepsis, while dexmedetomidine should be used with caution in patients with heart disease or gastrointestinal motility disorder. However, take species differences into consideration, this finding needs more clinic investigation to be extrapolated to the situation in humans.

Abbreviations
LPS: Lipopolysaccharide; ICU: Intensive care unit; GI: Gastrointestinal; ARRIVE: Animal research: reporting of in vivo experiments; GE: Gastric emptying; SIT: Small intestinal transit; CMMCs: Colonic migrating motor complexes; GIT: Gastrointestinal transit; WGTT: Whole gut transit time; SD: Standard deviation; CLP: Cecal ligation and puncture

Acknowledgments
Not applicable.

Authors' contributions
QW, YFG designed this study. HQC, YSL, JWM, BC, HG, HH conducted the experiments. HQC, YSL, SL, HH analysed data. HQC, YSL, SL interpreted the data. HQC, HLM Drafted the paper. All authors read and approved the final version of the manuscript.

Author details
[1]Department of Anesthesiology & Center for Brain Science, The First Affiliated Hospital of Xi'an Jiaotong University, Xi'an 710061, Shaanxi, China. [2]Department of Pharmacology, School of Basic Medical Sciences, Health Science Center, Xi'an Jiaotong University, Xi'an 710061, Shaanxi, China.

References
1. Fleischmann C, Scherag A, Adhikari NK, Hartog CS, Tsaganos T, Schlattmann P, Angus DC, Reinhart K. Assessment of global incidence and mortality of hospital-treated Sepsis. Current estimates and limitations. Am J Respir Crit Care Med. 2016;193(3):259–72.
2. Adike A, Quigley EMM. Gastrointestinal motility problems in critical care: a clinical perspective. J Dig Dis. 2014;15(7):335–44.
3. Bauer AJ, Schwarz NT, Moore BA, Türler A, Kalff JC. Ileus in critical illness: mechanisms and management. Curr Opin Crit Care. 2002;8(2):152–7.
4. Levy MM, Dellinger RP, Townsend SR, Linde-Zwirble WT, Marshall JC, Bion J, Schorr C, Artigas A, Ramsay G, Beale R, et al. The surviving Sepsis campaign: results of an international guideline-based performance improvement program targeting severe sepsis. Crit Care Med. 2010;38(2):367–74.
5. Cawcutt KA, Peters SG. Severe sepsis and septic shock: clinical overview and update on management. Mayo Clin Proc. 2014;89(11):1572–8.
6. Rhodes A, Evans LE, Alhazzani W, Levy MM, Antonelli M, Ferrer R, Kumar A, Sevransky JE, Sprung CL, Nunnally ME, et al. Surviving Sepsis campaign:

7. international guidelines for Management of Sepsis and Septic Shock: 2016. Intensive Care Med. 2017;43(3):304–77.
7. Herbert MK, Roth-Goldbrunner S, Holzer P, Roewer N. Clonidine and dexmedetomidine potently inhibit peristalsis in the Guinea pig ileum in vitro. Anesthesiology. 2002;97(6):1491–9.
8. Reintam Blaser A, Jakob SM, Starkopf J. Gastrointestinal failure in the ICU. Curr Opin Crit Care. 2016;22(2):128–41.
9. Mostafa SM, Bhandari S, Ritchie G, Gratton N, Wenstone R. Constipation and its implications in the critically ill patient. Br J Anaesth. 2003;91(6):815–9.
10. McKeage K, Perry CM. Propofol: a review of its use in intensive care sedation of adults. CNS Drugs. 2003;17(4):235–72.
11. Diss LB, Villeneuve S, Pearce KR, Yeoman MS, Patel BA. Region specific differences in the effect of propofol on the murine colon result in dysmotility. Auton Neurosci. 2019;219:19–24.
12. Inada T, Asai T, Yamada M, Shingu K. Propofol and midazolam inhibit gastric emptying and gastrointestinal transit in mice. Anesth Analg. 2004;99(4):1102.
13. Iirola T, Vilo S, Aantaa R, Wendelin-Saarenhovi M, Neuvonen PJ, Scheinin M, Olkkola KT. Dexmedetomidine inhibits gastric emptying and oro-caecal transit in healthy volunteers. Br J Anaesth. 2011;106(4):522–7.
14. Kim N, Yoo YC, Lee SK, Kim H, Ju HM, Min KT. Comparison of the efficacy and safety of sedation between dexmedetomidine-remifentanil and propofol-remifentanil during endoscopic submucosal dissection. World J Gastroenterol. 2015;21(12):3671–8.
15. Hong G-S, Zillekens A, Schneiker B, Pantelis D, de Jonge WJ, Schaefer N, Kalff JC, Wehner S. Non-invasive transcutaneous auricular vagus nerve stimulation prevents postoperative ileus and endotoxemia in mice. Neurogastroenterol Motil. 2019;31(3):e13501.
16. Li Y, Wu Y, Li R, Wang C, Jia N, Zhao C, Wen A, Xiong L. Propofol regulates the surface expression of GABAA receptors: implications in synaptic inhibition. Anesth Analg. 2015;121(5):1176–83.
17. De Winter BY, Bredenoord AJ, Van Nassauw L, De Man JG, De Schepper HU, Timmermans JP, Pelckmans PA. Involvement of afferent neurons in the pathogenesis of endotoxin-induced ileus in mice: role of CGRP and TRPV1 receptors. Eur J Pharmacol. 2009;615(1–3):177–84.
18. Nasser Y, Fernandez E, Keenan CM, Ho W, Oland LD, Tibbles LA, Schemann M, MacNaughton WK, Ruhl A, Sharkey KA. Role of enteric glia in intestinal physiology: effects of the gliotoxin fluorocitrate on motor and secretory function. Am J Physiol Gastrointest Liver Physiol. 2006;291(5):G912–27.
19. Hoffman JM, McKnight ND, Sharkey KA, Mawe GM. The relationship between inflammation-induced neuronal excitability and disrupted motor activity in the Guinea pig distal colon. Neurogastroenterol Motil. 2011;23(7): 673–e279.
20. Swaminathan M, Hill-Yardin E, Ellis M, Zygorodimos M, Johnston LA, Gwynne RM, Bornstein JC. Video imaging and spatiotemporal maps to analyze gastrointestinal motility in mice. J Vis Exp. 2016;108:53828.
21. Moore BA, Manthey CL, Johnson DL, Bauer AJ. Matrix metalloproteinase-9 inhibition reduces inflammation and improves motility in murine models of postoperative ileus. Gastroenterology. 2011;141(4):1283–92 1292 e1281–1284.
22. Nagakura Y, Naitoh Y, Kamato T, Yamano M, Miyata K. Compounds possessing 5-HT3 receptor antagonistic activity inhibit intestinal propulsion in mice. Eur J Pharmacol. 1996;311(1):67–72.
23. De Winter B-Y, De Man J-G. Interplay between inflammation, immune system and neuronal pathways: effect on gastrointestinal motility. World J Gastroenterol. 2010;16(44):5523–35.
24. Yoo JY, Kwak HJ, Kim YB, Park CK, Lee SY, Kim JY. The effect of dexmedetomidine pretreatment on the median effective bolus dose of propofol for facilitating laryngeal mask airway insertion. J Anesth. 2017;31(1): 11–7.
25. Nair AB, Jacob S. A simple practice guide for dose conversion between animals and human. J Basic Clinical Pharm. 2016;7(2):27–31.
26. Gargiulo S, Greco A, Gramanzini M, Esposito S, Affuso A, Brunetti A, Vesce G. Mice anesthesia, analgesia, and care, part I: anesthetic considerations in preclinical research. ILAR J. 2012;53(1):E55–69.
27. Coursin DB, Skrobik Y. What is safe sedation in the ICU? N Engl J Med. 2019; 380(26):2577–8.
28. Shehabi Y, Howe BD, Bellomo R, Arabi YM, Bailey M, Bass FE, Bin Kadiman S, McArthur CJ, Murray L, Reade MC, et al. Early sedation with Dexmedetomidine in critically ill patients. N Engl J Med. 2019;380(26):2506–17.
29. Alves HC, Valentim AM, Olsson IA, Antunes LM. Intraperitoneal propofol and propofol fentanyl, sufentanil and remifentanil combinations for mouse

anaesthesia. Lab Anim. 2007;41(3):329–36.

30. Li Lin A, Shangari N, Chan TS, Remirez D, O'Brien PJ. Herbal monoterpene alcohols inhibit propofol metabolism and prolong anesthesia time. Life Sci. 2006;79(1):21–9.

31. Chassard D, Lansiaux S, Duflo F, Mion F, Bleyzac N, Debon R, Allaouchiche B. Effects of subhypnotic doses of propofol on gastric emptying in volunteers. Anesthesiology. 2002;97(1):96–101.

32. Freye E, Sundermann S, Wilder-Smith OH. No inhibition of gastro-intestinal propulsion after propofol- or propofol/ketamine-N2O/O2 anaesthesia. A comparison of gastro-caecal transit after isoflurane anaesthesia. Acta Anaesthesiol Scand. 1998;42(6):664–9.

33. Lee TL, Ang SB, Dambisya YM, Adaikan GP, Lau LC. The effect of propofol on human gastric and colonic muscle contractions. Anesth Analg. 1999; 89(5):1246–9.

34. Auteri M, Zizzo MG, Serio R. GABA and GABA receptors in the gastrointestinal tract: from motility to inflammation. Pharmacol Res. 2015;93: 11–21.

35. Koutsoviti-Papadopoulou M, Akahori F, Kounenis G, Nikolaidis E. Propofol's biphasic effect on GABA(a)-receptor-mediated response of the isolated Guinea pig ileum. Pharmacol Res. 1999;40(4):313–7.

36. De Ponti F, Giaroni C, Cosentino M, Lecchini S, Frigo G. Adrenergic mechanisms in the control of gastrointestinal motility: from basic science to clinical applications. Pharmacol Ther. 1996;69(1):59–78.

37. Furness JB. Types of neurons in the enteric nervous system. J Auton Nerv Syst. 2000;81(1–3):87–96.

38. Fulop K, Zadori Z, Ronai AZ, Gyires K. Characterisation of alpha2-adrenoceptor subtypes involved in gastric emptying, gastric motility and gastric mucosal defence. Eur J Pharmacol. 2005;528(1–3):150–7.

39. Scheibner J, Trendelenburg AU, Hein L, Starke K, Blandizzi C. Alpha 2-adrenoceptors in the enteric nervous system: a study in alpha 2A-adrenoceptor-deficient mice. Br J Pharmacol. 2002;135(3):697–704.

17

Single nucleotide polymorphisms associated with postoperative inadequate analgesia after single-port VATS in chinese population

Xiufang Xing, Yongyu Bai, Kai Sun and Min Yan*🆔

Abstract

Background: Postoperative inadequate analgesia following video-assisted thoracoscopic surgery (VATS) is a common and significant clinical problem. While genetic polymorphisms may play role in the variability of postoperative analgesia effect, few studies have evaluated the associations between genetic mutations and inadequate analgesia after single-port VATS.

Methods: Twenty-eight single nucleotide polymorphisms (SNPs) among 18 selected genes involved in pain perception and modulation were genotyped in 198 Chinese patients undergoing single-port VATS. The primary outcome was the occurrence of inadequate analgesia in the first night and morning after surgery which was defined by a comprehensive postoperative evaluation. Multivariable logistic regression analyses were used to identify the association between genetic variations and postoperative inadequate analgesia.

Results: The prevalence of postoperative inadequate analgesia was 45.5% in the present study. After controlling for age and education level, association with inadequate analgesia was observed in four SNPs among three genes encoding voltage-gated sodium channels. Patients with the minor allele of rs33985936 (*SCN11A*), rs6795970 (*SCN10A*), and 3312G > T (*SCN9A*) have an increased risk of suffering from inadequate analgesia. While the patients carrying the minor allele of rs11709492 (*SCN11A*) have lower risk experiencing inadequate analgesia.

Conclusions: We identified that SNPs in *SCN9A*, *SCN10A*, and *SCN11A* play a role in the postoperative inadequate analgesia after single-port VATS. Although future larger and long-term follow up studies are warranted to confirm our findings, the results of the current study may be utilized as predictors for forecasting postoperative analgesic effect for patients receiving this type of surgery.

Keywords: Postoperative pain, Single nucleotide polymorphism, Single-port video-assisted thoracoscopic surgery

Background

Thoracotomy is considered to be one of the most painful of surgical procedures [1]. Even though video-assisted thoracoscopic surgery (VATS) is less invasive and is generally expected to induce lower pain intensity, the moderate to severe postoperative pain remains common after VATS [2, 3]. The postoperative pain not only causes respiratory complications but negatively affects long-term rehabilitation [4, 5].

Multiple factors have been reported to affect pain sensitivity after surgery, such as age, gender, ethnicity, and type of surgery [6]. Recent advances in genetic research have shown that genetic polymorphisms may also play a role in the variability of pain perception [7–9]. Opioid receptor mu 1 (*OPRM1*) encodes the mu opioid receptor in humans, and plays an important role in endogenous pain modulation and opioid analgesia. Four single nucleotide polymorphisms (SNPs) in *OPRM1* were found

* Correspondence: zryanmin@zju.edu.cn
Department of Anesthesiology and Pain Medicine, Second Affiliated Hospital, Zhejiang University School of Medicine, No.88 Jiefang Road, Hangzhou 310009, China

significantly associated with higher pain intensity after thoracotomy [8]. Zhonghai Zhao et al. indicated that patients with mutant homozygous rs2032582 and rs1128503 loci in the *ABCB1* gene consumed more sufentanil at 6 h, 24 h and 48 h after thoracoscopic-assisted radical resection [9]. Besides, patients with the UGT2B7*2/*2 genotype had a higher risk of suffering severe pain 48 h after surgery [10]. Jin Ma et al. found that rs1718125 polymorphism in *P2RX7* gene had significant association with postoperative pain intensity and the consumption of fentanyl in patients undergoing lung resection [11].

The mechanism of acute pain after thoracotomy has not been fully illuminated, but it is believed to be caused by a variety of factors including the local damage of rib and skin incision, the inflammation caused by injury, and the acute intercostal neuralgia [1, 12]. The multifactorial nature of postoperative pain suggests that a number of distinct genetic factors may contribute to the variability in pain perception and analgesic effect after thoracotomy. Although more and more genetic polymorphisms have been identified as risk factors for rare and common pain syndromes [13, 14], most of these genes have not been studied in thoracotomy subjects.

In the present study, except for *OPRM1, ABCB1, UGT2B7, and P2RX7*, we selected other 14 genes known to be involved in systems related to pain perception and modulation based on evidence in the literature. The selected genes have been related to the ion channels (*SCN9A, SCN10A, SCN11A, KCNJ6, TRPV1,* and *CACN A1E*) [15–20], dopaminergic system (*COMT, DRD2*) [21, 22], purinergic receptor (*P2RY12*) [23], adrenergic receptor (*ADRB1*) [24], estrogen receptor (*ESR1*) [25], serine/threonine kinase (*TAOK3*) [26], growth factors (*TGFB1*) [27], and transcription factor (*CREB1*) [28]. The aim of the present study was to evaluate the association of common SNPs among aforementioned genes with the inadequate analgesia after single-port VATS.

Methods

The current prospective study was approved by the Ethics Committee of the Second Affiliated Hospital of Zhejiang University School of Medicine, Hangzhou, Zhejiang, China, and the protocol was registered in the ClinicalTrials.gov Registry (NCT03916120). All subjects signed informed consent documents prior to enrollment.

Patient characteristics

Two hundred Thirty-two subjects were recruited from consecutive patients undergoing selective lung section with single-port VATS performed by one attending surgeon at the Second Affiliated Hospital of Zhejiang University School of Medicine between July 2018 and January 2019. The detailed surgical procedure was previously described [29]. The criteria for inclusion in the study were age from

18 to 70, ASA classification I to III, and voluntarily received patient-controlled intravenous (PCIA) treatment. The exclusion criteria included the following: (1) history of mental illness, chronic pain, and alcohol or drug abuse; (2) remarkably abnormal liver and/or kidney function (more than two times of the normal); (3) allergy to related opioid drugs; (4) women during pregnancy or lactation.

Anesthesia protocol

All patients received general anesthesia under standard protocol. Specifically, general anesthesia was induced with midazolam (0.2 mg*kg-1), sufentanil (10 μg*kg-1), and etomidate (0.3 mg*kg-1). Cisatracurium besilate (0.15 mg*kg-1) was administered to induce a neuromuscular blockade for tracheal intubation. Anesthesia was continuously maintained with sevoflurane, propofol, and remifentanil. Cisatracurium was bloused as needed. During the surgery, standardized monitoring and bispectral index were applied. Central venous catheterization (CVC) and A-line were implemented for each patient. Before closure of the thoracic incision, surgeons performed a three-site intercostal nerve block with 0.75% 10 mL ropivacaine under thoracoscope. At the end of surgery, pentazocine 5 mg and tropisetron 5 mg were administered by the anesthetist. Immediately after surgery, PCIA was connected to the CVC. Then, patients were transferred to postanesthesia care unit (PACU) for recovery where their vital signs were continuously monitored.

Postoperative pain management

Each subject was extubated at PACU when vital signs stabilized. Patients were asked every 10–15 min after they were awake enough whether they needed pain medication until they became conscious enough to use the PCIA. If the patients felt moderate or severe pain (visual analog scale [VAS] 40–100, 0 = no pain to 100 = intense pain), they were given 40 mg dynastat until their VAS was ≤30. Patients were excluded if they received dynastat as rescue analgesia at PACU. PCIA was administered with a bolus doses of 0.002 mg/kg hydromorphone permitted every 8 min. In case of PCIA analgesic inadequate (VAS ≥ 40), dynastat 40 mg would be administered as an alternative rescue modality. Tropisetron 5 mg or palonosetron 0.25 mg could be administered to combat postoperative nausea and vomiting.

Data collection and follow-up

During the preoperative interview, demographic characteristics, educational background, work type, and history of cigarette smoking and alcohol consumption were recorded. Besides, the general sleep quality within 1 month was recorded by a scale with three levels (poor, fair, and good). At the same time, patients were instructed on how to use the VAS to describe the pain they were experiencing, and how to use the PCIA device to control the pain when necessary. After surgery, the intraoperative parameters including surgery type and duration, anesthesia duration, lymphadenectomy, adhesion loosening, and pathologic diagnosis were also recorded.

During the follow-up period, VAS at rest and during coughing was recorded on the first morning (8:00 a.m.) after surgery. In the meantime, the use of rescue analgesia, postoperative sleep quality, and the degree of satisfaction (bad, fair, good, and excellent) to the pain management were recorded.

End-points

The primary outcome was the occurrence of postoperative inadequate analgesia. Once patient experience at least one of the following situations during the first night and morning after surgery: require extra analgesic drug; report moderate-to-severe pain (VAS ≥ 4) at rest; report poor sleep quality; report bad satisfaction with pain control, they were defined as postoperative inadequate analgesia.

Genotype analysis

Blood samples were collected in tubes containing ethylenediaminetetraacetic acid 1 h after CVC was implemented and were then stored at − 80 °C. Genomic DNA was extracted from whole blood for genetic analysis by using Blood Genomic DNA Mini Kit (Biomed Corporation, China) according to the manufacturer's recommendations. DNA samples were then stored at − 20 °C. SNPs were genotyped using a KASP™ genotyping assay (Rui Biotechnology, Beijing, China) as previously described [30, 31].

Quality control was performed to ensure the robust genetic association: SNPs with call rates of < 95%, Minor Allele Frequency (MAF) < 0.05, or Hardy-Weinberg equilibrium (HWE) of $p <$ 0.05 were excluded. Linkage disequilibrium (LD) was calculated from the patients' genotypes. When strong LD ($r^2 >$ 0.9) was present in one gene, we only included one SNP from each pairs of SNP in the association study. Finally, there were 28 SNPs among the 18 candidate genes passed all quality control filters. (See Table 1).

Statistical analysis

Statistical analysis was completed with the SPSS 24.0 (SPSS Inc., Chicago, IL). Continuous variables were expressed as means and standard deviations (SDs) or as medians and interquartile range, and categorical variables as counts and percentages. Differences between two groups were evaluated by Student's t-test or the Mann-Whitney test for continuous variables, and Chi-squared test or Fisher's exact test for categorical variables. For analyzing the association between SNPs and inadequate analgesia, odds ratios (ORs) and 95% confidence intervals (CI) were calculated by logistic regression analysis adjusted for potential risk factors. Four genetic models (co-dominant, dominant, recessive

and overdominant) were evaluated for association of polymorphisms with risk of inadequate analgesia. HWE was assessed by SNPStats software [32]. The linkage disequilibrium and pairwise LD coefficients were implemented with Haploview 4.2 (Daly Lab: Cambridge, MA, USA, 2008). P value < 0.05 was considered significant.

Power analysis was done using QUANTO (University of Southern California, Los Angeles, CA). For the analyses of associations with postoperative inadequate analgesia, with the sample size of 198 and a modest Type I error rate of 5%, the analysis had more than 90% power to detect an OR of 2.15 for SNPs with an MAF ≥ 0.11 under dominant model and more than 99% power to detect an OR of 0.41 for SNPs with an MAF ≥ 0.26 under recessive model.

Results

Patient characteristics

From July 2018 to January 2019, a total of 232 patients underwent single-port VATS at our center. Two hundred eleven patients met the inclusion criteria voluntarily participate in this study. Thirteen patients were withdrawn due to conversion to open surgery ($n =$ 3) or expectant treatment (n = 3), transferred to the intensive care unit after operation ($n =$ 2), and received rescue analgesics in PACU ($n =$ 5). Therefore, the data from 198 patients entered the final analysis as shown in Fig. 1.

The overall demographic and clinical characteristics are shown in Table 2 and Table 3. All enrolled patients were Chinese population. The baseline cohort comprised 115 females (58.1%) and 83 males (41.9%), aged 37 to 70 years (mean 58.0 years). Postoperative inadequate analgesia was observed in 90 patients (90/198, 45.5%), including 66 patients with moderate-to-severe pain at rest (VAS ≥ 4), 45 patients required extra analgesic drug, 68 patients had bad sleep quality, and 30 patients were unsatisfactory to the pain management. Except for age and education level, there were no significant differences regarding demographic variables and clinical characteristics between patients with and without inadequate analgesia. The patients with inadequate analgesia were significant younger, and had higher education level than patients without inadequate analgesia. These variables were included as covariates in the regression model of genetic association analysis.

Association analysis

The genotyping call rate was 100%. All the selected SNPs met the HWE criterion ($p <$ 0.05) and without low MAF ($p <$ 0.05). Strong LDs in *SCN11A* (Additional file 1: Figure S1) were identified in our sample, and we included only one SNP from each pair of SNP in the association study. Thus, 28 SNPs among 18 genes were assessed for further association analysis.

Table 1 Description of all single nucleotide polymorphisms analyzed

Gene	Polymorphism	Functional Consequence	Variant	Major/minor allele frequency	Hardy Weinberg p-value
ABCB1	rs1045642	Synonymous codon	A > G	0.62/0.38	0.37
	rs1128503	Synonymous codon	A > G	0.67/0.33	0.63
ADRB1	rs1801252	Missense	A > G	0.83/0.17	0.46
	rs1801253	Missense	G > C	0.74/0.26	1
CACNA1E	rs3845446	Intron variant	T > C	0.7/0.3	0.61
COMT	rs4633	Synonymous codon	C > T	0.72/0.28	0.86
	rs4680	Missense	G > A	0.72/0.28	1
DRD2	rs6277	Synonymous codon	G > A	0.94/0.06	0.55
ESR1	rs9340799	Intron variant	A > G	0.81/0.19	0.25
KCNJ6	rs6517442	Upstream variant	C > T	0.73/0.27	0.07
	rs2070995	synonymous codon	T > C	0.61/0.39	0.55
OPRM1	rs1799971	Intron variant	A > G	0.69/0.31	0.50
	rs677830	Intron variant	C > T	0.89/0.11	0.46
	rs540825	Intron variant	A > T	0.92/0.08	1
P2RX7	rs7958311	Intron variant	G > A	0.52/0.48	0.67
P2RY12	rs3732765	Intron variant	G > A	0.87/0.13	1
SCN11A	rs33985936	Missense	C > T	0.89/0.11	0.48
	rs11709492	Intron variant	C > T	0.74/0.26	0.71
SCN10A	rs6795970	Missense	A > G	0.86/0.14	0.38
SCN9A	rs6746030	Intron variant	A > G	0.95/0.05	0.36
	rs4286289	Intron variant	C > A	0.56/0.44	1
	3312G > T	Missense	G > T	0.9/0.1	0.69
TAOK3	rs795484	Intron variant	T > C	0.68/0.32	0.74
	rs1277441	Intron variant	G > A	0.59/0.41	0.14
TGFB1	rs1800469	Downstream variant	A > G	0.51/0.49	0.26
TRPV1	rs8065080	Missense	T > C	0.64/0.36	0.22
UGT2B7	rs7439366	Missense	T > C	0.69/0.31	0.87
CREB1	rs2952768	None	T > C	0.57/0.43	0.77

Abbreviations: *ABCB1* ATP binding cassette subfamily B member 1, *ADRB1* adrenoceptor beta 1, *CACNA1E* calcium voltage-gated channel subunit alpha1 E, *COMT* catechol-O-methyltransferase, CREB1 cAMP responsive element binding protein 1, *DRD2* dopamine receptor D2, *ESR1* estrogen receptor 1, *KCNJ6* potassium voltage-gated channel subfamily J member 6; *OPRM1* opioid receptor mu 1, *P2RX7* purinergic receptor P2X 7; *P2RY12* purinergic receptor P2Y12, *SCN11A* sodium voltage-gated channel alpha subunit 11; *SCN10A* sodium voltage-gated channel alpha subunit 10, *SCN9A* sodium voltage-gated channel alpha subunit 9, *TAOK3* TAO kinase 3, *TGFB1* transforming growth factor beta 1, *TRPV1* transient receptor potential cation channel subfamily V member 1, *UGT2B7* UDP glucuronosyltransferase family 2 member B7

The distribution of the allele and genotype frequencies of the remaining 28 SNPs in patients with and without inadequate analgesia is summarized in Additional file 2: Table S1. Significant associations between genetic mutations and postoperative inadequate analgesia were detected in six SNPs among five genes (*ESR1, P2RY12, SCN11A, SCN9A,* and *TAOK3*) by the logistic regression (see Table 4). After adjusting for potential confounders, four SNPs remained significant: rs33985936 (*SCN11A*), rs11709492 (*SCN11A*), rs6795970 (*SCN10A*), and 3312G > T (*SCN9A*).

For *SCN11A*, two SNPs (i.e., rs33985936, rs11709492) were associated with the occurrence of inadequate analgesia. For rs33985936, individuals who carried the rare T allele (TC + TT vs. CC) had a 2.15-fold increase in the odds of reporting

inadequate analgesia. The rare T allele carriers of rs11709492 were found to be associated with decreased risk of inadequate analgesia (OR = 0.41, 95% CI: 0.22–0.77, p = 0.005).

For *SCN10A* rs6795970, patients with GA/ AA genotype had a 2.14-fold increase in the odds of reporting inadequate analgesia compared to GG genotype.

For *SCN9A* 3312G > T, patients who were heterozygous or homozygous for the rare T allele (TG + TT vs. GG) had a 2.85-fold increase in the odds of reporting postoperative inadequate analgesia.

Discussion

In the present study, the incidence of postoperative inadequate analgesia in patients undergoing single-

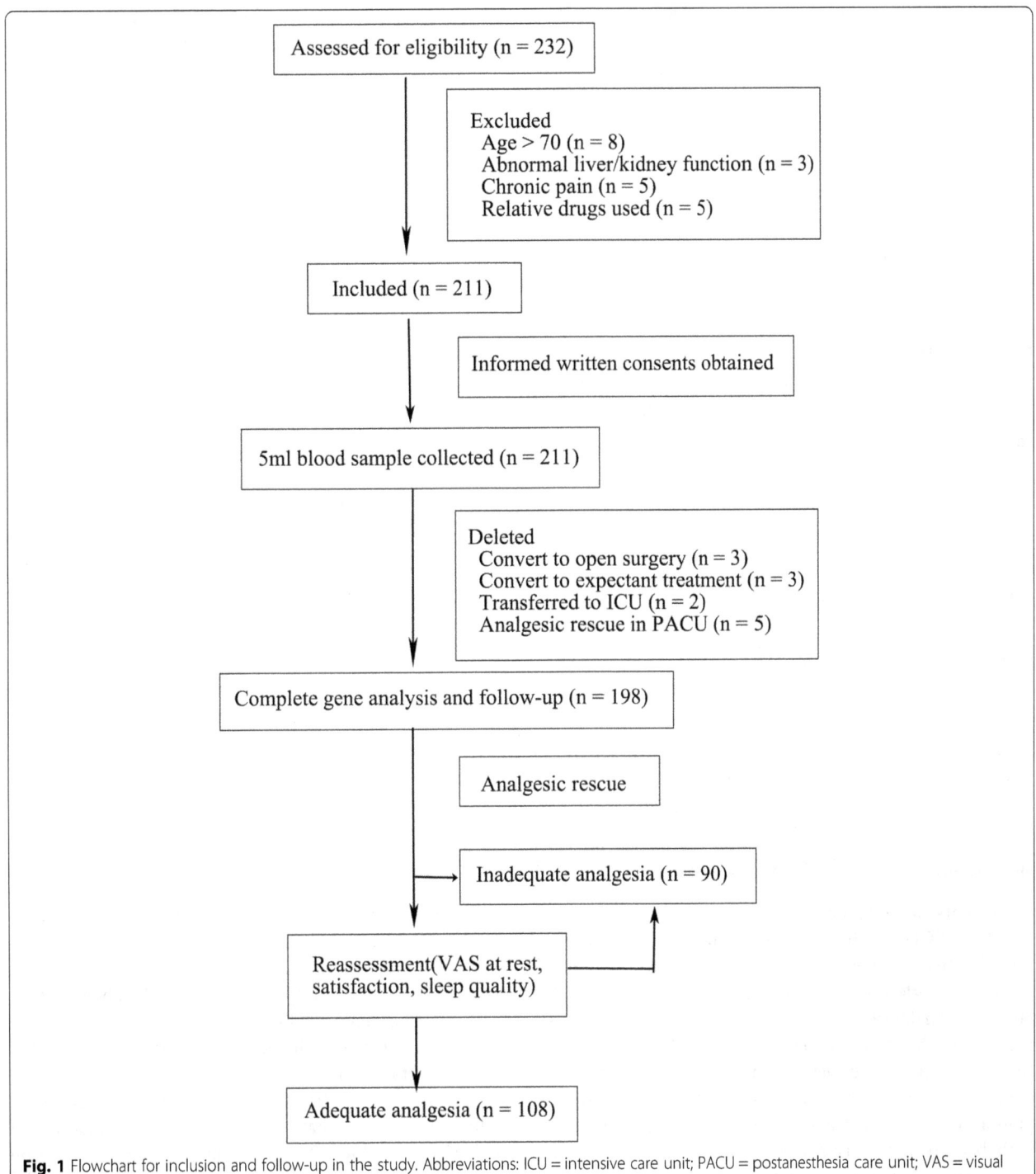

Fig. 1 Flowchart for inclusion and follow-up in the study. Abbreviations: ICU = intensive care unit; PACU = postanesthesia care unit; VAS = visual analog scale

port VATS was 45.5%. Twenty-eight SNPs among 18 genes involved in pain perception and modulation were selected to test the association between genetic polymorphisms and postoperative inadequate analgesia. After adjusting for confounding factors, significant association with inadequate analgesia was found in four SNPs (rs11709492, rs33985936, rs6795970, and 3312G > T) of genes encoding voltage-gated sodium channels.

Although numerous measures have been developed for the management of postoperative pain, the proportion of patient experience moderate to severe postoperative pain after thoracotomy was relatively high [2]. In the present study, the inadequate analgesia was happened in 45.5%

Table 2 Distribution of socio-demographic characteristics between patients with and without postoperative inadequate analgesia

Variables	Adequate analgesia (n = 108)	Inadequate analgesia (n = 90)	P-Value
Age (y) (mean ± SD)	60.08 ± 6.79	55.42 ± 9.03	< 0.001
Sex			0.11
Female	70 (63.1%)	45 (51.7%)	
Male	41 (36.9%)	42 (48.3%)	
BMI (mean ± SD)	22.86 ± 2.84	23.10 ± 2.57	0.54
Weight (mean ± SD)	60.92 ± 9.34	63.31 ± 9.30	0.07
History of Cigarette Smoking			0.62
Yes	22 (20.4%)	21 (24.1%)	
No	86 (79.6%)	69 (75.9%)	
History of Alcohol Consumption			1.00
Yes	24 (22.2%)	10 (22.2%)	
No	84 (77.8%)	70 (77.8%)	
Educational Level			< 0.001
Low	52 (48.1%)	23 (25.6%)	
Medium	46 (42.6%)	35 (38.9%)	
High	10 (9.3%)*	32 (35.6%)	
Exercise			0.26
Yes	49 (45.4%)	48 (53.3%)	
No	59 (54.6%)	42 (46.7%)	
Preoperative Sleep Quality			0.33
Poor	18 (16.7%)	21 (23.3%)	
Fair	43 (39.8%)	28 (31.1%)	
Good	47 (43.5%)	41 (45.6%)	
Major Surgery within 2 Years			0.51
Yes	9 (8.3%)	10 (11.1%)	
No	99 (91.7%)	80 (88.9%)	

Abbreviations: BMI = body mass index; SD = standard deviation

of patients who received intercostal nerve block and standard PCIA with hydromorphone after single-port VATS. This result was consistent with previous reports [3, 33]. Considering some patients were unwilling to take any extra analgesic drug even though they were unsatisfactory to the analgesia effect or their sleep was disturbed by pain, we defined postoperative inadequate analgesia as not only patients with moderate to severe pain and required extra analgesic drug, but also patients with bad sleep quality and low satisfaction. This definition comprehensively comprises the real patients with inadequate analgesia.

Our results indicated that four SNPs in genes encoding voltage-gated sodium channels (VGSCs) were associated with pain perception after sing-port VATS. VGSCs play a key role in the initiation and transmission of action potentials in excitable cells [34]. More than 1000 disease-related mutations have been discovered in nine VGSC-encoding genes [35]. It has been widely recognized that the changes of VGSC expression are involved

in the sensitization of sensory neurons in many acute and chronic pain conditions [36].

SCN11A encodes one member of the sodium channel alpha subunit gene family NaV1.9, and is highly expressed in nociceptive neurons of dorsal root ganglia and trigeminal ganglia. Mutations in this gene have been associated with hereditary pain syndromes [37]. In this study, we identified two SNPs (rs33985936, rs11709492) were associated with inadequate analgesia. The mutation of rs33985936 (2725C > T) causes amino acid substitution Val909Ile which leads to the changes in intermolecular force of Nav1.9 [17]. Previous study reported that subjects who carrying the minor allele of rs33985936 were more sensitive to pain, while patients carrying the minor allele of rs11709492 have lower pain sensitivity [17]. This was consistent with our results that individuals who carried the rare T allele of rs33985936 had a 2.3-fold increase in the odds of reporting inadequate analgesia, and the rare T allele of rs11709492 were found to be associated with decreased risk of inadequate analgesia.

Table 3 Distribution of clinical characteristics between patients with and without postoperative inadequate analgesia

Variables	Adequate analgesia ($n = 108$)	Inadequate analgesia ($n = 90$)	P-Value
Surgery time (median [IQR])	82.5 (60–105)	85 (65–100)	0.97
Anesthesia time (median [IQR])	110 (83.5–135)	110 (91.5–128.5)	0.89
Surgery end-time (median [IQR]	15.5 (13.3–18)	16 (14–18.6)	0.27
Section Parts			0.70
One part	90 (83.3%)	76 (84.4%)	
Two parts	15 (13.9%)	13 (14.4%)	
Three parts	3 (2.8%)	1 (1.1%)	
Surgery Type			0.49
Wedge resection	17 (15.7%)	8 (8.9%)	
Segmentectomy	21 (19.4%)	16 (17.8%)	
Lobectomy	69 (63.9%)	65 (72.2%)	
Pneumonectomy	1 (0.9%)	1 (1.1%)	
Lymph Node Dissection			0.35
Yes	91 (84.3%)	80 (88.9%)	
No	17 (15.7%)	10 (11.1%)	
Adhesion Loosening			0.28
Yes	54 (50.0%)	38 (42.2%)	
No	54 (50.0%)	52 (57.8%)	
Pathologic Diagnosis			0.47
Low-Grade	9 (8.3%)	12 (13.3%)	
High-Grade	73 (67.6%)	60 (66.7%)	
Benign	26 (24.1%)	18 (20.0%)	

Abbreviations: *IQR* interquartile range

Table 4 Logistic regression analyses of associations between SNPs and risk of postoperative inadequate analgesia

Gene	SNP	Model	Genotype	Adequate analgesia	Inadequate analgesia	OR (95% CI) unadjusted	P-Value unadjusted	OR (95% CI) adjusted	P-Value adjusted
ESR1	rs9340799	Recessive	A/A-G/A	99 (91.7%)	89 (98.9%)	1.00	0.01	1.00	0.020
			G/G	9 (8.3%)	1 (1.1%)	0.12 (0.02–0.99)		0.13 (0.02–1.08)	
P2RY12	rs3732765	Dominant	G/G	76 (70.4%)	75 (83.3%)	1.00	0.031	1.00	0.180
			G/A-A/A	32 (29.6%)	15 (16.7%)	0.48 (0.24–0.95)		0.61 (0.29–1.28)	
SCN11A	rs33985936	Dominant	C/C	89 (82.4%)	66 (73.3%)	1.00	0.12	1.00	0.042
			T/C-T/T	19 (17.6%)	24 (26.7%)	1.70 (0.86–3.37)		2.15 (1.02–4.52)	
	rs11709492	Dominant	C/C	51 (47.2%)	56 (62.2%)	1.00	0.03	1.00	0.005
			T/C-T/T	57 (52.8%)	34 (37.8%)	0.54 (0.31–0.96)		0.41 (0.22–0.77)	
SCN10A	rs6795970	Dominant	G/G	84 (77.8%)	59 (65.6%)	1.00	0.06	1.00	0.026
			G/A-A/A	24 (22.2%)	31 (34.4%)	1.84 (0.98–3.45)		2.14 (1.09–4.21)	
SCN9A	rs6746030	Dominant	G/G	94 (87%)	86 (95.6%)	1.00	0.032	1.00	0.067
			G/A-A/A	14 (13%)	4 (4.4%)	0.31 (0.10–0.99)		0.35 (0.10–1.16)	
	3312G > T	Dominant	G/G	96 (88.9%)	66 (73.3%)	1.00	0.005	1.00	0.011
			T/G-T/T	12 (11.1%)	24 (26.7%)	2.91 (1.36–6.22)		2.85 (1.25–6.51)	
TAOK3	rs1277441	Dominant	T/T	33 (30.6%)	40 (44.4%)	1.00	0.044	1.00	0.13
			T/C-C/C	75 (69.4%)	50 (55.6%)	0.55 (0.31–0.99)		0.61 (0.32–1.15)	

Abbreviations: *CI* confidence intervals, *ESR1* estrogen receptor 1, *OR* odds ratios, *P2RY12* purinergic receptor P2Y12, *SCN11A* sodium voltage-gated channel alpha subunit 11, *SCN10A* sodium voltage-gated channel alpha subunit 10, *SCN9A* sodium voltage-gated channel alpha subunit 9, *SNP* single nucleotide polymorphism, *TAOK3* TAO kinase 3

SCN10A and *SCN9A* encode Nav1.8 and Nav1.7 sodium channels, respectively. They are preferentially expressed in dorsal root ganglion sensory neurons and sympathetic ganglia and significantly influence nociceptor excitability [15, 38, 39]. Recent genetic studies have identified rare and common mutations in *SCN9A* and *SCN10A* as contributory both in chronic pain conditions and postoperative pain [15, 16, 39]. Guangyou Duan et al. reported that 3312G > T (*SCN9A*), a nonsynonymous SNP leading to the amino acid substitution V1104 L in human Nav1.7, was associated with postoperative inadequate analgesia [16]. Patients carrying the 3312G allele had a higher incidence of inadequate analgesia than those carrying the 3312 T allele. They also demonstrated an association between *SCN10A* rs6795970 and higher thresholds for mechanical pain in experimental pain testing [15]. However, in our study, we identified that patients with the 3312Tallele (3312G > T) and A allele (rs6795970) had a higher risk of presenting with inadequate analgesia.

As mentioned before, *OPRM1*and *COMT* play an important role in endogenous pain modulation and opioid analgesia. De Gregori M et al. found that genetic polymorphisms in *OPRM1* (rs540825), *COMT* (rs4680) and *ESR1* (rs9340799) have clinical effect on the morphine consumption and pain scores after major surgery [40]. The rs1799971 polymorphisms of the *OPRM1* gene is related to the analgesic effect and sufentanil consumption in Chinese Han patients after radical operation of lung cancer [9]. Nevertheless the correlations were not confirmed in our present study. For *ESR1* (rs9340799), the frequencies of G allele in patients with postoperative inadequate analgesia was less than in patients without (15% vs. 23%). Compared with the AA and AG genotypes, the homozygous genotype GG appeared to decrease the risk for postoperative inadequate analgesia (OR = 0.12, 95% CI: 0.02–0.99, p = 0.01). After adjusting for potential confounders, although the P-value of the correlation was statistically significant ($p < 0.05$), the odds ratio didn't have clinical significance (OR = 0.13, 95% CI: 0.02–1.08). So we didn't include the rs9340799 (*ESR1*) to the final results.

This inconsistence may partly due to the different subjects and different surgery type. The general situation of the patients included in the present study differed from previous studies, and it is known that factors such as age, race, and gender all may affect the patient's pain sensitivity [41, 42]. Then, the present study focused on patients undergoing single-port thoracoscopic surgery. The mechanisms (inflammatory pain, mechanical traction pain, and intercostal neuralgia) and degrees of postoperative pain may vary from the type of surgery. This difference may cause the same polymorphism to show inconsistent or even completely opposite results in different surgeries [20, 43]. Besides, the findings identified

by Guangyou Duan et al. were based on experimental pain tests performed on healthy volunteers [16]. This suggests that we should be rigorous to use these results in assessing pain sensitivity of patients after surgery. Therefore, further replication studies are warranted to confirm these findings.

There are some limitations in the present study. First, the postoperative inadequate analgesia was assessed within the first 24 h after surgery. In the previous study, we found that the intense pain after single-port VATS is sustained within 24 h especially during the first night and the first morning after surgery and majority of patients achieved satisfactory pain relief after 24 h [29]. So we only followed up until the first night and first morning after surgery. Second, these findings are specific to the patients underwent single-port VATS. The associations found in this study may differ in thoracotomy. Finally, due to the exploration nature of the study, the sample size was relative small and we did not replicate the study in a validation cohort. Future studies with a larger sample size may increase the power to detect differences in other candidate genes.

Conclusions

In summary, our findings suggest that polymorphisms in voltage-gated sodium channels genes play a role in the inadequate postoperative analgesia after single-port VATS. The genes and SNPs found in this study may help to identify, prevent, and targetedly treat patients with high risk of experiencing inadequate postoperative pain. This, in turn, may improve the postoperative rehabilitation and reduce short- and long-term morbidity. Future studies are warranted to confirm our findings and to determine if these associations are present in the opioid consumption analysis.

Supplementary information

Additional file 1: Figure S1. LD plots of SNPs of the *SCN11A* gene. Identifies the linkage disequilibrium of SNPs among *SCN11A* gene.

Additional file 2: Table S1. Genotype and allele distributions of polymorphisms in patients with and without postoperative inadequate analgesia.

Abbreviations
ABCB1: ATP binding cassette subfamily B member 1; ADRB1: Adrenoceptor beta 1; CACNA1E: Calcium voltage-gated channel subunit alpha1 E; CI: Confidence intervals; COMT: Catechol-O-methyltransferase; CREB1: CAMP responsive element binding protein 1; CVC: Central venous catheterization; DRD2: Dopamine receptor D2; ESR1: Estrogen receptor 1; HWE: Hardy-Weinberg equilibrium; KCNJ6: Potassium voltage-gated channel subfamily J member 6; LD: Linkage disequilibrium; MAF: Minor allele frequency; OPRM1: Opioid receptor mu 1; ORs: Odds ratios; P2RX7: Purinergic receptor P2X 7; P2RY12: Purinergic receptor P2Y12; PACU: Postanesthesia care unit; PCIA: Patient-controlled intravenous; SCN10A: Sodium voltage-gated channel alpha subunit 10; SCN11A: Sodium voltage-gated channel alpha subunit 11;

SCN9A: Sodium voltage-gated channel alpha subunit 9; SDs: Standard deviations; SNPs: Single nucleotide polymorphisms; TAOK3: TAO kinase 3; TGFB1: Transforming growth factor beta 1; TRPV1: Transient receptor potential cation channel subfamily V member 1; UGT2B7: UDP glucuronosyltransferase family 2 member B7; VAS: Visual analog scale; VATS: Video-assisted thoracoscopic surgery; VGSCs: Voltage-gated sodium channels

Acknowledgements
Not applicable.

Authors' contributions
XX helped to conduct the study, recruited patients, collected data, analyzed the data and prepared the manuscript. YB helped to design and conduct the study, analyzed the data and revised the manuscript. KS helped to design and revised the manuscript. MY designed the study and provided revision for intellectual content and final approval of the manuscript. All authors read and approved the final manuscript.

References

1. Gerner P. Postthoracotomy pain management problems. Anesthesiol Clin. 2008;26:355–67 vii.
2. Rizk NP, Ghanie A, Hsu M, Bains MS, Downey RJ, Sarkaria IS, Finley DJ, Adusumilli PS, Huang J, Sima CS, et al. A prospective trial comparing pain and quality of life measures after anatomic lung resection using thoracoscopy or thoracotomy. Ann Thorac Surg. 2014;98:1160–6.
3. Bayman EO, Parekh KR, Keech J, Larson N, Vander Weg M, Brennan TJ. Preoperative patient expectations of postoperative pain are associated with moderate to severe acute pain after VATS. Pain Med. 2019;20:543–54.
4. Muehling BM, Halter GL, Schelzig H, Meierhenrich R, Steffen P, Sunder-Plassmann L, Orend KH. Reduction of postoperative pulmonary complications after lung surgery using a fast track clinical pathway. Eur J Cardiothorac Surg. 2008;34:174–80.
5. Kolettas A, Lazaridis G, Baka S, Mpoukovinas I, Karavasilis V, Kioumis I, Pitsiou G, Papaiwannou A, Lampaki S, Karavergou A, et al. Postoperative pain management. J Thorac Dis. 2015;7:S62–72.
6. Zhang W, Chang YZ, Kan QC, Zhang LR, Lu H, Chu QJ, Wang ZY, Li ZS, Zhang J. Association of human micro-opioid receptor gene polymorphism A118G with fentanyl analgesia consumption in Chinese gynaecological patients. Anaesthesia. 2010;65:130–5.
7. Zhang F, Tong J, Hu J, Zhang H, Ouyang W, Huang D, Tang Q, Liao Q. COMT gene haplotypes are closely associated with postoperative fentanyl dose in patients. Anesth Analg. 2015;120:933–40.
8. Ochroch EA, Vachani A, Gottschalk A, Kanetsky PA. Natural variation in the mu-opioid gene OPRM1 predicts increased pain on third day after thoracotomy. Clin J Pain. 2012;28:747–54.
9. Zhao Z, Lv B, Zhao X, Zhang Y. Effects of OPRM1 and ABCB1 gene polymorphisms on the analgesic effect and dose of sufentanil after thoracoscopic-assisted radical resection of lung cancer. Biosci Rep. 2019;39: BSR20181211.
10. Sastre JA, Varela G, Lopez M, Muriel C, Gonzalez-Sarmiento R. Influence of uridine diphosphate-glucuronyltransferase 2B7 (UGT2B7) variants on postoperative buprenorphine analgesia. Pain Pract. 2015;15:22–30.
11. Ma J, Li W, Chai Q, Tan X, Zhang K. Correlation of P2RX7 gene rs1718125 polymorphism with postoperative fentanyl analgesia in patients with lung cancer. Medicine. 2019;98:e14445.
12. Semyonov M, Fedorina E, Grinshpun J, Dubilet M, Refaely Y, Ruderman L, Koyfman L, Friger M, Zlotnik A, Klein M, et al. Ultrasound-guided serratus anterior plane block for analgesia after thoracic surgery. J Pain Res. 2019;12: 953–60.
13. George SZ, Wu SS, Wallace MR, Moser MW, Wright TW, Farmer KW, Greenfield WH 3rd, Dai Y, Li H, Fillingim RB. Biopsychosocial influence on shoulder pain: influence of genetic and psychological combinations on twelve-month postoperative pain and disability outcomes. Arthritis Care Res. 2016;68:1671–80.
14. Li J, Wei Z, Zhang J, Hakonarson H, Cook-Sather SD. Candidate gene analyses for acute pain and morphine analgesia after pediatric day surgery: African American versus European Caucasian ancestry and dose prediction limits. Pharmacogenomics J. 2019;19:570–81.
15. Duan G, Han C, Wang Q, Guo S, Zhang Y, Ying Y, Huang P, Zhang L, Macala

L, Shah P, et al. A SCN10A SNP biases human pain sensitivity. Mol Pain. 2016;12:1744806916666083.
16. Duan G, Xiang G, Zhang X, Yuan R, Zhan H, Qi D. A single-nucleotide polymorphism in SCN9A may decrease postoperative pain sensitivity in the general population. Anesthesiology. 2013;118:436–42.
17. Sun J, Duan G, Li N, Guo S, Zhang Y, Ying Y, Zhang M, Wang Q, Liu JY, Zhang X. SCN11A variants may influence postoperative pain sensitivity after gynecological surgery in Chinese Han female patients. Medicine. 2017;96: e8149.
18. Nishizawa D, Nagashima M, Katoh R, Satoh Y, Tagami M, Kasai S, Ogai Y, Han W, Hasegawa J, Shimoyama N, et al. Association between KCNJ6 (GIRK2) gene polymorphisms and postoperative analgesic requirements after major abdominal surgery. PLoS One. 2009;4:e7060.
19. Kim H, Neubert JK, San Miguel A, Xu K, Krishnaraju RK, Iadarola MJ, Goldman D, Dionne RA. Genetic influence on variability in human acute experimental pain sensitivity associated with gender, ethnicity and psychological temperament. Pain. 2004;109:488–96.
20. Ide S, Nishizawa D, Fukuda K, Kasai S, Hasegawa J, Hayashida M, Minami M, Ikeda K. Association between genetic polymorphisms in Ca(v)2.3 (R-type) Ca2+ channels and fentanyl sensitivity in patients undergoing painful cosmetic surgery. PloS one. 2013;8:e70694.
21. Tan EC, Lim EC, Ocampo CE, Allen JC, Sng BL, Sia AT. Common variants of catechol-O-methyltransferase influence patient-controlled analgesia usage and postoperative pain in patients undergoing total hysterectomy. Pharmacogenomics J. 2016;16:186–92.
22. Jaaskelainen SK, Lindholm P, Valmunen T, Pesonen U, Taiminen T, Virtanen A, Lamusuo S, Forssell H, Hagelberg N, Hietala J, et al. Variation in the dopamine D2 receptor gene plays a key role in human pain and its modulation by transcranial magnetic stimulation. Pain. 2014;155:2180–7.
23. Sumitani M, Nishizawa D, Nagashima M, Ikeda K, Abe H, Kato R, Ueda H, Yamada Y. Japanese TRCPrg: association between polymorphisms in the Purinergic P2Y12 receptor gene and Severity of both Cancer pain and postoperative pain. Pain Med. 2018;19:348–54.
24. Moriyama A, Nishizawa D, Kasai S, Hasegawa J, Fukuda K, Nagashima M, Katoh R, Ikeda K. Association between genetic polymorphisms of the beta1-adrenergic receptor and sensitivity to pain and fentanyl in patients undergoing painful cosmetic surgery. J Pharmacol Sci. 2013;121:48–57.
25. An X, Fang J, Lin Q, Lu C, Ma Q, Qu H. New evidence for involvement of ESR1 gene in susceptibility to Chinese migraine. J Neurol. 2017;264:81–7.
26. Cook-Sather SD, Li J, Goebel TK, Sussman EM, Rehman MA, Hakonarson H. TAOK3, a novel genome-wide association study locus associated with morphine requirement and postoperative pain in a retrospective pediatric day surgery population. Pain. 2014;155:1773–83.
27. Somogyi AA, Sia AT, Tan EC, Coller JK, Hutchinson MR, Barratt DT. Ethnicity-dependent influence of innate immune genetic markers on morphine PCA requirements and adverse effects in postoperative pain. Pain. 2016;157: 2458–66.
28. Nishizawa D, Fukuda K, Kasai S, Hasegawa J, Aoki Y, Nishi A, Saita N, Koukita Y, Nagashima M, Katoh R, et al. Genome-wide association study identifies a potent locus associated with human opioid sensitivity. Mol Psychiatry. 2014; 19:55–62.
29. Bai Y, Sun K, Xing X, Zhang F, Sun N, Gao Y, Zhu L, Yao J, Fan J, Yan M. Postoperative analgesic effect of hydromorphone in patients undergoing single-port video-assisted thoracoscopic surgery: a randomized controlled trial. J Pain Res. 2019;12:1091–101.
30. Graves H, Rayburn AL, Gonzalez-Hernandez JL, Nah G, Kim DS, Lee DK. Validating DNA Polymorphisms Using KASP Assay in Prairie Cordgrass (Spartina pectinata Link) Populations in the U.S. Front Plant Sci. 2015;6:1271.
31. He C, Holme J, Anthony J. SNP genotyping: the KASP assay. Methods Mol Biol. 2014;1145:75–86.
32. Sole X, Guino E, Valls J, Iniesta R, Moreno V. SNPStats: a web tool for the analysis of association studies. Bioinformatics. 2006;22:1928–9.
33. Wang H, Li S, Liang N, Liu W, Liu H, Liu H. Postoperative pain experiences in Chinese adult patients after thoracotomy and video-assisted thoracic surgery. J Clin Nurs. 2017;26:2744–54.
34. Xu L, Ding X, Wang T, Mou S, Sun H, Hou T. Voltage-gated sodium channels: structures, functions, and molecular modeling. Drug Discov Today. 2019;24: 1389–97.
35. Huang W, Liu M, Yan SF, Yan N. Structure-based assessment of disease-related mutations in human voltage-gated sodium channels. Protein Cell. 2017;8:401–38.

36. Bennett DL, Clark AJ, Huang J, Waxman SG, Dib-Hajj SD. The role of voltage-gated sodium channels in pain signaling. Physiol Rev. 2019;99:1079–151.

37. Dib-Hajj SD, Black JA, Waxman SG. NaV1.9: a sodium channel linked to human pain. Nat Rev Neurosci. 2015;16:511–9.

38. Garrison SR, Weyer AD, Barabas ME, Beutler BA, Stucky CL. A gain-of-function voltage-gated sodium channel 1.8 mutation drives intense hyperexcitability of A- and C-fiber neurons. Pain. 2014;155:896–905.

39. Yang Y, Wang Y, Li S, Xu Z, Li H, Ma L, Fan J, Bu D, Liu B, Fan Z, et al. Mutations in SCN9A, encoding a sodium channel alpha subunit, in patients with primary erythermalgia. J Med Genet. 2004;41:171–4.

40. De Gregori M, Diatchenko L, Ingelmo PM, Napolioni V, Klepstad P, Belfer I, Molinaro V, Garbin G, Ranzani GN, Alberio G, et al. Human genetic variability contributes to postoperative morphine consumption. J Pain. 2016;17:628–36.

41. Riley JL 3rd, Cruz-Almeida Y, Glover TL, King CD, Goodin BR, Sibille KT, Bartley EJ, Herbert MS, Sotolongo A, Fessler BJ, et al. Age and race effects on pain sensitivity and modulation among middle-aged and older adults. J Pain. 2014;15:272–82.

42. Sato H, Droney J, Ross J, Olesen AE, Staahl C, Andresen T, Branford R, Riley J, Arendt-Nielsen L, Drewes AM. Gender, variation in opioid receptor genes and sensitivity to experimental pain. Mol Pain. 2013;9:20.

43. Amano K, Nishizawa D, Mieda T, Tsujita M, Kitamura A, Hasegawa J, Inada E, Hayashida M, Ikeda K. Opposite associations between the rs3845446 single-nucleotide polymorphism of the CACNA1E gene and Postoperative pain-related phenotypes in gastrointestinal surgery versus previously reported Orthognathic surgery. J Pain. 2016;17:1126–34.

18

Retrospective evaluation of pain in patients with coccydynia who underwent impar ganglion block

Ozlem Sagir* ⓘ, Hafize Fisun Demir, Fatih Ugun and Bulent Atik

Abstract

Background: We aimed to evaluate pain scores one year after impar ganglion block in patients with coccydynia who did not benefit from conservative treatment.

Methods: The medical records of 29 patients with coccydynia were reviewed. Patients who were referred to the algology clinic and underwent impar ganglion blocks were retrospectively evaluated. Demographic data, time to the onset of pain, causes of pain, X-ray findings, administered invasive procedures, and visual analog scale (pain) scores were recorded.

Results: A total of 29 patients were included in the study, 10 males (34%) and 19 females (66%). The average age and body mass index were 53.45 ± 9.6 and 29.55 ± 4.21 respectively. In 21 patients, the onset of pain was associated with trauma. Nineteen patients (65.5%) had anterior coccygeal angulation. The average visual analog scale score before undergoing an impar ganglion block was 7.4 ± 1. After the procedure, the scores at < 3 months, 3–6 months and 6 months-1 year follow-up intervals were significantly lower ($p < 0.05$). Furthermore, visual analog scale scores at the 3–6 months and 6 months-1 year periods were significantly lower in patients who received diagnostic blocks plus pulse radiofrequency thermocoagulation than in patients who underwent a diagnostic block only.

Conclusions: The impar ganglion block provides effective analgesia without complications in patients with coccydynia. Pulse radiofrequency thermocoagulation combined with a diagnostic block prolongs the analgesic effect of the procedure.

Keywords: Coccyx, Chronic pain, Sympathetic nerve block, Pain management, Pulsed radiofrequency treatment

Background

Coccydynia is defined as pain in the sacrococcygeal region. It is a disorder that not only reduces a patient's quality of life, but it is difficult to treat [1]. Numerous physiological and psychological causes can contribute to its etiology. Typically, it is related to chronic inflammation triggered by abnormal mobilization of the coccygeal structures. Childbirth as well as minor but repetitive and direct trauma are considered as possible causal factors. Coccydynia is rarely related to neoplasms or psychological conditions such as somatization [2, 3]. Its incidence is unknown, but female gender and obesity increase the risk [4].

Patients with coccydynia typically complain of pain in the coccyx. This pain increases with prolonged sitting, leaning backwards during sitting, prolonged standing and standing up after being in a sitting position. Conservative treatments such as non-steroidal, anti-inflammatory drugs (NSAIDs), levator ani relaxation exercises, sitting cushions and transcutaneous electrical simulation have all been used to alleviate the pain, however these methods are ineffective in 10% of patients [2].

* Correspondence: ozlemsagir@yahoo.com
Department of Anesthesiology, Balıkesir University Health Application and Research Hospital, 10100 Balikesir, Turkey

The impar ganglion, also known as the Walther ganglion, is the terminal pelvic division of the sympathetic chain and is located behind the rectum, anterior to the sacrococcygeal joint and coccyx. It provides nociceptive and sympathetic innervation to the perineum [5]. When conservative treatments fail to alleviate pain in patients with coccydynia, the impar ganglion can be blocked through the sacrococcygeal or the intercoccygeal junction with the help of screening techniques. After insertion and confirmation of the needle position, local anesthetic drugs, either with or without steroids are injected and thermal ablation via radiofrequency may be applied. However there is limited clinical evidence to support the efficacy of these interventions [6].

The aim of our study was to evaluate pain scores in patients with coccydynia who underwent an impar ganglion block in our algology department due to the failure of conservative treatment over the course of a 1-year follow-up period.

Methods

The medical records of 29 coccydynia patients treated with impar ganglion block at the algology department of Balikesir University Hospital were retrospectively reviewed. Age, gender, height, body weight, the onset of pain and its possible causes (falls, accidents, cancer, or idiopathic) were collected from medical records. X-ray images of the coccyx were examined to evaluate coccygeal structure and underlying physiology and potential pathologies. The images were classified as either normal or exhibiting anterior coccygeal angulation. Our study was approved by the institutional ethics committee (decision No: 2018/156).

The number of impar ganglion blocks used on patients, the 0.25% bupivacaine+ 40 mg methylprednisolone mixture used, and the application of radiofrequency thermocoagulation (RFT) were recorded. Visual analog scale (VAS) pain scores were acquired from the records both before and after the procedures. The VAS scores were obtained during policlinic check-ups and phone calls at < 3 months, 3–6 months and 6 months-1 year time intervals following the procedure. Patients who were referred to surgery after the procedure were also recorded, along with their VAS scores.

The impar ganglion block was performed using a 22-gauge needle from the midline. The tip of the needle and the spread of the radiopaque substance in front of the coccyx were observed using fluoroscopic lateral images with C-arm fluoroscopy assistance (Fig. 1). Blocks performed total 10 mL volume with 0.25% bupivacaine+ 40 mg methylprednisolone were classified as a diagnostic impar block (DB). After the DBs were performed, patients who subsequently underwent pulse RFT (NeuroTherm NT 1100, USA) at 42 °C for 2 min with a 22-G

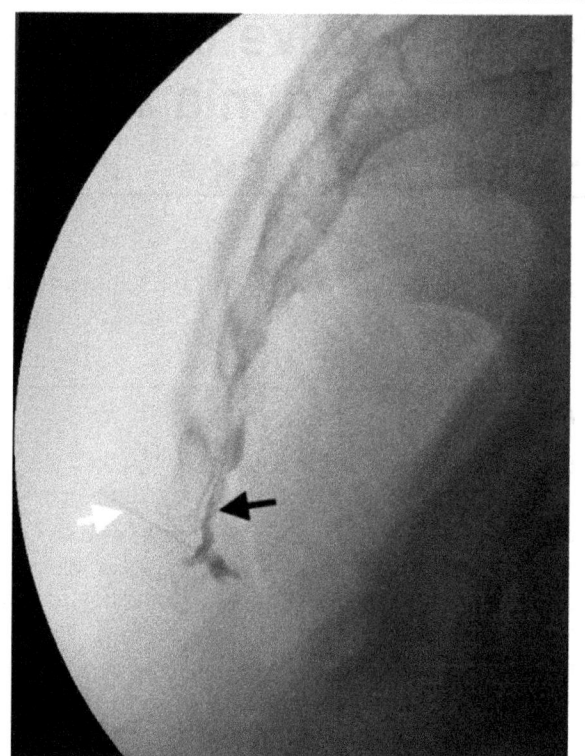

Fig. 1 Lateral fluoroscopy view of the impar ganglion block. Application of the needle from the sacrococcygeal junction (white arrow) and confirmation of the location of the needle tip and spreading of the radiopaque dye in the anterior part of the sacrococcygeal joint (black arrow)

insulated RFT needle with a 5 mm active tip were classified as DB + RFT.

Data was analyzed using IBM SPSS Statistics version 22 (IBM Corp., Armonk, NY, USA). Continuous data is expressed as averages and standard deviations and categorical data as frequencies and percentages. The Shapiro-Wilk test was used to evaluate the normal distribution of parameters. Comparisons of the data was performed using the Wilcoxon and Mann-Whitney U test. Parametric data is shown as average ± standard deviation (SD). Association among VAS score, gender, and body mass index was carried out using the Spearman's correlation test. A p-value < 0.05 was accepted as statistically significant.

Results

Twenty-nine patients, 10 males (34%) and 19 females (66%) were included in the study. The average age, weight, height and body mass index (BMI) of all patients was 53.45 ± 9.6 years, 82.59 ± 12.12 kg, 166.21 ± 8.8 cm and 29.55 ± 4.21, respectively. Body mass index was over 25 in 23 of 29 patients (79.3%). The onset of pain was greater than 1 year in 23 (79.3%) patients and less than 1 year in 6 patients (20.7%) (Table 1). Seventeen patients

Table 1 Examination findings from 29 patients with coccydynia

Weight characteristics	n (%)
BMI < 25	6 (20.7)
BMI 25–29.9	8 (27.6)
BMI ≥ 30	15 (51.7)
Time of pain onset	
< 1 year	6 (20.7)
> 1 year	23 (79.3)
Causes of pain	
Falling	17 (58.6)
Traffic accident	4 (13.8)
Neoplasm	2 (6.9)
Idiopathic	6 (20.7)
X-ray findings	
Normal	10 (34.5)
Anterior angulation	19 (65.5)

Table 2 Average VAS scores of impar ganglion block patients

Observation time	VAS (Mean ± SD)	P-value
Before the block	7.4 ± 1	
After the block	5.2 ± 1.5	< 0.001
< 3 months	4.7 ± 2.1	< 0.001
3–6 months	4.3 ± 2.4	< 0.001
6 months-1 year	4.2 ± 2.6	< 0.001

VAS Visual Analog Scale; Values compared with the average value before the block $p < 0.01$

(58.6%) reported pain after falling backwards, and 4 (13.8%) experienced pain following a traffic accident. In 2 patients (6.9%) the pain was due to cancer and in 6 patients (20.7%) it was idiopathic (Table 1). X-ray evaluations were normal in 10 patients (34.5%), while an anterior coccygeal angulation was found in 19 patients (65.5%) (Table 1).

Twenty patients (68.9%) underwent DB only, while 9 (31.1%) underwent DB+ pulse RFT. In all patients, a DB with a total of 10 ml of 0.25% bupivacaine+ 40 mg methylprednisolone was administered during the first procedure. The block was performed using either a transsacrococcygeal or intercoccygeal approach.

The average VAS score before undergoing the impar ganglion block was 7.4 ± 1 and decreased to 5.2 ± 1.5 following the procedure. At the 3-month evaluation period, the average VAS score was 4.7 ± 2.1, and at the 3–6 month and 6 month-1 year evaluations the scores were 4.3 ± 2.4 and 4.2 ± 2.6, respectively. VAS scores were found to be significantly lower in patients at the 3-month, 3–6 months and 6 months-1 year follow-up evaluations ($p < 0.05$) (Table 2). VAS scores before the block, after the block and in the first 3-month follow-up period were similar in both the DB block and DB+ pulse RFT block groups. However, patients who received RFT had significantly lower VAS scores at the 3–6 months and 6 months-1 year follow-up periods (Table 3). In these periods, VAS score was lower than 4 in 9 patients who received DB block and in 8 patients who received DB + pulse RFT block. Percentage of improvement in pain score after treatment were 40% in DB block and 72% DB + RFT block. The patients were allowed to take gabapentin, pregabalin or a single tablet of tramadol and paracetamol (37.5 mg + 325 mg) combination when

required. In 4 patients, the VAS scores remained ≥7 throughout all of the follow-up measurements (3 patients in the DB group and 1 patient in the DB + pulse RFT group). These patients were referred to surgery for coccyx excision.

There was no correlation between VAS scores and gender or BMI.

Discussion

A 1-year follow-up of coccydynia patients demonstrated that the impar ganglion block procedure effectively controlled pain and that a DB + pulse RFT further prolonged analgesic efficacy. Coccydynia is a symptom with different causal factors including twisting of the sacrococcygeal joint or intercoccygeal segment, fracture, infection, tumor or degenerative changes [2]. These factors can lead to localized pain at the coccygeal site, which increases while in a seated position. Pain is the diagnostic symptom, especially in the coccyx and sacrococcygeal areas, as demonstrated during physical examination and through radiologic screening. Conservative treatments include oral analgesic drugs, use of a sitting cushion, physiotherapy, massage, psychotherapy and manipulation [6]. An impar ganglion block is an option when conservative treatment is insufficient; therefore, in this study, we evaluated the efficacy of the impar ganglion block in patients who did not benefit from conservative treatment.

The impar ganglion is the terminal division of the sympathetic chain located in the midline and, in contrast to other divisions, is the only solitary autonomic

Table 3 Comparison of average VAS scores in diagnostic and radiofrequency impar ganglion block groups

Observation time	DB (n = 20)	DB + RFT (n = 9)	P-value
Before the block	7.4 ± 0,9	7.5 ± 1.1	0.729
After the block	5.5 ± 1.5	4.5 ± 1.4	0.127
< 3 months	5.2 ± 2.3	3.7 ± 1.2	0.085
3–6 months	5 ± 2.5	3 ± 1.8	0.044
6 months-1 year	5 ± 2.4	2.4 ± 2.1	0.010

DB Diagnostic block, RFT Radiofrequency thermocoagulation

division. The definitive anatomic location of the impar ganglion remains uncertain but is considered to be anterior to the sacrococcygeal joint, coccyx or distal end of the coccyx [7]. Different approaches to accessing the ganglion using screening techniques such as fluoroscopy, ultrasonography and computerized tomography to view the tip of the needle during the procedure have been described in the literature [8–10]. The sacrococcygeal joint is closed in 51% of patients, which makes access from the intercoccygeal area easier for the physician [11]. The blocks in this study were performed using transsacrococcygeal and intersacrococcygeal approaches with the assistance of fluoroscopy.

Coccydynia occurs more frequently in females. While it can occur at any age, the incidence increases in people over forty [12]. Consistent with the literature, 66% of our patients were female and the average age was 53.45 ± 9.6. A high BMI is also a known risk factor for coccydynia, and, in our study, the average patient had a BMI of 29.55 ± 4.21, which is close to the obesity cut-off value [13]. We observed a tendency of patients to be overweight and obese, but there was no association between the BMI and patient's VAS scores.

Gündüz et al. noted that trauma, especially after a backwards fall, was the cause of coccydynia in 50% of patients [14]. Similar to this finding, trauma was the leading cause of coccydynia in our study: 58.6% experienced a fall and for 13.8%, a traffic accident was the origin. X-rays and magnetic resonance imaging are useful tools for diagnosing sarcococcygeal hypermobility, hypomobility, fracture and luxation, especially in cases of trauma [15]. In our patients, only X-ray images could be evaluated and were found to be normal in 10 patients (34.5%), while coccygeal angulation at the distal end was observed in the remaining 19 patients (65.5%).

Pain relief can be achieved with conservative medical treatment in 90% of patients with coccydynia [16, 17]. Patients referred to our policlinic were treated with multiple analgesics including NSAIDs, paracetamol and seating cushions. An impar ganglion block was performed if the VAS score remained ≥4 despite conservative treatment. Under fluoroscopy, 20 patients (68.9%) received only DB, and 9 patients (31.1%) received DB + pulse RFT at 42 °C for 2 min at the impar ganglion area. Gonnade et al. reported a significant decrease in pain in 31 patients following impar ganglion blocks in a 1-year follow-up study [18]. We observed a similar significant reduction in pain scores in our patients. The average VAS score was 7.4 ± 1.6 before the block, which then significantly decreased in the first 3 months, 3–6 months and 6 months-1 year evaluations post-procedure.

Radiofrequency treatment is a percutaneous and minimally invasive procedure that can be used in coccydynia patients who do not benefit from appropriate medical treatment and physiotherapy. It is more selective compared to phenol and alcohol neurolysis and leads to fewer complications. Reig et al. reported impar ganglion blocks with RFT as useful for non-malignant perineal pain [8]. Similarly, Kırcelli et al. observed a significant decrease in pain scores, without complications, after impar ganglion block with RFT in patients with chronic coccydynia, except in 2 patients for whom the decrease in pain scores after RFT was no more than 50% [19]. In our study, 4 patients (3 in the DB and 1 in the DB+ pulse RFT group) did not benefit from treatment and were referred to coccyx-excision surgery.

Serious complications such as rectal perforation, hemorrhage and infection, along with difficulties in implementing the technique, restrict the popularity of this highly effective block [6]. In all of our patients, the blocks were performed after both the needle tip and the spread of the radiocontrast substance was confirmed at the relevant area under fluoroscopy. No complications occurred during or after the procedure.

Surgical excision of the coccyx for the treatment of coccydynia is the option of last resort and is performed only if all other treatments have failed. High complication rates and failure to relieve pain have been reported with this procedure, but its overall success rate is between 51 and 90% [15, 20]. In 4 of our patients who underwent surgical coccyx excision due to insufficient pain relief with conservative and interventional treatments, their VAS scores decreased to ≤2 following surgery in 2 patients but remained between 5 and 6 in the other 2.

Limitations to our study include its relatively small sample size and the retrospective nature of the review. The impar ganglion block provides effective pain relief without complications in patients with coccydynia. Diagnostic blocks combined with pulse RFT achieved prolonged analgesic efficacy. However, prospective randomized studies involving larger sample sizes are needed to reach more conclusive results regarding the effectiveness of these procedures.

Conclusions

İn conclusion, impar ganglion block is an effective procedure with low complication rate for pain relief in coccydynia. The analgesic effect can be prolonged by combining the DB with pulse RFT.

Abbreviations

NSAIDs: Non-steroidal, anti-inflammatory drugs; RFT: Radiofrequency thermocoagulation; VAS: Visual analog scale; DB: Diagnostic impar block; BMI: Body mass index

Acknowledgements

None.

Authors' contributions

Concept and design– OS. Materials - Data Collection and/or Processing – OS, HFD, FU. Analysis and/or Interpretation – OS., FU, BA. Literature Search – OS, HFD, FU, BA. Writing Manuscript - OS, HFD, BA. Revised the draft paper - OS, HFD, FU, BA. The authors have read and approved the manuscript.

References

1. Patijn J, Janssen M, Hayek S, Mekhail N, Zundert JV, Kleef MV. Coccygodynia. Pain Pract. 2010;10:554–9.
2. Lirette LS, Chaiban G, Tolba R, Eissa H. Coccydynia: an overview of the anatomy, etiology, and treatment of coccyx pain. Ochsner J. 2014;14:84–7.
3. Nathan ST, Fisher BE, Roberts CS. Coccydynia: a review of pathoanatomy, aetiology, treatment and outcome. J Bone Joint Surg Br. 2010;92:1622–7.
4. Maigne JY, Doursounian L, Chatellier G. Causes and mechanisms of common coccydynia: role of body mass index and coccygeal trauma. Spine (Phila Pa 1976). 2000;25:3072–9.
5. Peng P, Narouze S. Ultrasound-guided interventional procedures in pain medicine: a review of anatomy, sonoanatomy and procedures. Part I: non-axial structures. Reg Anesth Pain Med. 2009;34:458–74.
6. Elkhashab Y, Ng A. A review of current treatment options for Coccygodynia. Curr Pain Headache Rep. 2018;19:22–8.
7. Oh CS, Chung IH, Ji HJ, Yoon DM. Clinical implications of topographic anatomy on the ganglion impar. Anesthesiology. 2004;101:249–50.
8. Reig E, Abejón D, del Pozo C, Insausti J, Contreras R. Thermocoagulation of the ganglion impar or ganglion of Walther: description of a modified approach. Preliminary results in chronic, nononcological pain. Pain Pract. 2005;5:103–10.
9. Agarwal-Kozlowski K, Lorke DE, Habermann CR, Amm Esch JS, Beck H. CT-guided blocks and neuroablation of the ganglion impar (Walther) in perineal pain: anatomy, technique, safety and efficacy. Clin J Pain. 2009;25: 570–6.
10. Lin CS, Cheng JK, Hsu YW, Chen CC, Lao HC, Huang CJ, et al. Ultrasound-guided ganglion impar block: a technical report. Pain Med. 2010;11:390–4.
11. Postacchini F, Massobrio M. Idiopathic coccygodynia. J Bone Joint Surg Am. 1983;65A:1116–24.
12. Fogel GR, Cunningham PY, Esses SI. Coccygodynia: evaluation and management. J Am Acad Orthop Surg. 2004;12:49–54.
13. Maigne JY, Pigeau I, Aguer N, Doursounian L, Chatellier G. Chronic coccydynia in adolescents. A series of 53 patients. Eur J Phys Rehabil Med. 2011;47:245–51.
14. Gunduz OH, Sencan S, Kenis-Coskun O. Pain relief due to Transsacrococcygeal ganglion Impar block in chronic Coccygodynia: a pilot study. Pain Med. 2015;16:1278–81.
15. Pennekamp PH, Kraft CN, Stütz A, Wallny T, Schmitt O, Diedrich O. Coccygectomy for coccygodynia: does pathogenesis matter? J Trauma. 2005;59:1414–9.
16. Capar B, Akpinar N, Kutluay E, Müjde S, Turan A. Coccygectomy in patients with coccydynia [in Turkish]. Acta Orthop Traumatol Turc. 2007;41:277–80.
17. Trollegaard AM, Aarby NS, Hellberg S. Coccygectomy: an effective treatment option for chronic coccydynia: retrospective results in 41 consecutive patients. J Bone Joint Surg Br. 2010;92:242–5.
18. Gonnade N, Mehta N, Khera PS, Kumar D, Rajagopal R, Sharma PK. Ganglion impar block in patients with chronic coccydynia. Indian J Radiol Imaging. 2017;27:324–8.
19. Kırcelli A, Demirçay E, Özel Ö, Çöven I, Işık S, Civelek E, et al. Radiofrequency Thermocoagulation of the ganglion Impar for Coccydynia management: long-term effects. Pain Pract. 2019;19:9–15.
20. Foye PM. Coccydynia: tailbone pain. Phys Med Rehabil Clin N Am. 2017;28: 539–49.

19

Differences in pain treatment between surgeons and anesthesiologists in a physician staffed prehospital emergency medical service

Stefan J. Schaller[1]* (iD), Felix P. Kappler[1], Claudia Hofberger[1], Jens Sattler[1], Richard Wagner[1], Gerhard Schneider[1], Manfred Blobner[1] and Karl-Georg Kanz[2]

Abstract

Background: Although pain treatment is an important objective in prehospital emergency medicine the incidence of oligoanalgesia is still high in prehospital patients. Given that prehospital emergency medicine in Germany is open for physicians of any speciality, the prehospital pain treatment may differ depending on the primary medical education. Aim of this study was to explore the difference in pain treatment between surgeons and anaesthesiologists in a physician staffed emergency medical service.

Methods: Retrospective single centre cohort analysis in a physician staffed ground based emergency medical service from January 2014 until December 2016. A total of 8882 consecutive emergency missions were screened. Primary outcome measure was the difference in application frequency of prehospital analgesics by anaesthesiologist or surgeon. Univariate and multivariate logistic regression analysis was used for statistical analysis including subgroup analysis for trauma and acute coronary syndrome.

Results: A total of 8238 patients were included in the analysis. There was a significant difference in the application frequency of analgesics between surgeons and anaesthesiologists especially for opioids ($p < 0.001$, OR 0.68 [0.56–0.82]). Fentanyl was the most common administered analgesic in the trauma subgroup, but significantly less common used by surgeons ($p = 0.005$, OR 0.63 [0.46–0.87]). In acute coronary syndrome cases there was no significant difference in morphine administration between anaesthesiologists and surgeons ($p = 0.49$, OR 0.88 [0.61–1.27]).

Conclusions: Increased training for prehospital pain treatment should be implemented, since opioids were administered notably less frequent by surgeons than by anaesthesiologists.

Keywords: Prehospital pain management, Prehospital emergency medicine, Emergency physicians

* Correspondence: s.schaller@tum.de
[1]Klinik für Anästhesiologie und Intensivmedizin, Klinikum rechts der Isar,
School of Medicine, Technical University of Munich, Munich, Germany

Differences in pain treatment between surgeons and anesthesiologists in a physician staffed prehospital...

155

Background

Stabilization of vital functions and treatment of pain is essential in prehospital emergency medicine. Importantly, pain is the main indication for alerting the prehospital emergency medical service (EMS) in Germany [1]. Moreover, sufficient pain relief is a key marker of quality in health care supply. Nevertheless, insufficiently or even not treated pain referred to as oligoanalgesia, is a well-recognized problem in the prehospital setting [2, 3], in particular in trauma patients [4–7]. A meta-analysis has established major reasons for oligoanalgesia: (1) insufficient or impossible communication with the patient, (2) the physicians' presumption that analgesia could cover clinical symptoms and hence mislead the clinical diagnosis in the emergency department, and (3) fear of side effects, especially respiratory depression by opioids [8]. Furthermore, oligoanalgesia is accompanied by low quality of pain documentation being unclear if the latter is reason or part of the avoidance strategy [7]. Finally, prehospital oligoanalgesia occurs in different countries and systems, regardless the organisation of the EMS system [2–5, 7].

In Germany, the EMS is staffed with paramedics and supported by physicians working in any patient caring discipline, who have completed a postgraduate training and examination in prehospital medicine. If the rescue centre decides, based on severity, a physician is needed, or the paramedic on scene calls for reinforcement, the physician is dispatched. Administration of analgesics is allowed to physicians only by federal law and forbidden for paramedics and nurses.

To work in prehospital care, physicians require a minimum clinical experience of 24 months in any patient caring department, including at least six months in anaesthesiology, intensive care medicine or an emergency department. In addition, treatment of 50 prehospital emergency patients under supervision of a responsible prehospital physician, and a preparation course of 80 h in prehospital emergency medicine is necessary [9]. Physicians, who have then passed the prehospital emergency care examination, continue to work in their primal specialty working some shifts in prehospital care only. Given that prehospital emergency medicine is open for physicians of any medical speciality with its specific training and its specific in-hospital standard for pain treatment, the prehospital pain treatment including the problem of oligoanalgesia may differ depending on the primary medical education.

Aim of this study, therefore, is the exploration of differences in pain treatment between surgeons and anaesthesiologists in a physician staffed EMS service with a focus on the two most frequent subgroups with severe pain and opioid administration: chest pain and trauma [10, 11].

Methods

Study setting

After Ethics Committee approval (Ethics Committee of the Medical Faculty of the Technical University of Munich, Munich, Germany, No. 59/15), data were obtained from all prehospital emergency physician standardized forms of one dispatch location (fire department 10) in Munich, Germany between January 1st, 2014, to December 31st, 2016. The ethical committee waived the requirement for informed consent. This ground based EMS is a special equipped BMW X3 (Bayerische Motorenwerke, Munich, Germany) staffed with a paramedic from the Munich fire department who also serves as driver and a physician working at a university hospital (Klinikum rechts der Isar, Technische Universität München, Munich, Germany) mainly of the specialities anaesthesiology or surgery. The BMW X3 is equipped with different analgesics according to Bavarian standards: acetaminophen, butylscopolamine, metamizole, acetylsalicylic acid, ketamine and the opioids fentanyl and morphine.

Data points and definitions

Data was collected from standardized EMS forms (DIVI version 4.2 (see Additional file 1), DIVI version 5.0 (see Additional file 2) and DIVI version 5.1 (see Additional file 3) containing patient and field data. We stored and analysed anonymized data only: Gender, age, heart rate, intubation, Glasgow Coma Scale (GCS), pain assessment as numeric rating scale (NRS), National Advisory Committee for Aeronautics' (NACA) severity score, disease categories based on protocol classification, suspected diagnosis, specialty of the performing physician, assessment of injury and administered drugs.

Trauma cases were defined as cases where injuries were assessed in the protocols. Acute coronary syndrome (ACS) cases were defined with documentation of a suspected diagnosis of instable angina pectoris, ACS, non-ST segment elevation myocardial infarction (NSTEMI) and ST elevation myocardial infarction (STEMI).

Primary outcome measures were selection of prehospital analgesics and administration frequency by anaesthesiologist or surgeon. Prehospital analgesics selection and frequency was chosen as a measurement for the difference in prehospital pain treatment between members of these two medical specialities.

We further assessed documentation quality, that means documentation frequency of GCS, NRS, patient sex, age, heart rate and NACA severity score.

Statistical analysis

Statistical analysis was done in the anonymized dataset. Results are expressed as median [Interquartile Range

(IQR)] or frequencies with counts and percentages as appropriate. For statistical calculation we used logistic regression for binary outcomes and t-test or Mann-Whitney test as appropriate. For data points with adequate documentation frequency (> 90%) univariate analysis was performed. If significant, the variable was included in the multivariate analysis. Analyses were performed with IBM SPSS Premium Statistics for Windows v24.0 (IBM Corporation 2016, USA). All statistical tests were based on a 0.05 significance level and presented with 95% confidence intervals (CI). A subanalysis was performed for trauma and ACS cases.

Results

Study population

A total of 8882 protocols during January 1st 2014 and December 31st 2016 were evaluated and consequently 644 excluded due to false alerts, treatment by one specialist of internal medicine or missing documentation of the treating physician (Fig. 1). Consequently, 8238 cases were included in the analysis, performed by anaesthesiologists and surgeons. Patient characteristics are presented in Table 1, physicians characteristics in Table 2.

Documentation quality

Most consistently documented was age (99%), sex (99%) and initial GCS (95%, Table 3). NACA score and NRS documentation was inadequate. Anaesthesiologists documented the NRS less often at the beginning (37.3% vs. 41.2%) but not in the end (25.8% vs. 27.4%) of their care

of patients compared to surgeons. In the subgroups trauma and ACS, a higher compliance of NRS documentation for both disciplines was achieved, but was still poor in total. The highest documentation rate for NRS with above 50% documentation frequency was achieved if an opioid was administered.

Pain medication use

There was no significant difference in the administration frequency between surgeons and anaesthesiologists for any non-opioid: ketamine ($p = 0.27$), butylscopolamine ($p = 0.88$), acetaminophen ($p = 0.25$) and metamizole ($p = 0.34$, see Additional file 4). This was different for opioids with a highly significant difference in the univariate analysis ($p < 0.001$, see Additional file 4). Multivariate analysis showed that surgeons significantly less often administered opioids compared to anaesthesiologists ($p < 0.001$, OR 0.68 [0.56–0.82]; Table 4) independent if the patient was intubated (p < 0.001), of the initial GCS ($p < 0.001$), the disease category ($p < 0.001$), the physician's qualification ($p = 0.004$) and the physician's sex ($p < 0.001$). In the subgroup of fentanyl administration, the difference remained significant ($p < 0.001$, OR 0.59 [0.46–0.77]; see Additional file 5), but not for morphine administration ($p = 0.08$; see Additional file 6).

Subsequently, two sub-cohorts were tested: trauma (Table 4, details in see Additional file 5) and ACS (Table 4, details in see Additional file 6). In the trauma subgroup, surgeons administered fentanyl significantly less often ($p = 0.005$, OR 0.63 [0.46–0.87], see Additional file

Table 1 Patients Characteristics

Patient Characteristic	Study population (n = 8238)	Anaesthesiologists (n = 6492)	Surgeons (n = 1746)	p-values
Female, n (%)	3979 (48.7)	3131 (48.6)	848 (48.9)	0.84
Age, median (IQR)	64 (40–79)	64 (41–79)	63 (39–78)	0.12
Intubated, n (%)	280 (3.4)	212 (3.3)	68 (3.9)	0.20
GCS initial, median (IQR)	15 (14–15)	15 (14–15)	15 (14–15)	0.63
Disease Categories, n (%)				
Cardiovascular	2695 (32.7)	2106 (32.4)	589 (33.7)	0.31
subgroup ACS cases	947 (11.5)	761 (11.7)	186 (10.7)	0.21
Traumatic	1541 (18.7)	1199 (18.5)	342 (19.6)	0.29
subgroup Polytrauma	72 (0.9)	48 (0.7)	24 (1.4)	0.013
Neurologic	901 (10.9)	733 (11.3)	168 (9.6)	0.048
Respiratory	670 (8.1)	535 (8.2)	135 (7.7)	0.49
Visceral	564 (6.8)	449 (6.9)	115 (6.6)	0.63
Mental	495 (6.0)	385 (5.9)	110 (6.3)	0.56
Endocrinological	277 (3.4)	225 (3.5)	52 (3.0)	0.32
Paediatrical	185 (2.2)	144 (2.2)	41 (2.3)	0.75
Gynaecological/Obstetrical	54 (0.7)	44 (0.7)	10 (0.6)	0.63
Other	856 (10.4)	672 (10.4)	184 (10.5)	0.82

n (%), number (percentages), IQR Inter Quartile Range, GCS Glasgow Coma Scale, ACS acute coronary syndrome

Table 2 Physician characteristics

Physician characteristic		Study population (n = 8238)	Anaesthesiologists (n = 6492)	Surgeons (n = 1746)	p-value
Sex	female	2209 (26.8)	2209 (34.0)	0 (0.0)	n/a
	male	6029 (73.2)	4283 (66.0)	1746 (100)	
Qualification	resident	2574 (31.2)	2378 (36.6)	196 (11.2)	< 0.001
	specialist	5664 (68.8)	4114 (63.4)	1550 (88.8)	

n (%), number (percentages), n/a, not applicable

5). In the subgroup of ACS, morphine was administered in 40.2% (see Additional file 4). Although there was a trend that anaesthesiologists administered morphine more frequently (42.0%) than surgeons (32.8%) this was not significant in the multivariate analysis (p = 0.49, OR 0.88 [0.61–1.27], see Additional file 6).

Discussion

Our study suggests that specialization influences pain treatment in prehospital emergency cases, in particular between surgeons and anaesthesiologists. Especially the selection of opioids, in particular fentanyl, was more likely administered by anaesthesiologists than by surgeons.

There is no general European or German guideline for pain treatment in the prehospital setting for trauma patients. The level 3 (S3) evidence- and consensus-based guideline on the treatment of patients with severe and multiple injuries published [12], includes recommendations for emergency anaesthesia only. US recommendations for treatment of prehospital trauma patients

postulate that opioids should be used in moderate to severe pain, as long as there are no contraindications [13]. In our data, opioids were the most used analgesics, especially in trauma and ACS cases.

For ACS, however, distinct guidelines are available: According to the 2015 European Society of Cardiology (ESC) guidelines for NSTEMI patients, morphine administration is reasonable for patients with persisting severe chest pain if the ischaemic symptoms do not relieve by nitrates and beta-blockers [14]. This might explain why there was no difference in administration frequency of morphine between surgeons and anaesthesiologists. There were, however, concerns about administration of morphine and a probable delay on prasugrel and ticagrelor effect [15, 16]. Recently, it has been shown, that prehospital morphine use did not increase one-year mortality in STEMI patients [17]. In these studies, the frequency of morphine administration was much lower (32 and 19%, respectively) than in our study (40.2%), although prehospital morphine administration in STEMI patients is recommended [15, 17, 18].

Table 3 Documentation quality

	Study population (n = 8238)	Anaesthesiologists (n = 6492)	Surgeons (n = 1746)	p-value
GCS initial documented	7806 (94.8)	6143 (94.6)	1663 (95.2)	0.30
GCS end documented	3817 (46.3)	3133 (48.3)	684 (39.2)	< 0.001
NACA documented	3709 (45.0)	2787 (42.9)	922 (52.8)	< 0.001
Heartrate initial documented	6875 (83.5)	5392 (83.1)	1483 (84.9)	0.06
Heartrate end documented	4990 (60.6)	3932 (60.6)	1058 (60.6)	0.98
Age documented	8194 (99.5)	6456 (99.4)	1738 (99.5)	0.62
Sex documented	8177 (99.3)	6442 (99.2)	1735 (99.4)	0.55
NRS initial documented	3139 (38.1)	2419 (37.3)	720 (41.2)	0.002
trauma cases (n = 1541)	741 (48.1)	576 (48.0)	165 (48.2)	0.95
ACS cases (n = 947)	478 (50.5)	379 (49.8)	99 (53.2)	0.40
if pain drug was administered (n = 2067)	1112 (53.8)	904 (53.4)	208 (55.6)	0.44
if opioid was administered (n = 1287)	717 (55.7)	598 (54.7)	119 (61.7)	0.07
NRS end documented	2154 (26.1)	1676 (25.8)	478 (27.4)	0.19
trauma cases (n = 1541)	494 (32.1)	393 (32.8)	101 (29.5)	0.26
ACS cases (n = 947)	396 (41.8)	317 (41.7)	79 (42.5)	0.84
if pain drug was administered (n = 2067)	822 (39.8)	675 (39.9)	147 (39.3)	0.84
if opioid was administered (n = 1287)	554 (43.0)	468 (42.8)	86 (44.6)	0.65

n (%), number (percentages), *GCS* Glasgow Coma Scale, *NACA* National Advisory Committee for Aeronautics' severity score, *NRS* numeric rating scale

Table 4 Multivariate analysis of opioid use

Factor	OR$_{adj}$ (95% CI)		
	Total	Trauma	ACS
Surgeon	0.68 (0.56–0.82)	0.71 (0.52–0.96)	0.93 (0.64–1.34)
Physician qualification resident	1.23 (1.07–1.42)	–	1.80 (1.35–2.40)
Physician sex female	1.40 (1.20–1.63)	1.86 (1.42–2.44)	1.35 (1.00–1.83)
ACS	8.34 (7.01–9.91)	n/a	n/a
Trauma	5.93 (5.07–6.93)	n/a	n/a
Age > 65 yrs	–	1.77 (1.39–2.27)	–
Female Patient	–	1.20 (0.94–1.52)	–
Patient intubated	12.88 (8.67–19.11)	45.33 (12.92–159.05)	–
GCS < 13	0.29 (0.21–0.40)	0.07 (0.03–0.19)	–

Factors included in the multivariate analysis if $p < 0.05$ in univariate analysis, n/a not applicable, –, not significant in univariate analysis, OR$_{adj}$ adjusted Odds-Ratio in multivariate analysis, CI Confidence Interval, yrs., years, GCS Glasgow Coma Scale, ACS acute coronary syndrome

Pain treatment and sedation is an inherent part of speciality trainings in anaesthesiology as well as in surgery [9]. While anaesthesiologists, however, use powerful analgesics like fentanyl and morphine permanently, e.g. for narcosis induction, postoperative treatment and sedation in the intensive care unit, the daily routine of surgeons requires more often the constant training of other skills. Hence, anaesthesiologists might have a higher self-confidence in dosing and treatment of possible complications after administration of strong analgesics like fentanyl [19, 20]. Typical complications from side effects of opioids in the prehospital setting are nausea, vomiting (with the possibility of aspiration), decrease of the respiratory drive, the respiratory rate or tidal volume. The consequence of the described respiratory effects may lead to hypoventilation and upper airway obstruction in susceptible individuals.

While surgeons and anaesthesiologists built a team in operating theatre and use their different abilities synergistically, they are alone in the emergency field, that leads to different views depending on their speciality. Mechanical skills like splinting and positioning of fractures might be a common attempt of pain treatment by surgeons, maybe more common compared to anaesthesiologists. This could explain the difference in the use of fentanyl was highly significant ($p < 0.001$, see Additional file 5). Unfortunately, it was not possible to determine physical interventions, due to bad documentation compliance in this point.

Nevertheless, actions should be implemented to improve surgeons' prehospital pain treatment: (1) Sattler et al. [21] suggested, adding a weaker opioid like piritramide to the available drugs on the EMS system might be an option to improve pain treatment by surgeons who are used to administer such drugs on a daily basis on their wards. An additional weaker opioid, however, would have important disadvantages: the onset time is slower and the risk of oligoanalgesia in patients with moderate to severe pain would continue. (2) Tactical

Combat Casualty Care Guidelines from the US army [22] advise medical personnel to use fentanyl lozenges for moderate to severe pain without shock or respiratory distress [23]. In our system fentanyl lozenges are not available, but might be an option to raise fentanyl administration. (3) The most successful option in our point of view is to increase the training for prehospital physicians in knowledge and use of titrating pain medication.

In our comparison, the physicians' speciality influenced the frequency of pain treatment with opioids significantly. A study about prehospital care differences between male and female trauma patients in Stockholm showed, that nearly one third of these patients received analgesics [24]. In this study the majority of cases were performed by emergency medical technicians and registered nurses. This may explain why our frequency of trauma cases with at least one analgesic administered in our physician staffed EMS, is higher (49.8%, see Additional file 5). A similar phenomenon was determined by the comparison between different EMS systems in four countries. The paramedic based systems in Coventry and Richmond and also the physician staffed EMS in Cantabria (general practitioners or family doctors) administered significantly less drugs in chest pain cases than the EMS in Bonn staffed by anaesthesiologists only. In all patients with cardiac chest pain and in the subgroup of patients with severe pain, treatment was more effective by anaesthesiologists than in other EMS systems [25].

Frequency of pain assessment in our trauma cases (48.1%, Table 3) is comparable with published data, showing rates of pain assessment and opioid administration averaging about 50% and that patient condition affect the ability of providers to effectively and appropriately manage pain [7]. However, in our data there was no significant difference in the frequency of pain assessment in trauma cases between anaesthesiologists and surgeons. The underassessment and undertreatment of pain really seems to be an omnipresent problem. A mandatory handover sheet might be an option or electronic documentation might improve documentation and quality control in the future [26]. Maybe the application of mandatory fields will be useful, because incomplete documentation was associated with increased mortality [27].

Our study has some methodical limitations. First, data is collected on a single emergency service location in Munich, which is staffed by physicians of one university hospital only. Second, since the study is retrospective it cannot detect the cause for the differences in pain treatment between anaesthesiologists and surgeons. Furthermore, we do not have outcome parameters of the hospital stay or any questionnaires filled out by the physicians to learn more about potential consequences of different treatments. Third, although comparable with other published data, documentation compliance was low. Therefore, we were not able to calculate pain scores and changes in pain scores or vital signs after administration of pain medication or report side effects of pain medication used.

Conclusion

In summary, surgeons administered less opioids in the prehospital setting than anaesthesiologists, especially in trauma cases. However, no difference could be detected for morphine administration in ACS. Training for prehospital physicians in knowledge and use of titrating pain medication should be increased.

Additional files

Additional file 1: Standardized Bavarian EMS form for physicians DIVI version 4.2.

Additional file 2: Standardized Bavarian EMS form for physicians DIVI version 5.0.

Additional file 3: Standardized Bavarian EMS form for physicians DIVI version 5.1.

Additional file 4: Table Univariate analysis of pain medication use. Presented as no. (%), ACS, acute coronary syndrome; Opioids (total, fentanyl & morphine) and non-opioid pain medication (ketamine, butylscopolamine, acetaminophen and metamizole); n/a, not applicable.

Additional file 5: Table Multivariate analysis of Fentanyl use. Factors included in the multivariate analysis if $p < 0.05$ in univariate analysis; n/a, not applicable; –, not significant in univariate analysis; OR_{adj}, adjusted Odds-Ratio in multivariate analysis; CI, Confidence Interval; yrs., years; GCS, Glasgow Coma Scale; ACS, acute coronary syndrome.

Additional file 6: Table Multivariate analysis of Morphine use. Factors included in the multivariate analysis if $p < 0.05$ in univariate analysis; n/a, not applicable; –, not significant in univariate analysis, OR_{adj} adjusted Odds-Ratio in multivariate analysis, CI Confidence Interval, yrs. years, GCS Glasgow Coma Scale, ACS acute coronary syndrome.

Abbreviations

ACS: Acute coronary syndrome; CI: Confidence interval; EMS: Emergency medical service; GCS: Glasgow Coma Scale; IQR: Interquartile Range; NACA: National Advisory Committee for Aeronautics'; NRS: Numeric rating scale; NSTEMI: non-ST segment elevation myocardial infarction; OR: Odds-Ratio; STEMI: ST elevation myocardial infarction; yrs.: Years

Acknowledgements
Not applicable.

Authors' contributions
SJS: study design, analysis and interpretation of data and writing of the article, responsible for archiving the study files. FPK: data acquisition, analysis and interpretation of data and writing of the article. CH: data acquisition and analysis of data, contribution in revising the manuscript JS: data acquisition and analysis of data, contribution in revising the manuscript. RW: interpretation of data and contribution in revising the manuscript, GS: interpretation of data and contribution in revising the manuscript. MB: study design, analysis and interpretation of data, substantial contribution in revising the manuscript. KGK: study design, analysis and interpretation of data, substantial contribution in revising the manuscript. All authors have read and approved the final manuscript.

Author details
[1]Klinik für Anästhesiologie und Intensivmedizin, Klinikum rechts der Isar, School of Medicine, Technical University of Munich, Munich, Germany. [2]Klinik für Unfallchirurgie, Klinikum rechts der Isar, School of Medicine, Technical University of Munich, Munich, Bavaria, Germany.

References
1. Hossfeld B, Holsträter S, Bernhard M, et al. Prähospitale Analgesie beim Erwachsenen – Schmerzerfassung und Therapieoptionen. Anästhesiol Intensivmed Notfallmed Schmerzther. 2016;51(02):84–96.
2. Galinski M, Ruscev M, Gonzalez G, et al. Prevalence and Management of Acute Pain in prehospital emergency medicine. Prehospital Emergency Care. 2010;14(3):334–9.
3. Jennings PA, Cameron P, Bernard S. Epidemiology of prehospital pain: an opportunity for improvement. Emerg Med J. 2011;28(6):530–1.
4. Albrecht E, Taffe P, Yersin B, et al. Undertreatment of acute pain (oligoanalgesia) and medical practice variation in prehospital analgesia of adult trauma patients: a 10 yr retrospective study. Br J Anaesth. 2013;110(1):96–106.
5. Calil AM, Pimenta CAM, Birolini D. The "oligoanalgesia problem" in the emergency care. Clinics. 2007;62:591–8.
6. Eidenbenz D, Taffe P, Hugli O, et al. A two-year retrospective review of the determinants of pre-hospital analgesia administration by alpine helicopter emergency medical physicians to patients with isolated limb injury. Anaesthesia. 2016;71(7):779–87.
7. Spilman SK, Lechtenberg GT, Hahn KD, et al. Is pain really undertreated? Challenges of addressing pain in trauma patients during prehospital transport and trauma resuscitation. Injury. 2016;47(9):2018–24.
8. Stork B, Hofmann-Kiefer K. Analgesia as an important component of emergency care. Anaesthesist. 2009;58(6):639–48 quiz 649-650.
9. Landesärztekammer B: Weiterbildungsordnung für die Ärzte Bayerns vom 24. April 2004 – in der Fassung der Beschlüsse vom 25. Oktober 2015. In. Edited by Pflege BSfGu; 2015: 79.
10. Bakkelund KE, Sundland E, Moen S, et al. Undertreatment of pain in the prehospital setting: a comparison between trauma patients and patients with chest pain. Eur J Emerg Med. 2013;20(6):428–30.
11. Hofmann-Kiefer K, Praeger K, Fiedermutz M, et al. Quality of pain management in preclinical care of acutely ill patients. Anaesthesist. 1998;47(2):93–101.
12. Hilbert-Carius P, Wurmb T, Lier H, et al. Care for severely injured persons : update of the 2016 S3 guideline for the treatment of polytrauma and the severely injured. Anaesthesist. 2017;66(3):195–206.
13. Gausche-Hill M, Brown KM, Oliver ZJ, et al. An evidence-based guideline for prehospital analgesia in trauma. Prehosp Emerg Care. 2014;18(Suppl 1):25–34.
14. Roffi M, Patrono C, Collet JP, et al. 2015 ESC guidelines for the management of acute coronary syndromes in patients presenting without persistent ST-segment elevation: task force for the Management of Acute Coronary Syndromes in patients presenting without persistent ST-segment elevation of the European Society of Cardiology (ESC). Eur Heart J. 2015;37(3):267–315.
15. Parodi G, Bellandi B, Xanthopoulou I, et al. Morphine is associated with a delayed activity of oral antiplatelet agents in patients with ST-elevation acute myocardial infarction undergoing primary percutaneous coronary intervention. Circ Cardiovasc Interv. 2015;8(1).
16. Kubica J, Adamski P, Ostrowska M, et al. Morphine delays and attenuates

ticagrelor exposure and action in patients with myocardial infarction: the randomized, double-blind, placebo-controlled IMPRESSION trial. Eur Heart J. 2016;37(3):245–52.

17. Puymirat E, Lamhaut L, Bonnet N, et al. Correlates of pre-hospital morphine use in ST-elevation myocardial infarction patients and its association with in-hospital outcomes and long-term mortality: the FAST-MI (French registry of acute ST-elevation and non-ST-elevation myocardial infarction) programme. Eur Heart J. 2016;37(13):1063–71.

18. Ibanez B, James S, Agewall S, et al. 2017 ESC guidelines for the management of acute myocardial infarction in patients presenting with ST-segment elevation: the task force for the management of acute myocardial infarction in patients presenting with ST-segment elevation of the European Society of Cardiology (ESC). Eur Heart J. 2018;39(2):119–77.

19. Smith MD, Wang Y, Cudnik M, et al. The effectiveness and adverse events of morphine versus fentanyl on a physician-staffed helicopter. The Journal of emergency medicine. 2012;43(1):69–75.

20. Kanowitz A, Dunn TM, Kanowitz EM, et al. Safety and effectiveness of fentanyl administration for prehospital pain management. Prehosp Emerg Care. 2006;10(1):1–7.

21. Sattler PW: Analgetische Therapie durch Notärzte im Rettungsdienst [Dissertation]. *Diss.* Bonn: Rheinische Friedrich-Wilhelms-Universität; 2005.

22. updates TCCC. Tactic combat casualty care guidelines for medical personnel: 3 June 2015. Journal of special operations medicine : a peer reviewed journal for SOF medical professionals. 2015;15(3):129–35.

23. Butler FK, Kotwal RS, Buckenmaier CC 3rd, et al. A triple-option analgesia plan for tactical combat casualty care: TCCC guidelines change 13-04. Journal of special operations medicine : a peer reviewed journal for SOF medical professionals. 2014;14(1):13–25.

24. Rubenson Wahlin R, Ponzer S, Lovbrand H, et al. Do male and female trauma patients receive the same prehospital care?: an observational follow-up study. BMC Emerg Med. 2016;16:6.

25. Fischer M, Kamp J, Garcia-Castrillo Riesgo L, et al. Comparing emergency medical service systems--a project of the European emergency data (EED) project. Resuscitation. 2011;82(3):285–93.

26. Katzer R, Barton DJ, Adelman S, et al. Impact of implementing an EMR on physical exam documentation by ambulance personnel. Applied clinical informatics. 2012;3(3):301–8.

27. Laudermilch DJ, Schiff MA, Nathens AB, Rosengart MR. Lack of emergency medical services documentation is associated with poor patient outcomes: a validation of audit filters for prehospital trauma care. J Am Coll Surg. 2010; 210(2):220–7.

20

Premedication with oral paracetamol for reduction of propofol injection pain

Sasikaan Nimmaanrat* [iD], Manasanun Jongjidpranitarn, Sumidtra Prathep and Maliwan Oofuvong

Abstract

Background: To compare the effect of premedication with 2 different doses of oral paracetamol to prevent pain at propofol intravenous injection.

Methods: We conducted a double-blind randomized controlled trial in which patients scheduled for induction of general anesthesia with intravenous propofol received either a placebo, 500 mg or 1000 mg of oral paracetamol (P500 and P1000, respectively) 1 h prior to induction. Two mg/kg of propofol was injected at a rate of 600 ml/hr. After 1/4 of the full dose had been injected, the syringe pump was paused, and patients were asked to rate pain at the injection site using a verbal numerical rating score (VNRS) from 0 to 10.

Results: Three hundred and twenty-four patients were included. Pain intensity was lower in both P500 and P1000 groups (median VNRS [interquartile range] = 2 [0–3] and 4 [2–5], respectively) than in the placebo group (8 [7–10]; $P < 0.001$)*. The rate of pain was lower in the P1000 group (70.4%) than in both the P500 and the placebo group (86.1 and 99.1%, respectively; $P < 0.001$)*. The respective rates of mild (VNRS 1–3), moderate (VNRS 4–6) and severe pain (VNRS 7–10) were 47.2, 23.2 and 0% in the P1000 group, 28.7, 50 and 7.4% in the P500 group, and 0, 22.2 and 76.9% in the placebo group ($P < 0.001$* for between group comparisons). Tolerance was similar in the 3 groups.

Conclusions: A premedication with oral paracetamol can dose-dependently reduce pain at propofol intravenous injection. To avoid this common uncomfortable concern for the patients, this well-tolerated, available and cheap treatment appears as an option to be implemented in the current practice.

Keywords: Paracetamol, Propofol, Pain, Injection pain

Background

Propofol (di-isopropylphenol) is the most frequently used agent for the induction of general anesthesia because of its rapid onset and short duration of action. However, pain from the injection is a common problem [1]. The incidence of injection pain has been shown to vary between 28 and 90% which might be severe [2, 3] and the data from Songklanagarind Hospital found the high incidence of pain as 83%.

Pain upon injection of some anesthetic agents are thought to be a direct irritant effect by the non-physiological osmolality or pH of their preparations

[4]. Nonetheless, propofol is nearly isotonic, nonhyperosmolar and has a pH from 6 to 8.5. Hence, this concept cannot explain for the pain produced by the injection of propofol [1]. Propofol injection pain may be caused by an effect via the kinin cascade [5]. In addition, many factors seem to contribute to the incidence of injection pain including site [6] and speed of injection [7], size of vein [7, 8], rate of intravenous fluid infusion [9], concentration of propofol in the aqueous phase [4] as well as blood buffering effects [10].

A number of approaches have been proposed to lessen the injection pain such as injection of propofol at an antecubital fossa, fast injection [7] and pretreatment with lidocaine [11], opioids [12], or non-steroidal anti-inflammatory drugs (NSAIDs) [13]. The effective

* Correspondence: snimmaanrat@yahoo.com.au
Department of Anesthesiology, Faculty of Medicine, Prince of Songkla University, Hatyai, Songkhla 90110, Thailand

technique is a combination of lidocaine pretreatment together with venous occlusion (a modified Bier's block) [3]. However, this inflated arm tourniquet technique is quite difficult. From a systematic review and meta-analysis, the most 2 effective procedures to decrease propofol injection pain are injecting through an antecubital vein and pretreatment with lidocaine together with venous occlusion when a hand vein is used [14].

Canbay et al. [15] showed that intravenous acetaminophen (paracetamol) could diminish injection pain. The incidence of pain was significantly reduced to 22% as compared to a control group but less than lidocaine. Borazan et al. [16] compared the effect of injection of different paracetamol doses with lidocaine. They found that paracetamol 2 mg/kg administered intravenously 1 min before propofol was more effective than paracetamol 1 mg/kg and lidocaine in reducing propofol injection pain. The issue of pain at propofol injection pain should be addressed and managed accordingly. We hypothesized that oral paracetamol can reduce the severity of propofol injection pain. Our primary endpoint was pain intensity measured by verbal numerical rating score upon propofol injection. We used oral form of paracetamol because it is easier to administer and much cheaper in comparison to intravenous injection.

Additionally, Seymour et al. [17] demonstrated that a 1000-mg dose was more effective than 500 mg in reducing postoperative pain after third molar surgery. In regard to this study, we aimed to compare the efficacy of paracetamol 500 mg versus 1000 mg for reduction of propofol injection pain.

Methods

This study was a double-blinded randomized controlled trial (RCT). It was approved by the Faculty of Medicine, Prince of Songkla University Ethics Committee and registered with Thai Clinical Trial Registry (TCTR20150224002: prospectively registered on February 24, 2015). The principal investigator was Dr. Nimmaanrat. The data were collected from June 2015 until February 2016 at Songklanagarind Hospital (Faculty of Medicine, Prince of Songkla University). The authors prepared this trial report in accordance to the Consolidated Standards of Reporting Trials (CONSORT) guidelines. The full protocol is accessible on request.

We recruited 324 patients with the American Society Anesthesiologists (ASA) physical status I-III of who were aged between 18 and 65, scheduled for elective surgeries under general anesthesia, and having an intravenous catheter number 20G at a hand dorsum.

Exclusion criteria included weight less than 50 kg, chronic pain, hypertension, cardiovascular disease or cerebrovascular disease, difficulty in communicating, cirrhosis or abnormal liver function test result (aspartate transaminese (AST), alanine transaminase (ALT) ≥ 2 times of normal range), renal failure or creatinine clearance (CrCl) ≤ 10 umol/L, paracetamol and/or propofol allergy. Exclusion criteria also included patients who were not using propofol for an induction, using an intravenous catheter that was not on a hand dorsum, or whereas the size of the catheter was not 20G and had to have a rapid sequence induction.

After obtaining a written informed consent, a randomization was performed by using a block of 6 method. The drugs were prepared by one of the investigators (MJ), with both the patient and an independent assessor (anesthesiologist in-charge) blinded. The groups Pb, P500 and P1000, patients were premedicated with oral placebo, 500 or 1000 mg of paracetamol, respectively 1 h prior to transferal to the operating room. Each patient received either 2 tablets of placeco (Pb group), 1 tablet of placebo and 1 tablet of paracetamol 500 mg (P500), or 2 tablets of paracetamol 500 mg (P1000). Both placebo and paracetamol were identical in shape, size, color and weight. None of them received any other analgesic or sedative drug. A 20G intravenous catheter was inserted into a superficial vein on the hand dorsum and intravenous fluid at a rate of 80 ml/hr. was infused into each patient.

After preoxygenation, an emulsion of 1% propofol in a mixture of long-chain and medium-chain triglycerides (Lipuro®, B Braun) 2 mg/kg (for obese patients, dose was calculated by using lean body weight) was intravenously administered into each patient with a syringe pump at a rate of 600 ml/hr. (10 ml/min). After 1/4 of the calculated dose of propofol had been delivered, the infusion pump was temporarily paused and the patient was asked to rate his/her pain at the injection site using an 11-point verbal numerical rating score (VNRS) when 0 is not pain and 10 is the worst pain imaginable. None of them was heavily anesthetized and unable to give the VNRS. The residual dose of propofol was then given, followed by opioids and neuromuscular blocking agent as per usual.

In the operating room and postanesthesia care unit, each patient was carefully evaluated for paracetamol's side effects including rash, swelling, flushing, hypotension and tachycardia.

Statistical analysis was performed by using R software 2.14.1. Continuous variables were analyzed by ANOVA F- test or Kruskal-Wallis test. Categorical variables were analyzed by ANOVA F-test, Fisher's exact test or Chi-square test. Post-hoc analysis was carried out by using a Bonferroni correction. P value less than 0.05 was considered as statistical significant. Continuous variables were presented as median and interquartile range (IQR) or mean and standard deviation (SD). Categorical variables were presented as number of patients and percentages. The power of this study was 0.9.

For sample size calculation, we collected pain intensity by using the 11-point verbal numerical rating score (VNRS) in 30 patients who received propofol for an induction, without having paracetamol for premedication. The mean VNRS in this group of patients was 5.7. Anticipating that patients premedicated with paracetamol would have 25% less pain (VNRS of 4.2), a number of patients per each group was calculated to be 96. With 10% drop out, the definite number of patients per each group was 108.

Results

A total of 834 patients were assessed for eligibility from June 2015 to February 2016. Five hundred and ten patients were excluded and 324 patients were randomly allocated to each group. Each group equally had 108 patients. All participants were completely analyzed. (Fig. 1) There were no differences between the groups regarding gender, age, weight, height, body mass index (BMI), ASA physical classification and interval between ingestion of paracetamol and injection of propofol. (Table 1).

In all cases, it was possible to achieve a clear response from the patients before they became anesthetized. The overall incidence of pain during propofol injection among the 3 groups is shown in Fig. 2. The incidence of pain was less in the P1000 group (70.4%) compared with the P500 (86.1%) and the Pb groups (99.1%) ($P < 0.001$). The incidences of pain by categories of intensity (mild/moderate/severe) were lower in the P1000 group in comparison to those in the P500 and the Pb groups ($P < 0.001$). (Table 2).

The median pain score showed a significant reduction in the P1000 group compared with the P500, and the Pb groups. Those were 2 (0–3), 4 (2–5), and 8 (7–10), respectively ($P < 0.001$). (Fig. 3).

There was no incidence of complications such as; rashes or edema of the tissue in each group at the recovery room.

Discussion

In this study, we found that an oral paracetamol was effective in decreasing the incidence and severity of propofol injection pain when compared with a placebo. Premedication with 1000 mg of paracetamol was also more effective in reducing propofol injection pain than 500 mg.

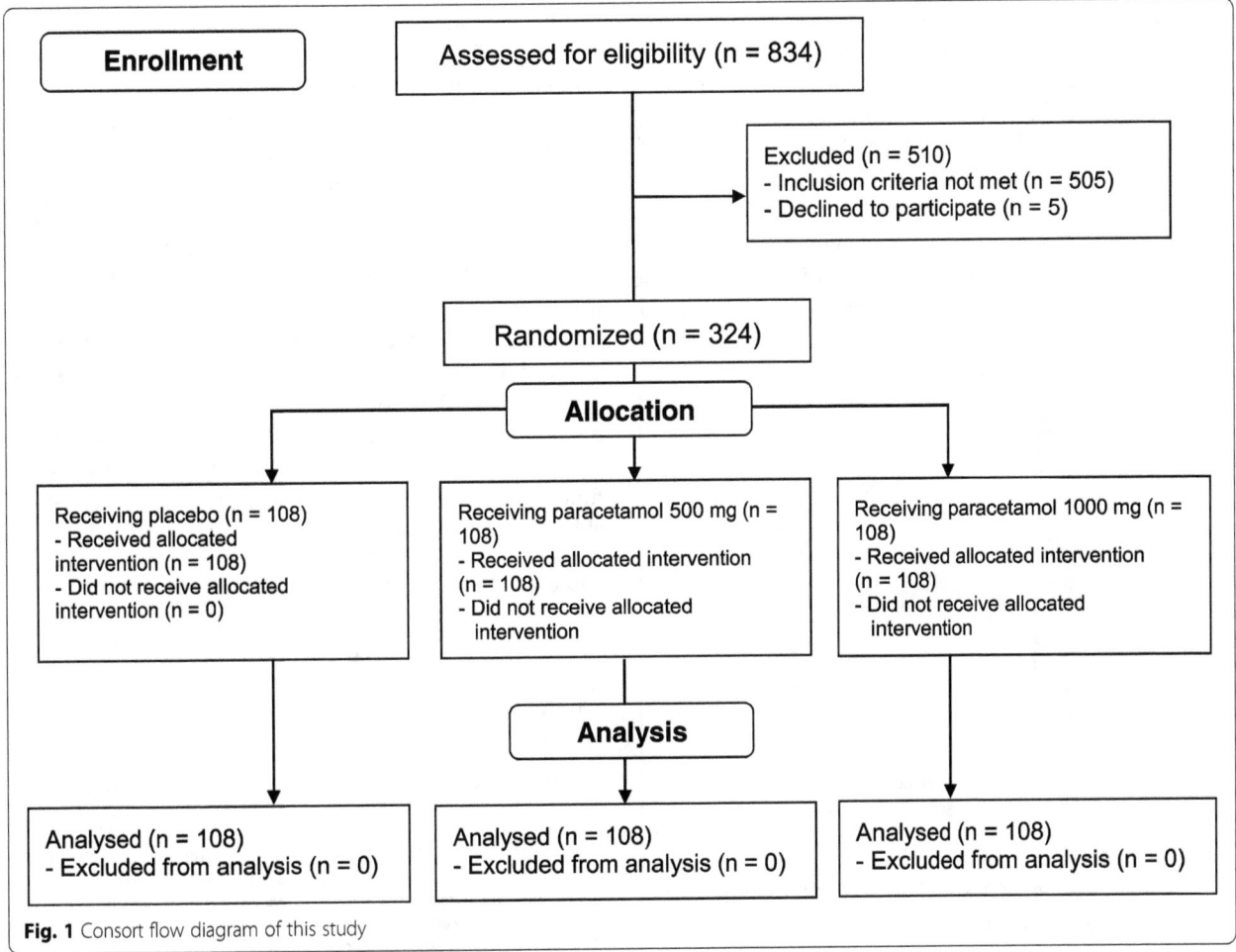

Fig. 1 Consort flow diagram of this study

Table 1 Patient demographic data. All data are n (%) or mean (SD)

Patients	Pb (n = 108)	P500 (n = 108)	P1000 (n = 108)	P-value
Gender, n (%)				
- Male	24 (22.2)	33 (30.5)	36 (33.3)	0.16
Age (yr), mean (SD)	42.7 (11.5)	43 (12.2)	44.3 (10.3)	0.54
Weight (kg), mean (SD)	62.5 (9.6)	62.8 (9.8)	62.8 (9.1)	0.96
Height (cm), mean (SD)	159.5 (7.4)	160.3 (7.3)	159.5 (8.2)	0.67
BMI (kg/m^2), mean (SD)	24.6 (3.6)	24.4 (3.4)	24.8 (3.5)	0.80
ASA classification, n (%)				0.19
- I	19 (17.6)	28 (25.9)	23 (21.3)	
- II	84 (77.8)	79 (73.1)	81 (75)	
- III	5 (4.6)	1 (1)	4 (3.7)	
IPP[a], mean (SD)	65.1 (32.1)	66.5 (28.3)	70.8 (28.9)	0.35

[a]IPP = interval between ingestion of paracetamol to injection of propofol (minutes)
Data are presented as the number of patients (%) and mean ± SD values

Paracetamol is one of the most popular and frequently used pain killer throughout the world. The mechanisms of action are sophisticated and cover both peripheral and central antinocciceptive manners. The pain relief effect provided by paracetamol is via inhibition of the cyclooxygenase pathway centrally and peripherally, reducing the production of prostaglandins [18]. Nevertheless, its antiinflammatory effects are weak, probably due to poor effectiveness when the concentration of peroxidases is high at the area of inflammation [19]. Paracetamol has been postulated to be classified to the group of the so-called atypical NSAIDs, determined as peroxide sensitive analgesic and antipyretic drugs (PSAAD) [20]. It has been shown that paracetamol is a selective cyclooxygenase-2 inhibitor in vivo [21]. Other proposed possible modes of action are an endogenous cannabinoid effect [22, 23], fatty acid amide hydrolase (FAAH)-dependent metabolism of acetaminophen into N-arachidonoylphenolamine (AM404) [23], and a modulatory effect on the descending serotoninergic bulbospinal inhibitory pathway [24, 25] as concurrent administration of granisetron or tropisetron with paracetamol completely blocks the analgesic effect of paracetamol [26]. Pain relieving effect of paracetamol might also be a result of inhibition of nitric oxide (NO) formation. The synthesis of NO is through activation of L-arginine/NO pathway by substance P (SP) and N-methyl-D-aspartate (NMDA) receptors. NO is an important neurotransmitter involved in nociceptive process of the spinal cord [27, 28]. Ohashi N, et al. suggest that paracetamol metabolite N-acylphenolamine induces analgesic effect directly via transient receptor potential vanilloid 1 (TRPV1) receptors expressed on central terminals of C-fibers in the spinal dorsal horn and leads to conduction block, shunt currents, and desensitization of these fibers [29]. Treatment with paracetamol within 24 h of intensive care unit admission may lessen oxidative injury and improve renal function in adult patients with severe sepsis and detectable plasma cell-free hemoglobin [30].

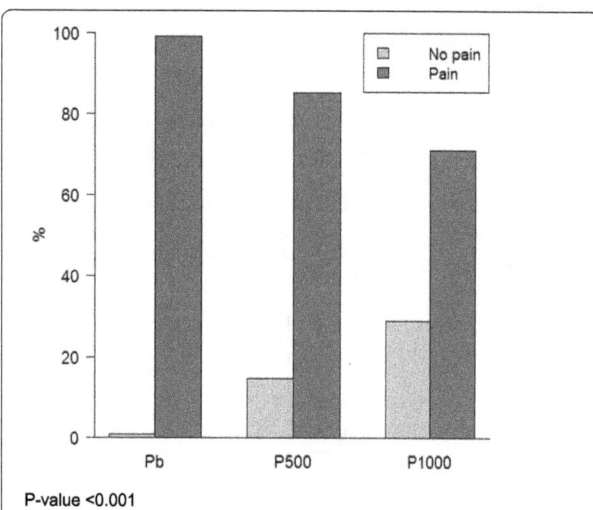

P-value <0.001

Pb = placebo, P500 = parecetamol 500 mg, P1000 = paracetamol 1000 mg

Fig. 2 Incidence of injection pain among the 3 groups

Table 2 Number of patients experiencing propofol injection pain among the 3 groups

Severity of pain n (%)	Pb group (n = 108)	P 500 group (n = 108)	P 1000 group (n = 108)
None (VNRS 0)	1 (0.9)	15 (13.9)	32 (29.6)
Mild (VNRS 1–2)	0 (0)	31 (28.7)	51 (47.2)
Moderate (VNRS 4–6)	24 (22.2)	54 (50)	25 (23.2)
Severe (VNRS 7–10)	83 (76.9)	8 (7.4)	0 (0)

P-value < 0.001 among the 3 groups and P-value < 0.001 for Pb vs P500, P-value < 0.001 for Pb vs P1000, P-value < 0.001 for P500 vs P1000
Pb placebo, P500 parecetamol 500 mg, P1000 paracetamol 1000 mg
VNRS verbal numerical rating score
Data are presented as the number of patients (%)

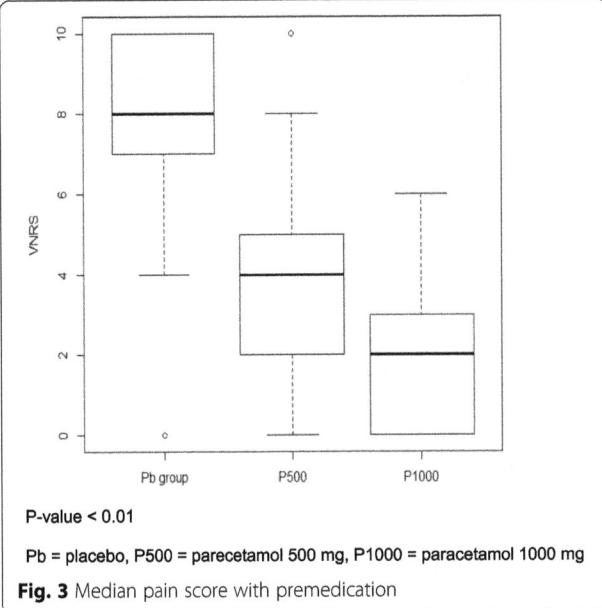

P-value < 0.01

Pb = placebo, P500 = parecetamol 500 mg, P1000 = paracetamol 1000 mg

Fig. 3 Median pain score with premedication

Paracetamol has been found as effective for reducing propofol injection pain. Canbay et al. [15] conducted a double-blinded RCT in 150 patients and showed that the incidence of propofol injection pain was 64% in the control group and 22% in the intravenous paracetamol pretreatment group. Khouadja et al. [31] performed a double-blinded RCT in 180 patients and also showed similar results, 85% in the control group and 36.6% in the intravenous paracetamol group. Our results revealed that premedication with oral paracetamol reduced the incidence and severity of propofol injection pain. It added more information that oral paracetamol was also effective for this type of pain.

In our study, the overall incidence of pain during propofol injection was higher than other studies. The previous 3 studies [15, 31, 32] used intravenous paracetamol, not oral tablet as we did. Oral form of paracetamol exerts different pharmacokinetics and pharmacodynamics in comparison to intravenous form. This is why our results (using oral paracetamol) somewhat differed from other previous studies (using intravenous paracetamol) in terms of incidence and severity of propofol injection pain. Singla et al. [33] has shown that intravenous paracetamol has earlier and higher plasma level compared with oral paracetamol. After administration, plasma concentration of intravenous paracetamol reaches its peak rapidly within 15 min as shown by a very steep part of its graph. Plasma concentration of oral paracetamol at any time of measurement (0.25, 0.5, 0.75, 1, 2, 3, 4 and 6 h) is much lower than that of intravenous paracetamol at 15 min. The intravenous route provides a 76% higher maximum concentration (C_{max}) than the oral route.

The other reasons that the incidence of propofol injection pain in the paracetamol group in previous studies was lower than ours may be from inserting a bigger venous catheter [31] and/or using a venous occlusion technique [15, 31]. It has been demonstrated that this tourniquet technique can help to increase the effectiveness of intravenous paracetamol in reducing propofol injection pain [32]. Canbay et al. [15] occluded their patient's vein and gave pretreatment of intravenous paracetamol over 10 s. The patient's vein was further occluded for 2 more minutes before releasing. Propofol was given after the patient's vein had been released. Pain was measured during 5 s of paracetamol injection. The patients in Canbay et al.'s study rated their pain within the period of the highest plasma concentration of paracetamol. Regarding analgesic effects provided by intravenous in comparison with oral paracetamol, Fenlon S. et al. performed a study in 128 patients scheduled for lower third molar extraction. It has been shown that oral paracetamol is not inferior than intravenous paracetamol for providing postoperative analgesia in patients undergoing dental surgery [34].

According to the severity of pain, the incidence of mild, moderate, and severe pain was also significantly different in our P1000, P500 and Pb groups. These findings indicate that premedication with oral paracetamol reduce propofol injection pain by means of a dose-dependent fashion.

Different method of assessing pain severity may also explain our different results on severity of propofol injection pain. We used a Verbal Numerical Rating Score (VNRS) ranging from 0 to 10 (11 points) to measure our patients' pain. All of our patients verbally reported their pain by themselves ('subjective' assessment). The other studies used a 4-point scale (0 = none, 1 = mild, 2 = moderate and 3 = severe). They did not mainly ask their patients to verbally rate the level of pain upon propofol injection but they principally observed their patients' pain behaviors ('observational' assessment): 0 = none (negative response to questioning), 1 = mild pain (pain reported only in response to questioning with no behavioral signs), 2 = moderate pain (pain reported in response to questioning and accompanied by a behavioral sign or pain reported spontaneously without questioning), and 3 = severe pain (strong vocal response or response accompanied by facial grimacing, arm withdrawals or tears). Measuring pain by the VNRS is reliable, valid, sensitive to change, and easy to administer [35]. We did not use behavioral assessment because it is not subjective and less reliable.

This study found no adverse consequence of paracetamol.

Strengths of this study are utilization of a simple analgesic (paracetamol) and administered it to the patients in a simple way (oral route). Considering that oral paracetamol has been shown to increase the incidence of no pain as well as to reduce the incidence of severe pain upon propofol injection, the results of this study are clinically useful and applicable to daily practice because oral paracetamol is readily and widely available, practically simple and convenient to use as well as economic wise. As our study's protocol is easy to apply and early administration or oral paracetamol is pharmacologically sensible, the result of this study can be clinically applied in general.

Limitations of this study are a subjective method of pain intensity measurement and the fractional dose of given propofol. The intensity of propofol injection pain was rated by using the verbal numerical rating score (VNRS), although patient's self-assessment is the gold standard of pain intensity measurement but it is subjective and depends of each individual. Because propofol is a powerful induction agent, we could not inject the entire dose of propofol to each patient before measuring the pain intensity as a significant number of them felt asleep and were unable to give the pain rating.

Conclusions

Premedication with oral paracetamol can reduce propofol injection pain on a dose-dependent basis, without causing any adverse effect. As propofol injection pain is common and remains a concern of anesthesia providers for the comfort of their patients, and early oral administration of paracetamol is pharmacologically sensible, easy to apply, well-tolerated, available and economic, the results of this study provide the basis for changing practice with a positive impact on patient care.

Abbreviations

ALT: Alanine transminase; ASA: American Society of Anesthesiologists; AST: Aspartate transaminase; BMI: Body mass index; C_{max}: Maximum concentration; COX: Cyclooxygenase; IQR: Interquartile range; NMDA: N-methyl-D-aspartate; NO: Nitric oxide; NSAIDs: Non-steroidal anti-inflammatory drugs; PSAAD: Peroxide sensitive analgesic and antipyretic drugs; SD: Standard deviation; SP: Substance P; VNRS: Verbal numerical rating score

Acknowledgements

Department of Anesthesiology, Faculty of Medicine, Prince of Songkla University.

Authors' contributions

SN and MJ participated in protocol writing, collecting data, statistical analysis, interpretation of results and manuscript writing. SP participated in protocol writing, interpretation of results and manuscript writing. MO did the statistical analysis and reviewed the manuscript. All authors read and approved the final manuscript.

References

1. Tan CH, Onsiong MK. Pain on injection of propofol. Anaesthesia. 1998; 53:468–76.
2. Stark RD, Binks SM, Dutka VN, O'Connor KM, Arnstein MJA, Glen JB. A review of the safety and tolerance of propofol (Diprivan). Postgrad Med J. 1985;61:152–6.
3. Manger D, Holak EJ. Tourniquet at 50 mmHg followed by intravenous lidocaine diminishes hand pain associated with propofol injection. Anesth Analg. 1992;74:250–2.
4. Klement W, Arndt JO. Pain on intravenous injection of some anaesthetic agents is evoked by the unphysiological osmolarity or pH of their formulations. Br J Anaesth. 1991;66:189–95.
5. Nakane M, Iwama H. A potential mechanism of propofol-induced pain on injection based on studies using nafamostat mesilate. Br J Anaesth. 1999;83:397–404.
6. McCulloch MJ, Lees NW. Assessment and modification of pain on induction with propofol (Diprivan). Anaesthesia. 1985;40:1117–20.
7. Scott RPF, Saunders DA, Norman J. Propofol: clinical strategies for preventing pain on injection. Anaesthesia. 1988;43:492–4.
8. Briggs LP, Clarke RSJ, Dundee JW, Moore J, Bahar M, Wright PJ. Use of di-isopropyl phenol as main agent for short procedures. Br J Anaesth. 1981;53:1197–201.
9. Huang CL, Wang YP, Cheng YJ, Susetio L, Liu CC. The effect of carrier intravenous fluid speed on the injection pain of propofol. Anesth Analg. 1995;81:1087.
10. McDonald DS, Jameson P. Injection pain with propofol. Reduction with aspiration of blood. Anaesthesia. 1996;51:878–80.
11. Ganta R, Fee JP. Pain on injection of propofol: comparison of lignocaine with metoclopramide. Br J Anaesth. 1992;69:316–7.
12. Kizilcik N, Menda F, Bilgen S, Keskin O, Koner O. Effects of a fentanyl-propofol mixture on propofol injection pain: a randomized clinical trial. Korean J Anesthesiol. 2015;68:556–60.
13. Bahar M, McAteer E, Dundee JW, Briggs LP. Aspirin in the prevention of painful intravenous injection of disoprofol (ICI 35, 868) and diazepam (valium). Anaesthesia. 1982;37:847–8.
14. Jalota L, Kalira V, George E, Shi YY, Hornuss C, Radke O, et al. Prevention of pain on injection of propofol: systematic review and meta-analysis. Cited as. BMJ. 2011;342:d1110.
15. Canbay O, Celebi N, Arun O, Karagoz H, Sarıcaoglu F, Ozgen S. Efficacy of intravenous acetaminophen and lidocaine on propofol injection pain. Br J Anaesth. 2008;100:95–8.
16. Borazan H, Erdem TB, Kececioglu M, Otelcioglu S. Prevention of pain on injection of propofol: a comparison of lidocaine with different doses of paracetamol. Eur J Anaesthesiol. 2010;27:253–7.
17. Seymour RA, Kelly PJ, Hawkesford JE. The efficacy of ketoprofen and paracetamol (acetaminophen) in postoperative pain after third molar surgery. Br J Clin Pharmacol. 1996;41:581–5.
18. Jozwiak-Bebenista M, Nowak JZ. Paracetamol: mechanism of action, applications, and safety concern. Acta Pol Pharm. 2014;71:11–23.
19. Candido KD, Perozo OJ, Knezevic NN. Pharmacology of acetaminophen, nonsteroidal antiinflammatory drugs, and steroid medications: implications for anesthesia or unique associated risks. Anesthesiol Clin. 2017;35:e145–62.
20. Graham GG, Scott KF. Mechanisms of action of paracetamol and related analgesics. Inflammopharmacology. 2003;11:401–13.
21. Lee YS, Kim H, Brahim JS, Rowan J, Lee G, Dionne RA. Acetaminophen selectively suppresses peripheral prostaglandin E_2 release and increases COX-2 gene expression in a clinical model of acute inflammation. Pain. 2007;129:279–86.
22. Mallet C, Barriera DA, Ermund A, Jonsson BAG, Eschalier A, Zygmunt PM, et al. TRPV1 in brain is involved in acetaminophen-induced antinociception. PLoS One. 2010;5:e12748.
23. Mallet C, Daulhac L, Bonnefont J, Ledent C, Etienne M, Chapuy E, et al. Endocannabinoid and serotonergic systems are needed for acetaminophen-induced analgesia. Pain. 2008;139:190–200.
24. Pickering G, Esteve V, Loriot MA, Eschalier A, Dubray C. Acetaminophen reinforces descending inhibitory pain pathways. Clin Pharmacol Ther. 2008;84:47–51.
25. Bonnefont J, Alloui A, Chapuy E, Clottes E, Eschalier A. Orally administered paracetamol does not act locally in the rat formalin test: evidence for a supraspinal, serotonin-dependent antinociceptive mechanism. Anesthesiology. 2003;99:976–81.
26. Pickering G, Loriot MA, Libert F, Eschalier A, Beaune P, Dubray C. Analgesic effect of acetaminophen in humans: first evidence of a central serotonergic mechanism. Clin Pharmacol Ther. 2006;79:371–8.
27. Bjorkman R. Central antinociceptive effects of non-steroidal anti-inflammatory drugs and paracetamol. Experimental studies in the rat. Acta Anaesthesiol Scand. 1995;103(Suppl.):1–44.
28. Bujalska M. Effect of nitric oxide synthase inhibitor on antinociceptive action of different doses of acetaminophen. Pol J Pharmacol. 2004;56:605–10.
29. Ohashi N, Uta D, Sasaki M, Ohashi M, Kamiya Y, Kohno T. Acetaminophen metabolite N-acylphenolamine induces analgesia via transient receptor

potential vanilloid 1 receptors expressed on the primary afferent terminals of C-fibers in the spinal dorsal horn. Anesthesiology. 2017;127:355–71.

30. Janz DR, Bastarache JA, Rice TW, Bernard GR, Warren MA, Wickersham N, et al. Randomized, placebo-controlled trial of acetaminophen for the reduction of oxidative injury in severe sepsis: the acetaminophen for the reduction of oxidative injury in severe Sepsis trial. Crit Care Med. 2015;43:534–41.

31. Khouadja H, Arnous H, Tarmiz K, Beletaifa D, Brahim A, Brahem W, et al. Pain on injection of propofol: efficacy of paracetamol and lidocaine. Open J Anesthesiol. 2014;4:81–7.

32. Ozkan S, Sen H, Sizlan A, Yanarates O, Mutlu M, Dagli G. Comparison of acetaminophen (with or without tourniquet) and lidocaine in propofol injection pain. Klinik Psikofarmakol Bülteni. 2011;21:100–4.

33. Singla NK, Parulan C, Samson R, Hutchinson J, Bushnell R, Beja EG, et al. Plasma and cerebrospinal fluid pharmacokinetic parameters after single dose administration of intravenous, oral or rectal acetaminophen. Pain Pract. 2012;12:523–32.

34. Fenlon S, Collyer J, Giles J, Bidd H, Lees M, Nicholson J, et al. Oral vs intravenous paracetamol for lower third molar extractions under general anaesthesia: is oral administration inferior? Br J Anaesth. 2013;110:432–7.

35. Bendinger T, Plunkett N. Measurement in pain medicine. BJA Education. 2016;16:310–5.

21

Ultrasound-guided erector spinae plane block for postoperative analgesia

Jiao Huang and Jing-Chen Liu[*]

Abstract

Background: Ultrasound-guided Erector Spinae Plane Block (ESPB) has been increasingly applied in patients for postoperative analgesia. Its effectiveness remain uncertain. This meta-analysis aimed to determine the clinical efficacy of ultrasound-guided ESPB in adults undergoing general anesthesia (GA) surgeries.

Methods: A systematic databases search was conducted in PubMed, Embase, and the Cochrane Library for randomized controlled trials (RCTs) comparing ESPB with control or placebo. Primary outcome was iv. opioid consumption 24 h after surgery. Standardized mean differences (SMDs) and risk ratios (RRs) with 95% confidence intervals (CIs) were calculated with a random-effects model.

Results: A total of 12 RCTs consisting of 590 patients were included. Ultrasound-guided ESPB showed a reduction of intravenous opioid consumption 24 h after surgery (SMD = -2.18; 95% confidence interval (CI) -2.76 to $-1.61, p < 0.00001$). Considerable heterogeneity was observed (87%). It further reduced the number of patients who required postoperative analgesia (RR = 0.41, 95% CI 0.25 to 0.66, $p = 0.0002$) and prolonged time to first rescue analgesia (SMD = 4.56, 95% CI 1.89 to 7.22, $p = 0.0008$).

Conclusions: Ultrasound-guided ESPB provides effective postoperative analgesic in adults undergoing GA surgeries.

Keywords: Erector Spinae plane block (ESPB), Postoperative analgesia, Regional blockade, Opioid, Pain score

Background

Ultrasound-guided Erector Spinae Plane Block (ESPB) is a novel regional anesthesia technique that local anesthetic (LA) injection is performed into the fascial plane situated between the transverse process of the vertebra and the erector spinae muscles it is considered a relatively safe simple technique to perform [1, 2]. Followed by first description by Forero et al. [1] in 2016, it has been demonstrated successfully to provide analgesia in thoracic and thoracoabdominal surgeries [3, 4] However, the use of ultrasound-guided

ESPB remained controversial. Recently, several randomized controlled trials (RCTs) [5–7] on this topic have been published, but the determine conclusions cannot be established owing to the modest sample size of these RCTs. We therefore conducted a meta-analysis to examine the efficacy of ultrasound-guided ESPB among adults undergoing general anesthesia (GA) surgery. Our primary outcome was intravenous opioid consumption 24 h after surgery. Secondly outcomes included pain scores, number of patients who need rescue analgesia, time to first rescue analgesic and postoperative nausea or vomiting (PONV).

* Correspondence: jingchenl@sina.com
Department of Anesthesiology, First Affiliated Hospital of Guangxi Medical University, 6 Shuangyong Road, Nanning 530021, Guangxi Zhuang Autonomous Region, People's Republic of China

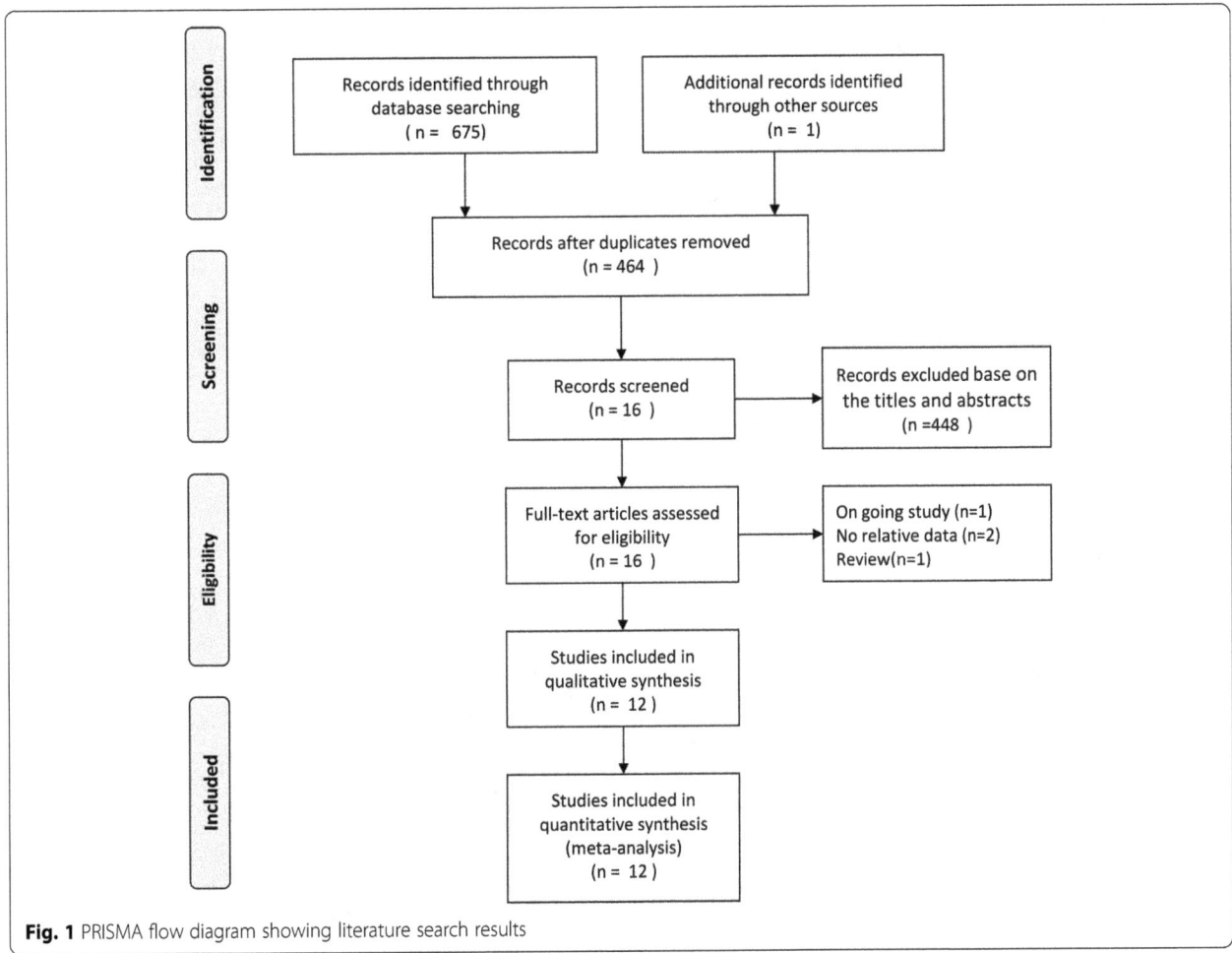

Fig. 1 PRISMA flow diagram showing literature search results

Methods
Literature search and selection criteria
This systematic review and meta-analysis of RCTs was reported abiding by the Preferred Reporting Items for Systematic Reviews and Meta Analyses (PRISMA) statement [8] and it was conducted base on the statement of the Cochrane Handbook for Systematic Reviews of Interventions [9]. No formal protocol was registered for this meta-analysis.

PubMed, EMBASE, and the Cochrane Library were searched from inception to August 2019 with no language restriction. The search terms used were: ('erector spinae plan block' OR 'erector spinae block' OR 'erector spinae plan blocks' OR 'erector spinae blocks'). The bibliographies of included trials were also manually searched for any eligible trials missed by the electronic search. This process was conducted iteratively until no extra reference could be verified.

Two of us independently performed the preliminary data search, after removing duplicate references, the titles and abstracts were screening for the eligible trials. We included all RCTs in adults who were undergoing GA surgery with the intervention of ultrasound-guided ESPB Trials were excluded for the following criteria: animal or cadaveric studies; reviews; did not report opioid consumption or pain scores as an outcome; Any discrepancies were resolved by discussion with coauthors.

Data extraction and quality assessment
Data collection was performed by two authors (JH and JCL). The following information was collected from each eligible trial: first author, publication year, patient number, patient characteristics, American Society of Anesthesiologists (ASA) physical status, surgical procedure, ESPB group (position, dosage and concentration), control group (placebo or no invention). Extracted data were entered into a predefined standardized Excel (Microsoft 6 Corporation, USA) file.. For continuous data, we calculated mean and SD, if not provided,

Table 1 Characteristics of included studies

	No. Of patients	Surgical procedure	ASA	Patient Characteristics	ESPB group	Control group	GA induction
Tulgar 2018 (1)	30 (15/15)	Laparoscopiccholecystectomy	I-II	18–65 years of age	Bilateral ultrasound-guided ESPB at the level of T9 transverse process using 10 mL of bupivacaine 0.375% on each side	Received no intervention	Propofol 2–3mgkg − 1, fentanyl100µg and rocuronium bromide 0.6 mg kg − 1
Gürkan 2018	50 (25/25)	Elective breast cancer surgery	I-II	Aged 20–65 years	Ultrasound (US)-guided ESPB with 20 ml 0.25% bupivacaine at the T4 vertebral level	Received no intervention	Propofol(2–3 mg kg − 1) and fentanyl(2 mg kg − 1) iv, rocuronium 0.6 mg kg − 1
Tulgar 2018 (2)	40 (20/20)	Hip and proximal femur surgery	I-III	Aged 18–65 years	Ultrasound-guided ESPB at T9 vertebrae level with 20 ml bupivacaine 0.5%, 10 ml lidocaine 2%,	Underwent thesame procedure but had no block	Propofol 2-3 mg/kg, fentanyl 100 µg and rocuronium bromide 0.6 mg/kg.
Singh 2019 (1)	40 (20/20)	Elective lumbarspine surgery	I-III	18–65 years of age	Ultrasound (US)-guided ESPB with total 20 ml 0.5% bupivacaine at the T10 vertebral level	Received no intervention	Propofol 2 to3 mg/kg, morphine 0.1 mg/kg and vecuronium 0.1 mg/kg
Gürkan 2019	50 (25/25)	Elective unilateral breast surgery	I-II	Aged 18–65 years	Ultrasound (US) guided ESP block with 20 ml 0.25% bupivacaine at the T4 vertebral level	Received no intervention	Propofol (2–3 mg kg − 1) and fentanyl (2 µg kg − 1) iv and rocuronium 0.6 mg kg − 1
Singh 2019 (2)	40 (20/20)	Modified radical mastectomy	I-II	Female patients between 20 and 55 years	Ultrasound (US)-guided ESP block with total 20 ml 0.5% bupivacaine at the T5 vertebral level	Received no intervention	Propofol 2–3 mg kg − 1, morphine 0.1 mg kg − 1, and vecuronium 0.1 mg kg − 1
Aksu 2019 (1)	46 (23/23)	LaparoscopicCholecystectomy	I-II	20–75 years of age	Ultrasound (US) guided ESP block with 20 ml 0.25% bupivacaine at the T5–6 vertebral level	Received no intervention	Propofol (2–3 mg kg-1) and fentanyl (2 mg kg-1) iv and Rocuronium (0.6 mg kg-1)IV
Ciftci 2019	60 (30/30)	Video-Assisted Thoracic surgery	I-II	18–65 years of age	Ultrasound guided Bilateral ESP block with20ml of 0.375% bupivacaine at the T5 vertebral level	Received no intervention	Propofol (2–2.5 mg/kg) and fentanyl (1–1.5 mg/kg) and rocuronium bromide (0.6 mg/kg)
Ciftci 2019	60 (30/30)	Video-Assisted Thoracic surgery	I-II	18–65 years of age	Ultrasound guided Bilateral ESP block with20ml of 0.375% bupivacaine at the T5 vertebral level	Received no intervention	Propofol (2–2.5 mg/kg) and fentanyl (1–1.5 mg/kg) and rocuronium bromide (0.6 mg/kg)
Yayik 2019	60 (30/30)	Lumbar Spinal Decompression Surgery	I-III	18–65 years of age	Ultrasound guided Bilateral ESP block with 0.25% bupivacaine 20 mL at the L3 vertebral level	No intervention was performed	2 mg/kg IV propofo, 0.6 mg/kg IV rocuronium and 2 mcg/kg IV fentanyl
Hamed 2019	60 (30/30)	Abdominal hysterectomy	I-III	Women aged 40–70 years old and weighed 50–90 kg	Ultrasound-guided ESPB at T9 vertebrae level with 20 ml bupivacaine 0.5%.	Underwent the same procedure but had a sham injection(20 ml of saline)	Fentanyl 2 mcg.kg − 1 and propofol 2 mg.kg1, followed by atracurium 0.5 mg.kg − 1
AKSU 2019 (2)	50 (25/25)	elective breast surgery	I-II	Aged between 25 and 70 years	Ultrasound-guided ESPB betweenT2 and T4 with 10 ml of 0.25% bupivacaine	No intervention was performed	Propofol (2–3 mg/kg) and fentanyl (2 mg/kg) iv and Rocuronium 0.6 mg/kg was administered iv

median and interquartile range were seen as means and standard deviation (SD) approximately as follows: the median was considered equal to the mean, and the SD was calculated as the interquartile range divided by 1.35 [10]. Any uncertainty arose were figured out though a consensus achieved.

Two authors (JH and JCL) evaluated the methodological quality of the trials according to the Cochrane risk-of-bias tool [11]. Each item was categorized as having a 'low', 'unclear', or 'high' risk of bias. Any uncertainty arose were resolve by discussion between two researches until a consensus was achieved.

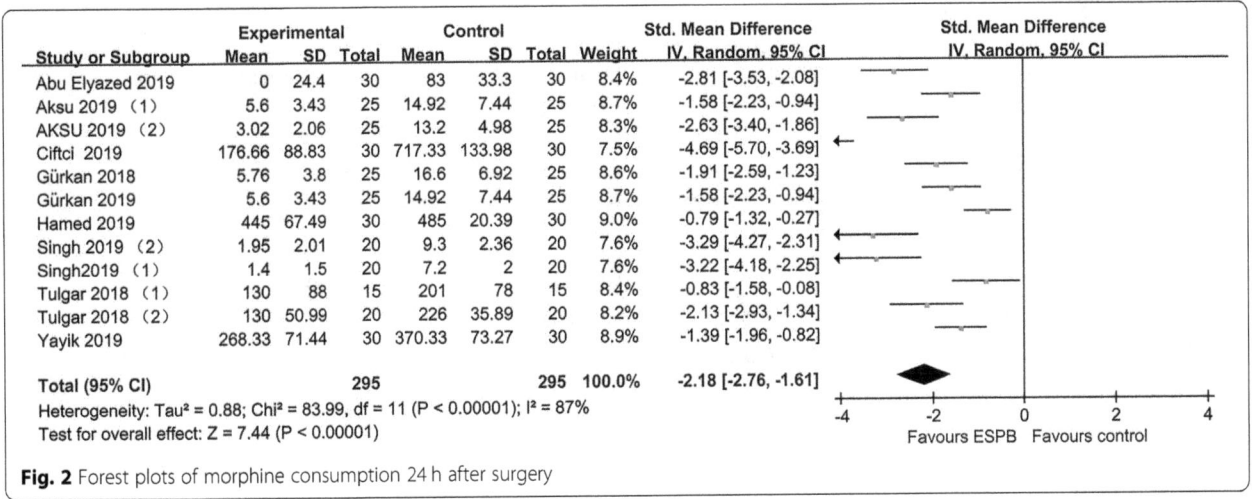

Fig. 2 Forest plots of morphine consumption 24 h after surgery

Statistical analysis

The relative risks (RRs) and standardized mean differences (SMDs) with 95% confidence intervals (CIs) were calculated. A random effects model was selected to acquire the most conservative effects estimate. An I^2 statistic of 25–50% were defined as low heterogeneity, an I^2 statistic of 50–75% were described as moderate heterogeneity, and those with an I^2 statistic of > 75% were considered as high heterogeneity [12], The heterogeneity was substantial when an I^2 value was over 50%. Subgroup analysis was conducted based on additional analgesia (patient-controlled analgesia device (PCA) versus not PCA). Publication bias was evaluated using funnel plots. Statistical analyses were calculated using the Review Manager Version 5.3 (Nordic Cochrane Centre, Cochrane Collaboration).

Results

Study identification and characteristics

A total of 675 studies were obtained by the literature search. One further citations were found by hand searching. 212 records were excluded for duplicate studies and a further 448 records removed by screening titles and abstracts. 16 full text publications remained were

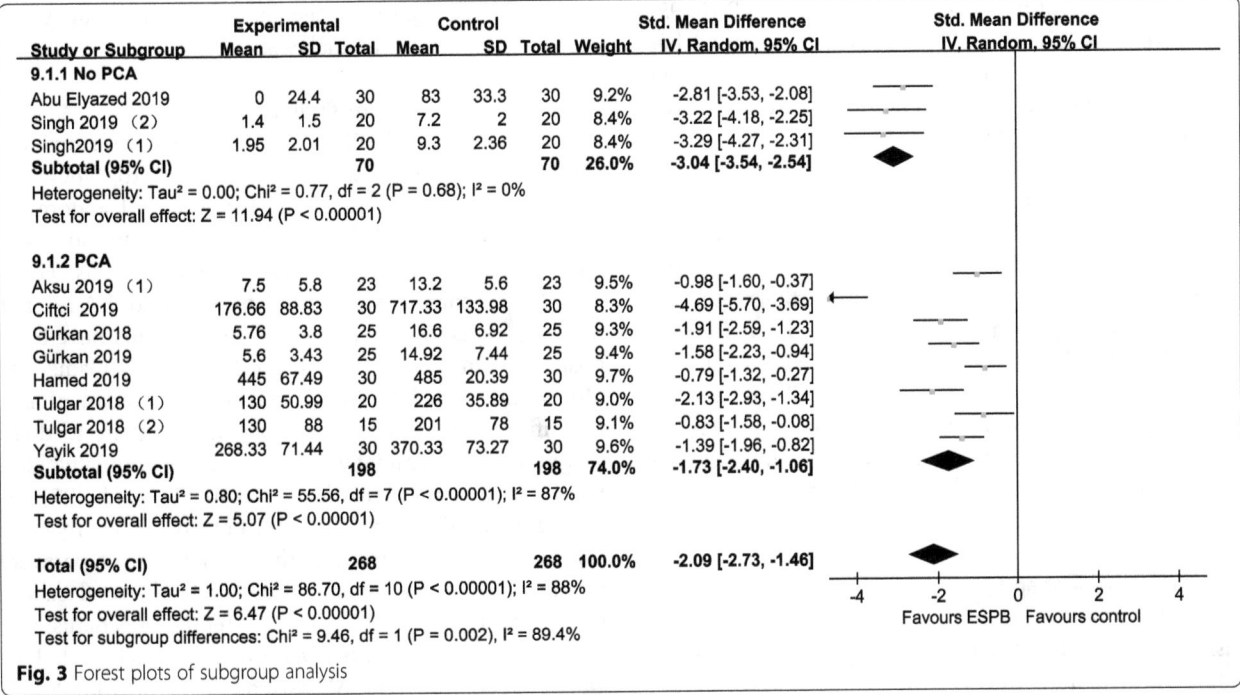

Fig. 3 Forest plots of subgroup analysis

Table 2 Outcome data of RCTs included in the meta-analysis

Outcome	Studies include	RR or Std.mean differance [95%CI]	P-value for statistical significance	P-value for heterogeneity	I^2 test for heterogeneity
Opiod consumption in the first 24 h (mg)	12	-2.18[-2.76,-1.61]	< 0.00001	< 0.00001	87%
VAS/NRS scores at the 1st hour	6	-0.80[-1.54,-0.06]	0.03	< 0.00001	88%
VAS/NRS scores at the 6th hour	8	-0.64[- 0.99,-0.30]	0.0003	0.03	58%
VAS/NRS scores at the 12th hour	6	-0.16[- 0.66,0.33]	0.51	0.0008	76%
VAS/NRS scores at the 24th hour	8	-0.83[-1.78,0.12]	0.09	0.00001	94%
Rescue analgesia requirement(n)	7	0.41 [0.25,0.66]	0.0002	0.006	67%
Time to first rescue analgesic (min)	3	4.56 [1.89,7.22]	0.0008	0.00001	95%
POVN(postoperative nausea and vomiting)	9	0.45 [0.20,1.00]	0.05	< 0.00001	84%

scrutinized for conclusive identified. 4 of them were excluded because 2 did not report data of interest [13, 14], one was currently ongoing study [15],one was review article [16].Finally,12 RCT [5–7, 17–25] satisfied our inclusion criteria. A flowchart of the literature search is shown in (Fig. 1).

All RCTs included in this meta-analysis were published between 2018 and 2019, with a total of 490. The main characteristics of the 12 RCTs included are presented in Table 1.

Primary outcomes

All RCTs [5–7, 17–25] reported data on intravenous opioid consumption 24 h after surgery. Pooled analysis showed that ultrasound-guided ESPB was associated with a reduction of opioid 24 h after surgery (– 2.18, 95% CI – 2.76 to – 1.61; P <.00001; Fig. 2). Substantial heterogeneity was observed among these studies (P for heterogeneity<.00001; I^2 = 87%). The finding was consistent in subgroup analysis. (Fig. 3).

Secondary outcomes

Ultrasound-guided ESPB significantly decrease pain scores at the 1 h(– 0.80, 95% CI – 1.54 to – 0.06;) and 6 h[– 0.64, 95% CI – 0.99 to – 0.30;).Furthermore, No. need rescue analgesia (0.41, 95% CI 0.25 to 0.66; P = .0002, I^2 = 67%) was lower in the ESPB group and time to first rescue analgesic (4.56, 95% CI 1.89 to 7.22) was longer in the ESPB group. Pain scores at 12 h,24 h after surgery and PONV did not achieve statistical significance. All outcomes of the identified trials are reported in Table 2.

Quality assessment and publication bias

Four trials at a low risk of bias, and 8 trials at an unclear risk of bias. The randomisation procedure was adequately generated in 11 trials [5–7, 17–20, 22–25].

Since we subjectively judge the outcome measurement was little prone to be changed by lacking of blinding, all RCTs included were classified as low risk of bias at blinding of outcome assessments. Assessment of risk-of-bias summary of all RCTs are presented in (Fig. 4). There was no evidence of publication bias by inspection of the funnel plot (Fig. 5).

Discussion
Main finding

The main finding of this meta-analysis is that ultrasound-guided ESPB significantly reduced opioid consumption 24 h after surgery. It further reduced pain scores and patients who need rescue analgesia, besides, it prolonged the time to first request of rescue analgesia. Despite of the high heterogeneity, the main finding was consistent in subgroup analyses.

Possible mechanisms for findings

Ultrasound-guided ESPB is a peri-paravertebral regional anesthesia technique which is supposed to block the dorsal and ventral rami of the thoracic and abdominal spinal nerves [1], and thereby to block the anterior, posterior, and lateral thoracic and abdominal walls. However, the mechanisms of action and spread of LA are not fully elucidated. Several potential mechanisms have been posited. One of the suggested mechanisms of ultrasound-guided ESPB is paravertebral spread of LA, LA infiltration was observed from injection site to three vertebral levels cranially and four levels caudally [26]. Based on this mechanism, Coşarcan SK et al. [27] reported a modification ESPB and got good pain relief in various surgeries. However, the mechanism of paravertebral spread of LA remained debated in several cadaveric studies [28–30]. Another potential mechanism is epidural spread of LA. Schwartzmann A et al. [31], Tulgar S, et al. [32] and Altıparmak B, et al. [33] found

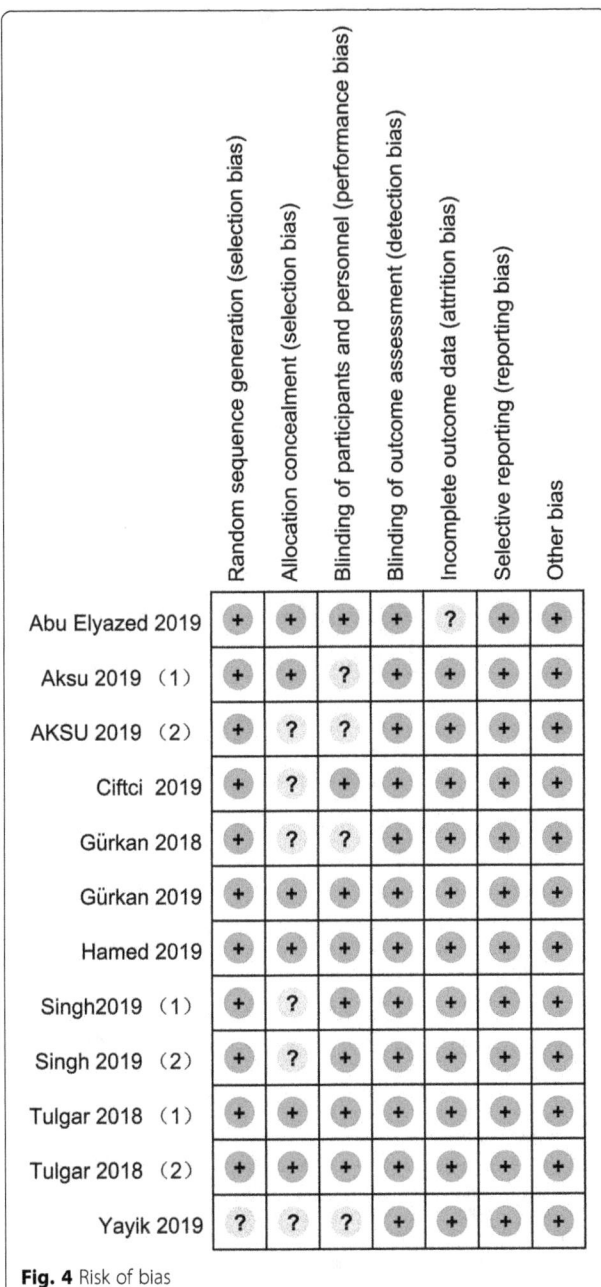

Fig. 4 Risk of bias

However, ultrasound-guided ESPB has only been utilized in clinical setting for about 3 years, several important issues have not been resolved yet. First, the optimal concentration, volume and type of LA in ESPB is not well established. Although 20 and 30 ml of 0.25% bupivacaine or 0.5% ropivacaine were recommended [36], concentrations of 0.25–0.5% bupivacaine 10-20 ml were used in ultrasound-guided ESPB among all 12 RCTs included in this meta-analysis. Is bupivacaine more preferred than ropivacaine? why? We tried to make a judgment but stop by the insufficient evidence. More researches of ultrasound-guided ESPB on concentration, volume, type of LA are necessary. Next, although no complications of ultrasound-guided ESPB have been reported in all included RCTs, risks such as LA toxicity, vascular puncture and pneumothorax still need our attention. Two studies have reported pneumothorax associated with ESPB [37, 38], and Selvi O et al. [39] reported unintended motor block linked to ESPB. More complications may appear as the increased use of ultrasound-guided ESPB in population. Last, compared to other regional block techniques such as transversus abdominis plane block (TAPB), serratus plane block (SPB), and Quadratus Lumborum Block (QLB), is the erector spine block more effective in some operations where the block areas overlap? Several RCTs on these topics published recently but far from achieving convincing conclusions [40–42].

Strengths and limitations

Our meta-analysis has several strengths. As far as we know, this is the first meta-analysis to evaluate the efficacy of ultrasound-guided ESPB in adults undergoing GA surgery. Besides, we performed this meta-analysis in compliance with the Cochrane Handbook and the PRISMA statement. Several notable limitations should be considered when interpreting the results. Firstly, the trials included have a modest sample size which could magnify the treatment effect. Secondly, the substantial heterogeneity was observed, one major factor result in heterogeneity is the diversity of surgery types (breast, lumbar spine, hip, abdominal etc). Parietal pain is more prominent in breast and lumbar spine, while visceral pain is the main component of postoperative pain following abdominal surgeries. The use of different types of opioid and supplementary analgesics such as paracetamol [23, 24] may also add an extra heterogeneity. Furthermore, owing to all patients were under GA surgeries, sensory blocking could not be evaluated adequately to exclude potential block failures of ESPB. Last, although we conducted a comprehensive literature search, it is hard to rule out the possibility of missing studies.

unilateral erector spinae plane block result in bilateral sensory blockade in some patients, epidural spread of the LA during ESPB may explain this result. Moreover, some evidence indicated that penetration of LA acted on dorsal and ventral rami through the connective tissues and branch communication leaded to visceral analgesia [34, 35].

Implications for clinical researches

Our findings demonstrated that ultrasound-guided ESPB was associated with a reduction of opioid consumption, which further proved the effectiveness of ESPB.

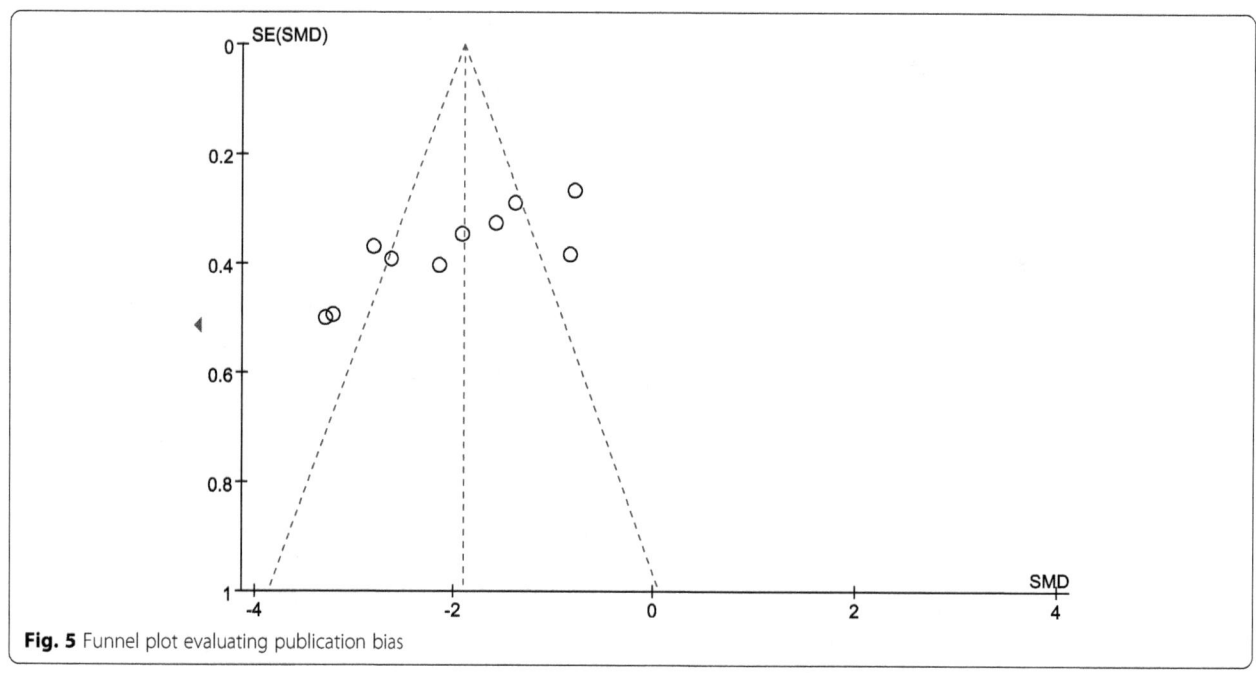

Fig. 5 Funnel plot evaluating publication bias

Conclusion

In summary, ESPB block provides an effective analgesic in adults. However, the results should be interpreted cautiously since insufficient evidence, although accumulating. Further large-scale RCTs are required to support our results.

Abbreviations
ESPB: Erector Spinae Plane Block; GA: General anesthesia; LA: Local anesthetic; RCTs: Randomized controlled trials; PRISMA: Preferred Reporting Items for Systematic Reviews and Meta Analyses; RCTs: American Society of Anesthesiologists; PONV: Postoperative nausea or vomiting; RRs: Relative risks; SD: Standard deviation; SMDs: Confidence intervals (CIs) standardized mean differences; PCA: Patient-controlled analgesia device

Acknowledgements
Not applicable.

Authors' contributions
JH and JC L participated in the entire procedure including the design and coordination of the study, the literature search, data extraction, performed the statistical analysis, drafted the manuscript, revised submitted the manuscript. All authors read and approved the final manuscript.

References
1. Forero M, Adhikary SD, Lopez H, Tsui C, Chin KJ. The erector Spinae plane block: a novel analgesic technique in thoracic neuropathic pain. Reg Anesth Pain Med. 2016;41(5):621–7.
2. El-Boghdadly K, Pawa A. The erector spinae plane block: plane and simple. Anaesthesia. 2017;72(4):434–8.
3. Chin KJ, Malhas L, Perlas A. The erector Spinae plane block provides visceral abdominal analgesia in bariatric surgery: a report of 3 cases. Reg Anesth Pain Med. 2017;42(3):372–6.
4. Bonvicini D, Tagliapietra L, Giacomazzi A, Pizzirani E. Bilateral ultrasound-guided erector spinae plane blocks in breast cancer and reconstruction surgery. J Clin Anesth. 2018;44:3–4.
5. Tulgar S, Kapakli MS, Senturk O, Selvi O, Serifsoy TE, Ozer Z. Evaluation of ultrasound-guided erector spinae plane block for postoperative analgesia in laparoscopic cholecystectomy: a prospective, randomized, controlled clinical trial. J Clin Anesth. 2018;49:101–6.
6. Tulgar S, Kose HC, Selvi O, Senturk O, Thomas DT, Ermis MN, Ozer Z. Comparison of ultrasound-guided lumbar erector Spinae plane block and Transmuscular Quadratus Lumborum block for postoperative analgesia in hip and proximal femur surgery: a prospective randomized feasibility study. Anesth Essays Res. 2018;12(4):825–31.
7. Singh S, Kumar G, Akhileshwar. Ultrasound-guided erector spinae plane block for postoperative analgesia in modified radical mastectomy: a randomised control study. Ind J Anaesth. 2019;63(3):200–4.
8. Moher D, Liberati A, Tetzlaff J, Altman DG. Preferred reporting items for systematic reviews and meta-analyses: the PRISMA statement. BMJ. 2009; 339:b2535.
9. Higgins JPT, Green S (editors). Cochrane handbook for systematic reviews of interventions version 5.1.0 [updated March 2011]. The Cochrane Collaboration. 2011. Available from www.handbook.cochrane.org.
10. Hozo SP, Djulbegovic B, Hozo I. Estimating the mean and variance from the median, range, and the size of a sample. BMC Med Res Methodol. 2005;5:13.
11. Higgins JP, Altman DG, Gotzsche PC, Juni P, Moher D, Oxman AD, Savovic J, Schulz KF, Weeks L, Sterne JA. The Cochrane Collaboration's tool for assessing risk of bias in randomised trials. BMJ. 2011;343:d5928.
12. Higgins JP, Thompson SG, Deeks JJ, Altman DG. Measuring inconsistency in meta-analyses. BMJ. 2003;327(7414):557–60.
13. Krishna SN, Chauhan S, Bhoi D, Kaushal B, Hasija S, Sangdup T, Bisoi AK. Bilateral erector Spinae plane block for acute post-surgical pain in adult cardiac surgical patients: a randomized controlled trial. J Cardiothorac Vasc Anesth. 2019;33(2):368–75.
14. Macaire P, Ho N, Nguyen T, Nguyen B, Vu V, Quach C, Roques V, Capdevila X. Ultrasound-guided continuous thoracic erector Spinae plane block within an enhanced recovery program is associated with decreased opioid consumption and improved patient postoperative rehabilitation after open cardiac surgery-a patient-matched, controlled before-and-after study. J Cardiothorac Vasc Anesth. 2019;33(6):1659–67.
15. Breebaart MB, Van Aken D, De Fre O, Sermeus L, Kamerling N, de Jong L, Michielsen J, Roelant E, Saldien V, Versyck B. A prospective randomized double-blind trial of the efficacy of a bilateral lumbar erector spinae block on the 24h morphine consumption after posterior lumbar inter-body fusion surgery. Trials. 2019;20(1):441.
16. Urits I, Charipova K, Gress K, Laughlin P, Orhurhu V, Kaye AD, Viswanath O. Expanding role of the erector Spinae plane block for postoperative and

chronic pain management. Curr Pain Headache Rep. 2019;23(10):71.

17. Singh S, Choudhary NK, Lalin D, Verma VK. Bilateral ultrasound-guided erector Spinae plane block for postoperative analgesia in lumbar spine surgery: a randomized control trial. J Neurosurg Anesthesiol 2019.

18. Ciftci B, Ekinci M, Celik EC, Tukac IC, Bayrak Y, Atalay YO. Efficacy of an ultrasound-guided erector Spinae plane block for postoperative analgesia management after video-assisted thoracic surgery: a prospective randomized study. J Cardiothorac Vasc Anesth. 2019.

19. Gurkan Y, Aksu C, Kus A, Yorukoglu UH. Erector spinae plane block and thoracic paravertebral block for breast surgery compared to IV-morphine: a randomized controlled trial. J Clin Anesth. 2019;59:84–8.

20. Hamed MA, Goda AS, Basiony MM, Fargaly OS, Abdelhady MA. Erector spinae plane block for postoperative analgesia in patients undergoing total abdominal hysterectomy: a randomized controlled study original study. J Pain Res. 2019;12:1393–8.

21. Yayik AM, Cesur S, Ozturk F, Ahiskalioglu A, Ay AN, Celik EC, Karaavci NC. Postoperative analgesic efficacy of the ultrasound-guided erector Spinae plane block in patients undergoing lumbar spinal decompression surgery: a randomized controlled study. World Neurosurg. 2019;126:e779–85.

22. Aksu C, Kuş A, Yörükoğlu HU, Kılıç CT, Gürkan Y. The effect of erector Spinae plane block on postoperative pain following laparoscopic cholecystectomy: a randomized controlled study. JARSS. 2019;27(1):9–14.

23. Gurkan Y, Aksu C, Kus A, Yorukoglu UH, Kilic CT. Ultrasound guided erector spinae plane block reduces postoperative opioid consumption following breast surgery: a randomized controlled study. J Clin Anesth. 2018;50:65–8.

24. Abu Elyazed MM, Mostafa SF, Abdelghany MS, Eid GM. Ultrasound-guided erector Spinae plane block in patients undergoing open Epigastric hernia repair: a prospective randomized controlled study. Anesth Analg. 2019; 129(1):235–40.

25. Aksu C, Kus A, Yorukoglu HU, Tor Kilic C, Gurkan Y. Analgesic effect of the bi-level injection erector spinae plane block after breast surgery: A randomized controlled trial. Agri. 2019;31(3):132–7.

26. Chin KJ, Adhikary S, Sarwani N, Forero M. The analgesic efficacy of pre-operative bilateral erector spinae plane (ESP) blocks in patients having ventral hernia repair. Anaesthesia. 2017;72(4):452–60.

27. Cosarcan SK, Gurkan Y, Dogan AT, Ercelen O. Targeted modification of erector spinae plane block. Acta Anaesthesiol Scand. 2020;64(2):276.

28. Ivanusic J, Konishi Y, Barrington MJ. A cadaveric study investigating the mechanism of action of erector Spinae blockade. Reg Anesth Pain Med. 2018;43(6):567–71.

29. Aponte A, Sala-Blanch X, Prats-Galino A, Masdeu J, Moreno LA, Sermeus LA. Anatomical evaluation of the extent of spread in the erector spinae plane block: a cadaveric study. Can J Anaesth. 2019;66(8):886–93.

30. Yang HM, Choi YJ, Kwon HJ, O J, Cho TH, Kim SH. Comparison of injectate spread and nerve involvement between retrolaminar and erector spinae plane blocks in the thoracic region: a cadaveric study. Anaesthesia. 2018; 73(10):1244–50.

31. Schwartzmann A, Peng P, Maciel MA, Forero M. Mechanism of the erector spinae plane block: insights from a magnetic resonance imaging study. Can J Anaesth. 2018;65(10):1165–6.

32. Tulgar S, Selvi O, Ahiskalioglu A, Ozer Z. Can unilateral erector spinae plane block result in bilateral sensory blockade? Can J Anaesth. 2019;66(8):1001–2.

33. Altiparmak B, Korkmaz Toker M, Uysal AI. Potential mechanism for bilateral sensory effects after unilateral erector spinae plane blockade in patients undergoing laparoscopic cholecystectomy. Can J Anaesth. 2020;67(1):161–2.

34. Hamilton DL, Manickam B. Erector spinae plane block for pain relief in rib fractures. Br J Anaesth. 2017;118(3):474–5.

35. Adhikary SD, Bernard S, Lopez H, Chin KJ. Erector Spinae plane block versus Retrolaminar block: a magnetic resonance imaging and anatomical study. Reg Anesth Pain Med. 2018;43(7):756–62.

36. Krishnan S, Cascella M: Erector Spinae plane block. In: StatPearls. Edn. Treasure Island (FL): StatPearls Publishing StatPearls Publishing LLC.; 2020.

37. Ueshima H. Pneumothorax after the erector spinae plane block. J Clin Anesth. 2018;48:12.

38. Hamilton DL. Pneumothorax following erector spinae plane block. J Clin Anesth. 2019;52:17.

39. Selvi O, Tulgar S. Ultrasound guided erector spinae plane block as a cause of unintended motor block. Rev Esp Anestesiol Reanim. 2018;65(10):589–92.

40. Altiparmak B, Korkmaz Toker M, Uysal AI, Kuscu Y, Gumus Demirbilek S. Ultrasound-guided erector spinae plane block versus oblique subcostal transversus abdominis plane block for postoperative analgesia of adult patients undergoing laparoscopic cholecystectomy: randomized, controlled trial. J Clin Anesth. 2019;57:31–6.

41. Aksu C, Sen MC, Akay MA, Baydemir C, Gurkan Y. Erector Spinae plane block vs Quadratus Lumborum block for pediatric lower abdominal surgery: a double blinded, prospective, and randomized trial. J Clin Anesth. 2019;57: 24–8.

42. Gaballah KM, Soltan WA, Bahgat NM. Ultrasound-guided Serratus plane block versus erector Spinae block for postoperative analgesia after video-assisted Thoracoscopy: a pilot randomized controlled trial. J Cardiothorac Vasc Anesth. 2019;33(7):1946–53.

22

The effect of various dilute administration of rocuronium bromide on both vascular pain and pharmacologic onset

Mayuko Kanazawa[1], Aiji Sato (Boku)[1]* ⓘ, Yoko Okumura[1], Mayumi Hashimoto[1], Naoko Tachi[1], Yushi Adachi[2] and Masahiro Okuda[1]

Abstract

Background: Rocuronium bromide (RB) is known to cause vascular pain. Although there have been a few reports that diluted administration causes less vascular pain, there have been no studies investigating diluted administration and the onset time of muscle relaxation. Therefore, we examined the influence of diluted administration of RB on the onset time of muscle relaxation and vascular pain.

Methods: 39 patients were randomly assigned to three groups: RB stock solution 10 mg/ml (Group 1), two-fold dilution 5 mg/ml (Group 2), or three-fold dilution 3.3 mg/ml (Group 3). After the largest vein of the forearm was secured, anesthesia was induced by propofol and 0.6 mg/kg of RB was administered. The evaluation method devised by Shevchenko et al. was used to evaluate the degree of vascular pain. The time from RB administration until the maximum blocking of T1 by TOF stimulation was measured.

Results: There was no significant difference in escape behaviors of vascular pain among the three groups, and the onset time of muscle relaxation was significantly slower in Group 3 than in Group 1 ($p = 0.033$).

Conclusion: Our results suggested that it is unnecessary to dilute RB before administration if a large vein in the forearm is used.

Keywords: Rocuronium bromide, Diluted administration, Onset time, Vascular pain

Background

Rocuronium bromide (RB) is the most commonly used non-depolarizing neuromuscular blocking drug (NMBD) due to its shorter onset time and duration of action, and good operability as compared with other NMBDs. However, unconscious body response [1], which is an escape behavior from the pain caused upon RB administration in a single dose, is often observed. The degree of pain can sometimes be severe, causing a burning sensation [2], and it is reported that aspiration pneumonia may be caused by vomiting due to escape behaviors [3]. Many previous studies focused on drug administration to eliminate vascular pain before administration of RB, but there have been few studies indicating that diluted administration causes less vascular pain [4–7]. Furthermore, to the best of our knowledge, there have been no reports on diluted administration and the onset time of muscle relaxation. Therefore, we investigated the influence of diluted administration of RB on the onset time of muscle relaxation and vascular pain.

* Correspondence: bokuaiji@dpc.aichi-gakuin.ac.jp; bokuaiji@dpc.agu.ac.jp
[1]Department of Anesthesiology, Aichi Gakuin University School of Dentistry, 2-11 Suemori-dori, Chikusaku, Nagoya 464-8651, Japan

Methods

Ethics approval and consent to participate

This study was approved by the Ethics Committee of the School of Dentistry, Aichi Gakuin University (approval number: 490). Clinical trial registration was performed at UMIN-CTR before the start of the study (approval number: 000026737). After providing an adequate explanation regarding the aims of the research to all subjects, we obtained written informed consent from all the patients.

Subjects

Overall, 45 ASA-PS 1–2 patients between 20 and 70 years of age who were scheduled to undergo general anesthesia at our hospital. Patients who did not give consent, who had neuromuscular diseases, or who had a BMI ≥25 were excluded from the study. Patients were randomly assigned to the following three groups: patients receiving RB the stock solution of 10 mg/ml (Group 1:13 patients), patients receiving the two-fold dilution of 5 mg/ml (Group 2:13 patients), or patients receiving the three-fold dilution of 3.3 mg/ml (Group 3: 13 patients) (Fig. 1). To dilute RB, 0.9% saline was used.

Methods of anesthesia

No premedication was used. After entering the operating room, the venous line was secured with a 20-G needle from the largest vein, excluding the cephalic vein, in the forearm. Furthermore, a TOF watch° was attached to the opposite arm. After induction of anesthesia with propofol at 1 to 2 mg/kg, it was visually confirmed that there was no residual propofol in the intravenous route, and RB at 0.6 mg/kg was administered in 10 s. The degree of vascular pain was evaluated based on the visual evaluation of escape behaviors from vascular pain. The time from RB administration until the maximum blocking of T1 by TOF stimulation was measured. In addition, the pH of the RB solution in Groups 1, 2, and 3 was measured using a pH meter (A&D AP-20).

Evaluation parameters

For the patient background, sex, age, height, and weight were evaluated. We also investigated the onset time of muscle relaxation using TOF and the escape behaviors from the vascular pain. The degree of vascular pain was evaluated using the scale devised by Shevchenko et al. as follows: grade 1 = no response, grade 2 = movement at the wrist only, grade 3 = withdrawal

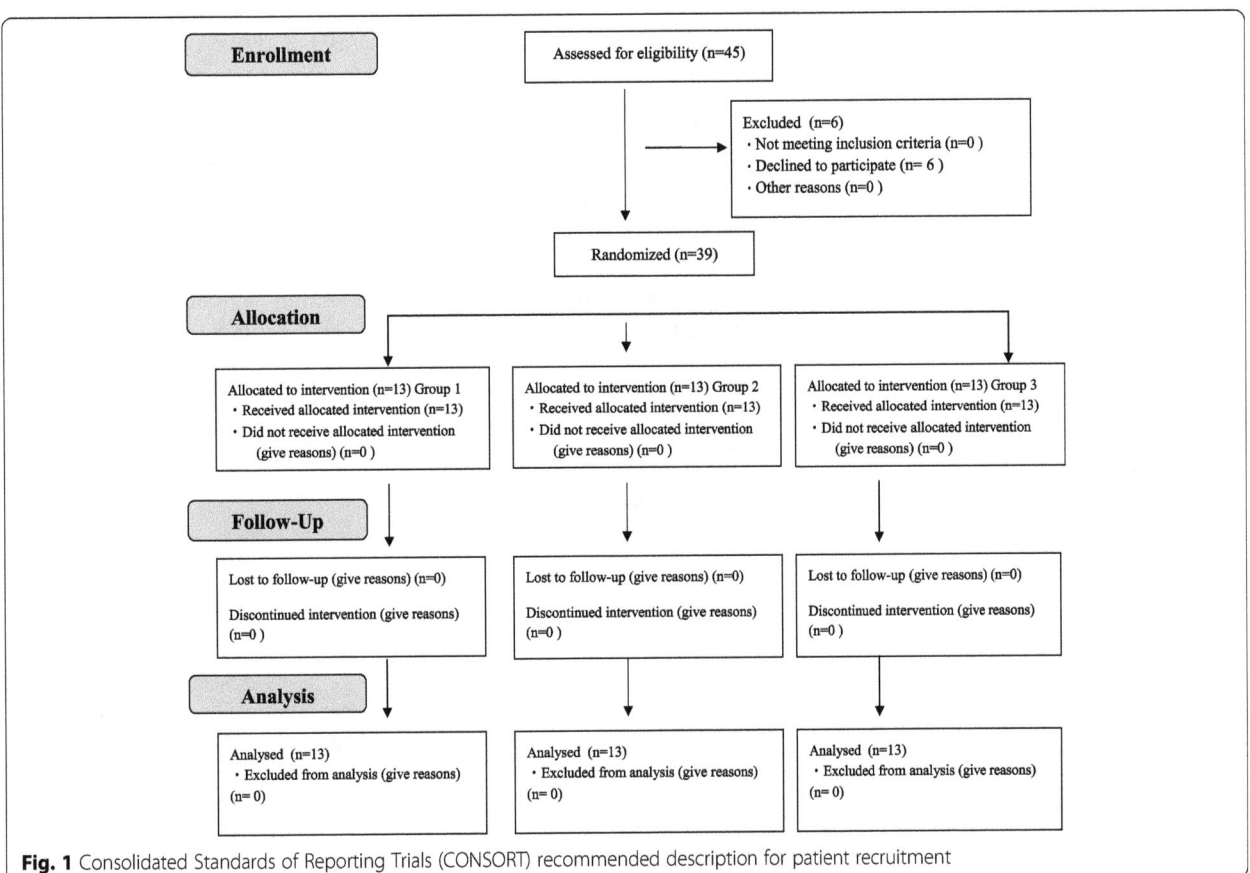

Fig. 1 Consolidated Standards of Reporting Trials (CONSORT) recommended description for patient recruitment

involving the arm only (elbow or shoulder), grade 4 = generalized response or withdrawal in more than one extremity. Pain of grade 2 or above was considered to indicate vascular pain [1].

Statistical analysis

The minimum sample size in total (30 patients) was calculated from a preliminary study based on the onset time of muscle relaxation (effect size 0.5, α-error level 0.05, and power 0.8).

The dropout rate in a preliminary study was 0.1. If an R dropout rate is expected, a simple but adequate adjustment is provided by $N_d = N/(1-R)^2$ where N is sample size calculated assuming no dropout and N_d that required with dropouts [8]. Therefor our adjustment was 37.5 and 39 patients were randomly assigned to the three groups.

Statistical analysis was performed for age, height, weight, and the onset time of muscle relaxation using one-way ANOVA and multiple comparison by Tukey's method. The chi-square test using the m × n division table was employed to investigate the impact of sex. In addition, escape behaviors from vascular pain were tested by the Kruskal-Willis test, and $p < 0.05$ was considered to indicate significance.

Results

A CONSORT Diagram is shown in Fig. 1. Among 45 patients, six who refused to participate were excluded from the study, and the remaining 39 patients were randomly assigned to three groups. There were no patients who were unable to be followed up and 13 patients in each group were examined.

The patient backgrounds are shown in Table 1. There was no significant difference among the three groups regarding sex, age, height, or weight. Escape behaviors from vascular pain did not significantly differ among the three groups (Table 2). In addition, the onset time of muscle relaxion were 93.4 ± 28.1 s in Group 1, 101.7 ± 39 s in Group 2, and 136.1 ± 55.4 s in Group 3. There were significant difference between the Group 1 and Group 3 ($p = 0.033$) (Table 3).

Grade 2 or higher escape behaviors from vascular pain were observed in 53% (7/13) in both Group 1 and Group 2, and in 46% (6/13) in Group 3 (Fig. 2).

The pH of the RB solution was 4.0 for Group 1, 3.9 for Group 2, and 3.9 for Group 3.

Discussion

In order for NMBD to induce muscle relaxation, it must bind to at least 70% of the nicotinic acetylcholine receptors. It has been reported that changes in the degree of binding of NMBD to the receptor may affect the time of onset of action [9], and that the nicotinic acetylcholine receptor consists of five units of adult-type α2βδε and fetal-type α2βδγ. The relationship between free molecules of NMBD that bind to the subunit and the time of onset of action has also been clarified [10]. In this study, RB was diluted with 0.9% physiological saline. The physiological saline used to dilute RB may have attenuated the affinity of RB to nicotinic acetylcholine receptors, and the change in free molecules due to dilution may have delayed the onset of muscle relaxation. In addition, as the onset time of NMBD and its titer are inversely correlated [9], it is necessary to increase the dose to accelerate the onset time of NMBD if the titer is low [11]. If the RB titer was decreased by dilution with 0.9% saline, the dose of diluted RB should be increased in order to accelerate the onset time of action. However, in this study, the dose of RB was fixed at 0.6 mg/kg in all three groups, which may explain why a difference was noted in the onset time of muscle relaxation between Group 1 and Group 3.

Table 1 Characteristics of patients in this study

		Group 1	Group 2	Group 3	P Value
Gender	Male	6	8	7	0.76NS
	Female	7	5	6	
Age yr		38.6±17.2	34.6±12.1	42.0±15.1	0.47NS
Height cm		165.3±5.5	164.0±7.3	163.6±6.3	0.78NS
Weight kg		63.7±13.1	62.1±11.0	58.9±9.1	0.54NS

Values are Mean ± SD or number.   Group 1: RB 10mg/ml,   Group 2: RB 5mg/ml,   Group 3: RB 3.3mg/ml
NS: Not Significant

Table 2 Grade of Withdrawal Movement Related to Rocuronium injection

	Group 1	Group 2	Group 3	P Value
No response	6	6	7	
Movement at the wrist only	4	3	3	
Withdrawal involving arm only	1	3	3	0.87 NS
Generalized response	2	1	0	

Values are number.　Group 1: RB 10mg/ml,　Group 2: RB 5mg/ml,　Group 3: RB 3.3mg/ml
The movement followe by rocuroniumu injection were graded according to the four point scale. NS: Not Significant

It has been reported that vascular pain due to single administration of RB is observed in approximately 50 to 80% of patients [12, 13]. Although the cause is not clear, the low pH and osmotic pressure of RB solution may stimulate chemical nociceptors on the vessel walls, and trigger the release of pain-inducing factors such as histamine and bradykinin [12, 14]. Regarding pH, it has been reported that RB solution with a pH of 4 does not cause vascular pain [12]. In this study, no difference was noted in vascular pain between Group 1 (RB solution pH 4.0) and Groups 2 and 3 (RB solution pH 3.9). Regarding osmotic pressure, Tuncali B et al. reported that the osmotic pressure of RB at 10 mg/ml is 308 mOsm/kg H_2O and the osmotic pressure of RB at 1 mg/ml is 306 mOsm/kg H_2O [6]; however, the osmotic pressure of RB at 10 mg/ml or 1 mg/ml did not cause vascular pain because these values were not different from the osmotic pressure of plasma (280–290 mOsm/kg H_2O) [6]. Although we did not measure the osmotic pressure, that of RB at 5 mg/ml in Group 2 and RB at 3.3 mg/ml in Group 3 used in this study likely falls between the osmotic pressure of RB at 10 mg/ml of 308 mOsm/kg H_2O and that of RB at 1 mg/ml of 306 mOsm/kg H_2O. Taken together, the pH and osmotic pressure values of RB solution used are consistent with those reported in previous studies and are

unlikely to affect vascular pain, which may be why there was no difference in escape behaviors from vascular pain noted in our study.

In our study, Group 2 and Group 3 did not exhibit differences in escape behaviors from vascular pain as compared with Group 1, which was inconsistent with previous studies [6, 7] demonstrating that diluted RB decreased vascular pain. When evaluating the reason for this different result, we focused on the position where the venous route was secured and vessel diameters. Similar to RB, propofol is known to cause vascular pain upon injection. Scott RP et al. demonstrated that administration of propofol through the median cubital vein can minimize pain due to decreased contact between the vessel wall and the drug [15]. In addition, Dalgleish DJ reported that RB administration through the median cubital vein did not cause vascular pain in 18 out of 20 patients [16]. This suggests that administrating RB through a larger vein can eliminate vascular pain due to less contact between the vessel wall and the drug. In the previous studies in which administration of diluted RB reduced vascular pain [6, 7], RB was injected through the dorsal digital veins in the hand. In contrast, we administered RB using the largest vein in the forearm. Thus, diluting RB is effective when administrating through relatively smaller veins but not when using a large

Table 3 Onset Time of Neuromuscular Blockade

Group 1	Group 2	Group 3	P Value
93.4±28.1	101.7±39	136.1±55.4	0.033 ※

Values are Mean ± SD.　Group 1: RB 10mg/ml,　Group 2: RB 5mg/ml,　Group 3: RB 3.3mg/ml
※ Group 1 vs Group 3

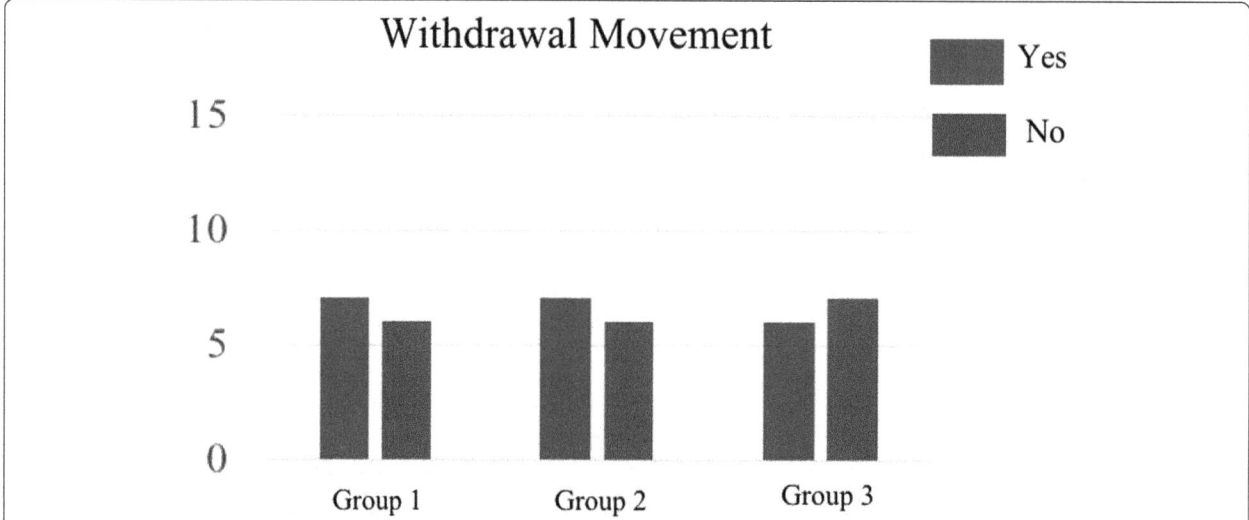

Fig. 2 Overall incidence of withdrawal movement related to rocuronium injection. Group 1: RB 10 mg/ml, Group 2: RB 5 mg/ml, Group 3: RB 3.3 mg/ml. Values indicate the number of patients. There was no difference among the groups

vein, and no significant difference in escape behaviors from vascular pain is expected in such cases.

Conclusion

We investigated the influence of diluted administration of RB on the onset time of muscle relaxation and vascular pain. We found that when diluted RB was administered through a large vein, there was no significant difference in escape behaviors from vascular pain. However, it should be noted that the onset time of muscle relaxation is delayed by dilution.

Abbreviation
NMBD: Non-depolarizing neuromuscular blocking drug; RB: Rocuronium bromide

Acknowledgements
The authors would like to thank the Department of Anesthesiology at Aichi Gakuin University Dental Hospital for their help in recruiting patients for this study.

Authors' contributions
MK and AS wrote this manuscript under supervision of MO. AS, YO and MH designed the study. AS, MK, MH and NT performed the investigation and analyzed the data. AS,NT and YA made substantial contribution to the interruption of the data. MO was responsible for the study design, writing of the manuscript, analysis and interpretation of the data. All authors have read and approved the final manuscript.

Author details
[1]Department of Anesthesiology, Aichi Gakuin University School of Dentistry, 2-11 Suemori-dori, Chikusaku, Nagoya 464-8651, Japan. [2]Department of Anesthesiology, Nagoya University Graduate School of Medicine, 65 Tsurumaicho, Showaku, Nagoya 466-8550, Japan.

References
1. Shevchenko Y, Jocson JC, McRae VA, Stayer SA, Schwartz RE, Rehman M, Choudhry DK. The use of lidocaine for preventing the withdrawal associated with the injection of rocuronium in children and adolescents. Anesth Analg. 1999;88:746–8.
2. Moorthy SS, Dierdorf SF. Pain on injection of rocuronium bromide. Anesth Analg. 1995;80:1067.
3. Lui JT, Huang SJ, Yang CY, Hsu JC, Lui PW. Rocuronium-induced generalized spontaneous movements cause pulmonary aspiration. Chang Gung Med J. 2002;25:617–20.
4. Memis D, Turan A, Karamanlioglu B, Sut N, Pamukçu Z. The prevention of pain from injection of rocuronium by ondansetron, lidocaine, tramadol and fentanyl. Anesth Analg. 2002;94:1517–20.
5. Jung KT, Kim HJ, Bae HS, Lee HY, Kim SH. So KY, LimKJ, Yu BS, Jung JD, an TH, park HC. Effects of lidocaine, ketamine, and remifentanil on withdrawal response of rocuronium. Korean J Anesthesiol. 2014;67:175–80.
6. Tuncali B, Karci A, Tuncali BE, Mavioglu O, Olguner CG, Ayhan S, Elar Z. Dilution of rocuronium to 0. 5 mg/mL with 0. 9% NaCl eliminates the pain during intravenous injection in awake patients. Anesth Analg. 2004;99:740–3.
7. Shin YH, Kim CS, Lee JH, Sim WS, Ko JS, Cho HS, Jeong HY, Lee HW, Kim SH. Dilution and slow injection reduces the incidence of rocuronium-induced withdrawal movements in children. Korean J Anesthesiol. 2011;61:465–9.
8. Lachin JM. Introduction to sample size determination and power analysis for clinical trials. Control Clin Trials. 1981;2:93–113.
9. Kopman AF. Pancuronium, gallamine, and d-tubocurarine compared: is speed of onset inversely related to drug potency? Anesthesiology. 1989; 70:915–20.
10. Shear TD, Martyn JA. Physiology and biology of neuromuscular transmission in health and disease. J Crit Care. 2009;24:5–10.
11. Bhatt SB, Amann A, Nigrovic V. Onset-potency relationship of nondepolarizing muscle relaxants: a reexamination using simulations. Can J Physiol Pharmacol. 2007;85:774–82.
12. Borgeat A, Kwiatkowski D. Spontaneous movements associated with rocuronium is pain on injection the cause? Br J Anaesth. 1997;79:382–3.
13. Lee YC, Jang YH, Kim JM, Lee SG. Rapid injection of rocuronium reduces withdrawal movement on injection. J Clin Anesth. 2009;21:427–30.
14. Lockey D, Coleman P. Pain during injection of rocuronium bromide. Anaesthesia. 1995;50:474.
15. Scott RPF, Saunders DA, Norman J. Propofol: clinical strategies for preventing pain on injection. Anaesthesia. 1988;43:492–4.
16. Dalgleish DJ. Drugs which cause pain on intravenous injection. Anaesthesia. 2000;55:828–9.

23

Comparison of postoperative pain between patients who underwent primary and repeated cesarean section

Guangyou Duan[†], Guiying Yang[†], Jing Peng, Zhenxin Duan, Jie Li, Xianglong Tang and Hong Li[*] [iD]

Abstract

Background: The differences in post-operative pain are unclear between the primiparas who underwent a primary cesarean section and multiparas who underwent their first repeat cesarean section. The study aimed to explore the possible differences in postoperative pain between primiparas and multiparas.

Methods: A prospective cohort study was performed only including women who underwent cesarean deliveries under spinal anesthesia. Postoperative patient-controlled intravenous analgesia (PCIA) was administered to all subjects with 0.2 mg/kg hydromorphone and 4 mg/kg flurbiprofen; the pump was programmed as 2.0 mL/h background infusion with a loading dose of 1 mL and a lockout period of 15 min. Postoperative incision and visceral pain intensity were evaluated using the visual analogue scale, and inadequate analgesia was defined as a visual analogue scale score $\geq$ 40 during 48 h post-operation. Additionally, the patients' pain statuses in postoperative week 1 and week 4 were also assessed during follow-up via telephone.

Results: From January to May 2017, a total of 168 patients (67 primiparas and 101 multiparas) were included. The relative risk for multiparas to experience inadequate analgesia on incision pain was 0.42 (95% CI: 0.25 to 0.74) compared to primiparas. In patients aged < 30 years, inadequate analgesia on visceral pain was higher in multiparas than in primiparas (RR, 3.56 [1.05 to 12.04], $P = 0.025$). There was no significant difference in the combined incidence of inadequate analgesia in both types of pain between the multiparas and primiparas (33.7% vs. 40.2%, $P = 0.381$). No difference was found in PCIA use between the two groups (111.1 ± 36.0 mL vs. 110.9 ± 37.3 mL, $P = 0.979$). In addition, a significantly higher incidence of pain was noted 4 weeks post-surgery in primiparas than that in multiparas (62.2% vs. 37.7%, $P = 0.011$).

Conclusion: Multiparas who underwent their first repeat cesarean section have a lower for inadequate analgesia on incision pain during the first 48 h after surgery than primiparas. Multiparas aged under 30 years may be more prone to experiencing postoperative inadequate analgesia on visceral pain.

Keywords: Cesarean section, Postoperative pain, Analgesia, Primiparas, Multiparas

* Correspondence: lh78553@163.com
[†]Guangyou Duan and Guiying Yang contribute equally to the project and both are considered as first authors.
Department of Anesthesiology, Xinqiao Hospital, Army Medical University, Chongqing 400037, China

Background

Cesarean section is the most common impatient surgical procedure globally. In 2016, the cesarean delivery rate in the United States was 31.9% [1]. In China, the annual cesarean delivery rate reached 41.1% in 2016 after relaxation of the one child policy [2]. However, despite the numerous measures that have been developed to manage postoperative pain, inadequate analgesia after cesarean section is common, with an incidence of nearly 50% [3–6]. Therefore, post-operative pain treatment remains a considerable clinical challenge in acute postoperative care during cesarean section. Inadequate postoperative pain management is associated with persistent pain, delayed functional recovery, and a longer hospital stay, which increase medical expenses, and is becoming a public health issue [7, 8]. Therefore, the treatment of pain after a cesarean section remains unresolved.

In China, a new clinical challenge for the treatment of pain after a cesarean section has emerged, following the implementation of China's new national two-child policy [9, 10]. Many obstetric patients with known history of previous cesarean section are scheduled to undergo repeated cesarean section. Because repeated cesarean sections is common in very aged individuals and are known to have higher operative difficulties and longer surgical times due to severe adhesions [11, 12], we speculated that there would be a difference in pain control during the postoperative period between the patients who underwent repeated and primary cesarean sections; and that the multiparas may have a higher risk of receiving inadequate analgesia.

Intravenous or intrathecal analgesia with opioids is recommended and is a commonly used method for pain treatment after cesarean delivery. However, currently, most female patients receive a one-size-fits-all approach for analgesia after cesarean section, regardless of primiparas or multiparas. In the recent Practice Guidelines for Obstetric Analgesia and Anesthesia, there was no specific explanation for the possible difference in postoperative pain between the patients who underwent repeat and primary cesarean sections [13, 14]. There are limited studies focusing on this issue. In addition, exploring the inter-individual variability in the degree of pain, and accurately targeting treatment in women who may experience inadequate analgesia may improve clinical outcomes [15, 16]. Therefore, the current prospective cohort study included patients who were scheduled to undergo primary or repeated cesarean sections to investigate the potential difference in postoperative pain between them.

Methods

Patients

This study was conducted according to the STROBE recommendations [17, 18]. The study protocol was approved by the Institutional Ethics Committee of Xinqiao Hospital, Third Military Medical University, Chongqing, China. Prior to the enrollment of patients, written informed consent was obtained from all the patients, and the study was registered on Clinicaltrial.gov (ID: NCT03009955).

Patients were included according to established inclusion and exclusion criteria. From January to May 2017, 168 Chinese patients, aged 20 to 40 years scheduled to undergo elective cesarean section with a transverse incision were recruited for this study (Fig. 1). Patients who had a gestational age of 37 to 40 weeks and singleton pregnancy, voluntarily receiving intravenous patient-controlled intravenous analgesia (PCIA) treatment, and classified as having ASA physical status scale I-II were eligible for participation. The reasons for an elective cesarean section in a primipara included the patient's own choice, preoperative complications including malpresentation (breech and transverse positions and compound presentation), placenta previa, uterine inertia, gestational diabetes, chronic or gestational hypertension, and preeclampsia. For the multiparas, the indication for a cesarean section was a previously scarred uterus. Only those who were undergoing their first repeat cesarean deliveries were included. Exclusion criteria included a history of chronic pain disorder, recent or chronic opioid use, substance abuse, heavy smoking (> 30 pack-years) [19] or alcohol dependence, absolute or relative contraindication to subarachnoid space block anesthesia, history of prior pelvic or abdominal surgery, or severe pregnancy complications, such as heart disease, brain disease, liver disease and kidney disease, that were life-threatening and required emergency treatment prior to the cesarean section.

Anesthesia and Analgesia Management

Cardiac rhythm via electrocardiography, mean arterial pressure, and pulse oxygen saturation were monitored after the patients entered the operating room. Standardized anesthesia was administered by an experienced anesthetist, and the operations were conducted by a single surgical team using the same standardized technique. Spinal anesthesia, via a subarachnoid space block at the L3–4 interspace, was administered using 0.66% ropivacaine (20 mg).

After the fetal section and once daily after the surgery, oxytocin (20 IU in 500 mL of saline) was routinely administered while the patient was admitted to the obstetrics ward. PCIA was started immediately after surgery with a mixture of hydromorphone (0.2 mg/kg), flurbiprofen (4 mg/kg), and 0.9% normal saline at a dose volume of 200 mL, using a controlled infusion pump. The pump was programmed to a loading dose of 2 mL, background infusion rate of 2.0 mL/h, and PCIA dose of 1 mL, with a lockout period of 15 min. For the prevention of the postoperative nausea and vomiting, 3 mg of droperidol was administered at the outset of PCIA.

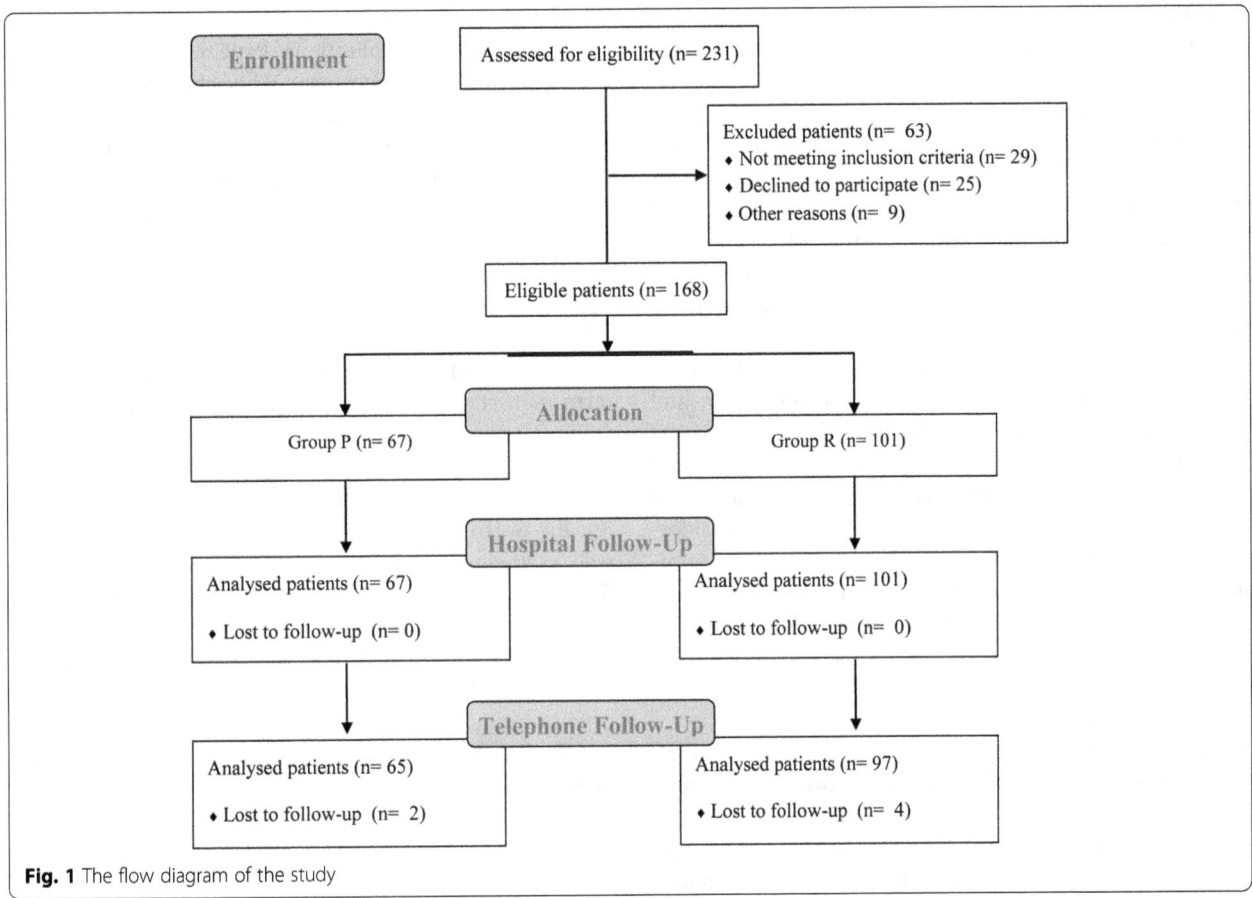

Fig. 1 The flow diagram of the study

Patients were monitored for 6 h in the postanesthesia care unit of the obstetrics ward after surgery. When pain was treated inadequately, the patients were administered additional pain treatment with tramadol 50 mg in a timely manner.

Outcome Measurements

Standardized training for follow-up assessment was performed for all included investigators. A pain visual analogue scale (VAS score; 0–100, where 0 is defined as no pain and 100 as maximum pain) was used to evaluate postoperative pain at 4, 8, 12, 24, and 48 h. The primary outcome was the incidence of inadequate analgesia (defined as a pain VAS score ≥ 40) [20] during the postoperative 48 h. Pain caused by abdominal incision at rest and during mobilization (during coughing) was assessed using the VAS. Visceral pain was also assessed using the VAS. For visceral pain, the subjects were asked to report the pain induced by uterine contractions and were informed that the visceral pain could be enhanced when oxytocin was given. The duration of pain according to the patient's self-reported time and PCIA consumption for 48 h after surgery were recorded.

Assessment with the hospital anxiety and depression scale (HADS) before the operation was performed in all

patients. The HADS includes 14 assessments, including the symptoms of anxiety and depression (seven items scored 0 to 3 in each subscale, yielding a range of 0–21) with subscale scores of 8 indicating possible anxiety or depression [21, 22]. The intraoperative amount of blood loss, neonatal Apgar score, weight and height of the newborn, and surgery time were recorded. The Ramsay sedation score, respiratory rate, pulse oxygen saturation, systolic pressure, diastolic pressure, and heart rate were recorded before surgery and during the postoperative 48 h. Early walking time (determined by the time point when patients could ambulate) was also recorded. The sleep quality (rated as good or poor) on the day of and 1 day after surgery was evaluated. Postoperative adverse events including nausea, vomiting, and pruritus were also noted. Additionally, the patients' duration of hospital stay was recorded.

The results of routine blood examinations before and 24 h after the surgery were retrospectively collected for all patients. The leukocyte and neutrophil counts were analyzed. At 1 week and 4 weeks after surgery, patients were interviewed by telephone and asked the following questions from a standardized questionnaire: Was there an existing pain? Was the location of pain at the incision, viscera, both, or none? Was sleep affected? Were they able to perform the activities of daily life with full autonomy, partial dependency, or absolute dependence?

Sample size determination

The sample size was calculated according to the design of chi-square test for four-fold table data in a cohort study. Since previous studies reported the incidence of moderate to severe pain under postoperative analgesia for primipara as approximately 50% [4, 5], the current study hypothesized that the relative risk (RR) value for multiparas was 1.5 compared to that for primiparas. The anticipated incidence for multiparas was 75%. Therefore, based on a significance level of 0.05, power of 0.9, and an estimated ratio between the number of multiparas and primiparas of 1.5, according to the retrospective analysis based on the data from our hospital Electronic Medical Records System of the past 1 year, and considering about 3% loss of follow-up, the total required minimum sample size was determined to be 168 individuals using the sample size calculation software PASS, version 11.0 (NCSS, Kayesville, UT).

Statistical Analysis

Statistical analysis was performed using SPSS for Windows version 19.0 (SPSS Inc., Chicago, IL). A two-tailed P-value less than 0.05 was considered statistically significant. The mean ± standard deviation (SD), median (interquartile range), and number (frequency) were used to summarize the variables. The patients who were scheduled to undergo a primary cesarean section were designated as group P in the final analysis, while the patients scheduled to undergo repeat cesarean section were designated as group R. The primary outcomes (postoperative inadequate analgesia on incision or visceral pain) were respectively described and analyzed. Logistic regression analysis using enter model was performed to evaluate the role of group P or group R in the prediction of postoperative inadequate analgesia. The presence of postoperative inadequate analgesia on incisional and visceral pain was considered as the outcome variable. BMI, age, gestational age, surgery time, preoperative complications (yes/no), depression (yes/no), and anxiety (yes/no) were also considered in the model. Odds ratios (OR) with 95% confidence intervals (CIs) were determined based on the logistic regression analysis.

An independent-sample t test was used to compare the differences in demographic and preoperative data between group P and R. Due to abnormal distribution, HAD scale, incision pain VAS at rest, and visceral pain VAS were compared using a Mann-Whitney U test. Propensity score matching (PSM) analysis was performed using STATA version 12 (Stata Corp, College Station, TX). Group P and group R were matched by propensity scores, and factors used to generate the propensity scores were those preoperative factors which had significant difference between

the two groups. These factors included age, gestational age, and preoperative complications. Patients were matched in a 1:1 ratio without replacement. The caliper was defined as 0.2. The absolute standardized difference was calculated, and the absolute standardized difference less than 10% was considered to support the assumption of balance between the two groups. Then, other postoperative outcomes including the start time to feel pain, early walking time, hospital stays and PCIA administration were compared between groups P and R.

Differences in the incidence of postoperative inadequate analgesia, sleep quality, adverse events, and long-term pain status between the two groups were analyzed using Pearson's chi-squared test. Furthermore, RR values and 95% CI for the probability of the occurrence of inadequate analgesia on incision pain and visceral pain during the postoperative 48-h follow-up were calculated, as well as the postoperative pain status at 1 and 4 weeks. Subgroup analysis according to age group (≤30 years or > 30 years) was performed. Two-way repeated analysis of variance (ANOVA) with post hoc LSD testing was used to compare the preoperative and postoperative systolic pressure, diastolic pressure, heart rate, respiratory rate, and leukocyte and neutrophil counts between the two groups.

Results

General results

Among the 67 primiparas who were scheduled to undergo cesarean section, 54 underwent the procedure due to preoperative complications (maternal or fetal factors) and 13 due to social factors. For the 101 multiparas, all underwent the procedure due to the history of a previous cesarean section. Fifty-four also had accompanying preoperative complications. As shown in Fig. 1, all patients completed the postoperative 48-h follow-up. However, six patients (two in group P and 4 in group R, $P = 0.739$) could not complete the study either because they could not be contacted or they withdrew from the study. The demographic and preoperative data of all patients are shown in Table 1. The results showed that the incidence of severe bleeding (≥ 500 mL) was 5.9% (6/101) in group R and was 7.5% (5/67) in group P and that there was no difference between the two groups ($P = 0.696$).

Logistic regression analysis

Enter logistic regression models were applied to explore the possible predictors for postoperative inadequate analgesia on incisional pain and visceral pain. For the model of incisional pain, the statistical test for the overall model was significant ($P = 0.001$), and the predicted accuracy rate based on this model was 80.8%, while the overall model was not significant ($P = 0.589$) for visceral pain. As summarized in Table 2, patient group and

Table 1 Demographic, preoperative and intraoperative data

	Group P ($n = 67$)	Group R ($n = 101$)	Statistics
Age (year)	29.5 ± 3.9	31.3 ± 3.4	$t = 3.112, P = 0.002$
Age group (> 30)	20 (29.9%)	57 (56.4%)	$\chi^2 = 11.467, P = 0.001$
BMI (kg/m^2)	26.7 ± 1.9	26.9 ± 1.9	$t = 0.820, P = 0.415$
Gestational age (week)	38.9 ± 0.9	38.4 ± 0.6	$t = 103, P < 0.001$
Preoperative complications	54 (80.6%)	54 (53.5%)	$t = 12.912, P < 0.001$
HADS-A(score)	2 (0, 5)	1 (0, 4)	$U = 0.887, P = 0.375$
HADS-D (score)	0 (0, 2)	0 (0, 2)	$U = 0.129, P = 0.897$
Surgery duration (min)	62.1 ± 15.3	71.1 ± 16.2	$t = 3.782, P < 0.001$
Weight of newborn (g)	3278 ± 481	3443 ± 1074	$t = 1.185, P = 0.238$
Height of newborn (cm)	49.7 ± 2.1	49.9 ± 1.7	$t = 0.820, P = 0.505$
Blood loss (mL)	286 ± 94	306 ± 92	$t = 0.668, P = 0.889$

Group P and R mean patients who received primary and repeated cesarean delivery, respectively; Data were presented as Means±SD, median (interquartile range) or as numbers (percentage); BMI = Body mass index; HADS-A = Hospital anxiety scale; HADS-D = Hospital depression scale

preoperative complications were identified as significant factors for inadequate analgesia on incision pain. This showed that patients in group P or with accompanying preoperative complications would have higher odds of inadequate pain control.

Postoperative Data

The distribution of pain VAS is shown in Fig. 2. The incidence of inadequate postoperative analgesia on incision or visceral pain at different times is shown in Fig. 3. In total, 24.4% (41/168) of patients were found to have inadequate treatment for their incision pain (Fig. 3a). The total incidence of inadequate analgesia on incision pain in group P

was significantly higher than that in group R, and the RR for multiparas to experience inadequate analgesia on incision pain was 0.42 (95% CI: 0.25 to 0.74; $P = 0.001$) compared to primiparas. As shown in Fig. 3b, the total incidence of inadequate analgesia on visceral pain in group P was lower than that in group R, and the RR for patients in group R to experience inadequate analgesia on visceral pain was 1.75 (95% CI: 0.82 to 3.70; $P = 0.078$) compared to that for patients in group P. In addition, no significant difference was found in the total combined incidence of inadequate analgesia between groups P and R (Fig. 3c).

The results of subgroup analysis showed that group R was associated with a lower incidence of inadequate control on

Table 2 Logistic regression analysis of inadequate analgesia on incision pain and visceral

Outcome	Predictors	Wals	P value	OR	95% CI
Inadequate analgesia on incision pain	Age (year)	0.543	0.461	1.043	0.932 to 1.169
	BMI (kg/m^2)	0.193	0.660	1.048	0.850 to 1.293
	Gestational age (week)	0.035	0.853	1.048	0.637 to 1.727
	Preoperative complications (yes/no)	4.721	0.030	0.365	0.147 to 0.906
	Surgery duration (min)	3.610	0.057	1.000	0.999 to 1.000
	Patient group(P/R)	10.790	0.001	0.191	0.071 to 0.513
	Anxiety (yes/no)	0.000	0.999	0.000	NA
	Depression (yes/no)	0.000	0.999	0.000	NA
Inadequate analgesia on visceral pain	Age	3.463	0.063	0.897	0.801 to 1.006
	BMI	0.002	0.968	1.005	0.804 to 1.256
	Gestational age (week)	0.175	0.675	0.885	0.498 to 1.570
	Preoperative complications (yes/no)	0.277	0.599	1.273	0.519 to 3.124
	Surgery duration (min)	0.586	0.444	1.000	0.999 to 1.000
	Patient group(P/R)	0.599	0.439	1.515	0.529 to 4.340
	Anxiety (yes/no)	0.133	0.715	1.462	0.190 to 11.219
	Depression (yes/no)	0.423	0.515	0.403	0.026 to 6.228

BMI = Body mass index; CI = Confidence interval; OR = Odds rate

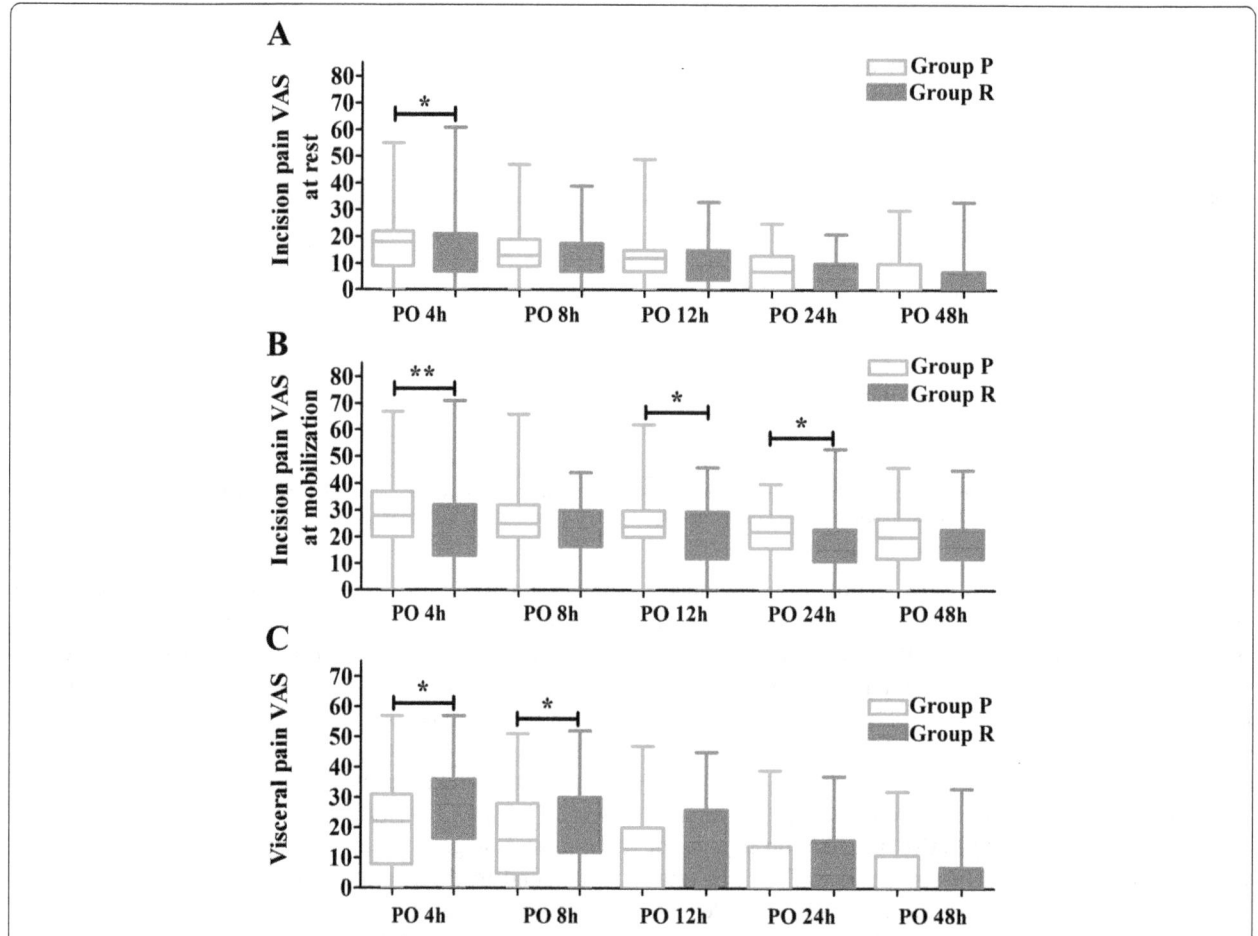

Fig. 2 The distribution of postoperative incision pain VAS at rest (**a**) incision pain VAS at mobilization (**b**) and visceral pain VAS (**c**) at different time points. Means of groups P and R patients who received primary and repeated cesarean section, respectively; VAS = visual analogue scale; PO = postoperative; * $P < 0.05$; ** $P < 0.01$

incision pain in both age groups (≤30 and > 30 years; RR, 0.47 [0.23 to 0.98], $P = 0.033$ and 0.40 [0.17 to 0.96], $P = 0.042$, respectively, Table 3). Group R was associated with a higher incidence of inadequate control on viscera pain in the age group ≤30 years (RR, 3.56 [1.05 to 12.04], $P = 0.025$).

After propensity score matching according to preoperative factors, including age, gestational age, and preoperative complications, no significant differences remained between the two groups, and a total of 45 pairs of subjects were included for comparison of other postoperative outcomes (Table 4). As shown in Table 5, the pain VAS score at different time points were listed, and the distributions were similar to that in the non-matched cohort. Furthermore, the RR in multiparas for inadequate analgesia on incision pain was 0.35 (95% CI: 0.15 to 0.79; $P = 0.007$) compared to primiparas in this matched cohort. There was no significant difference in the incidence of inadequate analgesia on visceral pain between the two groups ($P > 0.05$). In addition, there was no significant difference in the incidence of adverse effects between the two groups. No respiratory depression, excessive sedation, or agitation was found in the present study. In

addition, no significant difference was found in the time elapsed prior to the onset of pain, early waking time, sleep quality, and PCIA administration between the two groups. The results showed the mean hospital stay for primiparas was longer than that for multiparas.

Changes of serum leukocyte count and neutrophil count

Two-way repeated ANOVA for leukocyte count showed a group effect ($P = 0.004$), time effect ($P < 0.001$), and group and time interaction effect ($P = 0.024$). For the neutrophil count, the group effect ($P = 0.012$) and time effect ($P < 0.001$) were significant, while group and time interaction effects were not significant ($P = 0.023$). As shown in Fig. 4, there was no difference in the absolute leukocyte ($9.03 \pm 2.19 \times 10^9$/L vs. $8.38 \pm 2.57 \times 10^9$/L, $P = 0.202$) and neutrophil ($6.81 \pm 2.02 \times 10^9$/L vs. $6.41 \pm 2.39 \times 10^9$/L, $P = 0.388$) counts between the different groups before the surgery, while both leukocyte ($10.76 \pm 2.40 \times 10^9$/L vs. $8.97 \pm 1.81 \times 10^9$/L, $P < 0.001$) and neutrophil ($8.33 \pm 2.31 \times 10^9$/L vs. $6.78 \pm 1.61 \times 10^9$/

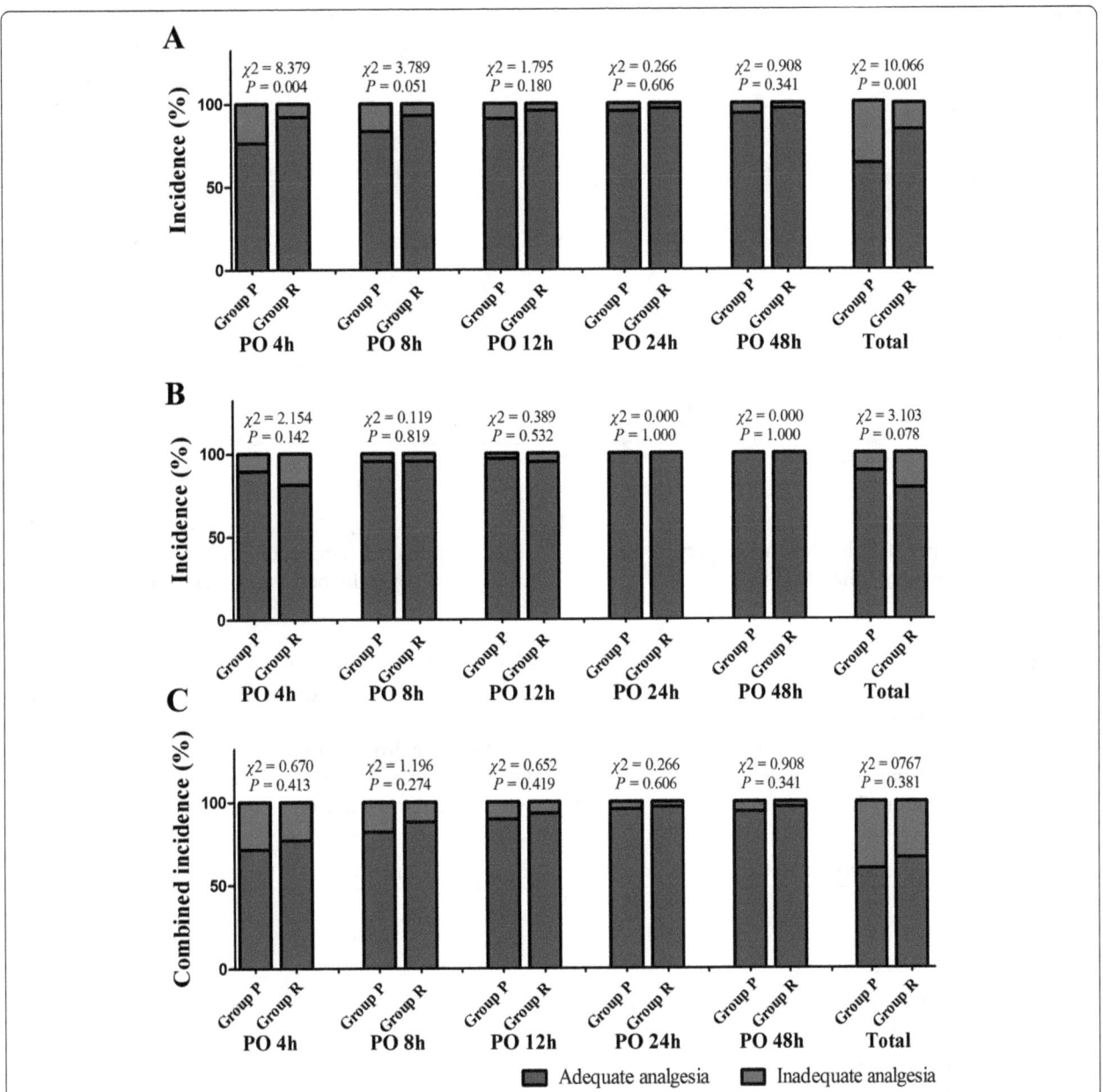

Fig. 3 The incidence of postoperative inadequate treatment on incision pain (**a**), visceral pain (**b**) and the combined incidence (**c**) Groups P and R represent patients who underwent primary and repeated cesarean sections, respectively; VAS = visual analogue scale; PO = postoperative.

Table 3 Subgroup analysis for different age groups

Age group	Outcomes	Group P	Group R	Statistics
≤30 years	Inadequate control on incision pain	18 (38.3%)	8 (18.2%)	$\chi 2 = 4.506, P = 0.033$
	Inadequate control on viscera pain	3 (6.4%)	10 (22.7%)	$\chi 2 = 4.958, P = 0.025$
	Inadequate control on both incision and viscera pain	18 (38.3%)	16 (36.4%)	$\chi 2 = 0.036, P = 0.849$
> 30 years	Inadequate control on incision pain	7 (35.0%)	8 (14.0%)	$\chi 2 = 4.149, P = 0.042$
	Inadequate control on viscera pain	5 (25.0%)	11 (19.3%)	$\chi 2 = 0.292, P = 0.588$
	Inadequate control on both incision and viscera pain	9 (45.0%)	18 (31.6%)	$\chi 2 = 1.171, P = 0.279$

Group P and R mean patients who received primary and repeated cesarean delivery, respectively; Data were presented as numbers (percentage)

Table 4 The postoperative short-term outcomes in different groups after propensity score matching

Outcomes	Group P (n = 45)	Group R (n = 45)	Statistics
Age (year)	30.3 ± 4.3	30.8 ± 3.4	t = 0.555, P = 0.580
Gestational age (week)	38.6 ± 1.0	38.5 ± 0.7	t = 0.569, P = 0.571
Preoperative complications	5 (11.1%)	3 (6.7%)	χ2 = 0.548, P = 0.458
Time to feel pain (hour)	3 (2, 6)	4 (2, 7)	U = 0.858, P = 0.391
Early walking time (hour)	28.9 ± 8.8	28.5 ± 9.6	t = 0.213, P = 0.832
Nausea or vomiting	3 (6.7%)	4 (8.9%)	χ2 = 0.155, P = 0.693
Pruritus	2 (4.5%)	3 (6.7%)	χ2 = 0.212, P = 0.645
Sleep quality PO 0d (poor)	16 (35.6%)	13 (28.9%)	χ2 = 0.457, P = 0.498
Sleep quality PO 1d (poor)	5 (11.1%)	3 (6.7%)	χ2 = 0.548, P = 0.458
PCIA consumption (mL)	111.1 ± 36.0	110.9 ± 37.3	t = 0.026, P = 0.979
Hospital stays (day)	3.5 ± 1.1	3.0 ± 0.8	t = 2.513, P = 0.014

Group P and R mean patients who received primary and repeated cesarean delivery, respectively; Data were presented as means ± SD, median (interquartile range) or as numbers (percentage); PO = Postoperative; PCIA = Patient controlled intravenous analgesia

L, $P < 0.001$) counts at 24 h after the surgery in group P were significantly higher than that in group R.

Long-term follow-up
As shown in Table 6, no significant difference in pain status was found between the two groups 1 week after surgery. The results showed that at 4 weeks after surgery, the incidence of existing pain in group P was significantly higher than that in group R.

In additional, a significant difference was noted in the location of pain between patients in group P and group R.

Discussion
Our results show that the total incidence of inadequate postoperative pain control was 36.3% using PCIA combined with hydromorphone and flurbiprofen, which was demonstrated as an effective combination for postoperative pain control [23]. One previous prospective cohort

Table 5 The patients' postoperative pain in different groups after propensity score matching

Outcomes	Group P (n = 45)	Group R (n = 45)	Statistics
Rest incision pain VAS at PO 4 h	18 (11, 20)	11 (7, 16)	U = 2.508, P = 0.012
Moving incision pain VAS at PO 4 h	29 (21, 39)	23 (13, 30)	U = 2.705, P = 0.007
Visceral pain VAS at PO 4 h	22 (6, 32)	27 (17, 36)	U = 1.690, P = 0.091
Rest incision pain VAS at PO 8 h	13 (9, 19)	9 (4, 13)	U = 2.423, P = 0.015
Moving incision pain VAS at PO 8 h	25 (21, 34)	22 (12, 29)	U = 1.922, P = 0.055
Visceral pain VAS at PO 8 h	21 (8, 28)	20 (11, 30)	U = 0.342, P = 0.732
Rest incision pain VAS at PO 12 h	12 (6, 15)	9 (3, 12)	U = 1.973, P = 0.048
Moving incision pain VAS at PO 12 h	24 (21, 32)	15 (10, 26)	U = 3.198, P = 0.001
Visceral pain VAS at PO 12 h	13 (0, 25)	11 (0, 24)	U = 0.470, P = 0.638
Rest incision pain VAS at PO 24 h	6 (0, 13)	4 (0, 6)	U = 1.482, P = 0.138
Moving incision pain VAS at PO 24 h	22 (17, 29)	14 (9, 20)	U = 3.408, P = 0.001
Visceral pain VAS at PO 24 h	0 (0, 13)	5 (0, 15)	U = 0.373, P = 0.709
Rest incision pain VAS at PO 48 h	0 (0, 8)	0 (0, 4)	U = 1.043, P = 0.297
Moving incision pain VAS at PO 48 h	20 (12, 27)	14 (10, 20)	U = 1.804, P = 0.071
Visceral pain VAS at PO 48 h	0 (0, 8)	0 (0, 5)	U = 0.096, P = 0.924
Inadequate analgesia on incision pain	17 (37.8%)	6 (13.0%)	χ2 = 7.368, P = 0.007
Inadequate analgesia on visceral pain	7 (15.6%)	9 (19.6%)	χ2 = 0.252, P = 0.615

Group P and R mean patients who received primary and repeated cesarean delivery, respectively; Data were presented as median (interquartile range) or as numbers (percentage); PO = Postoperative; VAS = Visual analogue scale

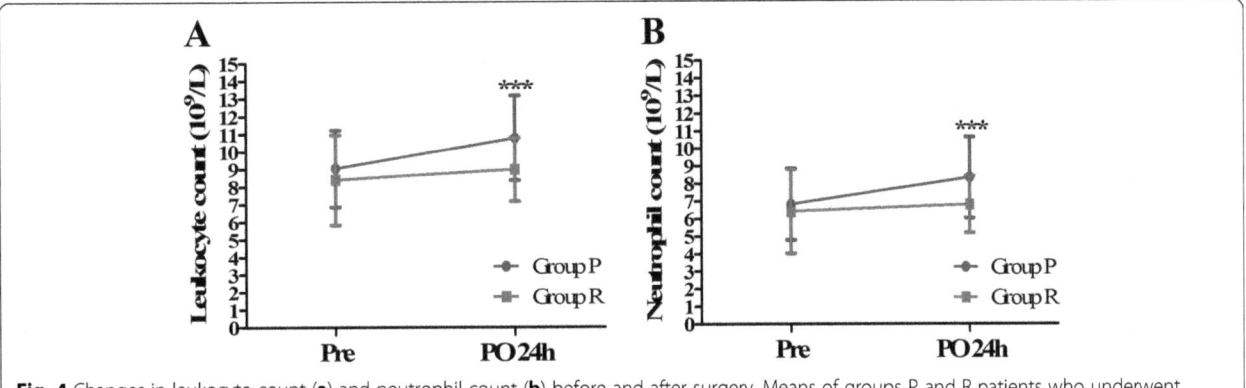

Fig. 4 Changes in leukocyte count (**a**) and neutrophil count (**b**) before and after surgery. Means of groups P and R patients who underwent primary and repeated cesarean sections, respectively; Pre = preoperative; PO = postoperative; *** compared to group R, $P < 0.001$.

study [4] demonstrated that postoperative pain after a cesarean section reached 6 (interquartile range: 4 to 8), and the incidence of moderate to severe pain or requirement of extra analgesia was reported to range from 40 to 60% [5, 6]. Therefore, the analgesia strategy in this study might be effective for postoperative pain control. Nevertheless, the incidence of 36.3% remains relatively high, and more effective analgesia strategies should be explored in the future.

As we know, a high proportion of female patients are scheduled to undergo secondary cesarean section because of a previous cesarean section. In the United States, a repeat cesarean section due to a previous uterine scar contributed to more than 30% of all cesarean sections [24, 25]. Severe adhesions induced by previous surgery were often inevitable and thus, would cause higher operative difficulties [26, 27]. In this study, surgery duration in

group R was significantly longer than that in group P, which is also indicative of higher operative difficulties in patients with repeat cesarean sections. In addition, previous surgery history might increase the patients' pain sensitivity [28, 29]. Therefore, based on the above information, it was speculated that multiparas might experience more postoperative pain than primiparas.

For patients undergoing cesarean section, oxytocin, which can induce contraction pain, was routinely used to reduce intraoperative and postoperative hemorrhage [30, 31]. Thus, postoperative visceral pain induced by uterine contraction must frustrate the patients and should not be ignored. Although numerous previous studies have focused on the improvement of postoperative analgesia for cesarean section [32–35], many of these studies did not differentiate incision pain from visceral pain. However, a previous study found that the analgesic effects of the same analgesics on incision

Table 6 The long-term postoperative outcomes in different groups after propensity score matching

Time point	Outcomes	Group P (n = 45)	Group R (n = 45)	Statistics
PO 1 week	Experiencing pain	38 (84.4%)	35 (77.7%)	χ2 = 0.653, P = 0.419
	location of pain (abdominal incision/viscera /both)	26 (57.8%)/5 (11.1%)/3 (6.7%)	26 (57.8%)/3 (6.7%)/0 (0.0%)	χ2 = 4.426, P = 0.219
	Affect sleep	14 (31.1%)	10 (22.2%)	χ2 = 0.909, P = 0.340
	Ability of daily life (partial dependency/fully autonomy)	19 (42.2%)/26 (57.8%)	18 (40.0%)/27 (60.0%)	χ2 = 0.046, P = 0.830
PO 4 week	Experiencing pain	28 (62.2%)	17 (37.7%)	χ2 = 6.403, P = 0.011
	location of pain (abdominal incision/ viscera/both)	18 (40.0%)/7 (15.6%)/1 (2.2%)	8 (17.8%)/4 (8.9%)/0 (0%)	χ2 = 9.434, P = 0.024
	Affect sleep	8 (17.8%)	4 (8.9%)	χ2 = 1.538, P = 0.215
	Ability of daily life (partial dependency/ fully autonomy)	45 (100%)/0 (0%)	45 (100%)/0 (0%)	χ2 = 0.000, P = 1.000

Group P and R mean patients who received primary and repeated cesarean delivery, respectively; Data were presented as numbers (percentage); PO = Postoperative

and uterine cramping pain varied [36]. Therefore, postoperative abdominal incision and visceral pain were evaluated in this study.

One previous study demonstrated that compared to primiparous women, the analgesic effect on post-cesarean uterine cramping pain is less in multiparous women [37]. The current results also showed that the incidence of inadequate treatment on visceral pain in group R was higher than that in group P, with the RR for multipara being 3.56 (95% CI: 1.05 to 12.04) in the patients aged ≤30 years. In addition, of all patients in the two groups, few were found to experience inadequate analgesia 8 h after the surgery, indicating that visceral pain might mainly appear at an early postoperative stage. Therefore, for the multipara, the focus should be on postoperative visceral pain at the early stage, especially for young patients.

In contrast, this study showed that multiparas were less likely to experience inadequate treatment on incision pain. The RR for multiparas was 0.42 (95% CI: 0.25 to 0.74), and the mean incision pain VAS score in group R was significantly lower than that in group P at several time points, including 4, 12, and 24 h after surgery. Based on the results of the current study, several reasons might account for this phenomenon. First, as shown in the study, the rate of preoperative complications in group P was higher than that in group R (80.6% vs. 53.5%) and was identified as a significant risk factor for inadequate treatment on incision pain. Second, through retrospective analysis, we found that both the leukocyte count and neutrophil count were significantly increased 24 h post-operation compared to that prior to surgery, and these elevations were higher in group P than in group R. Previous studies [38, 39] have also reported that there was a significant difference between preoperative and postoperative leukocyte and neutrophil counts for patients undergoing cesarean deliveries. However, it remains unclear whether this difference varied between primiparas and multiparas after cesarean deliveries. Increases in white blood cell and neutrophil counts have been demonstrated to be positively associated with inflammatory responses in previous studies [40–42]. Therefore, this indicated that different physiological responses to surgery or analgesia might exist between multiparas and primiparas. For primiparas, an effective analgesia strategy, e.g., combination of perioperative anti-inflammatory agents on incision pain should be considered.

In summary, because of the difference between postoperative control on visceral and incision pain, there was no significant difference in the combined incidence of inadequate analgesia on both types of pain between patients in groups P and R. Regarding the other postoperative outcomes during the hospital stay, no significant difference was found in the incidence of adverse events, time to feel pain, early walking time, sleep quality, and PCIA administration between the two groups. However,

we found that the mean hospital stay for primiparas was longer than that for multiparas. This indicated that primiparas might need more care after cesarean section. Furthermore, the current study demonstrated that primiparas might experience a longer duration of pain, because higher incidences of existing pain and affected sleep were found in group P than in group R 4 weeks after surgery. This might be due to the higher incidence of inadequate incision pain control in patients of group P, because a previous study has identified inadequately controlled acute postoperative pain as a risk factor for the development of chronic pain post-operation [43].

Several limitations should be noted in the study. First, the study only included Chinese women from urban areas; thus, race and socio-economic status should be considered when interpreting the current results [44, 45]. Second, although a significant difference in postoperative pain status was found between primiparas and multiparas, the current sample size was relatively small. Third, in the current study, all multiparas were undergoing secondary surgery; thus, the differences for those who underwent two or more cesarean deliveries were not known. Thus, to address these potential limitations, a multicenter study with a larger sample size might be needed, and more studies including other populations should be performed in the future.

Conclusion

Multiparas under 30 years of age may be more prone to experiencing moderate to severe visceral pain under PCIA with opioids during the first 48 h after surgery compared to primiparas; however, primiparas have a higher incidence of inadequate treatment on incision pain and possibly a higher incidence of existing pain 4 weeks after surgery. Based on the results of the current study, individual differences between primipara and multipara should be considered in postoperative analgesia in the future.

Abbreviations
ANOVA: analysis of variance; CI: confidence intervals; HADS: hospital anxiety and depression scale; OR: Odds ratios; PCIA: patient-controlled intravenous analgesia; RR: Relative Risk; SD: standard deviation; VAS: visual analogue scale

Acknowledgements
Not Applicable.

Authors' Contributions
Conceptualization, JP; Data curation, GY, JP, ZD, JL, and XT; Formal analysis, GD, GY, and HL; Funding acquisition, GD and HL; Investigation, ZD, JL, and XT; Supervision, HL; Writing original draft, GD and GY; Writing – review and editing, HL. All authors have read and approved the manuscript.

References
1. Martin JA, Hamilton BE, Osterman MJK. Births in the United States 2016. NCHS Data Brief. 2017;287:1–8.
2. Liang J, Mu Y, Li X, et al. Relaxation of the one child policy and trends in caesarean section rates and birth outcomes in China between 2012 and

2016: observational study of nearly seven million health facility births. BMJ. 2018;360:k817.

3. Raja SN, Jensen TS. Predicting postoperative pain based on preoperative pain perception: are we doing better than the weatherman? Anesthesiology. 2010;112:1311–2.

4. Gerbershagen HJ, Aduckathil S, van Wijck AJ, Peelen LM, Kalkman CJ, Meissner W. Pain intensity on the first day after surgery: a prospective cohort study comparing 179 surgical procedures. Anesthesiology. 2013; 118:934–44.

5. Patel R, Carvalho JC, Downey K, Kanczuk M, Bernstein P, Siddiqui N. Intraperitoneal Instillation of Lidocaine Improves Postoperative Analgesia at Cesarean Delivery: A Randomized, Double-Blind, Placebo-Controlled Trial. Anesth Analg. 2017;124:554–9.

6. Ortner CM, Granot M, Richebe P, Cardoso M, Bollag L, Landau R. Preoperative scar hyperalgesia is associated with post-operative pain in women undergoing a repeat Caesarean delivery. Eur J Pain. 2013;17:111–23.

7. Eisenach JC, Pan PH, Smiley R, Lavand'Homme P, Landau R, Houle TT. Severity of acute pain after childbirth, but not type of delivery, predicts persistent pain and postpartum depression. Pain. 2008;140:87–94.

8. Lavand'Homme P. Chronic pain after vaginal and cesarean delivery: a reality questioning our daily practice of obstetric anesthesia. Int J Obstet Anesth. 2010;19:1–02.

9. Zeng Y, Hesketh T. The effects of China's universal two-child policy. Lancet. 2016;388:1930–8.

10. Wang L, Xu X, Baker P, et al. Factors associated with intention to have caesarean delivery in pregnant women in China: a cross-sectional analysis. Lancet. 2016;388 Suppl 1:S2.

11. Gasim T, Al JF, Rahman MS, Rahman J. Multiple repeat cesarean sections: operative difficulties, maternal complications and outcome. J Reprod Med. 2013;58:312–8.

12. Elbohoty AE, Gomaa MF, Abdelaleim M, Abd-El-Gawad M, Elmarakby M. Diathermy versus scalpel in transverse abdominal incision in women undergoing repeated cesarean section: A randomized controlled trial. J Obstet Gynaecol Res. 2015;41:1541–6.

13. Practice Guidelines for Obstetric Anesthesia. An Updated Report by the American Society of Anesthesiologists Task Force on Obstetric Anesthesia and the Society for Obstetric Anesthesia and Perinatology. Anesthesiology. 2016;124:270–300.

14. Practice Bulletin No. 177: Obstetric Analgesia and Anesthesia. Obstert Gynecol. 2017;129:e73–e89.

15. Pan PH, Tonidandel AM, Aschenbrenner CA, Houle TT, Harris LC, Eisenach JC. Predicting acute pain after cesarean delivery using three simple questions. Anesthesiology. 2013;118:1170–9.

16. Ip HY, Abrishami A, Peng PW, Wong J, Chung F. Predictors of postoperative pain and analgesic consumption: a qualitative systematic review. Anesthesiology. 2009;111:657–77.

17. von Elm E, Altman DG, Egger M, Pocock SJ, Gotzsche PC, Vandenbroucke JP. The Strengthening the Reporting of Observational Studies in Epidemiology (STROBE) statement: guidelines for reporting observational studies. PLoS Med. 2007;4:e296.

18. Eisenach JC, Kheterpal S, Houle TT. Reporting of Observational Research in ANESTHESIOLOGY: The Importance of the Analysis Plan. Anesthesiology. 2016;124:998–1000.

19. Pietzak EJ, Mucksavage P, Guzzo TJ, Malkowicz SB. Heavy Cigarette Smoking and Aggressive Bladder Cancer at Initial Presentation. Urology. 2015;86:968–72.

20. Duan G, Xiang G, Zhang X, Yuan R, Zhan H, Qi D. A single-nucleotide polymorphism in SCN9A may decrease postoperative pain sensitivity in the general population. Anesthesiology. 2013;118:436–42.

21. de Miranda S, Pochard F, Chaize M, et al. Postintensive care unit psychological burden in patients with chronic obstructive pulmonary disease and informal caregivers: A multicenter study. Crit Care Med. 2011;39:112–8.

22. Zigmond AS, Snaith RP. The hospital anxiety and depression scale. Acta Psychiatr Scand. 1983;67:361–70.

23. Oh E, Ahn HJ, Sim WS, Lee JY. Synergistic Effect of Intravenous Ibuprofen and Hydromorphone for Postoperative Pain: Prospective Randomized Controlled Trial. Pain Physician. 2016;19:341–8.

24. Zhang J, Troendle J, Reddy UM, et al. Contemporary cesarean delivery practice in the United States. Am J Obstet Gynecol. 2010;203:321–6.

25. Molina G, Weiser TG, Lipsitz SR, et al. Relationship Between Cesarean Delivery Rate and Maternal and Neonatal Mortality. JAMA. 2015;314:2263–70.

26. Tulandi T, Agdi M, Zarei A, Miner L, Sikirica V. Adhesion development and morbidity after repeat cesarean delivery. Am J Obstet Gynecol. 2009;201:51–6.

27. Arlier S, Seyfettinoglu S, Yilmaz E, et al. Incidence of adhesions and maternal and neonatal morbidity after repeat cesarean section. Arch Gynecol Obstet. 2017;295:303–11.

28. Valdes AM, Suokas AK, Doherty SA, Jenkins W, Doherty M. History of knee surgery is associated with higher prevalence of neuropathic pain-like symptoms in patients with severe osteoarthritis of the knee. Semin Arthritis Rheum. 2014;43:588–92.

29. Duan G, Guo S, Zhang Y, et al. The effects of epidemiological factors and pressure pain measurement in predicting postoperative pain: A prospective survey of 1002 Chinese patients. Pain Physician. 2017;20:903–14.

30. De Bonis M, Torricelli M, Leoni L, et al. Carbetocin versus oxytocin after caesarean section: similar efficacy but reduced pain perception in women with high risk of postpartum haemorrhage. J Matern Fetal Neonatal Med. 2012;25:732–5.

31. Rath W. Prevention of postpartum haemorrhage with the oxytocin analogue carbetocin. Eur J Obstet Gynecol Reprod Biol. 2009;147:15–20.

32. Schewe JC, Komusin A, Zinserling J, Nadstawek J, Hoeft A, Hering R. Effects of spinal anaesthesia versus epidural anaesthesia for caesarean section on postoperative analgesic consumption and postoperative pain. Eur J Anaesthesiol. 2009;26:52–9.

33. Booth JL, Harris LC, Eisenach JC, Pan PH. A Randomized Controlled Trial Comparing Two Multimodal Analgesic Techniques in Patients Predicted to Have Severe Pain After Cesarean Delivery. Anesth Analg. 2016;122:1114–9.

34. Kagwa S, Hoeft MA, Firth PG, Ttendo S, Modest VE. Ultrasound guided transversus abdominis plane versus sham blocks after caesarean section in an Ugandan village hospital: a prospective, randomised, double-blinded, single-centre study. Lancet. 2015;385 Suppl 2:S36.

35. Moriyama K, Ohashi Y, Motoyasu A, Ando T, Moriyama K, Yorozu T. Intrathecal Administration of Morphine Decreases Persistent Pain after Cesarean section: A Prospective Observational Study. PLoS One. 2016;11:e155114.

36. Hsu HW, Cheng YJ, Chen LK, et al. Differential analgesic effect of tenoxicam on the wound pain and uterine cramping pain after cesarean section. Clin J Pain. 2003;19:55–8.

37. Yeh YC, Chen SY, Lin CJ, Yeh HM, Sun WZ. Differential analgesic effect of tenoxicam on post-cesarean uterine cramping pain between primiparous and multiparous women. J Formos Med Assoc. 2005;104:647–51.

38. Partlow DB Jr, Chauhan SP, Justice L, et al. Diagnosis of postpartum infections: clinical criteria are better than laboratory parameter. J Miss State Med Assoc. 2004;45:67–70.

39. Hartmann KE, Barrett KE, Reid VC, et al. Clinical usefulness of white blood cell count after cesarean delivery. Obstet Gynecol. 2000;96:295–300.

40. Csendes A, Burgos AM, Roizblatt D, Garay C, Bezama P. Inflammatory response measured by body temperature, C-reactive protein and white blood cell count 1, 3, and 5 days after laparotomic or laparoscopic gastric bypass surgery. Obes Surg. 2009;19:890–3.

41. Chen SB, Lee YC, Ser KH, et al. Serum C-reactive protein and white blood cell count in morbidly obese surgical patients. Obes Surg. 2009;19:461–6.

42. Kim SY, Koo BN, Shin CS, Ban M, Han K, Kim MD. The effects of single-dose dexamethasone on inflammatory response and pain after uterine artery embolisation for symptomatic fibroids or adenomyosis: a randomised controlled study. BJOG. 2016;123:580–7.

43. Jin J, Peng L, Chen Q, et al. Prevalence and risk factors for chronic pain following cesarean section: a prospective study. BMC Anesthesiol. 2016;16:99.

44. Dorner TE, Muckenhuber J, Stronegger WJ, Rasky E, Gustorff B, Freidl W. The impact of socio-economic status on pain and the perception of disability due to pain. Eur J Pain. 2011;15:103–9.

45. Ng B, Dimsdale JE, Rollnik JD, Shapiro H. The effect of ethnicity on prescriptions for patient-controlled analgesia for post-operative pain. Pain. 1996;66:9–12.

24

Effects of ultrasound-guided paravertebral block on MMP-9 and postoperative pain in patients undergoing VATS lobectomy

Haichen Chu[1†], He Dong[1†], Yongjie Wang[2] and Zejun Niu[1*]

Abstract

Background: Local anesthesia can reduce the response to surgical stress and decrease the consumption of opioids, which may reduce immunosuppression and potentially delay postoperative tumor recurrence. We compared paravertebral block (PVB) combined with general anesthesia (GA) and general anesthesia regarding their effects on postoperative pain and matrix metalloproteinase-9 (MMP-9) after video-assisted thoracoscopic surgery (VATS) lobectomy.

Methods: 54 patients undergoing elective VATS lobectomy at a single tertiary care, teaching hospital located in Qingdao between May 2, 2018 and Sep 28, 2018 were randomised by computer to either paravertebral block combined with general anesthesia or general anesthesia. The primary outcomes were pain scores at rest and on cough at 1, 4, 24, and 48 h after surgery. The secondary outcome were plasma concentrations of MMP-9, complications, and length of postoperative hospital stay.

Results: 75 were enrolled to the study, of whom 21 were excluded before surgery. We analyzed lobectomy patients undergoing paravertebral block combined with general anesthesia ($n = 25$) or general anesthesia ($n = 24$). Both groups were similar regarding baseline characteristics. Pain scores at rest at 4 h and 24 h, on cough at 4 h were lower in PVB/GA group, compared with GA group ($P < 0.05$). There were no difference in pain scores at rest at 1 h, 48 h and on cough at 1 h, 24 h, and 48 h between groups. Patients in the PVB/GA group showed a greater decrease in plasma MMP-9 level at T1 and T2 after VATS lobectomy ($P < 0.05$). Postoperative complications and length of stay did not differ by anesthetic technique.

Conclusions: The paravertebral block/general anesthesia can provide statistically better pain relief and attenuate MMP-9 response to surgery and after VATS lobectomy. This technique may be beneficial for patients to recover rapidly after lung surgery and reduce postoperative tumor recurrence.

Keywords: Video-assisted thoracoscopic lobectomy, Paravertebral anesthesia, Pain, Operative, Matrix metalloproteinase-9

* Correspondence: nzj16niu@sina.com
†Haichen Chu and He Dong contributed equally to this work.
[1]Department of Anesthesiology, The Affiliated Hospital of Qingdao University, No.16 Jiangsu Road, Shinan District, Qingdao, China

Background

In recent decades, lung cancer is the most common malignant tumor from the worldwide. The most common type of lung cancer that causes death is non-small cell lung cancer (NSCLC), which has caused serious burden on patients and society [1]. Surgery is still the effective treatment for lung cancer. Even if the tumors are complete resected including systemic lymph node dissection, the chance of tumor recurrence is still high due to undetected micro-metastasis [2–4]. Although general anesthesia is the most commonly used anesthetic method for lung cancer surgery, it has higher levels of inflammation and stronger immunosuppressive effects in comparison with regional anesthesia [5]. Nerve block anesthesia such as paravertebral nerve block has many advantages such as reducing opioids and general anesthetic consumption, reducing the inflammatory response and immunosuppression caused by surgical trauma, and can improve the long-term survival rate of postoperative patients with lung cancer [6].

The matrix metalloproteinase (MMP) family plays an important role in tumor recurrence. MMP-9 is the most detected in a variety of malignant tissues and is associated with tumor metastasis and recurrence potential [7]. Immunohistochemical expression and increased plasma levels of MMP-9 have been demonstrated in NSCLC patients [8]. However, to the best of our knowledge, a comparision of the effects of ultrasound-guided paravertebral block combined with general anesthesia and general anesthesia on postoperative pain scores and MMP-9 in VATS lobectomy is rare. Therefore, we compared the effect of PVB/general anesthesia and general anesthesia on pain scores, MMP-9, postoperative complications and length of stay after VATS lobectomy.

Methods

The study was approved by the Medical Ethics Committee of the Affiliated Hospital of Qingdao University and was performed between May 2018 and Sep 2018. Informed written consent was signed by every patient prior to enrollment in this study. Our study was registered with Chinese Clinical Trial Registry (ChiCTR1800016379). All study procedures were completed at the affiliated hospital of Qingdao university, a tertiary care, teaching hospital located in Qingdao, China. The surgical procedures performed included VATS lobectomy and systematic mediastinal lymphadenectomy.

The inclusion criteria included the following: patients with lung tumors who were undergoing VATS lobectomy, aged 18–70 years, of both genders, American Society of Anesthesiologists physiological statusIto III. The exclusion criteria were used: body mass index $\geq 30\,\mathrm{kg/m^2}$, anatomical abnormalities of the thoracic spine identified by chest computed tomography, spontaneous pneumothorax in the medical history, known allergy or hypersensitivity against amino-amide local anesthetics (LA), use of nonsteroidal anti-inflammatory drugs 2 weeks before surgery, coagulopathies in the medical history. Seventy-five patients scheduled for VATS lobectomy completed. 54 patients undergoing elective VATS lobectomy were randomized by computer to either PVB/GA ($n = 27$) or GA ($n = 27$). Two PVB patients who was with failed PVB and converted to open surgery did not participate in the final analysis. Three GA patients dropped out after randomization. We finally analyzed patients undergoing PVB/GA ($n = 25$) or GA ($n = 24$). Perioperative data were collected by anesthesia personnel (residents, nurse anesthetists and attendings).

Thoracic paravertebral block technique

We performed ultrasound-guided two-shot paravertebral blocks with 20 ml of 0.375% ropivacaine (AstraZeneca AB, PS05070, Sweden) at the thoracic interspace T4–5 and T7–8. We used long-axis (transverse approach) in-plane techniques for thoracic paravertebral nerve block. Using the ultrasound system (SonoSite M-Turbo, SonoSite Inc., Bothell, WA) to determine the thoracic paravertebral space (TPVS) of T4 and T7 levels in the lateral position, we visualized that the needle tip (Stimuplex D Plus, 0.71 × 80 mm, 22G × 3 1/8," B.Braun Melsungen AG, Germany) was between the superior costotransverse ligament and the pleura and placed it inside the TPVS, 20 ml of 0.375% ropivacaine (each injection point) was administered after negative aspiration under direct ultrasound imaging [9].

Intraoperative and postoperative management

On the day of surgery, investigators generated the randomization sequence using a computerized program. The allocation was concealed until shortly before anesthesia. An anesthesiologist who was not involved in this study placed the assignment numbers in opaque sealed envelopes to conceal the randomization sequence. All cases were allocated at random to one of two group: a control group (group GA), receiving general anesthesia and postoperative patient-controlled intravenous analgesia (PCIA), and a treatment group (group PVB), receiving thoracic paravertebral anesthesia combined general anesthesia and postoperative PCIA. Medical Ethics Committee approval and written informed consent were obtained. All patients were conducted by same anesthesiologist who had considerable prior experience with use of PVB.

In both groups, induction of anesthesia was performed with propofol (1–2 mg/kg), sufentanil (0.4–0.5 μg/kg), and cisatracurium (0.15–0.2 mg/kg) for muscle paralysis. After tracheal intubation, maintenance of anesthesia was performed with sevoflurane (1%) in a mixed oxygen/air fresh gas, and cisatracurium as needed in both groups. Analgesia was assured by the ropivacaine solution (0.375%) in the PVB group and by sufentanil as needed in the GA group.

Flurbiprofen 50 mg was intravenous injection at 30 min before the end of surgery in the both groups. When the surgery is finished, all patients were transferred to the postanesthesia care unit (PACU). All patients who were awake were connected with the PCIA pump with sufentanil and ondansetron. Sufentanil was inserted with 1-2 μg/h. A bolus of 2 mL was allowed at every 15 min up to a maximal dose of 10 μg/h.

All patients were treated with IV flurbiprofen in 50–100 mg increments for a Visual Analog Scale (VAS) score of 4/10 or greater or patient request for analgesia. Patients were monitored in the PACU until they met discharge criteria.

Outcomes

Our primary end point was pain scores at rest and on cough. A VAS was used to assess pain intensity at 1, 4, 24 and 48 h after completion of surgery. The secondary outcomes were plasma concentrations of MMP-9, postoperative complications and postoperative hospital stay. Postoperative complications including pneumonia, atelectasis, air leak, atrial fibrillation, hypotension and postoperative nausea and vomiting (PONV).

Blood samples were obtained 10 min before anesthesia (T0), at the end of surgery (T1), and at 12 h after operation (T2). Blood was collected into EDTA tubes and centrifuged at 4000 g for 15 min at 4 °C immediately after sampling. Thereafter, plasma was stored at − 70 °C until all the samples were collected. Plasma concentrations of MMP-9 were measured with commercially quantitative sandwich ELISA kits (Wuhan USCN Business Co., Ltd., Wuhan, China). Standards were prepared, and the appropriate volume of sample or standard was added to a 96-well polystyrene microtitre plate, and incubated for 1 h at 37 °C. Unbound material was removed. Detection Reagent A (biotin-conjugated antibody specific to target protein) was added to each well, and the incubation was continued for 37 °C. After washing with wash buffer 3 times, Detection Reagent B (avidin conjugated HRP) was added to each well, and the incubation was continued for 0.5 h at 37 °C. After washing with wash buffer 5 times, TMB substrate was added to each well, and the incubation was continued for 10–20 min at 37 °C. Once 50 μl stop solution was added to each well, and the absorbance at 450 nm was measured.

Seven known concentrations, ranging from 0.156 to 10 ng/ml was measured for MMP-9. Samples values was used for further statistical analysis. The concentration of target protein in the samples is then determined by comparing the O.D. of the sample to the standard curve.

Demographic information (age, sex, body mass index, and the American Society of Anesthesiologists grade) and pertinent surgical information (operation time, estimated blood loss, type of surgery, histology and stage of tumor) were recorded.

Prospectively collected data included pain scores at 1, 4, 24 and 48 h after completion of surgery, complications (pneumonia, atelectasis, air leak, atrial fibrillation, hypotension, PONV), and length of stay. Both groups received PCA using a mixture of 1 μg/mL sufentanil and 0.08 mg/mL ondansetron with the pump set to deliver doses of 1-2 μg/h intravenous sufentanil with a 15-min lockout time. If the VAS score is greater than 3, 50–100 mg of flurbiprofen was injected intravenously. Nausea and vomiting were treated with intravenous 8 mg ondansetron. Ambulation early after VATS lobectomy was a postoperative ERAS element. The patients were made to walk along the bedside, if possible, walk around the ward always accompanied by family member and the nursing staff on the following day after surgery. Oral liquid on the first day after surgery, and a semi-liquid diet after flatus passage were started at postoperative day 1. The early postoperative intake of solids was initiated at postoperative passage of flatus. All patients were subjected to enforced early mobilization. Perioperative management was similar in both groups.

Statistical analysis

The sample size calculation was based on mean VAS scores (2.53 ± 0.83) from our hospital in the pilot study. To have a greater than 90% power with an overall 2-sided typeIerror rate of 5%, and consider withdrawal and loss of follow-up (cases of 10%), at least 22 patients were required in each group.

Continuous variables were expressed as the mean (± 1 standard deviation) or median (95% confidence interval (CI)) when data were not normally distributed and were compared between the two groups using the Mann-Whitney U test. $P < 0.05$ was considered significant for all data. Data were analyzed by use of the statistical package for the social sciences (SPSS 23.0).

Results

Between May 2, 2018 and September 28, 2018, 75 consecutive patients were assessed for eligibility. Twenty-one patients did not meet the inclusion criteria or refused to participate. The remaining 54 patients provided written consent to participate and were randomized to either group PVB ($n = 27$) or group GA (n = 27). Two PVB patients who was with failed PVB and converted to open surgery did not participate in the final analysis. Three GA patients dropped out after randomization. Final analysis compared therefore 25 PVB patients with 24 GA patients (Fig. 1). All subjects were included in the primary outcome analysis. There were no clinically significant differences in demographic data and surgical data between groups, except for the intraoperative consumption of sufentanil (Table 1).

Pain scores and consumption of flurbiprofen

VAS pain scores at rest and on cough after VATS lobectomy are shown in Figs. 2 and 3. Compared with the GA group, postoperative VAS pain scores at rest at 4 h [2.53 ± 0.83 (95%CI: 2.20 to 2.86) vs 3.4 ± 0.91 (3.04 to 3.76) respectively, $P = 0.011$] and 24 h [2.2 ± 0.94 (1.83 to 2.57) vs 3.0 ± 0.93 (2.63 to 3.37), $P = 0.026$] were lower in the PVB group. Although there were no difference in VAS on cough at 1 h, 24 h, and 48 h ($P > 0.05$), VAS scores on cough at 4 h was significantly lower in the PVB group than in the GA group (2.6 $\pm$0.65 vs 3.00 $\pm$0.59 respectively, $P = 0.028$). There was no statistically significant difference in VAS scores at rest and on cough between the two groups at 1 h and 48 h after surgery. Total postoperative flurbiprofen consumption was significantly lower in the PVB group compared to GA group. The consumption of flurbiprofen postoperatively was 20 ± 32 mg in the PVB group and 48 ± 43 mg in the GA group respectively, $P = 0.013$.

Plasma concentrations of MMP-9

Mean plasma MMP-9 concentrations at three different time points are shown in Fig. 4. Preoperative MMP-9 did not differ between the PVB group and the GA group [94 ± 24 (95%: 85 to103) vs 99 ± 13 (94 to 104) respectively, $P = 0.743$]. Plasma MMP-9 concentrations increased significantly after surgery compared to preoperative values. Plasma MMP-9 concentrations at T1 and T2 in the PVB group were significantly lower after surgery than in the GA group [142 ± 53 ng/mL(95%CI: 140 to 144) vs 236 ± 69 ng/mL(208 to 264) at T1 respectively, $P = 0.019$; 238 ± 53 ng/mL(95%CI: 217 to 259) vs 307 ± 16 ng/mL(301 to 313) at T2 respectively, $P = 0.032$].

Complications and length of stay

Postoperative complications are shown in Table 2. Composite complications were uncommon (0–12.5% frequency) and didn't differ between groups. Although GA group has an increasing trend in postoperative nausea and vomiting (PONV), there was no difference between groups. Mean postoperative hospital stay was not statistically different between the groups (5.3 ± 1.3 days in the PVB group vs. 5.1 ± 1.6 days in the GA group; $P = 0.647$).

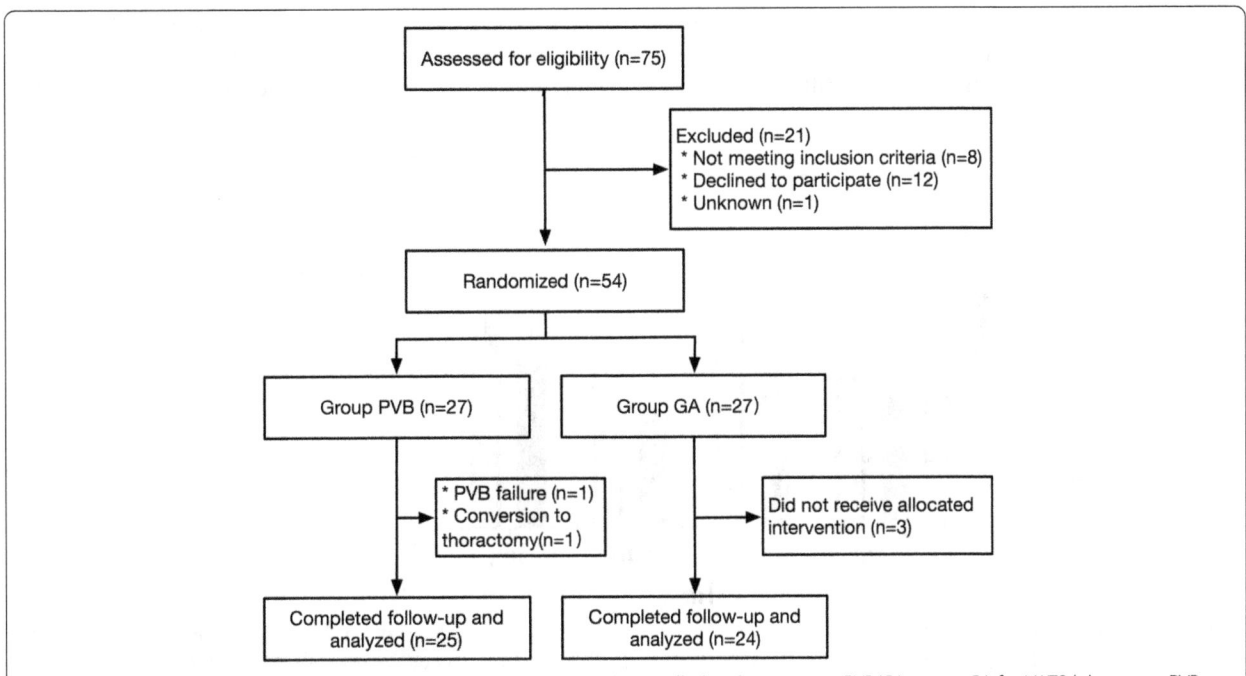

Fig. 1 Protocol for patient enrolment in the study groups. Randomized controlled trial comparing PVB/GA versus GA for VATS lobectomy. PVB = paravertebral block; GA = general anesthesia; VATS = video-assisted thoracoscopic surgery

Table 1 Demographic Data

Characteristics	Group PVB(n = 25)	Group GA(n = 24)	P Value
Age (yr)	58 ± 11	59 ± 9	0.767
Male, n (%)	20 (54)	16 (42)	0.329
BMI	24 ± 3.6	25 ± 3.2	0.126
ASA I/II/III	5/30/2	8/27/3	0.595
Operation time (min)	138 ± 57	129 ± 60	0.571
Estimated blood loss (mL)	33 ± 12	36 ± 13	0.558
Sufentanil dosage (µg)	37 ± 16	68 ± 19	< 0.001
Type of surgery n (%)			0.502
Lobectomy	17 (68)	20 (83)	
Segmentectomy	7 (28)	3 (13)	
Wedge resection	1 (4)	1 (4)	
Histology, n (%)			0.189
Adenocarcinoma	24 (96)	20 (83)	
Squamous	1 (4)	4 (17)	
Others	0 (0)	0 (0)	
Stage, n (%)			0.869
I	21 (84)	19 (79)	
II	3 (12)	3 (13)	
III	1 (4)	2 (8)	
IV	0 (0)	0 (0)	

Values are shown as mean ± standard deviation or number (n) and %. BMI indicates body mass index; ASA, American Society of Anesthesiologists

Discussion

Our results showed that VAS pain scores at rest at postoperative 4 h and 24 h and on cough at 4 h were lower in the PVB/GA group. There was no difference in VAS between the groups at other time points. At the same time, plasma MMP-9 levels at the end of surgery and at postoperative 12 h were also significantly decreased in the PVB/GA group after VATS lobectomy. Postoperative complications and the length of hospital stay were not different between the two groups. Although there was an increasing trend in PONV in GA group, there's no statistics difference in PVB group and GA group.

Surgery is the most effective treatment for lung cancer. However, effective analgesia allows patients to recover quickly. Paravertebral nerve block combined with general anesthesia reduces patients' immunosuppression and the consumption of sufentanil. Ropivacaine is a long-acting local anesthetic, and its action time can reach 12–24 h. This study showed that patients at the end of surgery had similar VAS scores between groups and that the analgesia effect of paravertebral block was similar to that of sufentanil. Similar pain scores at 1 h were associated with intravenous injection of flurbiprofen at 30 mins before the end of surgery in the both groups. The other reason why VAS at 1 h between the both groups were not difference is that sufentanil has the residual analgesic effect. But the analgesia scores at rest at 4 and 24 h after surgery were lower in the PVB group. The low operative VAS score at 4 h and 24 h in the PVB group may be attributed to the effect of ropivacaine on the paravertebral space for up to 24 h. Analgesia on cough is very important for the patients who have undergone thoracic or upper abdominal surgeries. Our results showed that VAS on cough at 4 h in the PVB group were lower than in the GA group. The reason that PVB patients didn't have longer analgesia on cough is that we didn't use continuing PVB analgesia after surgery. If we choose to continue PVB analgesia after lobectomy, it may provide better analgesia when patients were coughing.

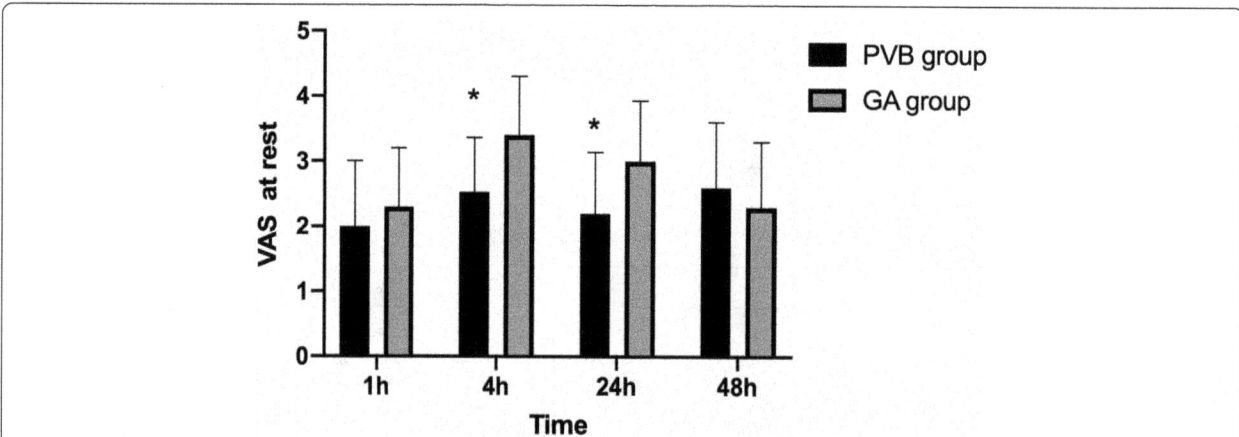

Fig. 2 Postoperative pain scores at rest. Pain was assessed by the use of a VAS ranging from 0 to 10 at 1, 4, 24, 48 h after surgery for PVB patients (black bar) and GA patients (gray bar), respectively. VAS scores at rest at 4, 24 h after lobectomy were significantly lower in the PVB group than in the GA group. *Statistical significance (P < 0.05). Data are expressed as mean ± standard deviation. VAS = visual analogue scale; PVB = paravertebral block; GA = general anesthesia

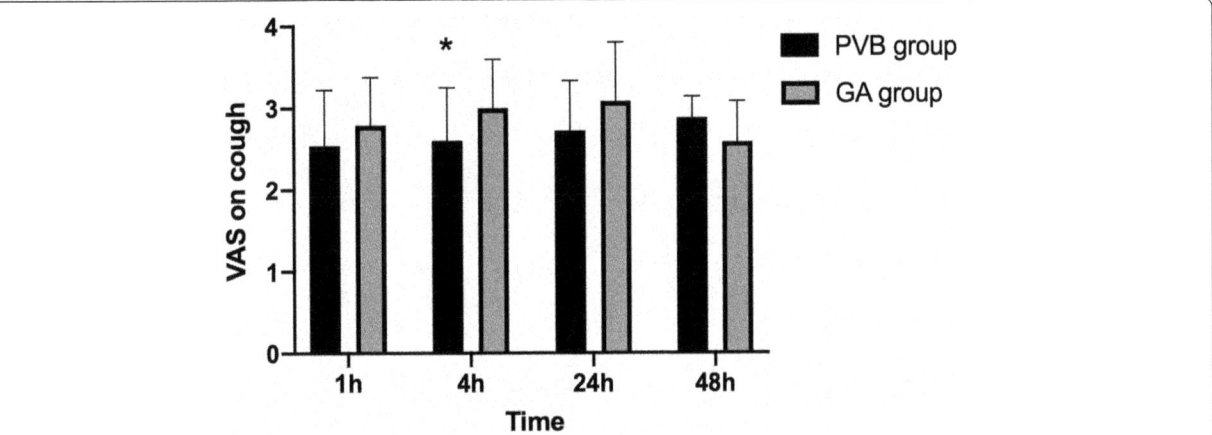

Fig. 3 Postoperative pain scores on cough. Pain was assessed by the use of a VAS ranging from 0 to 10 at 1, 4, 24, 48 h after surgery for PVB patients (black bar) and GA patients (gray bar), respectively. VAS scores on cough at 4 h after lobectomy were significantly lower in the PVB group than in the GA group. *Statistical significance ($P < 0.05$). Data are expressed as mean ± standard deviation. VAS = visual analogue scale; PVB = paravertebral block; GA = general anesthesia

Although the tumor is surgically removed, micro-metastasis is inevitable, especially when the patient's immune function is suppressed. Retrospective studies suggest regional anesthesia including nerve block reduces tumor metastasis and recurrence in various cancers [10–12]. Paravertebral block and postoperative analgesia can reduce the risk of recurrence and metastasis in breast cancer patients during the initial years of follow-up after mammectomy [10].MMP-9 that is a member of the MMP superfamily plays an important role in many pathophysiological processes, such as bone development, wound healing, cell migration, cancer invasion and metastasis [13]. The surgery trauma resulted in increased plasma MMP-9. Our results supported the notion that plasma MMP-9 level increased after VATS lobectomy. PVB inhibited surgical stress and decreased postoperative MMP-9 level. There may be several reasons that PVB decreased plasma MMP-9 level at T1 and T2. First of all, vitro experiments showed local anesthetics have antiproliferative and cytotoxic effects on cancer cells [14–16]. Second, paravertebral nerve block and analgesia reduced the risk of breast cancer recurrence or metastasis 4-fold during a four-year follow-up [10]. Moreover, our observations that reductions in MMP-9 at T1and T2 were greater when patients received combined paravertebral anesthesia with general anesthesia seem consistent with the hypothesis that PVB has little effect on immune function, thus strengthens immune defenses against tumor progression. Thereby, MMP-9 level in the PVB/GA group was lower during VATS lobectomy. Another possible mechanism by which PVB may decrease MMP-9 is that thoracic paravertebral block reduced the level of inflammatory factors and the surgical stress response. Therefore, general anesthesia combined with PVB methods undergoing VATS lobectomy can reduce MMP-9 levels, provide better postoperative analgesia, and should be recommended.

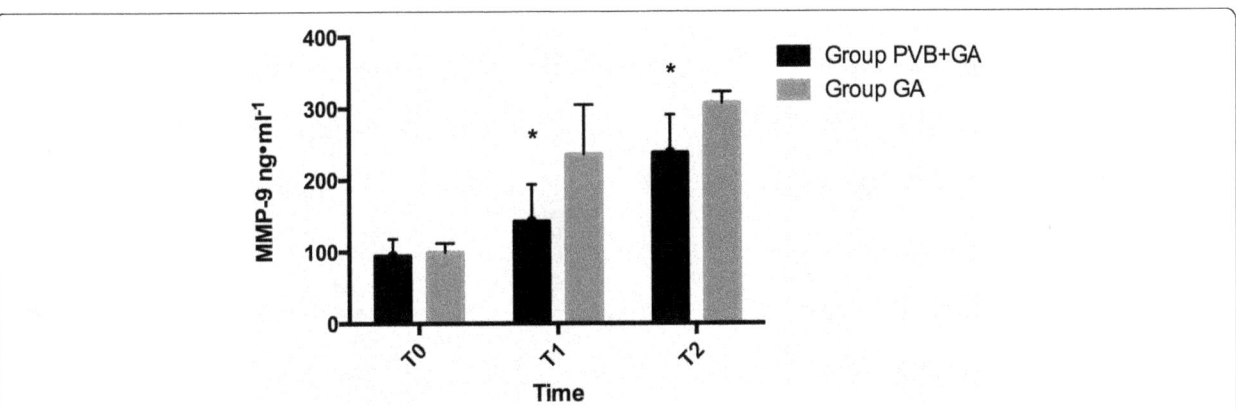

Fig. 4 Plasma concentration of measured MMP-9 in lung cancer patients receiving PVB combined general anesthesia or only general anesthesia. *$P < 0.05$ in the PVB group compared with GA group. MMP-9 = matrix metalloproteinase-9; PVB = paravertebral block; GA = general anesthesia

Table 2 Postoperative complications

Parameter	Group PVB n (%)	Group GA n (%)	P-value
Pneumonia	0	1 (4.2)	0.490
Atelectasis	1 (4.0)	2 (8.3)	0.527
Air leak	0	0	
AF	2 (8.0)	1 (4.2)	0.576
Hypotension	3 (12.0)	2 (8.3)	0.672
PONV	1 (4.0)	3 (12.5)	0.277

AF atrial fibrillation. *PONV* postoperative nausea and vomiting

Better analgesia (for example combined PVB) reduces intraoperative consumption of sufentanil. It is well known that opioids can suppress immune function, which may affect tumor metastasis and recurrence. The reasons that opioids promote tumor growth and metastasis are based on the modulation of cellular and humoral responses leading to immunosuppression [17] and the direct action on tumor cells and immune or endothelial cells [18]. The immunosuppressive effect of opioids is independent of their antinociceptive effect. Therefore, it is essential to individually evaluate the effect of opioids on the immune system. During thoracoscopic lobectomy we choosed paravertebral nerve block combined GA so that we can decrease the dose of sufentanil and potentially reduced the inhibition of immune function. If we choose postoperative PVB analgesia, patients in PVB group will have a better recovery.

Although GA group had a high consumption of sufentanil during lobectomy, postoperative complications such as nausea, vomiting, and respiratory depression were not different between the two groups. Previous studies [19, 20] demonstrated the PVB group had a significant reduction in the use of opioids and nerve block can reduce postoperative complications caused by opioids. There could be several reasons for the difference. First, because we did not use PVB as a postoperative analgesia method, the benefits of PVB were not fully shown, such as less pulmonary complications, hypotension, nausea and vomiting, and urinary retention etc. [21]. Second, enhanced recovery after VATS lobectomy protocols we used can prevent factors that delay postoperative recovery and issues that cause complications. Similar results from other studies [22]. Although previous investigations [23] have demonstrated that PVB is associated with shorter hospitalizations, the length of stay was similar in both groups in our study. Hospital stay is affected by various factors, and different postoperative analgesia methods may also affect the length of hospital stay [23].

Our study has several limitations. First, the surgical procedures carried out were not homogeneous. Although the lobectomy is performed by the same group of surgeons, the individual differences and anatomical abnormalities of the surgical patients will cause slight different degrees of surgical injuries. Secondly, postoperative paravertebral analgesia should be adopted in the PVB group, which can better show the difference between the two groups. Third, we should standardize the depth of anesthesia, the time to discharge and use a validated quality of recovery tool such as PosropQRS so that we can better observe the impact of different anesthetic methods on patient recovery. Lastly, we should collect samples of the bio-marker for longer periods to observe the effect of nerve block on the level of MMP-9.

Conclusions

In conclusion, in this prospective randomized clinical trial, PVB combined general anesthesia is accompanied with an attenuation of MMP-9 response to surgery and provided statistically better pain relief after VATS lobectomy. This technique may be beneficial for patients to recover rapidly after lung surgery and reduce tumor recurrence. Further studies are required to investigate this effect could be extended beyond immediate postoperative period by utilizing a continue paravertebral analgesia technique.

Abbreviations
GA: General anesthesia; MMP-9: Matrix metalloproteinase-9; NSCLC: Non-small cell lung cancer; PACU: Postanesthesia care unit; PCIA: Patient-controlled intravenous analgesia; PONV: Postoperative nausea and vomiting; PVB: Paravertebral block; TPVS: Thoracic paravertebral space; VAS: Visual analog scale; VATS: Video-assisted thoracoscopic surgery

Acknowledgements
The authors would like to thank Dr. Xianfei Yan and Guishen Miao for data collection.

Authors' contributions
HC contributed to study design, interpretation of data, and drafted the manuscript, and approved the final version. HD contributed to study design, acquisition of data, and approved the final version. HD and YW were primarily responsible for the processing and analysis of blood samples. YW contributed to study design, critically revised the manuscript, and approved the final version. ZN was responsible for the majority of ELISA experiments, contributed to study design, analysis, and interpretation of the data, revised the manuscript, and approved the final version.

Author details
¹Department of Anesthesiology, The Affiliated Hospital of Qingdao University, No.16 Jiangsu Road, Shinan District, Qingdao, China. ²Department of Thoracic Surgery, The Affiliated Hospital of Qingdao University, Qingdao, China.

References
1. Hong QY, Wu GM, Qian GS, Hu CP, Zhou JY, Chen LA, Li WM, Li SY, Wang K, Wang Q, et al. Prevention and management of lung cancer in China. Cancer. 2015;121(Suppl 17):3080–8.
2. Kim AW. Lymph node drainage patterns and micrometastasis in lung cancer. Semin Thorac Cardiovasc Surg. 2009;21(4):298–308.
3. Koulaxouzidis G, Karagkiouzis G, Konstantinou M, Gkiozos I, Syrigos K. Sampling versus systematic full lymphatic dissection in surgical treatment of non-small cell lung cancer. Oncol Rev. 2013;7(1):e2.
4. Merchant NN, McKenna R Jr, Onugha O. Is there a role for VATS sleeve lobectomy in lung Cancer? Surg Technol Int. 2018;32:225–9.
5. Perez-Gonzalez O, Cuellar-Guzman LF, Soliz J, Cata JP. Impact of regional

anesthesia on recurrence, metastasis, and immune response in breast Cancer surgery: a systematic review of the literature. Reg Anesth Pain Med. 2017;42(6):751–6.

6. Lee EK, Ahn HJ, Zo JI, Kim K, Jung DM, Park JH. Paravertebral block does not reduce Cancer recurrence, but is related to higher overall survival in lung Cancer surgery: a retrospective cohort study. Anesth Analg. 2017;125(4): 1322–8.

7. Shou Y, Hirano T, Gong Y, Kato Y, Yoshida K, Ohira T, Ikeda N, Konaka C, Ebihara Y, Zhao F, et al. Influence of angiogenetic factors and matrix metalloproteinases upon tumour progression in non-small-cell lung cancer. Br J Cancer. 2001;85(11):1706–12.

8. Ding G, Liu Y, Liang C. Efficacy of radiotherapy on intermediate and advanced lung cancer and its effect on dynamic changes of serum vascular endothelial growth factor and matrix metalloproteinase-9. Oncol Lett. 2018; 16(1):219–24.

9. Marhofer D, Marhofer P, Kettner SC, Fleischmann E, Prayer D, Schernthaner M, Lackner E, Willschke H, Schwetz P, Zeitlinger M. Magnetic resonance imaging analysis of the spread of local anesthetic solution after ultrasound-guided lateral thoracic paravertebral blockade: a volunteer study. Anesthesiology. 2013;118(5):1106–12.

10. Exadaktylos AK, Buggy DJ, Moriarty DC, Mascha E, Sessler DI. Can anesthetic technique for primary breast cancer surgery affect recurrence or metastasis? Anesthesiology. 2006;105(4):660–4.

11. Mao L, Lin S, Lin J. The effects of anesthetics on tumor progression. Int J Physiol Pathophysiol Pharmacol. 2013;5(1):1–10.

12. Sekandarzad MW, van Zundert AAJ, Lirk PB, Doornebal CW, Hollmann MW. Perioperative anesthesia care and tumor progression. Anesth Analg. 2017; 124(5):1697–708.

13. Raffetto JD, Khalil RA. Matrix metalloproteinases in venous tissue remodeling and varicose vein formation. Curr Vasc Pharmacol. 2008;6(3): 158–72.

14. Bundscherer A, Malsy M, Gebhardt K, Metterlein T, Plank C, Wiese CH, Gruber M, Graf BM. Effects of ropivacaine, bupivacaine and sufentanil in colon and pancreatic cancer cells in vitro. Pharmacol Res. 2015;95-96:126–31.

15. Jose C, Bellance N, Chatelain EH, Benard G, Nouette-Gaulain K, Rossignol R. Antiproliferative activity of levobupivacaine and aminoimidazole carboxamide ribonucleotide on human cancer cells of variable bioenergetic profile. Mitochondrion. 2012;12(1):100–9.

16. Jurj A, Tomuleasa C, Tat TT, Berindan-Neagoe I, Vesa SV, Ionescu DC. Antiproliferative and apoptotic effects of Lidocaine on human Hepatocarcinoma cells. A preliminary study. J Gastrointestin Liver Dis. 2017; 26(1):45–50.

17. Brack A, Rittner HL, Stein C. Immunosuppressive effects of opioids–clinical relevance. J NeuroImmune Pharmacol. 2011;6(4):490–502.

18. Afsharimani B, Doornebal CW, Cabot PJ, Hollmann MW, Parat MO. Comparison and analysis of the animal models used to study the effect of morphine on tumour growth and metastasis. Br J Pharmacol. 2015;172(2): 251–9.

19. Clendenen SR, Wehle MJ, Rodriguez GA, Greengrass RA. Paravertebral block provides significant opioid sparing after hand-assisted laparoscopic nephrectomy: an expanded case report of 30 patients. J Endourol. 2009; 23(12):1979–83.

20. Fortier S, Hanna HA, Bernard A, Girard C. Comparison between systemic analgesia, continuous wound catheter analgesia and continuous thoracic paravertebral block: a randomised, controlled trial of postthoracotomy pain management. Eur J Anaesthesiol. 2012;29(11):524–30.

21. Davies RG, Myles PS, Graham JM. A comparison of the analgesic efficacy and side-effects of paravertebral vs epidural blockade for thoracotomy--a systematic review and meta-analysis of randomized trials. Br J Anaesth. 2006;96(4):418–26.

22. Ljungqvist O, Scott M, Fearon KC. Enhanced recovery after surgery: a review. JAMA Surg. 2017;152(3):292–8.

23. Parikh RP, Sharma K, Guffey R, Myckatyn TM. Preoperative paravertebral block improves postoperative pain control and reduces hospital length of stay in patients undergoing autologous breast reconstruction after mastectomy for breast Cancer. Ann Surg Oncol. 2016;23(13):4262–9.

25

Delayed remnant kidney function recovery is less observed in living donors who receive an analgesic, intrathecal morphine block in laparoscopic nephrectomy for kidney transplantation

Jaesik Park[1], Minju Kim[1], Yong Hyun Park[2], Misun Park[3], Jung-Woo Shim[1], Hyung Mook Lee[1], Yong-Suk Kim[1], Young Eun Moon[1], Sang Hyun Hong[1] and Min Suk Chae[1*] (iD)

Abstract

Background: This study analyzed remnant kidney function recovery in living donors after laparoscopic nephrectomy to establish a risk stratification model for delayed recovery and further investigated clinically modifiable factors.

Patients and methods: This retrospective study included 366 adult living donors who underwent elective donation surgery between January 2017 and November 2019 at our hospital. ITMB was included as an analgesic component in the living donor strategy for early postoperative pain relief from November 2018 to November 2019 ($n = 116$). Kidney function was quantified based on the estimated glomerular filtration rate (eGFR), and delayed functional recovery of remnant kidney was defined as eGFR < 60 mL/min/1.73 m^2 on postoperative day (POD) 1 ($n = 240$).

Results: Multivariable analyses revealed that lower risk for development of eGFR < 60 mL/min/1.73 m^2 on POD 1 was associated with ITMB, female sex, younger age, and higher amount of hourly fluid infusion (area under the receiver operating characteristic curve = 0.783; 95% confidence interval = 0.734–0.832; $p < 0.001$). Propensity score (PS)-matching analyses showed that prevalence rates of eGFR < 60 mL/min/1.73 m^2 on PODs 1 and 7 were higher in the non-ITMB group than in the ITMB group. ITMB adjusted for PS was significantly associated with lower risk for development of eGFR < 60 mL/min/1.73 m^2 on POD 1 in PS-matched living donors. No living donors exhibited severe remnant kidney dysfunction and/or required renal replacement therapy at POD 7.

Conclusions: We found an association between the analgesic impact of ITMB and better functional recovery of remnant kidney in living kidney donors. In addition, we propose a stratification model that predicts delayed functional recovery of remnant kidney in living donors: male sex, older age, non-ITMB, and lower hourly fluid infusion rate.

Keywords: Intrathecal morphine block, Remnant kidney function, Laparoscopic donor nephrectomy

* Correspondence: shscms@gmail.com
[1]Department of Anesthesiology and Pain Medicine, Seoul St. Mary's Hospital, College of Medicine, The Catholic University of Korea, 222, Banpo-daero, Seocho-gu, Seoul 06591, Republic of Korea

Background

Kidney transplantation (KT) is a preferred definitive cure for patients with end-stage kidney disease, as it is associated with better survival rate, and improved quality of life, compared to renal replacement therapy methods (e.g., dialysis) [1]. The substantial increase in prevalence of patients requiring renal replacement therapy has augmented the demand for grafts, and the kidney graft survival rates from deceased donors have been shown to be significantly inferior to those from living related or unrelated donors. This may be due to the very short cold ischemic time and better-functioning nephron mass of kidneys from healthy living donors. Thus, living donor KT has emerged as an effective clinical option to resolve graft shortage [2, 3]. Although the safety of living donor KT has been established, living donors undergoing nephrectomy may have long-term risks of cardiovascular events and/or progression to remnant kidney dysfunction [4].

Compensation and recovery of remnant kidney function after donation surgery require a baseline level of clinical suitability. Perioperative contributors for delayed recovery of remnant kidney function include hypertension, diabetes mellitus (DM), history of smoking, and obesity [5]. However, few studies have investigated the role of analgesic treatment, which might affect the sympathetic stress response and influence the degree of recovery in remnant kidney function. Kidney function can be compromised by many factors, including hypoxic and inflammatory damage, hormonal alterations (including in cortisol, catecholamine, anti-diuretic hormone, and renin-angiotensin-aldosterone), and inadequate repair mechanisms. These deleterious effects seem to be triggered and activated by surgical nociceptive/noxious stimuli, and are ultimately associated with decreased intra- and postoperative vascular flow [6–8]. Healthy living donors undergoing nephrectomy may be more susceptible to postoperative pain than ill patients undergoing nephrectomy. Because appropriate pain control is recommended after donation, intrathecal morphine block (ITMB) is an acceptable treatment for significantly reducing the severity of postoperative pain on post-operative day (POD) 1 [9–12].

This study primarily assessed remnant kidney function recovery in living donors undergoing laparoscopic nephrectomy to establish a risk stratification model for delayed recovery, and further investigated risk factors that were clinically modifiable, including ITMB.

Methods

Ethical considerations

The study protocol was approved by the Institutional Review Board of Seoul, St. Mary's Hospital Ethics Committee (approval no. KC19RISI0911; December 26, 2019). The study was performed in accordance with the principles of the Declaration of Helsinki. The requirement for informed consent was waived because of the retrospective nature of the study.

Study population

Electronic medical records were retrospectively reviewed for 380 living donors (> 19 years of age) who underwent elective laparoscopic nephrectomy for KT between January 2017 and November 2019 at Seoul St. Mary's Hospital. Using the clinical practice guideline [13], a multidisciplinary consult team regularly assessed the clinical and psychological condition of the living kidney donors. Donors in our study population had American Society of Anesthesiologists physical status I or II, a tolerable estimated glomerular filtration (eGFR) rate (i.e., ≥ 60 mL/min/1.73 m^2), and no evidence of a pathological renal lesion on abdominal computed tomography (CT). Because of missing or incomplete data, 14 living donors were excluded; finally, 366 adult living donors were enrolled in this study. A study flow chart is shown in Fig. 1.

Surgery and anesthesia

Laparoscopic living donor nephrectomy was performed by an experienced urologic surgeon (Y.H.P.), using a method described in detail elsewhere [14]. Experienced attending anesthesiologists provided balanced anesthesia, with electrocardiography and standard vital monitoring of systolic blood pressure (SBP) and diastolic blood pressure (DBP), heart rate (HR), O$_2$ saturation, body temperature, and capnography. Induction of anesthesia was performed using 1–2 mg/kg propofol (Fresenius Kabi, Bad Homburg, Germany) and 0.6 mg/kg rocuronium (Merck Sharp & Dohme Corp., Kenilworth, NJ, USA); maintenance of anesthesia was then performed using 2.0–6.0% desflurane (Baxter, Deerfield, IL, USA) with medical air/oxygen. Remifentanil (Hanlim Pharm. Co., Ltd., Seoul, Republic of Korea) was administered at a rate of 0.1–0.5 µg/kg/min, as appropriate. The Bispectral Index™ measurement (Medtronic, Minneapolis, MN, USA) was maintained between 40 and 50 to assure suitable hypnotic depth. Rocuronium was routinely infused under train-of-four monitoring (> one twitch). End-tidal CO$_2$ was set between 30 and 40 mmHg through adjustment of the ventilator mode. Liberal fluid was administered during surgery, and mannitol (25 g) was administered immediately before ligation of the renal artery.

All living donors were administered postoperative intravenous (IV) patient-control analgesia (IV-PCA) (AutoMed 3200; Acemedical, Seoul, Republic of Korea), which included 1000 µg fentanyl (Dai Han Pharm. Co., Ltd., Seoul, Republic of Korea), 90 mg ketorolac (Hanmi Pharm. Co., Ltd., Seoul, Republic of Korea), which was supplied as an analgesic adjuvant at a low infusion rate to reduce the opioid requirement and thus avoid serious

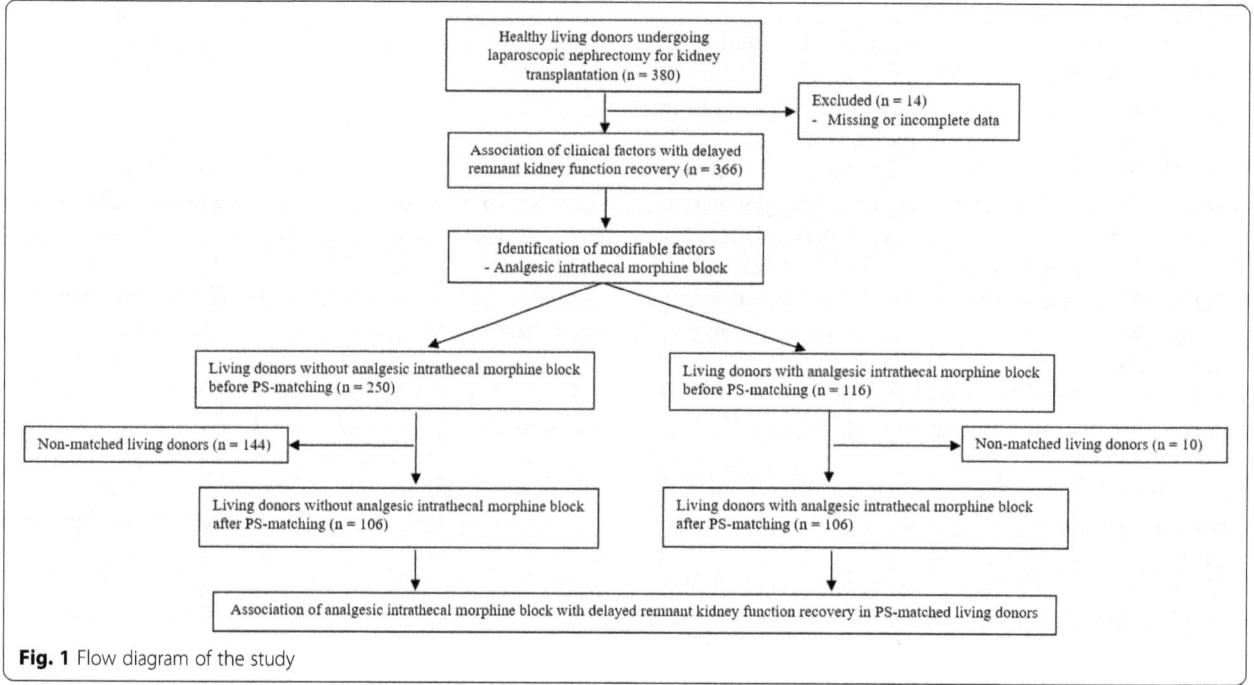

Fig. 1 Flow diagram of the study

side effects (such as nephrotoxicity and bleeding) [15–18], and 0.3 mg ramosetron as an anti-emetic adjuvant (Naseron; Boryung Co., Ltd., Seoul, Republic of Korea). The IV-PCA program consisted of a 1-mL bolus injection and a 1-mL basal infusion of the IV-PCA solution, with a lockout time of 10 min. When living donors experienced acute severe postoperative pain (pain score ≥ 7 on a numeric rating scale [NRS]), rescue IV drugs for pain relief were administered based on preferences and discretion of the attending physicians in the post-anesthesia care unit and ward.

ITMB intervention

Depending on the condition of healthy living donors, pain tolerance may be low [19, 20]. Therefore, ITMB, which is recognized as a safe and effective method of pain relief for living donors [12, 21], was included as an analgesic component in the living donor treatment strategy for early postoperative pain relief from November 2018 to November 2019. The day before donation surgery, informed consent for ITMB intervention was obtained from the living donors. Living donors who preferred to receive no ITMB intervention were provided with conventional analgesic service, including IV-PCA and rescue IV analgesic drugs.

To allow immediate identification of any nerve injury during the intrathecal practice performed before the induction of general anesthesia, living donors were provided no sedative medication in the operating room. Under standard vital sign monitoring, the living donors were positioned in the right or left lateral decubitus

position, and the skin over the lumbar region was cleaned with chlorhexidine and draped. The donors received 0.2 mg (0.2 mL) intrathecal morphine sulfate (BCWORLD Pharm. Co., Ltd., Seoul, Republic of Korea) with normal saline (0.8 mL) using a sterile 25G Quincke type-spinal needle (TAE-CHANG Industrial Co., Ltd., Chungcheongnam-do, Republic of Korea) between lumbar vertebrae 3 and 4. Morphine sulfate and normal saline (total 1.0 mL) were administered as a single injection after cerebrospinal fluid had been obtained.

Estimated glomerular filtration rate

Kidney function was quantified based on the eGFR, calculated using the Modification of Diet in Renal Disease formula: $eGFR = 175 \times standardized\ serum\ creatinine^{-1.154} \times age^{-0.203} \times 1.212$ (if black) $\times 0.742$ (if female) [22]. The baseline eGFR was estimated on the day before surgery, and serial eGFRs were measured on PODs 1 and 7. Based on the eGFR [23], the degree of kidney function was classified as normal function (eGFR ≥ 90 mL/min/1.73 m^2); mild dysfunction (eGFR 89–60 mL/min/1.73 m^2); and moderate dysfunction (eGFR 59–30 mL/min/1.73 m^2). In our study, delayed functional recovery of remnant kidney was defined as eGFR < 60 mL/min/1.73 m^2 on POD 1.

Clinical variables

Preoperative findings included sex, age, body mass index (BMI) (divided into ≥ 25 kg/m^2 [overweight] and < 25 kg/m^2 [normal weight]) [24], and hypertension, which was controlled to achieve the blood pressure goal (which is usually < 140/90 mmHg, but is < 130/80 mmHg for those with diabetes or chronic kidney disease) with or without anti-hypertensive drugs [25], eGFR, laboratory variables (white blood cell count, hemoglobin, platelet count, glucose, albumin, sodium, potassium, chloride, international normalized ratio, and activated partial thrombin time), and remnant kidney volume estimated using abdominal CT images and volume software (AW VolumeShare 4; General Electric Healthcare, Chicago, IL, USA). Intraoperative findings included a time effect, thus the serial order of the living donors from the first (no. 1) to the most recent (no. 366), ITMB status, total surgery duration, average vital signs (i.e., SBP, DBP, HR, and body temperature), hourly fluid infusion, hourly urine output, and total blood loss. Postoperative findings included eGFR, peak NRS, cumulative IV-PCA consumption, peak hemodynamic parameters (i.e., SBP, DBP, and HR), laboratory variables (i.e., white blood cell count, hemoglobin, platelet count, sodium, potassium, and chloride), ITMB-associated complications (i.e., intrathecal site infection, post-dural puncture headache, lower limb numbness, respiratory depression, and bleeding), and surgical complications assessed using the Clavien-Dindo classification [26].

Statistical analyses

The normal distribution of continuous findings was estimated using the Shapiro–Wilk test. Continuous data are expressed as means ± standard deviations (SDs) or medians (interquartile ranges). Categorical data are expressed as numbers and proportions. Perioperative findings were compared using the Mann–Whitney U test and χ^2 test or Fisher's exact test, as appropriate. The associations of pre- and intraoperative findings with delayed functional recovery of remnant kidney were evaluated by univariable and multivariable logistic regression analyses. Potentially significant findings ($p < 0.1$) in univariable analyses were entered into the multivariable analysis. The accuracy of the risk stratification model for delayed functional recovery of remnant kidney was estimated according to the area under the receiver operating characteristic curve. Preoperative and intraoperative findings in the non-ITMB and ITMB groups were assessed by propensity score (PS)-matching analysis. PS-matching analysis was performed to reduce the effect of potential confounding findings on intergroup differences according to the ITMB intervention. PSs were derived to match living donors at a 1:1 ratio using greedy matching algorithms without replacement. After the PS-matching had been completed, we assessed the balance in baseline covariates through paired t-tests and McNemar's tests, as appropriate for continuous and categorical variables. The association of ITMB intervention with delayed functional recovery of remnant kidney was evaluated by

multivariable logistic regression analyses with PS adjustment. The values are expressed as odds ratios with 95% confidence intervals (CIs). All tests were two sided, and $p < 0.05$ was considered to indicate statistical significance. All statistical analyses were performed using R software version 2.10.1 (R Foundation for Statistical Computing, Vienna, Austria) and SPSS for Windows (ver. 24.0; IBM Corp., Armonk, NY, USA).

Results

Perioperative baseline findings in living donors undergoing laparoscopic nephrectomy

Table 1 shows the pre-, intra-, and postoperative patient characteristics. No living donors had a history of DM. On PODs 1 and 7, there were no living donors with eGFR < 30 mL/min/1.73 m^2 and/or requiring renal replacement therapy.

Comparison of pre- and intraoperative findings between living donors with eGFR ≥60 mL/min/1.73 m^2 and those with eGFR < 60 mL/min/1.73 m^2 on POD 1

In the preoperative findings (Table 2), living donors with eGFR < 60 mL/min/1.73 m^2 on POD 1 had a higher proportion of male sex, older age, and higher incidence of hypertension than living donors with eGFR ≥60 mL/min/1.73 m^2 on POD 1. The laboratory variables revealed that living donors with eGFR < 60 mL/min/1.73 m^2 on POD 1 had higher hemoglobin and sodium levels, but lower international normalized ratio, compared to living donors with eGFR ≥60 mL/min/1.73 m^2 on POD 1. Intraoperative findings revealed that living donors with eGFR < 60 mL/min/1.73 m^2 on POD 1 had a lower proportion of ITMB intervention and lower HR and body temperature levels, compared with living donors with eGFR ≥60 mL/min/1.73 m^2 on POD 1.

Association of pre- and intraoperative findings with eGFR < 60 mL/min/1.73 m^2 on POD 1

Multivariable logistic regression analyses (Table 3) suggested that the analgesic intervention of ITMB played a critical and independent role in reducing the potential risk for development of eGFR < 60 mL/min/1.73 m^2 on POD 1. Additionally, male sex, older age, and a lower hourly fluid infusion rate were significantly associated with a higher risk for development of an eGFR < 60 mL/min/1.73 m^2 on POD 1. Our risk stratification model for donors with eGFR < 60 mL/min/1.73 m^2 on POD 1 showed association with non-ITMB, male sex, older age, and lower hourly fluid infusion rate (area under the receiver operating characteristic curve = 0.783; 95% CI = 0.734–0.832; $p < 0.001$).

In living donors with preoperative eGFRs ≥90 mL/min/1.73 m^2 ($n = 197$; Additional file 1), preoperative findings of male sex and older age, and several

Table 1 Perioperative baseline characteristics in living donors undergoing laparoscopic nephrectomy

	Living donors
n	**366**
Preoperative characteristics	
Sex (male)	154 (42.1%)
Age (years)	46 ± 12
Body mass index ≥25 kg/m^2	122 (33.3%)
Hypertension	21 (5.7%)
Remnant kidney volume (mL)	176.0 ± 35.4
Estimated glomerular filtration rate (mL/min/1.73 m^2)	
≥ 90	197 (53.8%)
89–60	169 (46.2%)
Laboratory variables	
White blood cell count (× 10^9/L)	6.1 ± 1.7
Hemoglobin (g/dL)	14.1 ± 1.5
Platelet count (× 10^9/L)	250.9 ± 58.0
Glucose (mg/dL)	97 ± 10
Albumin (g/dL)	4.4 ± 0.3
Sodium (mEq/L)	142 ± 2
Potassium (mEq/L)	4.3 ± 0.3
Chloride (mEq/L)	105 ± 3
International normalized ratio	1.00 ± 0.06
Activated partial thrombin time (s)	27.7 ± 3.1
Intraoperative findings	
Total surgery duration (min)	171 ± 29
Intrathecal morphine block	116 (31.7%)
Average vital signs	
Systolic blood pressure (mmHg)	123 ± 13
Diastolic blood pressure (mmHg)	77 ± 9
Heart rate (beats/min)	73 ± 10
Body temperature (°C)	36.4 ± 0.5
Hourly fluid infusion (mL/kg/h)	5.1 ± 2.9
Hourly urine output (mL/kg/h)	1.3 ± 1.1
Total blood loss (mL)	95 ± 98
Postoperative findings	
Total days of hospitalization	4 ± 1
Estimated glomerular filtration rate on POD 1	
≥ 60 mL/min/1.73 m^2	126 (34.4%)
< 60 mL/min/1.73 m^2	240 (65.6%)
Estimated glomerular filtration rate on POD 7	
≥ 60 mL/min/1.73 m^2	125 (34.2%)
< 60 mL/min/1.73 m^2	241 (65.8%)

Values are expressed as means (± SDs) and numbers (percentages)
Abbreviations: *POD* postoperative day

intraoperative findings (i.e., non-ITMB, a higher average DBP, and lower hourly fluid infusion and urine output rates) were associated with a higher risk for development of an eGFR < 60 mL/min/1.73 m^2 on POD 1. In those with preoperative eGFRs of 89–60 mL/min/1.73 m^2 ($n =$ 169; Additional file 2), a preoperative finding of older age and an intraoperative finding (non-ITMB) were associated with a higher risk for development of an eGFR < 60 mL/min/1.73 m^2 on POD 1.

Comparison of pre- and intraoperative findings between the non-ITMB and ITMB groups in PS-matching analysis

Pre- and intraoperative findings in the non-ITMB and ITMB groups were assessed by PS-matching analysis (Table 4). Significant differences were observed in preoperative findings (i.e., sex, an eGFR of 89–60 mL/min/1.73 m^2, hemoglobin level, and sodium level) and intraoperative findings (i.e., total surgery duration, average DBP and body temperature, hourly fluid infusion rate, and total blood loss), according to ITMB intervention status before PS matching. After PS-matching analysis, no significant differences in pre- or intraoperative findings were observed according to the ITMB intervention.

Comparison of remnant kidney function according to eGFR status on PODs 1 and 7 between PS-matched non-ITMB and ITMB groups

The prevalence rates in living donors with eGFR < 60 mL/min/1.73 m^2 on PODs 1 and 7 were significantly higher in the non-ITMB group than in the ITMB group (Fig. 2).

After adjustment for PS, ITMB was significantly associated with eGFR < 60 mL/min/1.73 m^2 on POD 1

After adjustment for PS, the ITMB group was significantly associated with lower risk for development of eGFR < 60 mL/min/1.73 m^2 on POD 1 in PS-matched living donors (Table 5).

Comparisons of postoperative peak NRS and laboratory variables between PS-matched living donors with and without ITMB

On POD 1 (Additional file 3), a high percentage of living donors with ITMB experienced a mild degree of pain (peak NRS ≤3 in 83.0% [$n = 88$] of donors); however, living donors without ITMB generally experienced a severe degree of pain (peak NRS ≥7 in 77.4% [$n = 82$] of donors). Cumulative IV-PCA consumption was higher in the non-ITMB group than in the ITMB group. The peak SBP, DBP and HR values were higher in the non-ITMB group than in the ITMB group.

Laboratory variables (Additional file 4) were comparable between the non-ITMB and ITMB groups on PODs 1 and 7. Although the chloride level on POD 7 differed between the two groups, the levels were within normal limits [27].

Table 2 Comparisons of pre- and intraoperative findings between living donors with eGFR ≥60 mL/min/1.73 m^2 and those with eGFR < 60 mL/min/1.73 m^2 on POD 1

Group	eGFR ≥ 60 mL/min/1.73 m^2 on POD 1	eGFR < 60 mL/min/1.73 m^2 on POD 1	p
n	126	240	
Preoperative findings			
Male sex: n (%)	39 (31.0%)	115 (47.9%)	0.002
Age (years)	43 (29–53)	51 (42–58)	< 0.001
Body mass index ≥25 kg/m^2	34 (27.0%)	88 (36.7%)	0.062
Hypertension n (%)	2 (1.6%)	19 (7.9%)	0.013
Remnant kidney volume (mL)	173.0 (149.5–203.5)	170.0 (148.5–200.0)	0.717
eGFR			
≥ 90 mL/min/1.73 m^2	64 (50.8%)	133 (55.4%)	0.399
89–60 mL/min/1.73 m^2	62 (49.2%)	107 (44.6%)	
Laboratory variables			
White blood cell count (× 10^9/L)	5.9 (5.0–7.0)	5.8 (5.1–6.7)	0.796
Hemoglobin (g/dL)	13.7 (12.8–14.9)	14.1 (13.3–15.3)	0.004
Platelet count (× 10^9/L)	246.5 (216.8–304.8)	243.0 (213.3–280.8)	0.115
Glucose (mg/dL)	95 (90–101)	97 (92–103)	0.109
Albumin (g/dL)	4.5 (4.3–4.6)	4.5 (4.3–4.6)	0.724
Sodium (mEq/L)	141 (140–142)	142 (141–143)	0.001
Potassium (mEq/L)	4.3 (4.1–4.4)	4.3 (4.1–4.5)	0.519
Chloride (mEq/L)	104 (103–106)	105 (104–106)	0.125
International normalized ratio	1.01 (0.97–1.04)	0.99 (0.96–1.03)	0.010
aPTT (s)	27.4 (26.0–29.1)	27.1 (25.6–28.5)	0.156
Intraoperative findings			
Intrathecal morphine block	63 (50.0%)	53 (22.1%)	< 0.001
Total surgery duration (min)	170 (155–190)	170 (147–190)	0.214
Average vital signs			
Systolic blood pressure (mmHg)	120 (112–130)	120 (115–130)	0.596
Diastolic blood pressure (mmHg)	80 (70–80)	80 (70–80)	0.298
Heart rate (beats/min)	76 (70–82)	72 (64–80)	< 0.001
Body temperature (°C)	36.5 (36.3–36.8)	36.4 (36.1–36.6)	< 0.001
Hourly fluid infusion (mL/kg/h)	4.7 (3.3–7.0)	4.4 (2.9–6.2)	0.144
Hourly urine output (mL/kg/h)	1.0 (0.7–1.7)	0.9 (0.6–1.6)	0.084
Total blood loss (mL)	50 (50–100)	70 (50–100)	0.353

Values are expressed as medians (interquartile ranges) and numbers (percentages)
Abbreviations: *eGFR* estimated glomerular filtration rate, *aPTT* activated partial thrombin time, *POD* postoperative day

During the follow-up period, there were no ITMB-associated complications, such as puncture site infection, post-dural puncture headache, lower limb numbness, respiratory depression, or bleeding, and all living donors were determined to be grade I on the Clavien-Dindo classification.

Discussion

This study showed that 65.6% (*n* = 240) of living donors undergoing laparoscopic nephrectomy for kidney transplantation exhibited delayed functional recovery of remnant kidney (eGFR < 60 mL/min/1.73 m^2 on POD 1). Our proposed risk stratification model showed association with preoperative findings (male sex and older age) and intraoperative findings (non-ITMB and lower hourly fluid infusion rate). PS-matching analysis revealed that living donors with ITMB had lower incidences of eGFR < 60 mL/min/1.73 m^2 on PODs 1 and 7, compared to living donors without ITMB. The analgesic impact of ITMB appeared to lower the risk for delayed functional recovery of remnant kidney (0.257-fold lower than risk in the non-ITMB group) on POD 1.

Table 3 Associations of pre- and intraoperative findings with eGFR < 60 mL/min/1.73 m^2 on postoperative day 1

	Univariable logistic regression analysis				Multivariable logistic regression analysis			
	ß	Odds ratio	95% CI	p	ß	Odds ratio	95% CI	p
Preoperative findings								
Female sex	−0.719	0.487	0.309–0.768	0.002	−0.987	0.373	0.214–0.65	0.001
Age (years)	0.055	1.057	1.037–1.077	< 0.001	0.071	1.074	1.05–1.098	< 0.001
Body mass index ≥25 kg/m^2	−0.449	0.638	0.398–1.024	0.063				
Hypertension	1.673	5.330	1.221–23.265	0.026				
Remnant kidney volume (mL)	−0.001	0.999	0.993–1.005	0.725				
eGFR ≥90 mL/min/1.73 m^2	−0.186	0.83	0.539–1.279	0.399				
Laboratory variables								
White blood cell count (× 10^9/L)	−0.041	0.960	0.844–1.092	0.535				
Hemoglobin (g/dL)	0.219	1.245	1.072–1.447	0.004				
Platelet count (× 10^9/L)	−0.005	0.995	0.991–0.999	0.007				
Glucose (mg/dL)	0.012	1.012	0.991–1.035	0.267				
Albumin (g/dL)	−0.286	0.751	0.316–1.786	0.518				
Sodium (mEq/L)	0.205	1.227	1.076–1.399	0.002				
Potassium (mEq/L)	0.396	1.485	0.689–3.202	0.313				
Chloride (mEq/L)	0.079	1.083	0.965–1.215	0.177				
International normalized ratio	−3.633	0.026	0.001–1.172	0.06				
Activated partial thrombin time (s)	−0.054	0.948	0.885–1.015	0.127				
Intraoperative findings								
Time effect[a]	0.000	1.000	0.997–1.002	0.639				
Analgesic intervention								
No ITMB	Reference				Reference			
ITMB	−1.261	0.283	0.178–0.451	< 0.001	−1.341	0.262	0.154–0.445	< 0.001
Total surgery duration (min)	−0.004	0.996	0.989–1.003	0.280				
Average vital signs								
Systolic blood pressure (mmHg)	0.006	1.006	0.990–1.024	0.458				
Diastolic blood pressure (mmHg)	0.018	1.018	0.994–1.043	0.135				
Heart rate (beats/min)	−0.041	0.960	0.939–0.981	< 0.001				
Body temperature (°C)	−0.765	0.466	0.257–0.843	0.012				
Hourly fluid infusion (mL/kg/h)	−0.065	0.937	0.871–1.009	0.084	−0.105	0.9	0.826–0.981	0.017
Hourly urine output (mL/kg/h)	−0.147	0.864	0.714–1.045	0.131				
Total blood loss (mL)	0.000	1.000	0.998–1.003	0.795				

Abbreviations: eGFR, estimated glomerular filtration rate; ITMB, intrathecal morphine block
[a]Time effect was determined by the serial order of the living donors from the first (no. 1) to the most recent (no. 366)

Although the mechanism connecting analgesia to remnant kidney function remains unclear, good analgesia may safely and effectively enhance remnant kidney function recovery after kidney donation. In our model of risk stratification, ITMB, an analgesic intervention, is clinically modifiable; after PS-matched adjustment, ITMB pain relief attenuated the eGFR loss during the early postoperative period. Effective preoperative pain-relief, such as ITMB, can promote postoperative recovery in patients undergoing abdominal surgery [11]. In patients undergoing aortic valve replacement surgery,

ITMB provided appropriate analgesic effects (lower opioid consumption and pain score), hemodynamic stability (tolerable cardiac output), and early postoperative recovery (earlier endotracheal extubation and shorter ICU administration) [28]. In organ transplantation settings, ITMB resulted in predominantly lower pain score on POD 1, compared to other analgesic practices (i.e., IV-PCA, wound infiltration, and peripheral nerve block) [10, 12, 21, 29]. The results of a small KT study by Sener et al. [30] suggested that analgesic care played a role in postoperative organ function recovery, including that of

Table 4 Comparisons of pre- and intraoperative findings between non-ITMB and ITMB groups using propensity score-matching analysis

Group	Before propensity score matched analysis				After propensity score matched analysis			
	non-ITMB	ITMB	p	SD	non-ITMB	ITMB	p	SD
n	250	116			106	106		
Preoperative findings								
Female sex (%)	133 (53.2%)	79 (68.1%)	0.007	0.318	65 (61.3%)	70 (66.0%)	0.475	0.101
Age (years)	50 (38–57)	48 (37–55)	0.258	−0.114	48 (36–56)	48 (37–56)	0.835	0.039
Body mass index ≥25 kg/m²	88 (35.2%)	34 (29.3%)	0.266	0.129	32 (30.2%)	33 (31.1%)	0.882	−0.021
Hypertension	18 (7.2%)	3 (2.6%)	0.077	−0.289	2 (1.9%)	3 (2.8%)	> 0.999	0.059
Remnant kidney volume (mL)	170.0 (148.0–202.0)	170.0 (150.0–200.0)	0.938	−0.025	170.0 (148.0–202.0)	170.0 (150.0–200.0)	0.721	0.014
eGFR (89–60 mL/min/1.73 m²)	136 (54.4%)	33 (28.4%)	< 0.001	−0.573	41 (38.7%)	33 (31.1%)	0.249	−0.167
Laboratory variables								
WBC count (× 10⁹/L)	5.9 (5.0–6.9)	5.8 (5.1–6.8)	0.836	0.009	5.8 (5.0–6.8)	5.9 (5.0–6.8)	0.881	0.012
Hemoglobin (g/dL)	14.1 (13.3–15.3)	13.7 (12.7–14.9)	0.003	−0.323	14.0 (13.2–15.2)	13.8 (12.8–14.9)	0.215	−0.184
Platelet count (× 10⁹/L)	243.0 (211.8–281.8)	248.0 (220.5–294.0)	0.216	0.149	242.5 (215.0–291.3)	243.5 (218.0–294.0)	0.937	−0.029
Glucose (mg/dL)	96 (91–103)	97 (91–103)	0.655	0.083	97 (92–103)	97 (91–102)	0.703	−0.055
Albumin (g/dL)	4.5 (4.2–4.6)	4.5 (4.3–4.7)	0.067	0.245	4.5 (4.3–4.7)	4.5 (4.3–4.7)	0.641	−0.045
Sodium (mEq/L)	142 (141–143)	141 (141–143)	0.024	−0.219	142 (141–143)	142 (141–143)	0.766	−0.028
Potassium (mEq/L)	4.3 (4.1–4.4)	4.3 (4.1–4.5)	0.942	−0.016	4.3 (4.1–4.4)	4.3 (4.1–4.5)	0.57	0.067
Chloride (mEq/L)	105 (104–106)	104 (103–106)	0.090	−0.243	104 (103–106)	105 (103–106)	0.713	−0.133
INR	1.00 (0.96–1.03)	1.00 (0.96–1.04)	0.350	0.096	1.00 (0.97–1.03)	1.00 (0.96–1.04)	0.561	−0.065
aPTT (s)	27.5 (25.6–29.1)	27.0 (25.8–28.2)	0.118	−0.271	27.0 (25.6–28.5)	26.9 (25.8–28.3)	0.686	−0.124
Intraoperative findings								
Surgery duration (min)	175 (160–190)	155 (140–180)	< 0.001	−0.531	165 (150–185)	160 (140–185)	0.108	−0.188
Average of vital signs								
SBP (mmHg)	120 (116–130)	120 (112–130)	0.727	−0.056	120 (120–130)	121 (112–131)	0.884	0.029
DBP (mmHg)	80 (70–80)	80 (72–88)	0.002	0.339	80 (71–80)	80 (74–87)	0.137	0.158
Heart rate (beats/min)	74 (67–80)	72 (63–80)	0.266	−0.086	74 (64–80)	72 (63–80)	0.455	−0.06
Body temperature (°C)	36.5 (36.3–36.7)	36.3 (36.1–36.6)	0.002	−0.275	36.5 (36.2–36.7)	36.4 (36.1–36.6)	0.311	−0.091

208   Assessment and Multimodal Management of Pain

Table 4 Comparisons of pre- and intraoperative findings between non-ITMB and ITMB groups using propensity score-matching analysis (*Continued*)

Group	Before propensity score matched analysis				After propensity score matched analysis			
	non-ITMB	ITMB	*p*	SD	non-ITMB	ITMB	*p*	SD
n	250	116			106	106		
Hourly fluid infusion (mL/kg/h)	4.86 (3.35–7.03)	3.80 (2.56–5.67)	<0.001	−0.348	4.79 (2.84–6.19)	3.82 (2.62–5.85)	0.215	−0.079
Hourly urine output (mL/kg/h)	0.98 (0.67–1.71)	0.96 (0.63–1.52)	0.261	−0.284	0.86 (0.65–1.39)	0.96 (0.62–1.51)	0.655	0.039
Total blood loss (mL)	95 (50–100)	50 (50–100)	0.017	−0.451	50 (50–100)	50 (50–100)	0.48	−0.068

Values are expressed as median (interquartile) and numbers (proportions)

Abbreviations: ITMB intrathecal morphine block, eGFR estimated glomerular filtration, WBC white blood cell, INR international normalized ratio, aPTT activated partial thrombin time, SBP systolic blood pressure, DBP diastolic blood pressure

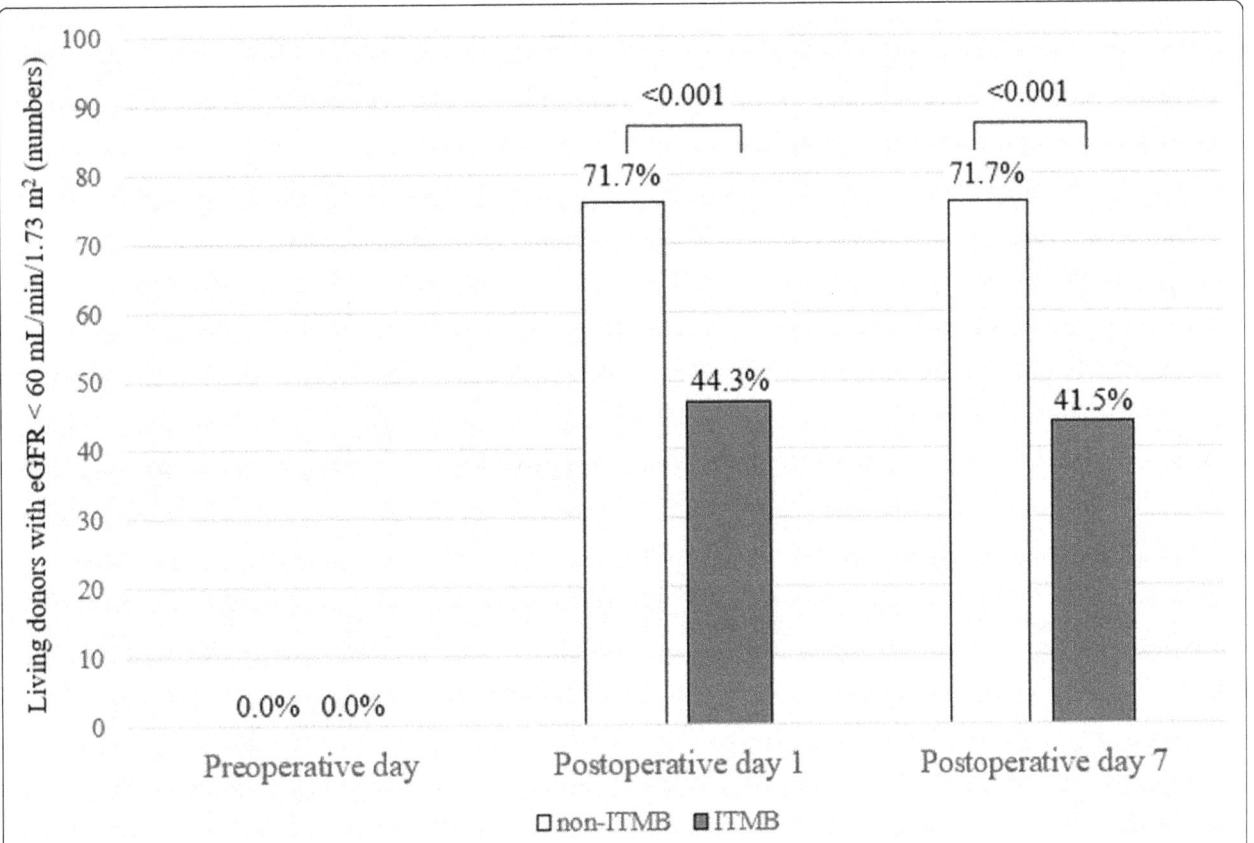

Fig. 2 Comparison of remnant kidney function in living donors with eGFRs < 60 mL/min/1.73 m² on the preoperative day and postoperative days 1 and 7 between PS-matched non-ITMB and ITMB groups. Values are expressed as numbers with proportions (%)

kidneys. However, the authors reported that parameters of kidney graft function (i.e., glomerular filtration rate, microalbuminuria, or creatinine clearance rate) for 2 days postoperatively were similar between grafts from living donors with and without combined spinal-epidural anesthesia. However, a larger KT study by Baar et al. [31] revealed that the incidence of delayed graft function, defined as the requirement of any renal replacement therapy within 1 week postoperatively, was significantly lower in patients who received grafts from living donors with epidural analgesic care than in patients who received grafts from living donors without epidural analgesic care. Potentially, the delayed graft function originates from complex cascades, including hypoxia/ischemia-reperfusion injury and impaired repair mechanisms, which may become aggravated by surgical trauma related to activation of the sympathetic stress response [7, 32]. Therefore, the effective prevention of

nociceptive pathways during/after surgery may lead to reduction in overactivity of the sympathetic stress response and subsequent improvement in organ microcirculation and recovery of function [33, 34]. In our study, PS-matched living donors who received ITMB prior to surgery showed markedly improved pain score (i.e., lower peak pain score and cumulative IV-PCA consumption) and more stable hemodynamic parameters (i.e., acceptable SBP, DBP and HR) during the first 24 h postoperatively, compared to those who did not receive ITMB, suggesting that ITMB may attenuate severe pain-related stress responses (i.e., sympathetic activation and vasoconstriction) and maintain homeostasis for optimal function of remnant kidney [35].

In this study, male sex was associated with a higher risk for delayed function recovery of remnant kidney. These findings were supported by Bellini et al. [36], who showed that the reduction in eGFR between pre- and

Table 5 Association of ITMB with eGFR < 60 mL/min/1.73 m² on postoperative day 1

	ß	Odds ratio	95% CI	p
PS-matched living donors (n = 212)				
ITMB adjusted for PS	−1.358	0.257	0.14–0.474	< 0.001

Abbreviations: ITMB intrathecal morphine block, eGFR estimated glomerular filtration rate, PS propensity score

post-donation was greater in male donors, whereas postoperative recovery of kidney function was greater in female donors. Massie et al. [37] reported that male donors had a 1.88-fold greater risk (95% CI = 1.50–2.35; $p < 0.001$) for post-donation renal failure, compared to female donors. Previous studies found that female sex showed stronger protective effects against kidney injury after donor nephrectomy. The authors suggested that sex differences in vulnerability of kidney injury were potentially due to sex hormonal modulation [38–40]. In an experimental model of ischemic kidney injury, rates of severe dysfunction and histologic damage were lower in females than males, and oophorectomy or testosterone administration exacerbated poor renal outcomes. However, estrogen infusion had kidney-protective effects [41, 42]. However, female sex has been regarded as a risk factor for acute kidney injury associated with cardiac surgery, aminoglycoside nephrotoxicity, contrast-induced nephropathy, and rhabdomyolysis [43–46]. The risk to male and female individuals might differ according to the sex-specific impact of factors, such as comorbidities and drug use history.

In this study, older donor age was associated with a higher risk of delayed functional recovery of the remnant kidney. In a European living kidney donor study, younger donors showed a higher post-donation eGFR and better recovery of remnant kidney function compared to older donors (> 60 years) [36]. In a living kidney donor study from the US, older age was also associated with increased risk of delayed functional recovery of the remnant kidney (hazard ratio = 1.40; 95% CI = 1.23–1.59; $p < 0.001$). Donor age is associated with comorbidities of the natural aging process; therefore, the postoperative reserve capacity of kidney function may gradually decrease over time. Nevertheless, the overall safety of living donors at older ages has been acceptable with respect to perioperative outcomes (i.e., operation duration, hemorrhage, hospital admission period, and potential risk for long-term kidney failure) [47, 48]. Additionally, young donors, who are expected to live for more than 60 years, may be more vulnerable to injuries or comorbidities in the future, such as hypertension and DM, compared to older healthy donors and younger individuals who have not undergone organ transplantation [5]. Therefore, a living donation strategy should not be discouraged on the basis of age alone.

In our study, lower hourly fluid infusion rate during surgery was associated with a higher risk for early remnant kidney dysfunction. Clinically, adequate correction of intravascular hypovolemia is a critical component for the prevention and treatment of acute kidney injury [49]. During surgery, optimal maintenance of intravascular volume by intravascular fluid administration is necessary to avoid volume deficiency caused by osmotic loss,

evaporation, and hemorrhage. Excessive fluid restriction is associated with an increased risk of organ hypoperfusion and subsequent dysfunction [50–52]. In particular, kidney function is vulnerable to acute changes in volume status, with low volume posing a potential hazard of postoperative kidney damage [49, 53]. Intraoperative pneumoperitoneum during laparoscopic surgery may aggravate the effect of intravascular hypovolemia on systemic circulation, eventually leading to lower renal blood flow and glomerular filtration rate [54]. However, fluid overload is also associated with adverse clinical outcomes, and may directly contribute to kidney injury related to intrarenal compartment syndrome and venous congestion due to encapsulation of the kidneys [55–57]. Aggressive fluid therapy may lead to an imbalance of the renal oxygen supply-demand relationship as a result of increased glomerular filtration rate and sodium reabsorption [58]. Therefore, to maintain appropriate euvolemia, organ perfusion, and oxygen delivery, meticulous monitoring of intraoperative fluid input is essential, in combination with regular estimation of fluid responsiveness and hemodynamic status.

This study had several limitations. First, we were unable to directly measure the analgesic effect of ITMB on systemic/renal hemodynamics. Although our findings regarding severity of pain are consistent with overactivity of the sympathetic stress response, further studies are needed to investigate the role of severe pain on systemic/renal vascular flow and/or perfusion [59, 60]. Second, we were unable to investigate long-term outcomes because of the short analgesic duration of ITMB (within 24 h). However, our donors with ITMB showed better renal recovery in the early (POD 1) and intermediate (POD 7) postoperative periods, compared to donors without ITMB. Because most patients undergoing surgery experience the peak pain level on the first day postoperatively, appropriate and immediate pain relief control may be necessary to achieve enhanced postoperative recovery [61]. Third, we were unable to determine optimal cut-off levels for donor age and hourly fluid infusion. Further prospective studies are needed to investigate such levels for guidance in donation and management. Fourth, we were unable to measure total IV opioid consumption, because various rescue IV opioids were selected based on the preferences and discretion of the attending physicians. The direct effect of IV opioid on remnant kidney function remains unclear; thus, further investigations are needed to determine the role of IV opioid administration, as a component of a multimodal pain-relief approach, on systemic/renal hemodynamics in living donors. Lastly, the ITMB group contained a larger proportion of females, and had a lower BMI and higher baseline eGFR after PS-matching analysis, where all of these factors are associated with improved renal function independent of any effects of ITMB.

Conclusions

The clinical safety and satisfaction of living donors during the perioperative period are key issues in living donor KT. After nephrectomy, enhanced recovery of remnant kidney function in living donors is critical for preventing the development of chronic kidney dysfunction. This study revealed an association between ITMB and better functional recovery of remnant kidney in living kidney donors. In addition to conferring favorable analgesic results, the use of ITMB resulted in enhanced renal function recovery in living kidney donors. To identify living kidney donors at potential risk for delayed renal function recovery, we propose a stratification model that includes male sex, older age, non-ITMB, and lower hourly fluid infusion rate. Further investigations are needed to confirm our findings in larger populations and in the context of long-term outcomes.

Supplementary information

Additional file 1. Association of pre- and intraoperative findings with eGFR < 60 mL/min/1.73 m^2 on postoperative day 1 in living donors with preoperative eGFR ≥90 mL/min/1.73 m^2 ($n = 197$).

Additional file 2. Association of pre- and intraoperative findings with eGFR < 60 mL/min/1.73 m^2 on postoperative day 1 in living donors with preoperative eGFR of 89–60 mL/min/1.73 m^2 ($n = 169$).

Additional file 3. Comparison of pain and hemodynamic outcomes on postoperative day 1 between propensity score-matched living donors with and without intrathecal morphine block.

Additional file 4. Comparison of laboratory variables on postoperative days 1 and 7 between propensity score-matched living donors with and without intrathecal morphine block.

Abbreviations

KT: Kidney transplantation; RRT: Renal replacement therapy; DM: Diabetes mellitus; ITMB: Intrathecal morphine block; IV: Intravenous; SBP: Systolic blood pressure; DBP: Diastolic blood pressure; HR: Heart rate; BT: Body temperature; IV-PCA: Intravenous patient-control analgesia; NRS: Numeric rating scale; PACU: Post-anesthesia care unit; POD: Postoperative day; eGFR: Estimated glomerular filtration rate; BMI: Body mass index; PS: Propensity score

Acknowledgements

All authors thank Eunju Choi, Hyeji An, and Hyunsook Yoo (Anesthesia Nursing Unit, Seoul St. Mary's Hospital, The Catholic University of Korea, Seoul, Republic of Korea) for participating in our study.

Authors' contributions

JP and MSC designed the study, wrote the manuscript, and analyzed and interpreted the data. JP, MK, YHP, JWS, HML, YSK, YEM, SHH, and MSC collected the data and provided critical comments. MP performed the statistical analyses. All authors revised the manuscript critically for important intellectual content. All authors read and approved the final manuscript.

Author details

^{1}Department of Anesthesiology and Pain Medicine, Seoul St. Mary's Hospital, College of Medicine, The Catholic University of Korea, 222, Banpo-daero, Seocho-gu, Seoul 06591, Republic of Korea. ^{2}Department of Urology, Seoul St. Mary's Hospital, College of Medicine, The Catholic University of Korea, Seoul, Republic of Korea. ^{3}Department of Biostatistics, Clinical Research Coordinating Center, Catholic Medical Center, The Catholic University of Korea, Seoul, South Korea.

References

1. Kasiske BL, Snyder J, Matas A, Collins A. The impact of transplantation on survival with kidney failure. Clin Transpl. 2000:135–43.
2. Cecka JM. Kidney transplantation in the United States. Clin Transpl. 2008:1–18.
3. Terasaki PI, Cecka JM, Gjertson DW, Takemoto S. High survival rates of kidney transplants from spousal and living unrelated donors. N Engl J Med. 1995;333:333–6.
4. Muzaale AD, Massie AB, Wang MC, Montgomery RA, McBride MA, Wainright JL, et al. Risk of end-stage renal disease following live kidney donation. JAMA. 2014;311:579–86.
5. Grams ME, Sang Y, Levey AS, Matsushita K, Ballew S, Chang AR, et al. Kidney-failure risk projection for the living kidney-donor candidate. N Engl J Med. 2016;374:411–21.
6. Schroppel B, Legendre C. Delayed kidney graft function: from mechanism to translation. Kidney Int. 2014;86:251–8.
7. Warltier DC, Pagel PS, Kersten JR. Approaches to the prevention of perioperative myocardial ischemia. Anesthesiology. 2000;92:253–9.
8. Zubrzycki M, Liebold A, Skrabal C, Reinelt H, Ziegler M, Perdas E, et al. Assessment and pathophysiology of pain in cardiac surgery. J Pain Res. 2018;11:1599–611.
9. Menjivar A, Torres X. Assessment of donor satisfaction as an essential part of living donor kidney transplantation: an eleven-year retrospective study. Transplant Int. 2018;31:1332–44.
10. Jun JH, Kim GS, Lee JJ, Ko JS, Kim SJ, Jeon PH. Comparison of intrathecal morphine and surgical-site infusion of ropivacaine as adjuncts to intravenous patient-controlled analgesia in living-donor kidney transplant recipients. Singap Med J. 2017;58:666–73.
11. Koning MV, Teunissen AJW, van der Harst E, Ruijgrok EJ, Stolker RJ. Intrathecal morphine for laparoscopic segmental colonic resection as part of an enhanced recovery protocol: a randomized controlled trial. Reg Anesth Pain Med. 2018;43:166–73.
12. Ko JS, Choi SJ, Gwak MS, Kim GS, Ahn HJ, Kim JA, et al. Intrathecal morphine combined with intravenous patient-controlled analgesia is an effective and safe method for immediate postoperative pain control in live liver donors. Liver Transpl. 2009;15:381–9.
13. Lentine KL, Kasiske BL, Levey AS, Adams PL, Alberu J, Bakr MA, et al. KDIGO clinical practice guideline on the evaluation and Care of Living Kidney Donors. Transplantation. 2017;101:S1–s109.
14. Seo SI, Kim JC, Hwangbo K, Park YH, Hwang TK. Comparison of hand-assisted laparoscopic and open donor nephrectomy: a single-center experience from South Korea. J Endourol. 2005;19:58–62.
15. Tabrizian P, Giacca M, Prigoff J, Tran B, Holzner ML, Chin E, et al. Renal safety of intravenous ketorolac use after donor nephrectomy. Prog Transplant. 2019;29:283–6.
16. Campsen J, Call T, Allen CM, Presson AP, Martinez E, Rofaiel G, et al. Prospective, double-blind, randomized clinical trial comparing an ERAS pathway with ketorolac and pregabalin versus standard of care plus placebo during live donor nephrectomy for kidney transplant. Am J Transplant. 2019;19:1777–81.
17. Freedland SJ, Blanco-Yarosh M, Sun JC, Hale SJ, Elashoff DA, Rajfer J, et al. Effect of ketorolac on renal function after donor nephrectomy. Urology. 2002;59:826–30.
18. Freedland SJ, Blanco-Yarosh M, Sun JC, Hale SJ, Elashoff DA, Litwin MS, et al. Ketorolac-based analgesia improves outcomes for living kidney donors. Transplantation. 2002;73:741–5.
19. Rege A, Leraas H, Vikraman D, Ravindra K, Brennan T, Miller T, et al. Could the use of an enhanced recovery protocol in laparoscopic donor nephrectomy be an incentive for live kidney donation? Cureus. 2016;8:e889.
20. Cywinski JB, Parker BM, Xu M, Irefin SA. A comparison of postoperative pain control in patients after right lobe donor hepatectomy and major hepatic resection for tumor. Anesth Analg. 2004;99:1747–52 table of contents.
21. Kang R, Chin KJ. Bilateral single-injection erector spinae plane block versus intrathecal morphine for postoperative analgesia in living donor laparoscopic hepatectomy: a randomized non-inferiority trial; 2019.

22. Levey AS, Coresh J, Greene T, Stevens LA, Zhang YL, Hendriksen S, et al. Using standardized serum creatinine values in the modification of diet in renal disease study equation for estimating glomerular filtration rate. Ann Intern Med. 2006;145:247–54.

23. Levey AS, Coresh J, Balk E, Kausz AT, Levin A, Steffes MW, et al. National Kidney Foundation practice guidelines for chronic kidney disease: evaluation, classification, and stratification. Ann Intern Med. 2003;139:137–47.

24. Flegal KM, Kit BK, Orpana H, Graubard BI. Association of all-cause mortality with overweight and obesity using standard body mass index categories: a systematic review and meta-analysis. JAMA. 2013;309:71–82.

25. Elliott WJ. Systemic hypertension. Curr Probl Cardiol. 2007;32:201–59.

26. Clavien PA, Barkun J, de Oliveira ML, Vauthey JN, Dindo D, Schulick RD, et al. The Clavien-Dindo classification of surgical complications: five-year experience. Ann Surg. 2009;250:187–96.

27. Alam MN, Uddin MJ, Rahman KM, Ahmed S, Akhter M, Nahar N, et al. Electrolyte changes in stroke. Mymensingh Med J. 2012;21:594–9.

28. Elgendy H, Helmy HAR. Intrathecal morphine improves hemodynamic parameters and analgesia in patients undergoing aortic valve replacement surgery: a prospective, double-blind, randomized trial. Pain Physician. 2017;20:405–12.

29. Lee SH, Gwak MS, Choi SJ, Park HG, Kim GS, Kim MH, et al. Prospective, randomized study of ropivacaine wound infusion versus intrathecal morphine with intravenous fentanyl for analgesia in living donors for liver transplantation. Liver Transpl. 2013;19:1036–45.

30. Sener M, Torgay A, Akpek E, Colak T, Karakayali H, Arslan G, et al. Regional versus general anesthesia for donor nephrectomy: effects on graft function. Transplant Proc. 2004;36:2954–8.

31. Baar W, Goebel U, Buerkle H, Jaenigen B, Kaufmann K, Heinrich S. Lower rate of delayed graft function is observed when epidural analgesia for living donor nephrectomy is administered. BMC Anesthesiol. 2019;19:38.

32. Perico N, Cattaneo D, Sayegh MH, Remuzzi G. Delayed graft function in kidney transplantation. Lancet. 2004;364:1814–27.

33. Daudel F, Freise H, Westphal M, Stubbe HD, Lauer S, Bone HG, et al. Continuous thoracic epidural anesthesia improves gut mucosal microcirculation in rats with sepsis. Shock. 2007;28:610–4.

34. Nygard E, Kofoed KF, Freiberg J, Holm S, Aldershvile J, Eliasen K, et al. Effects of high thoracic epidural analgesia on myocardial blood flow in patients with ischemic heart disease. Circulation. 2005;111:2165–70.

35. Grassi G, Bertoli S, Seravalle G. Sympathetic nervous system: role in hypertension and in chronic kidney disease. Curr Opin Nephrol Hypertens. 2012;21:46–51.

36. Bellini MI, Charalampidis S, Stratigos I, Dor F, Papalois V. The effect of donors' demographic characteristics in renal function post-living kidney donation. analysis of a UK single centre cohort. J Clin Med. 2019;8:883.

37. Massie AB, Muzaale AD, Luo X, Chow EKH, Locke JE, Nguyen AQ, et al. Quantifying postdonation risk of ESRD in living kidney donors. J Am Soc Nephrol. 2017;28:2749–55.

38. Okumura K, Yamanaga S. Prediction model of compensation for contralateral kidney after living-donor donation. BMC Nephrol. 2019;20:283.

39. Neugarten J, Golestaneh L, Kolhe NV. Sex differences in acute kidney injury requiring dialysis. BMC Nephrol. 2018;19:131.

40. Neugarten J, Golestaneh L. Gender and the prevalence and progression of renal disease. Adv Chronic Kidney Dis. 2013;20:390–5.

41. Hutchens MP, Dunlap J, Hurn PD, Jarnberg PO. Renal ischemia: does sex matter? Anesth Analg. 2008;107:239–49.

42. Metcalfe PD, Meldrum KK. Sex differences and the role of sex steroids in renal injury. J Urol. 2006;176:15–21.

43. Neugarten J, Sandilya S, Singh B, Golestaneh L. Sex and the risk of AKI following cardio-thoracic surgery: a meta-analysis. Clin J Am Soc Nephrol. 2016;11:2113–22.

44. McMahon GM, Zeng X, Waikar SS. A risk prediction score for kidney failure or mortality in rhabdomyolysis. JAMA Intern Med. 2013;173:1821–8.

45. Mehran R, Aymong ED, Nikolsky E, Lasic Z, Iakovou I, Fahy M, et al. A simple risk score for prediction of contrast-induced nephropathy after percutaneous coronary intervention: development and initial validation. J Am Coll Cardiol. 2004;44:1393–9.

46. Moore RD, Smith CR, Lipsky JJ, Mellits ED, Lietman PS. Risk factors for nephrotoxicity in patients treated with aminoglycosides. Ann Intern Med. 1984;100:352–7.

47. Dols LF, Kok NF, Roodnat JI, Tran TC, Terkivatan T, Zuidema WC, et al. Living kidney donors: impact of age on long-term safety. Am J Transplant. 2011;11:737–42.

48. Stevens LA, Coresh J, Greene T, Levey AS. Assessing kidney function--measured and estimated glomerular filtration rate. N Engl J Med. 2006;354:2473–83.

49. Ostermann M, Liu K, Kashani K. Fluid management in acute kidney injury. Chest. 2019;156:594–603.

50. Shin CH, Long DR, McLean D, Grabitz SD, Ladha K, Timm FP, et al. Effects of intraoperative fluid management on postoperative outcomes: a hospital registry study. Ann Surg. 2018;267:1084–92.

51. Varadhan KK, Lobo DN. A meta-analysis of randomised controlled trials of intravenous fluid therapy in major elective open abdominal surgery: getting the balance right. Proc Nutr Soc. 2010;69:488–98.

52. Bundgaard-Nielsen M, Secher NH, Kehlet H. 'Liberal' vs. 'restrictive' perioperative fluid therapy--a critical assessment of the evidence. Acta Anaesthesiol Scand. 2009;53:843–51.

53. Prowle JR, Kirwan CJ, Bellomo R. Fluid management for the prevention and attenuation of acute kidney injury. Nat Rev Nephrol. 2014;10:37–47.

54. Mertens zur Borg IR, Di Biase M, Verbrugge S, Ijzermans JN, Gommers D. Comparison of three perioperative fluid regimes for laparoscopic donor nephrectomy : A prospective randomized dose-finding study. Surg Endosc. 2008;22:146–50.

55. Raimundo M, Crichton S, Martin JR, Syed Y, Varrier M, Wyncoll D, et al. Increased fluid administration after early acute kidney injury is associated with less renal recovery. Shock. 2015;44:431–7.

56. Finfer S, Myburgh J, Bellomo R. Intravenous fluid therapy in critically ill adults. Nat Rev Nephrol. 2018;14:541–57.

57. Prowle JR, Echeverri JE, Ligabo EV, Ronco C, Bellomo R. Fluid balance and acute kidney injury. Nat Rev Nephrol. 2010;6:107–15.

58. Skytte Larsson J, Bragadottir G, Krumbholz V, Redfors B, Sellgren J, Ricksten SE. Effects of acute plasma volume expansion on renal perfusion, filtration, and oxygenation after cardiac surgery: a randomized study on crystalloid vs colloid. Br J Anaesth. 2015;115:736–42.

59. Schlereth T, Birklein F. The sympathetic nervous system and pain. NeuroMolecular Med. 2008;10:141–7.

60. Hoiseth LO, Hisdal J, Hoff IE, Hagen OA, Landsverk SA, Kirkeboen KA. Tissue oxygen saturation and finger perfusion index in central hypovolemia: influence of pain. Crit Care Med. 2015;43:747–56.

61. Ljungqvist O. ERAS--enhanced recovery after surgery: moving evidence-based perioperative care to practice. JPEN J Parenter Enteral Nutr. 2014;38:559–66.

26

The combination of transversus abdominis plane block and rectus sheath block reduced postoperative pain after splenectomy

Jing-li Zhu[1], Xue-ting Wang[2], Jing Gong[2], Hai-bin Sun[2], Xiao-qing Zhao[2] and Wei Gao[3*]

Abstract

Background: Splenectomy performed with a curved incision results in severe postoperative pain. The aim of this study was to evaluate the effect of transversus abdominis plane block and rectus sheath block on postoperative pain relief and recovery.

Methods: A total of 150 patients were randomized into the control (C), levobupivacaine (L) and levobupivacaine/morphine (LM) groups. The patients in the C group received only patient-controlled analgesia. The patients in the L and LM groups received transversus abdominis plane block and rectus sheath block with levobupivacaine or levobupivacaine plus morphine. The intraoperative opioid consumption; postoperative pain score; time to first analgesic use; postoperative recovery data, including the times of first exhaust, defecation, oral intake and off-bed activity; the incidence of postoperative nausea and vomiting and antiemetics use; and the satisfaction score were recorded.

Results: Transversus abdominis plane block and rectus sheath block reduced intraoperative opioid consumption. The patients in the LM group showed lower postoperative pain scores, opioid consumption, postoperative nausea and vomiting incidence and antiemetic use and presented shorter recovery times and higher satisfaction scores.

Conclusions: The combination of transversus abdominis plane block and rectus sheath block with levobupivacaine and morphine can improve postoperative pain relief, reduce the consumption of analgesics, and partly accelerate postoperative recovery.

Keywords: Splenectomy, Transversus abdominis plane block, Rectus sheath block

Background

Splenectomy performed via a curved incision from the subxiphoid region to the anterior axillary line along the left subcostal margin results in injury to muscles, such as the rectus abdominis muscle, the external oblique muscle, the internal oblique muscle and the transversus abdominis muscle, etc. [1]. These broad injuries of the upper abdominal wall are the main contributors to severe postoperative pain [2], resulting in postoperative complications and a prolonged duration of recovery after the operation [3]. Sufficient analgesia could ameliorate postoperative nausea and vomiting (PONV), promote intestinal peristalsis, and enhance the recovery of patients [4]. Although patient-controlled analgesia (PCA) achieves higher patient satisfaction than epidural analgesia, PCA is the less effective of the two [5], while epidural analgesia is contraindicated because of coagulation disorders. Nerve block with the guidance of ultrasound can increase the success, safety and quality of regional nerve blocks [6]. Ultrasound-guided rectus sheath block (RSB) and transversus abdominis plane block (TAPB) were confirmed to reduce

* Correspondence: gaowei20055@126.com
[3]Department of Anesthesiology, the Second Affiliated Hospital of Harbin Medical University, 246 Xuefu Road, Nangang District, Harbin, Heilongjiang, China

postoperative pain and consumption of analgesics, decrease the incidence of postoperative complications and enhance recovery after the operation [7–9]. However, no study has investigated the analgesic efficacy of RSB or TAPB in splenectomy because neither the block range of RSB nor that of TAPB alone is sufficient for the surgical incision. Recently, some studies have applied both RSB and TAPB to reduce postoperative pain [10, 11]. Therefore, in this study, we performed ultrasound-guided RSB and TAPB and investigated their effect on postoperative pain and recovery after splenectomy.

Methods

Patients

This prospective, single-centre, randomized, parallel-group, double-blinded trial (Chinese Clinical Trial Registry: ChiCTR 1,800,015,141) was approved by the Ethics Committee of Harbin Medical University. The study adhered to the CONSORT guidelines and informed written consent was obtained from all patients.

After institutional review board approval (Harbin Medical University Institutional Research Board: KY2018–003), 150 Chinese patients aged 20–70 years who had an American Society of Anesthesiologists (ASA) Physical Status of II-III and underwent open splenectomy were included in this trial between March 2018 and July 2018. Patients with an ASA Physical Status of IV or higher, an allergy to local anaesthetics, a history of abdominal surgery, a body mass index < 15 kg.m^{-2} or > 40 kg.m^{-2} or severe cardiac and/or pulmonary dysfunction were excluded. Patients with acute or chronic preoperative opioid consumption or any other analgesic treatment for chronic pain before surgery, psychiatric or neurological factors (language barrier, neuropsychiatric disorder) were excluded. Patients who required postoperative mechanical ventilation, had sustained excessive haemorrhage (> 1 L of estimated blood loss) or required a massive transfusion and patients with failed nerve block (the needle could not be positioned in the anatomic structure and the drugs failed to enter the interspace) were also excluded.

Study design

The 150 patients for whom TAPB and RSB were successfully established were randomly divided into 3 groups: a control group (C), a levobupivacaine group (L) and a levobupivacaine/morphine group (LM) (n = 50). Patients in group C received general anaesthesia combined with RSB and TAPB with saline, and intravenous PCA for postoperative pain. Patients in groups L and LM received general anaesthesia combined with RSB and TAPB with levobupivacaine 0.2% alone or levobupivacaine 0.2% with morphine 30 μg.kg^{-1}. The dosage of morphine was adjusted according to paravertebral block [12].

All patients were monitored by continuous electrocardiography (ECG) and pulse oximetry (SpO$_2$). After local infiltration of lidocaine, the radial artery cannula was inserted to monitor the invasive blood pressure (BP). After induction with 0.03 mg.kg^{-1} midazolam, 1 mg.kg^{-1} lidocaine, 0.4 μg.kg^{-1} sufentanil, 0.5 mg.kg^{-1} atracurium, and 0.2 mg.kg^{-1} etomidate, the tracheal intubation was performed. After intubation, the patients were randomized into the groups C, L and LM. On the basis of our clinical experience, the patients in group C received intravenous PCA with sufentanil (0.04 μg.kg^{-1} h^{-1}) diluted into 150 ml of saline with a PCA device at a rate of 2 ml.h^{-1} continuously, a 2-ml bolus injection, and PCA with a 15-min lockout interval for postoperative analgesia. Patients in groups L and LM received levobupivacaine (60 ml of levobupivacaine 0.2%) or levobupivacaine combined with morphine (60 ml of levobupivacaine 0.2% and morphine 30 μg.kg^{-1}) for postoperative analgesia. Anaesthesia was maintained with sevoflurane (expiratory concentration 1.5%) and remifentanil. Patients in group C received remifentanil (10 μg.kg^{-1} h^{-1}), and patients in group L and group LM received remifentanil to maintain their BP and heart rate within the range of 20% from the baseline. If the change in BP and/or heart rate (HR) exceeded 20% of baseline, 1 μg.kg^{-1} remifentanil or 6 mg ephedrine was injected.

Patients were randomly allocated to group C, L or LM according to a random sequence generated using Stata version 11 software (StataCorp; TX, USA). An independent anaesthesiologist who did not participate in the perioperative evaluation prepared the drug for each group according to the allocation results. The second anaesthesiologist only performed the nerve block and anaesthesia. Another independent anaesthesiologist who was blinded to the randomization and anaesthesia results only investigated and recorded the peri-operative data.

All patients received RSB and TAPB after intubation in a supine position.

Ultrasound-guided rectus sheath block

We performed RSB at the first and second segments of the rectus abdominis muscle. In brief, under ultrasound guidance (M-Turbo- Ultrasound system; SonoSite, Bothell, WA, USA), a 38-mm broadband linear array ultrasound probe (5–10 MHz) was positioned at the level of the first segment of the subxiphoid region in the transverse plane. The needle was inserted into the skin from the left lateral side to the midline under the middle of the ultrasound probe using an in-plane technique at an angle of approximately 30 degrees to the skin. Under direct vision, we inserted the needle as described above, and after confirmation of the rectus abdominis muscle, we pierced the posterior rectus sheath. Saline was injected to confirm the placement of the needle at the posterior rectus sheath. When the needle placement into the rectus sheath was confirmed, 15 ml of saline, levobupivacaine 0.2% or levobupivacaine 0.2% combined with morphine was injected for the 3 groups after confirmation that no blood was withdrawn, leading to the appearance of a hypoechoic space. Then, RSB of the next segment was performed using the same method and the same volume of anaesthetic solution (Fig. 1a and b).

Ultrasound-guided transversus abdominis plane block

The ultrasound probe (5–10 MHz) was placed perpendicular to the rectus abdominis muscle and positioned laterally in the left rectus abdominis muscle between the subcostal margin and the iliac crest to obtain the classic view of abdominal layers, including the external oblique muscle, the internal oblique muscle, the transversus abdominis muscle, and the peritoneum. The needle was inserted into the skin from the left rectus abdominis muscle under the middle of the ultrasound probe using an in-plane technique at an angle of approximately 30 degrees to the skin. Under direct vision, after confirmation that no blood was withdrawn, we slowly moved the ultrasound probe from the left rectus abdominis muscle laterally to the left midaxillary line while advancing the needle in transversus abdominis plane. In order to expand the blockade area, when the tip of the needle had been advanced to the beginning of the transabdominal plane, the needle was inserted along the transabdominal plane, and 30 ml of saline, levobupivacaine 0.2% or levobupivacaine 0.2% combined with morphine was injected stepwise as the needle was advanced further; the goal of this technique was to ensure that the whole transabdominal plane was filled with anaesthetics. (Fig. 1c, d and e).

Procedures and measurements

Blood was collected at completion of the TAPB and then at 10, 20, 30, 60, 90, 120 and 150 min after injection of local anaesthetics so that the concentration of levobupivacaine could be measured using high-performance liquid chromatography (HPLC). Briefly, plasma was collected by centrifugation at 3000 rpm.min^{-1} for 10 min and kept frozen at $-20\,°C$ for subsequent HPLC (CBM-20A HPLC, Kyoto, Japan) test. The sample flow rate was set to 1.0 ml.min^{-1}, and the detection wavelength was 210 nm. The levobupivacaine concentration was calculated according to the concentration curve of levobupivacaine hydrochloride (Hengrui, Jiangsu, China). The calculated curve of levobupivacaine showed good linearity over a range of 0.5–2000 ng.ml^{-1} (correlation coefficient ≥ 0.99).

After RSB and TAPB, the right subclavian vein was cannulated to collect blood and infuse blood or fluids, and all patients underwent standard open splenectomy [13]. To avoid the influence of the surgical procedure on postoperative pain, all enrolled patients received RSB and TAPB by the same surgery team. All patients received a left subcostal incision in the supine position. Postoperative analgesia was induced with PCA using sufentanil (0.04 $\mu g.kg^{-1}h^{-1}$) in the C group.

All patients received 40 $\mu g.kg^{-1}$ granisetron to prevent PONV [14]. After extubation, all patients were transferred to the post-anaesthesia care unit (PACU). When a patient's SpO$_2$ was over 95% without the use of supplemental oxygen, the patient was transferred to the ward.

Blood loss, infusion (red blood cells [RBCs] and plasma) and consumption of remifentanil were recorded. Postoperative pain at rest and upon coughing was evaluated with a visual analogue scale (VAS) at 0, 2, 4, 6, 24, 48 and 72 h after the operation. The postoperative pain was evaluated by incision and visceral pain (0 = no pain, 10 = worst pain). If the VAS score of any patient was greater than 4, a 3 mg intravenous (i.v.) bolus of morphine was administered, and pain was reassessed after

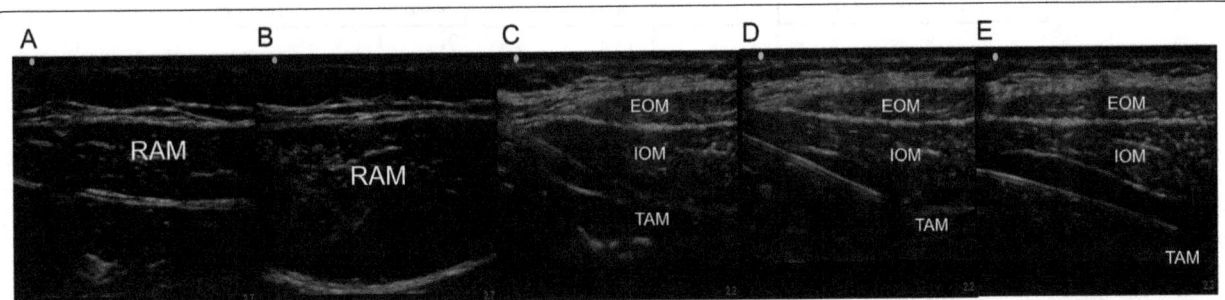

Fig. 1 Ultrasound-guided TAPB and RSBExternal oblique muscle, internal oblique muscle, transversus abdominis muscle, and peritoneum. A and B show ultrasound-guided RSB. The needle tip was positioned in the posterior rectus sheath, and saline was injected. Uniform hydrodissection of the muscle tissue and sheath was critical for the success of RSB, and then, the anaesthetics were injected. *RSB* rectus sheath block, *RAM* rectus abdominis muscle. C, D and E represent ultrasound images of TAPB. The needle tip was positioned in the plane between the internal oblique muscle and the transversus abdominis muscle. After dissection of the plane by injection of saline, the anaesthetics were injected. During the injection of anaesthetics, the needle was advanced further along the transabdominal plane, and the regional anaesthetics were injected step by step to ensure that the entire transabdominal plane was filled with anaesthetics. *TAPB* transversus abdominis plane block, *EOM* external oblique muscle, *IOM* internal oblique muscle, *TAM* transversus abdominis muscle.

10–15 min [7]. Other variables were recorded, including time to first exhaust, time to first defecation, time to first oral intake, time to first off-bed activity and incidence of PONV (scored from 0 to 10). Before discharge, all patients scored their satisfaction with postoperative analgesia (poor = 0; fair = 1; good = 2; excellent = 3).

Metoclopramide (10 mg) was intravenously injected if the patients reported a severe episode of nausea (> 7) or any episode of vomiting. The primary outcome was the use of analgesics over 24 h. The pain score, sedation score, satisfaction score postoperative recovery time and PONV were secondary outcomes. To guarantee objective results, the investigator was blinded to the randomization and anaesthesia.

Sample size

According to our preliminary pilot study and our own experience, the amount of morphine used during the first 72 h after surgery was approximately 15.8 (6.4) mg in patients who received no other analgesics. Approximately 46 patients in each group were required to detect a 25% reduction in morphine between the control and LM groups at 80% power with a two-sided alpha of 0.05.

Statistical analysis

The normality of the data was analysed with the Shapiro-Wilk test. Normally distributed data are presented as the mean (SD). Non-normally distributed data are presented as the median [interquartile range (IQR)]. Continuous data were analysed with repeated-measures analysis of variance. Normally distributed data were analysed with Student's t-test, and non-normally distributed data were analysed with the Mann-Whitney U test. Categorical data were analysed with the chi-squared test.

Results

Images of TAPB and RSB are shown in Fig. 1. A total of 155 patients were enrolled in this study. Five patients were excluded from the study because of failure of successful block (Fig. 2). There was no difference in demographic characteristics among the 3 groups (Table 1).

The postoperative pain scores at rest in the LM group were significantly lower than those in the C group. The

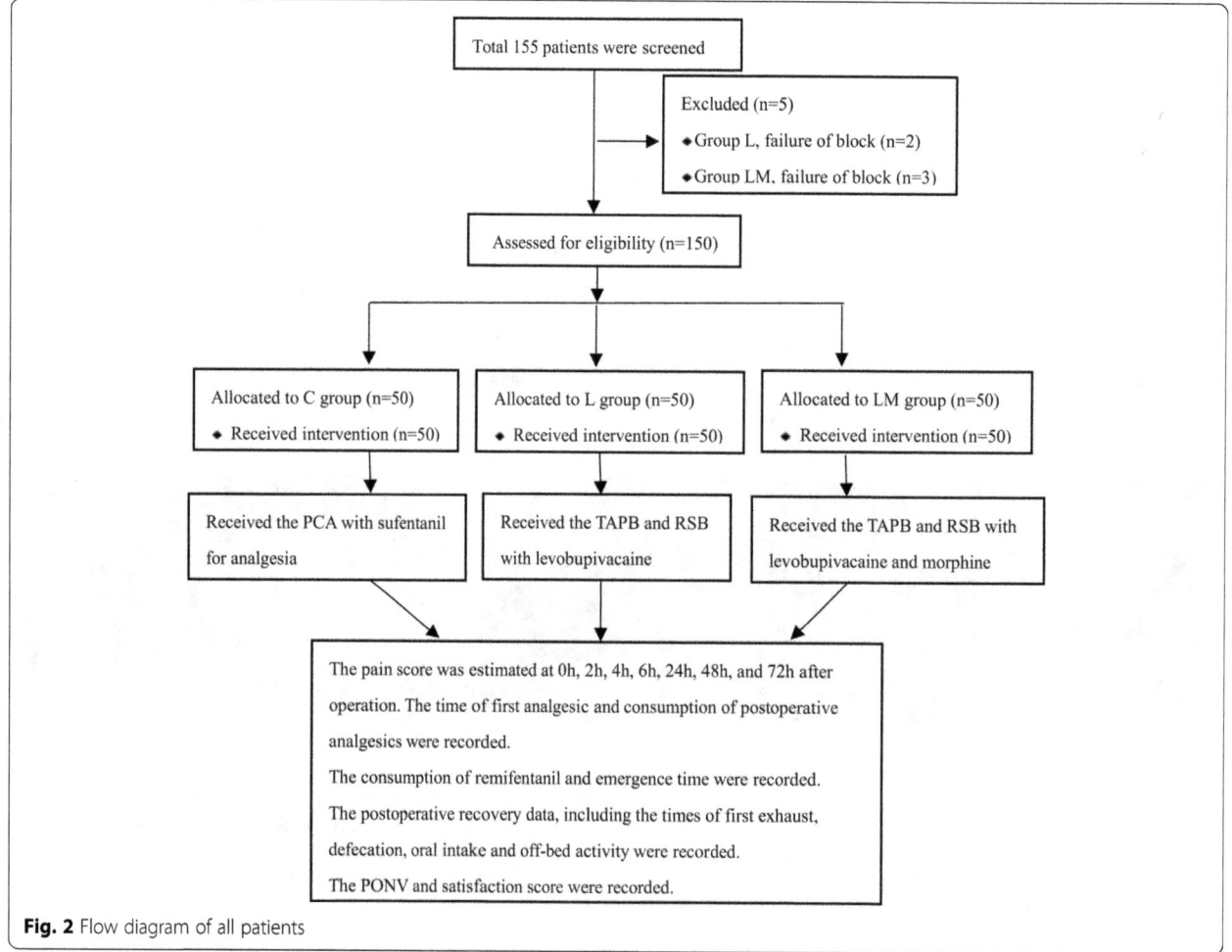

Fig. 2 Flow diagram of all patients

Table 1 The demographic data of patients in the 3 groups

	C	L	LM	P value
Age (year)	54.3 (10.6)	57.1 (10.1)	52.5 (9.3)	0.07
Gender (male n)	26	28	27	0.92
Height (cm)	166.2 (7.8)	164.8 (7.2)	165.3 (8.0)	0.65
Weight (kg)	64.5 (13.7)	64.6 (10.1)	64.5 (11.8)	0.98
Smoking (n)	12	15	17	0.54
Hypertension (n)	14	12	15	0.79
ASA				0.67
II	32	35	36	
III	18	15	14	
HBV	34	36	32	0.69
Hct (%)	36.8 (5.5)	36.9 (6.1)	36.3 (5.5)	0.85
Diagnosis				0.70
Hepatic cirrhosis	32	28	27	
Hypersplenism	11	10	13	
Thrombocytopenic purpura	7	12	10	
Bleeding volume (ml)	349 (192)	318 (192)	332 (133)	0.67
Transfusion volume (ml)	370 (134)	358 (147)	353 (87)	0.78
Operation time (h)	3.0 (1.3)	3.1 (0.9)	3.1 (1.0)	0.86
Anesthesia time (h)	3.8 (1.4)	3.5 (1.0)	3.4 (1.1)	0.21
With pericardial vascular dissection	32	28	27	0.56

Data are expressed as mean (SD) or number
ASA the American society of anesthesiologists, *HBV* hepatitis B virus, *Hct* hematocrit

pain scores at rest from 6 to 72 h were significantly lower in the LM group than in the L group. The postoperative pain scores at coughing in the LM group were significantly lower than those in the C group. The pain scores at coughing from 4 to 72 h were significantly lower in the LM group than in the L group (all $P < 0.05$) (Fig. 3). The time to first use of analgesics in the C group was significantly shorter than that in the L and LM groups ($P < 0.05$). The time to first analgesic use in the LM group was longer than that in the L group ($P < 0.05$). The total consumption of morphine in the LM group was less than that in the L group, and the consumption of morphine in the C group was less than that in the L group ($P < 0.05$ for all) (Table 2).

The intraoperative consumption of remifentanil in the L and LM groups was significantly less than that in the

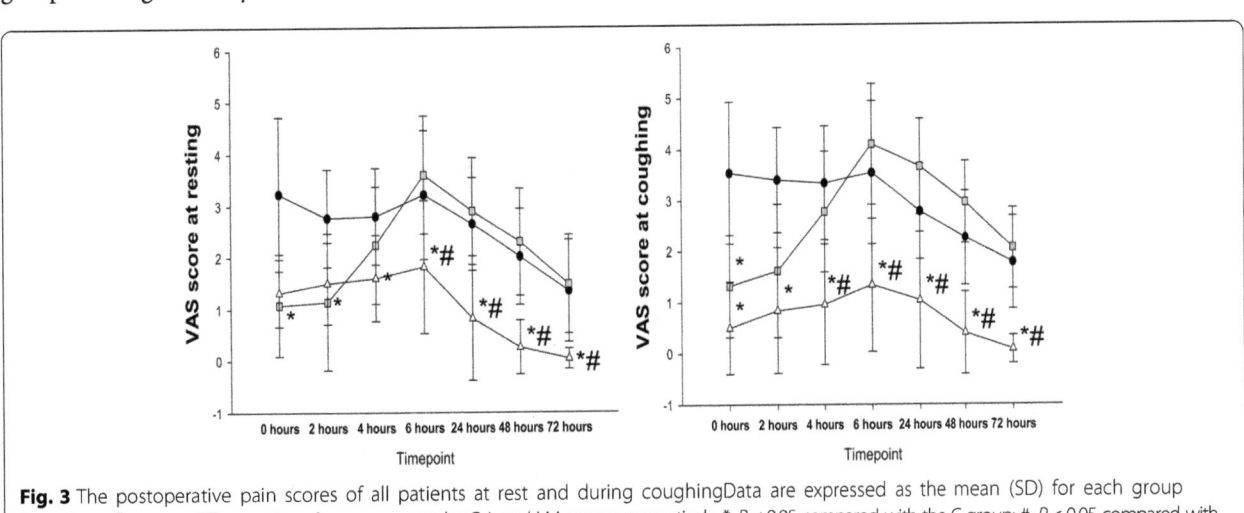

Fig. 3 The postoperative pain scores of all patients at rest and during coughingData are expressed as the mean (SD) for each group ($n = 50$). ——●——, ——■—— and ——△—— represent the C, L and LM groups, respectively. *, $P < 0.05$ compared with the C group; #, $P < 0.05$ compared with the L group.

Table 2 Comparison of postoperative recovery of patients in the 3 groups

	C	L	LM	P(C vs L)	P(C vs LM)	P(L vs LM)
Remifentanil consumption (mg)	2.97 (0.77)	1.91 (0.73)	1.62 (0.81)	< 0.0001	< 0.0001	0.047
Awaken time (min)	24.04 (6.04)	19.72 (4.83)	18.04 (4.84)	0.0001	< 0.0001	0.083
First analgesic (h)	2.00 (0.50–7.12)	4.65 (2.87–6.82)	13.00 (8.50–17.62)	0.048	< 0.0001	< 0.0001
Total morphine consumption (mg)	12.30 (5.22)	16.68 (5.29)	9.96 (4.51)	< 0.0001	0.0184	< 0.0001
First exhaust (h)	60.4 (14.1)	59.1 (25.4)	54.7 (22.9)	0.76	0.13	0.35
First defecation (h)	85.9 (19.4)	76.1 (23.1)	71.9 (24.1)	0.023	0.0019	0.38
First oral intake (h)	72.6 (13.8)	68.2 (29.1)	65.2 (23.0)	0.32	0.048	0.57
First off-bed (h)	52.8 (22.6)	49.7 (26.6)	46.4 (24.5)	0.53	0.18	0.52
PONV (%)	22%	28%	12%	0.48	0.29	0.04
Metoclopramide (mg)	13.6 (5.1)	15.7 (5.1)	11.4 (3.7)	0.019	0.007	< 0.0001
Satisfaction score	1.8 (0.6)	1.6 (0.6)	2.9 (0.7)	0.51	< 0.0001	< 0.0001

Data are expressed as mean (SD), number (%) or median (IQR)
PONV postoperative nausea and vomiting

C group ($P < 0.05$). The emergence time in the L and LM groups was significantly shorter than that in the C group ($P < 0.05$), but the difference in emergence time between the L and LM groups was not significant ($P > 0.05$) (Table 2).

Compared with the C group, the times to first exhaust and first off-bed activity time were shortened in the L and LM groups, but the differences among groups were not statistically significant (all $P > 0.05$). The time to first defecation was shorter in the L and LM groups than in

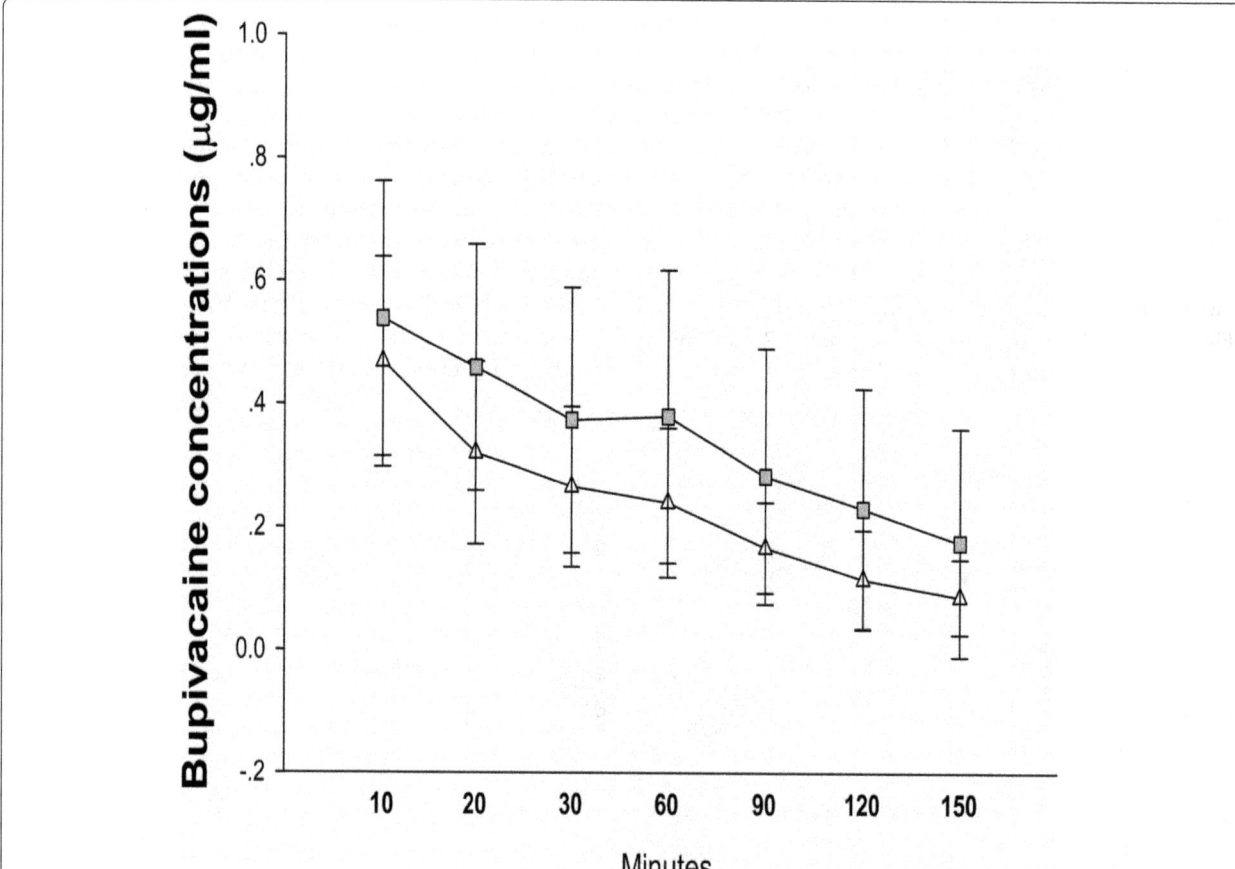

Fig. 4 Changes in plasma concentration of levobupivacaine between the L and LM groups. Data are expressed as the mean (SD) for each group ($n = 50$). ─■─ and ─△─ represent the L and LM groups, respectively

the C group ($P < 0.05$), but the difference between the L and LM groups was not statistically significant ($P > 0.05$). The time to oral intake was shorter in the LM group than in the C group ($P < 0.05$) but not the L group ($P > 0.05$). The incidence of PONV and consumption of antiemetic agents were significantly lower in the LM group ($P < 0.05$) than in the C group but not in the L group ($P > 0.05$). The satisfaction score of the LM group was significantly higher than that of the C and L groups ($P < 0.05$). There was no significant difference in satisfaction scores between the C and L groups ($P > 0.05$) (Table 2).

The levobupivacaine concentrations were significantly different among the groups at 10 min and 30 min after peripheral nerve block. However, no significant difference in the mean maximum plasma concentration of levobupivacaine was observed between the LM group and the L group (Fig. 4). No patient developed clinically severe side effects.

Discussion

In this study, we found that the combination of RSB and TAPB significantly ameliorated postoperative pain, reduced analgesic consumption, inhibited PONV, and partly promoted postoperative recovery. An enhanced effect of levobupivacaine by concurrent morphine treatment underlies this improvement in outcome.

Postoperative pain can cause a severe stress response [15], respiratory deterioration [16, 17] and neuroendocrine dysfunction [18], preventing early mobilization [17] and even prolonging hospitalization [19]. Moreover, abdominal surgery and consumption of analgesics contribute to PONV [20]. In contrast, sufficient postoperative analgesia is associated with the prevention of postoperative complications and the development of chronic pain, faster postoperative recovery, and a shorter duration of hospitalization [21].

In clinical work, local infiltration and PCA are usually applied in patients with coagulation disorders. However, PCA and local infiltration cannot provide sufficient analgesia [22, 23]. It has been reported that subcostal curve invasion of splenectomy surgery affects multiple nerves and results in severe postoperative pain and the use of many analgesics [13, 24]. Although TAPB can theoretically block the T6-L1 nerves [25], TAPB alone cannot block nerves beyond the costal margins. In our clinical experience, subxiphoid RSB can reduce local somatic pain. Therefore, we hypothesized that the combination of TAPB and RSB could block a more extensive region and provide better postoperative analgesia than either procedure performed alone. Considering its analgesic benefifits in the neuraxial space, we added 30 μg/kg morphine [12]. In this study, we found that TAPB and RSB significantly decreased intraoperative remifentanil consumption. This result was consistent with that of a previous study [26]. There are many afferent nerves that transfer invasive signals from the anterior abdominal wall and lie in potential spaces of the sheath of the rectus abdominis, internal oblique and transversus abdominis muscles. Local anaesthetics injected into these spaces can block the transfer of these invasive signals, further reducing the need for opioids for somatic pain during an operation. Moreover, in this study, we injected anaesthetics step-by-step to fill the entire space of the transversus abdominis plane. In our preliminary study, we found that the combination of TAPB and RSB, with the same method used in this study, can maintain the absence of pain in the entire area of skin of the subcostal curve.

We also found that TAPB and RSB significantly reduced postoperative pain and analgesic consumption and prolonged the time to first analgesia use. Postoperative pain is a serious problem for patients after splenectomy. The curved incision damages many muscles and afferent nerves, contributing to postoperative pain [1, 2]. Postoperative pain not only leads to discomfort and inhibits recovery but also prolongs hospitalization.

The patients underwent splenectomy, which is often combined with coagulation disorders, and were forbidden to receive epidural analgesia. Local infiltration and PCA can provide analgesia for somatic pain, but their efficacy is still debated. TAPB or RSB alone has been shown to provide more effective somatic analgesia for abdominal surgery [7, 11, 27]. However, considering the large range of invasion and the range of blockade from TAPB and RSB alone, we administered a combination of TAPB and RSB to increase the external blockade range. The results suggested that the combination of TAPB and RSB significantly reduced postoperative pain and postoperative analgesic consumption and prolonged the time to first analgesia use. In this study, we found that the VAS score in group C was consistently higher than those in groups L and LM, although the patients in groups L and LM received additional analgesics. In contrast, the patients who received nerve block had lower VAS scores, especially those in the LM group. The time to first analgesic use in the LM group was significantly longer than those in groups C and L. This result may be associated with the metabolic time of levobupivacaine. Without adjuvant drugs, the half-life of levobupivacaine is only approximately 5–7 h, even in muscle spaces. In this study, we added morphine because of its analgesic benefits in the neuraxial space [12]. The synergistic or additive effect of these drugs may prolong the duration of postoperative analgesia [28]. Therefore, the time to first analgesic use in the LM group was significantly longer than that in groups C and L. In this study, the time to first analgesia use in group LM was approximately 14.5 h postoperatively, which was significantly longer than that in groups C and L.

PONV was the most common postoperative complication and was an independent risk factor in postoperative recovery after abdominal surgery. Abdominal surgery and the application of opioids are key risk factors for PONV [20]. In this study, the incidence and severity of PONV were significantly reduced by levobupivacaine plus morphine but not by levobupivacaine alone. This result may be due to the reductions in remifentanil and morphine use. The patients in groups C and L received greater doses of morphine to provide postoperative analgesia than the patients in group LM. Although the LM group also received morphine in local anaesthetics, the absorption of morphine was slow, and the blood concentration of morphine was lower than that in the other two groups. Therefore, morphine had reduced side effects in the LM group. In addition, the inhibition of PONV in the LM group was also attributed to the improvement in postoperative bowel recovery.

In this study, the times to first oral intake, off-bed activity, exhaust and defecation in the LM group were significantly shorter than those in the C and L groups. These results suggest that levobupivacaine plus morphine significantly promoted the postoperative recovery of patients. The promotion of recovery by levobupivacaine plus morphine was not only associated with the effectiveness of the analgesia and the reduction in PONV but also with the reduction in postoperative analgesic use. Due to the effectiveness of analgesia, mobilization can be restored in patients as early as possible [29]. Early mobilization further promotes intestinal peristalsis and early oral intake. Moreover, opioids can lead to bowel dysfunction when they combine with receptors in the bowel wall, thus decreasing bowel peristalsis [30]. In contrast, TAPB had been indicated to promote the postoperative recovery of bowel function [27]. In this study, we found similar results in the LM group but not the L group. The bowel recovery in group L was improved compared with that in group C, but the difference was not statistically significant. We hypothesized that this difference may be due to postoperative opioid consumption. Although the patients received TAPB and RSB, the half-life of levobupivacaine contributed to the short-term analgesia of bupivacaine because the nerve block was performed preoperatively [31, 32]. After the efficacy of levobupivacaine was lost, the patients in group L received more morphine to relieve pain than patients in group C because PCA can continuously provide sufentanil for 75 h.

The novelty of this study is that we developed a new TAPB method to improve the success and efficacy of the procedure. The rate of TAPB failure has been reported to be approximately 10–12% [33, 34], and the efficacy of TAPB remains controversial [35, 36], possibly due to block failure or insufficient block range. In this study, to provide better nerve block efficacy, we administered TAPB via an amended method. We positioned the needle at the beginning of the transverse fascia and then injected the anaesthetics along the path of the advancing needle, proceeding over the entire transverse fascia. With this method, we injected levobupivacaine into the entire transverse fascia, and the success rate was nearly 100%.

Although TAPB and RSB reduced the quantity of opioids needed for postoperative pain relief, the adverse effects of levobupivacaine, including central and cardiac toxicity, must be carefully considered. The systemic toxicity of the anaesthetic is mainly determined by the plasma concentration. It has been indicated that a levobupivacaine plasma concentration exceeding $2620 \, ng.ml^{-1}$ can lead to central nervous system toxicity [37]. In this study, we found that the highest plasma levobupivacaine concentration was less than $800 \, ng.ml^{-1}$, which is significantly lower than the toxic concentration. This result suggests that the dose and injection are safe [38]. Although the application of morphine in nerve block has not been approved, morphine was applied in paravertebral blocks in a previous study [12], and no side effects were reported. In this study, we also did not observe any nerve complications in patients.

Conclusions
In this study, we found that the combination of TAPB and RSB with levobupivacaine plus morphine significantly reduced postoperative pain and analgesic consumption and promoted postoperative recovery.

Abbreviations
ASA: American Society of Anesthesiologists; BP: Blood pressure; ECG: Electrocardiography; HPLC: High-performance liquid chromatography; HR: Heart rate; PACU: Post-anaesthesia care unit; PCA: Patient-controlled analgesia; PONV: Postoperative nausea and vomiting; RSB: Rectus sheath block; SpO$_2$: Pulse oximetry; TAPB: Transversus abdominis plane block; VAS: Visual analogue scale

Acknowledgements
Not applicable.

Authors' contributions
Concept/design: J-lZ, WG; Data analysis/interpretation: X-tW, JG, H-bS, X-qZ; Drafting article: J-lZ; Critical revision of article: J-lZ, WG, X-tTW, JG; Approval of the article: J-lZ, X-tW, JG, H-bS, X-qZ, WG; Statistics: J-lZ, WG, X-tW; Data collection: JG, H-bS, X-qZ. All authors read and approved the final manuscript. accordance with the Declaration of Helsinki. Informed written consent was obtained from all patients.

Author details
[1]Department of Anesthesiology, the Second Affiliated Hospital of Harbin Medical University, Harbin, Heilongjiang, China. [2]Department of Anesthesiology, the Second Affiliated Hospital of Harbin Medical University, Harbin, Heilongjiang, China. [3]Department of Anesthesiology, the Second Affiliated Hospital of Harbin Medical University, 246 Xuefu Road, Nangang District, Harbin, Heilongjiang, China.

References

1. Sun JX, Bai KY, Liu YF, Du G, Fu ZH, Zhang H, et al. Effect of local wound infiltration with ropivacaine on postoperative pain relief and stress response reduction after open hepatectomy. World J Gastroenterol. 2017;23:6733–40.

2. Velanovich V, Shurafa MS. Clinical and quality of life outcomes of laparoscopic and open splenectomy for haematological diseases. Eur J Surg. 2001;167:23–8.

3. Nimmo SM, Foo ITH, Paterson HM. Enhanced recovery after surgery: pain management. J Surg Oncol. 2017;116:583–91.

4. Kamiya Y, Hasegawa M, Yoshida T, Takamatsu M, Koyama Y. Impact of pectoral nerve block on postoperative pain and quality of recovery in patients undergoing breast cancer surgery: a randomised controlled trial. Eur J Anaesthesiol. 2018;35:215–23.

5. Werawatganon T, Charuluxanun S. Patient controlled intravenous opioid analgesia versus continuous epidural analgesia for pain after intra-abdominal surgery. Cochrane Database Syst Rev. 2005;(1):CD004088.

6. Hopkins PM. Ultrasound guidance as a gold standard in regional anaesthesia. Br J Anaesth. 2007;98:299–301.

7. Bakshi SG, Mapari A, Shylasree TS. REctus sheath block for postoperative analgesia in gynecological ONcology surgery (RESONS): a randomized-controlled trial. Can J Anaesth. 2016;63:1335–44.

8. Xu L, Hu Z, Shen J, McQuillan PM. Efficacy of US-guided transversus abdominis plane block and rectus sheath block with ropivacaine and dexmedetomidine in elderly high-risk patients. Minerva Anestesiol. 2018;84:18–24.

9. Faiz SHR, Alebouyeh MR, Derakhshan P, Imani F, Rahimzadeh P, Ghaderi AM. Comparison of ultrasound-guided posterior transversus abdominis plane block and lateral transversus abdominis plane block for postoperative pain management in patients undergoing cesarean section: a randomized double-blind clinical trial study. J Pain Res. 2018;11:5–9.

10. Hamada T, Tsuchiya M, Mizutani K, Takahashi R, Muguruma K, Maeda K, et al. Levobupivacaine-dextran mixture for transversus abdominis plane block and rectus sheath block in patients undergoing laparoscopic colectomy: a randomised controlled trial. Anaesthesia. 2016;71:411–6.

11. Takebayashi K, Matsumura M, Kawai Y, Hoashi T, Katsura N, Fukuda S, et al. Efficacy of transversus abdominis plane block and rectus sheath block in laparoscopic inguinal hernia surgery. Int Surg. 2015;100:666–71.

12. Pintaric TS, Potocnik I, Hadzic A, Stupnik T, Pintaric M, Novak JV. Comparison of continuous thoracic epidural with paravertebral block on perioperative analgesia and hemodynamic stability in patients having open lung surgery. Reg Anesth Pain Med. 2011;36:256–60.

13. Jiang XZ, Zhao SY, Luo H, Huang B, Wang CS, Chen L, et al. Laparoscopic and open splenectomy and azygoportal disconnection for portal hypertension. World J Gastroenterol. 2009;15:3421–5.

14. Oksuz H, Zencirci B, Ezberci M. Comparison of the effectiveness of metoclopramide, ondansetron, and granisetron on the prevention of nausea and vomiting after laparoscopic cholecystectomy. J Laparoendosc Adv Surg Tech A. 2007;17:803–8.

15. Kehlet H, Holte K. Effect of postoperative analgesia on surgical outcome. Br J Anaesth. 2001;87:62–72.

16. Vassilakopoulos T, Mastora Z, Katsaounou P, Doukas G, Klimopoulos S, Roussos C, et al. Contribution of pain to inspiratory muscle dysfunction after upper abdominal surgery: a randomized controlled trial. Am J Respir Crit Care Med. 2000;161:1372–5.

17. Arici E, Tastan S, Can MF. The effect of using an abdominal binder on postoperative gastrointestinal function, mobilization, pulmonary function, and pain in patients undergoing major abdominal surgery: a randomized controlled trial. Int J Nurs Stud. 2016;62:108–17.

18. Yardeni IZ, Shavit Y, Bessler H, Mayburd E, Grinevich G, Beilin B. Comparison of postoperative pain management techniques on endocrine response to surgery: a randomised controlled trial. Int J Surg. 2007;5:239–43.

19. Zhu Z, Wang C, Xu C, Cai Q. Influence of patient-controlled epidural analgesia versus patient-controlled intravenous analgesia on postoperative pain control and recovery after gastrectomy for gastric cancer: a prospective randomized trial. Gastric Cancer. 2013;16:193–200.

20. Leslie K, Myles PS, Chan MT, Paech MJ, Peyton P, Forbes A, et al. Risk factors for severe postoperative nausea and vomiting in a randomized trial of nitrous oxide-based vs nitrous oxide-free anaesthesia. Br J Anaesth. 2008; 101:498–505.

21. Wu CL, Raja SN. Treatment of acute postoperative pain. Lancet. 2011;377: 2215–25.

22. Jørgensen H, Wetterslev J, Møiniche S, Dahl JB. Epidural local anaesthetics versus opioid-based analgesic regimens on postoperative gastrointestinal paralysis, PONV and pain after abdominal surgery. Cochrane Database Syst Rev. 2000;(4):CD001893.

23. Gasanova I, Alexander J, Ogunnaike B, Hamid C, Rogers D, Minhajuddin A, et al. Transversus Abdominis plane block versus surgical site infiltration for pain management after open Total abdominal hysterectomy. Anesth Analg. 2015;121:1383–8.

24. Abelson AL, Armitage-Chan E, Lindsey JC, Wetmore LA. A comparison of epidural morphine with low dose bupivacaine versus epidural morphine alone on motor and respiratory function in dogs following splenectomy. Vet Anaesth Analg. 2011;38:213–23.

25. Suresh S, Chan VW. Ultrasound guided transversus abdominis plane block in infants, children and adolescents: a simple procedural guidance for their performance. Paediatr Anaesth. 2009;19:296–9.

26. Erdogan MA, Ozgul U, Ucar M, Yalin MR, Colak YZ, Colak C, et al. Effect of transversus abdominis plane block in combination with general anesthesia on perioperative opioid consumption, hemodynamics, and recovery in living liver donors: The prospective, double-blinded, randomized study. Clin Transplant. 2017;31(4). https://doi.org/10.1111/ctr.12931.

27. Fusco P, Cofini V, Petrucci E, Scimia P, Pozone T, Paladini G, Carta G, Necozione S, Borghi B, Marinangeli F. Transversus Abdominis plane block in the Management of Acute Postoperative Pain Syndrome after caesarean section: a randomized controlled clinical trial. Pain Physician. 2016;19:583–91.

28. Yang Y, Zeng C, Wei J, Li H, Yang T, Deng ZH, et al. Single-dose intra-articular bupivacaine plus morphine versus bupivacaine alone after arthroscopic knee surgery: a meta-analysis of randomized controlled trials. Knee Surg Sports Traumatol Arthrosc. 2017;25:966–79.

29. Nagata J, Watanabe J, Sawatsubashi Y, Akiyama M, Arase K, Minagawa N, et al. A novel transperitoneal abdominal wall nerve block for postoperative pain in laparoscopic colorectal surgery. Asian J Surg. 2018;41:417–21.

30. Webster LR. Opioid-induced constipation. Pain Med. 2015;16(Suppl 1):S16–21.

31. Kanazi GE, Aouad MT, Abdallah FW, Khatib MI, Adham AM, Harfoush DW, et al. The analgesic efficacy of subarachnoid morphine in comparison with ultrasound-guided transversus abdominis plane block after cesarean delivery: a randomized controlled trial. Anesth Analg. 2010;111:475–81.

32. Sivapurapu V, Vasudevan A, Gupta S, Badhe AS. Comparison of analgesic efficacy of transversus abdominis plane block with direct infiltration of local anesthetic into surgical incision in lower abdominal gynecological surgeries. J Anaesthesiol Clin Pharmacol. 2013;29:71–5.

33. Niraj G, Kelkar A, Hart E, Kaushik V, Fleet D, Jameson J. Four quadrant transversus abdominis plane block and continuous transversus abdominis plane analgesia: a 3-year prospective audit in 124 patients. J Clin Anesth. 2015;27:579–84.

34. Markic D, Vujicic B, Ivanovski M, Krpina K, Grskovic A, Zivcic-Cosic S, et al. Peritoneal Dialysis catheter placement using an ultrasound-guided Transversus Abdominis plane block. Blood Purif. 2015;39:274–80.

35. Freir NM, Murphy C, Mugawar M, Linnane A, Cunningham AJ. Transversus abdominis plane block for analgesia in renal transplantation: a randomized controlled trial. Anesth Analg. 2012;115:953–7.

36. Griffiths JD, Middle JV, Barron FA, Grant SJ, Popham PA, Royse CF. Transversus abdominis plane block does not provide additional benefit to multimodal analgesia in gynecological cancer surgery. Anesth Analg. 2010; 111:797–801.

37. Bardsley H, Gristwood R, Baker H, Watson N, Nimmo W. A comparison of the cardiovascular effects of levobupivacaine and rac-bupivacaine following intravenous administration to healthy volunteers. Br J Clin Pharmacol. 1998; 46:245–9.

38. Yasumura R, Kobayashi Y, Ochiai R. A comparison of plasma levobupivacaine concentrations following transversus abdominis plane block and rectus sheath block. Anaesthesia. 2016;71:544–9.

27

Epidural analgesia and avoidance of blood transfusion are associated with reduced mortality in patients with postoperative pulmonary complications following thoracotomic esophagectomy

Kai B. Kaufmann[1]*[iD], Wolfgang Baar[1], Torben Glatz[2], Jens Hoeppner[2], Hartmut Buerkle[1], Ulrich Goebel[1] and Sebastian Heinrich[1]

Abstract

Background: Postoperative pulmonary complications (PPCs) represent the most frequent complications after esophagectomy. The aim of this study was to identify modifiable risk factors for PPCs and 90-days mortality related to PPCs after esophagectomy in esophageal cancer patients.

Methods: This is a single center retrospective cohort study of 335 patients suffering from esophageal cancer who underwent esophagectomy between 1996 and 2014 at a university hospital center. Statistical processing was conducted using univariate and multivariate stepwise logistic regression analysis of patient-specific and procedural risk factors for PPCs and mortality.

Results: The incidence of PPCs was 52% (175/335) and the 90-days mortality rate of patients with PPCs was 8% (26/335) in this study cohort. The univariate and multivariate analysis revealed the following independent risk factors for PPCs and its associated mortality. ASA score ≥ 3 was the only independent patient-specific risk factor for the incidence of PPCs and 90-days mortality of patients with an odds ratio for PPCs being 1.7 (1.1–2.6 95% CI) and an odds ratio of 2.6 (1.1–6.2 95% CI) for 90-days mortality. The multivariate approach depicted two independent procedural risk factors including transfusion of packed red blood cells (PRBCs) odds ratio of 1.9 (1.2–3 95% CI) for PPCs and an odds ratio of 5.0 (2.0–12.6 95% CI) for 90-days mortality; *absence of* thoracic epidural anesthesia (TEA) revealed the highest odds ratio 2.0 (1.01–3.8 95% CI) for PPCs and an odds ratio of 3.9 (1.6–9.7 95% CI) for 90-days mortality.

Conclusion: In esophageal cancer patients undergoing esophagectomy via thoracotomy, epidural analgesia and the avoidance of intraoperative blood transfusion are significantly associated with a reduced 90-days mortality related to PPCs.

Keywords: Esophagectomy, Postoperative pulmonary complications, Thoracic epidural anesthesia, Blood transfusion, Independent risk factors, 90-days mortality

* Correspondence: kai.kaufmann@uniklinik-freiburg.de
[1]Department of Anesthesiology and Critical Care Medicine, University of Freiburg, – University of Freiburg, Hugstetter Strasse 55, 79106 Freiburg, Germany

Epidural analgesia and avoidance of blood transfusion are associated with reduced mortality in patients...

223

Introduction

Esophagectomy for esophageal cancer treatment is associated with increased rates of up to 50% for postoperative morbidity and of 12% for postoperative mortality [1–4]. Postoperative pulmonary complications (PPCs) represent the most frequent adverse events after esophagectomy with an incidence of up to 38% affecting patients' short- and long-term outcome [1]. PPCs are the major cause of early death after esophagectomy, especially when the transthoracic approach via thoracotomy was taken [1, 5, 6]. Several risk factors for PPCs after esophagectomy have been identified. These are increased age, female gender, preoperative comorbidities (diabetes, arterial hypertension, chronic obstructive lung disease), neoadjuvant radio- or chemotherapy, low preoperative forced expiratory volume in 1 s (FEV_1), low diffusion capacity of the lung for carbon monoxide (DLCO), smoking, transthoracic resection, high ASA score, high amounts of intraoperative fluids and increased blood loss [1, 7–9]. Whereas most of the risk factors have to be considered as non-adjustable, current research focuses on procedural risk factors that may be optimized. According to current literature it appears evident that intraoperative fluid overload is one of the major risk factors for PPCs and mortality after esophagectomy [10–12]. However, data on the quality of intraoperative fluids (for example colloids, PRBCs, FFPs) and its influence on PPCs and the subsequent mortality are scarce [13]. TEA is another procedural and anesthesia-related factor potentially reducing the incidence of PPCs after esophagectomy. Results on this topic appear contradictory [2, 14–20]. Although it has been shown that perioperative TEA in patients after esophagectomy significantly decreases time on ICU, there is no study that provides data on superior oncological results and mortality decrease among patients with PPCs due to TEA [19]. De la Gala and colleagues showed that the use of sevoflurane instead of propofol for anesthesia maintenance in lung surgery with thoracotomy led to a decrease of PPCs [21]. To our best knowledge there is no study that examined this effect in esophageal cancer patients undergoing esophagectomy.

The aim of this study was to identify further modifiable risk factors and to validate existing risk factors for mortality related to PPCs after esophagectomy in esophageal cancer patients. This is the first study that focuses on mortality related to PPCs after esophagectomy.

Methods

This retrospective cohort study was approved by the local Ethics Committee, University of Freiburg, Germany (EK569/14 December 9th 2014). The study was conducted at the Department of Anesthesiology and Intensive Care and the Department of General and Visceral Surgery, University Medical Center, Freiburg, Germany.

The study was planned and designed in accordance with the initiative for Strengthening the Reporting of Observational Studies in Epidemiology STROBE, using the suggested checklist for epidemiological cohort studies [22]. Patients' data were only entered into the cancer registry, if formal informed consent was obtained. In this retrospective cohort study 335 esophageal cancer patients, who underwent open esophagectomy between January 1st 1996 and March 31st 2014, were analyzed. A priori sample size calculation was not applicable due to the retrospective study design. Figure 1 shows the underlying data collection and statistical process of this study.

Surgery

The majority of patients underwent open esophagectomy via the Ivor-Lewis thoraco-abdominal approach. This included a right-sided thoracotomy and a median laparotomy. Only 26 (8%) patients had a transhiatal esophagectomy via laparotomy. For reconstruction the formation of a pulled-up gastric tube was the preferred technique, only 14 (4%) patients underwent colon interposition.

Anesthesia

The intraoperative anesthesia management was not standardized by study protocol. Whenever feasible a combination of thoracic epidural and general anesthesia was used. The epidural pain catheter was placed at interspaces T4/5, T5/6 or T6/7 prior to general anesthesia. After negative test dose injection epidural analgesia was induced by injection of a total of 8–10 ml of ropivacaine 0.2% plus epidural sufentanil (0.2–0.3 µg/kg) or fentanyl (2–3 µg/kg), followed by a continuous epidural infusion of ropivacaine 0.2% and sufentanil (0.5 µg/ml) or fentanyl (5 µg/ml) at 8 ml/h during surgery until the third postoperative day. A total of 49 patients (49/335, 15%) did not have an epidural pain catheter. These patients were treated with a systemic opioid therapy. The postoperative pain control for patients without epidural analgesia followed a standardized procedure: On ICU, analgesia was provided nurse controlled by using intravenous and if possible enteral opioids. If patients were transferred from ICU to the normal care ward and standard oral opioid analgesia was insufficient, an intravenous patient-controlled analgesia system was established. These patients were visited daily by the institutional acute pain service. In 24 patients (24/49, 49%) the placement of the epidural pain catheter was described as unsuccessful. In the remaining 25 patients, epidural analgesia was not provided because of patient refusal.

Mostly, anesthesia was maintained by isoflurane, desflurane or sevoflurane. The minority of patients had total intravenous anesthesia with propofol. Patients' radial artery was cannulated for continuous blood pressure and intermittent blood gas monitoring.

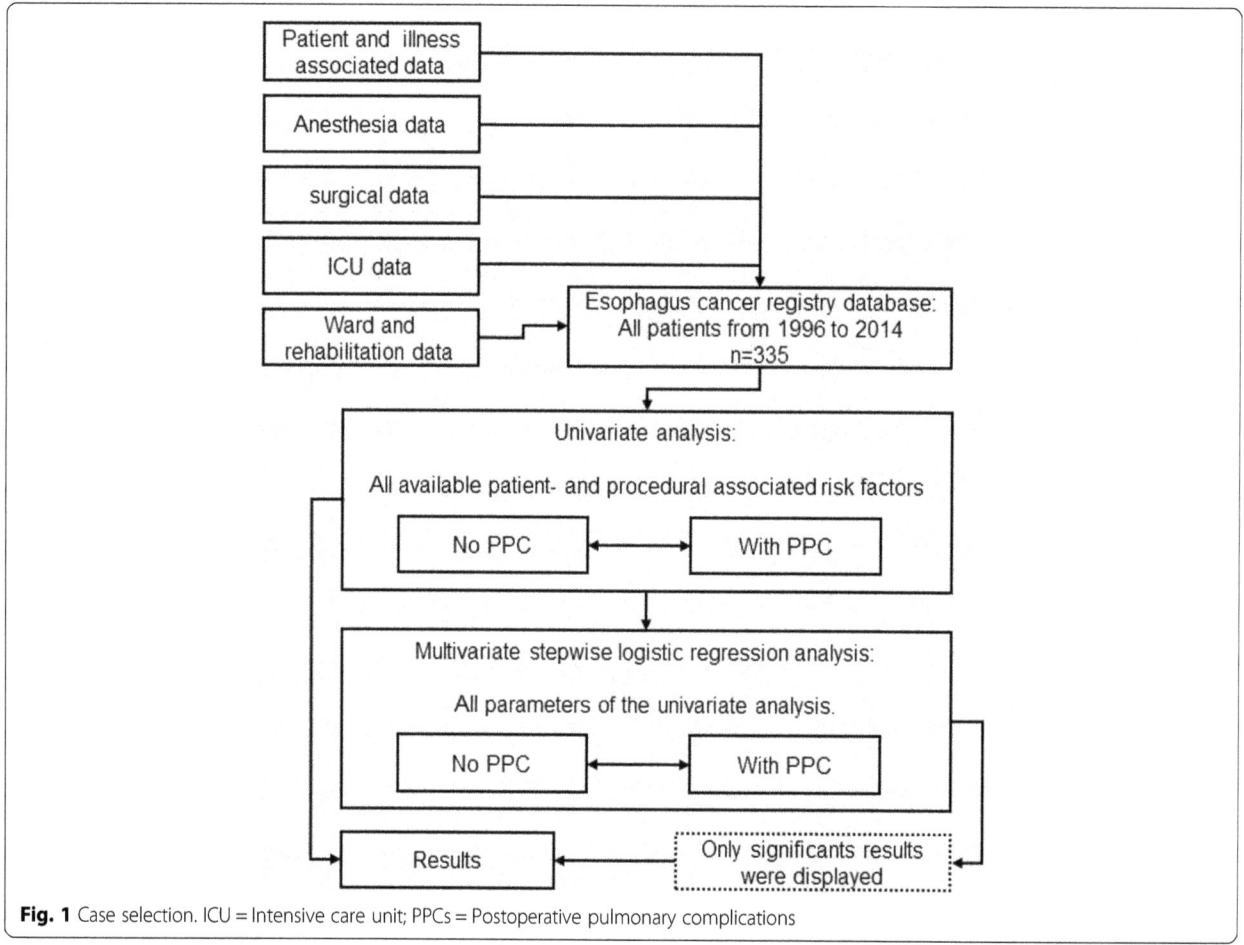

Fig. 1 Case selection. ICU = Intensive care unit; PPCs = Postoperative pulmonary complications

For endotracheal intubation with the double-lumen tube muscle relaxant was used. During surgery depth of muscle relaxation was continuously monitored. Adequate muscle relaxation was defined as 1 twitch out of 4 in the train-of-four technique. If patients were extubated in the operation room muscle relaxation was completely reversed by using neostigmine until four equal twitches were present. In all patients a left sided double-lumen endobronchial tube (35–39 Fr/Ch (11.7–13 mm)) was used. Positioning of the double-lumen endotracheal tube was checked visually by fiberoptic bronchoscope. The ventilator settings were standardized in accordance with an in-house standard operating procedure for single-lung ventilation. Pressure-controlled ventilation with a positive endexspiratory pressure of 5–7 cm H_2O and peak pressure less than 30 cm H_2O for both, double-lung and single-lung ventilation was chosen. Inspiratory oxygen fraction was set as low as possible to avoid hypoxia with a peripheral oxygen fraction above 90%. This resulted in an oxygen fraction of 0.4 for double-lung and usually 0.8 for single-lung ventilation. Lung protective ventilator settings were applied. These included tidal volumes up to 8 ml/kg and a respiratory

frequency of 10–15/min for double-lung ventilation, while for single-lung ventilation tidal volumes of 6–7 ml/kg with a respiratory frequency of 10–15 /min were applied. Re-inflating of the previously non-ventilated lung was restarted by a manual recruitment manoeuvre for 10 s to 30 cm H_2O five times. Norepinephrine, balanced electrolyte solutions (either Jonosteril® [Fresenius Kabi, Bad Homburg Germany] or Normofundin® [Braun, Melsungen Germany]) and hydroxyethyl starch 6% [Voluven® or Volulyte® [Fresenius Kabi, Bad Homburg Germany] were used to keep the arterial blood pressure within physiological ranges. According to the in-house standard operating procedure a hemoglobin level below 8 g/dl was considered as a threshold for PRBC administration during surgery. Intraoperative fluid administration was extracted from anesthetic protocols.

Definition of PPCs

All PPCs were defined according to the International Consensus on Standardization of Data Collection for Complications Associated with Esophagectomy (*Esophagectomy Complications Consensus Group (ECCG)*) [23]. The Re-intubation rate was documented. The indication for re-intubation was hypercapnia or hypoxia. Hypercapnia was defined as an arterial CO_2 partial pressure leading to a decrease of pH below 7,25 or unconsciousness. Hypoxia as an indication for re-intubation was defined as an arterial O_2 partial pressure below 55 mmHg. Pleural effusion was defined as new chest-tube insertion in addition to those placed in the operation room or delayed removal of intraoperatively placed chest tubes after the 10th postoperative day. The rate of postoperative chylothorax and pleural empyema was also defined according ECCG. Tracheostomy was performed due to prolonged respiratory weaning either after re-intubation or because the initial placed endotracheal tube in the OR could not be removed. Pneumonia was defined as new pulmonary infiltrate on chest X-ray with associated leukocytosis, fever, new purulent sputum, need for antibiotic therapy and increased oxygen demand via face mask. The assessment of chest X-rays was performed by two independent radiologists. We collected all parameters by chart review to diagnose postoperative pneumonia [23].

Statistical analysis

For parameters that were distributed normally, mean value and standard deviation were calculated. Median and interquartile range were calculated due to the fact that parameters were not normally distributed. Univariate statistical analysis was performed by dividing the cohort into two groups, with and without PPCs. Statistical analyses of continuous variables were calculated using the Mann-Whitney U test for not-normally distributed parameters and the Students T-test was used for normally distributed values. Categorical variables were analyzed with χ2 test. All parameters included in the univariate analysis were used for the multivariate stepwise logistic regression analysis to assess the impact of these on the incidence of PPCs and 90-days mortality of patients with PPCs. Continuous variables were dichotomized. The following parameters were included in the multivariate stepwise logistic regression analysis: Surgical approach (transhiatal versus thoracoabdominal); reconstruction (gastric tube versus colon interponate); duration of surgery ≥430 min (3. quartile of the study cohort); blood loss ≥1000 ml; norepinephrine ≥0.07 µg/kg/min (3. quartile of the study cohort); total amount of intraoperative crystalloids ≥7000 ml (3. quartile of the study cohort); intraoperative use of colloids, packed red blood cells, fresh frozen plasma; epidural anesthesia; total intravenous anesthesia versus gas to maintain intraoperative general anesthesia; age ≥ 65 years; gender; alcohol abuse; nicotine dependency; neoadjuvant therapy; ASA score ≥ 3 or 4; BMI ≤ 18.5; UICC grade ≥ 3 or 4; hemoglobin level preoperative ≤11 mg/dl; extubation in the OR. The significant results of the multivariate stepwise logistic regression analysis are highlighted. A P value of ≤0.05 was considered

statistically significant. IBM SPSS Statistics for Windows, (Version 23.0 Armonk, NY USA: IBM Corp.) was used for statistical analysis.

Results

Table 1 highlights the results of patient-specific and procedural (surgery- and anesthesia-related) parameters of the entire study cohort. The majority of patients had neoadjuvant therapy 78% (262/335), most of them were male 87% (290/335) and underwent thoracoabdominal esophagectomy 92% (309/335) reconstructed by gastric tube 96% (321/335). Apart from that, most patients had perioperative thoracic epidural anesthesia (TEA) 85% (286/335). The overall 30- and 90-days mortality rate in this study cohort was 5% (17/335) and 11% (37/335). The 90-days-mortality rate of patients with PPCs was 8% (26/335). One hundred seventy-five patients (52%) developed PPCs. The most frequent complication was pneumonia 34% (114/335), followed by pleural effusion 31% (104/335), re-intubation 20% (66/335) and tracheostomy 12% (39/335). Pleural effusion was diagnosed in 104 patients, of these 51 patients received a new chest tube after surgery. Twenty-three patients (23/335, 7%) developed a chylothorax, whereas 18 patients (18/335, 5%) showed postoperative pleural empyema. A total of 66 patients (66/335, 20%) were re-intubated. Of these, 37 patients (37/66, 56%) had a tracheostomy in their further clinical course. Tracheostomy was performed in a total of 39 patients. Of these, 37 (37/39, 95%) were re-intubated on ICU and only 2 had a tracheostomy due to delayed weaning from the endotracheal tube placed in the operation room. The total amount of PPCs differs from the amount of patients with PPCs as some patients suffered from more than one PPC. As PPCs are linked to each other and the occurrence of one predisposes for another, the numbers highlighted in the following tables refer to the number of patients.

Table 2 shows the results of the univariate analysis comparing patient-specific risk factors of patients with and without PPCs. Among patient-specific risk factors only the ASA score ≥ 3 showed a significantly higher rate in the PPC group (55/157 (35%) versus 87/178 (49%), $P = 0.01$)). All the other patient-specific risk factors including age, gender, alcohol abuse, smoking, neoadjuvant radio- and/or chemotherapy, body-mass-index (BMI), UICC (Union Internationale Contre Cancer) ≥3 and hemoglobin level before surgery showed no difference between patients with and without PPCs.

Table 3 shows the results of the univariate analysis comparing procedural risk factors of patients with and without PPCs. There were no differences with respect to surgery-related risk factors. Among anesthesia-related risk factors patients of the PPC group received a higher amount of crystalloids, more packed red blood cells

Table 1 Baseline patient-specific and procedural characteristics of the entire cohort

	Entire cohort ($n = 335$)
Patient-specific parameters	
Age (years)	62 ± 10
Gender (male/female)	290 (87%)/ 45 (13%)
Alcohol abuse	117 (35%)
Smoking	170 (51%)
Neoadjuvant RCT	262 (78%)
ASA 1/ 2/ 3/ 4 (n)	10 (3%)/183 (55%)/137 (41%)/5 (2%)
BMI (kg/m^2)	24 (5)
UICC I/ II	251 (75%)
UICC III/ IV	84 (25%)
Procedural parameters	
Surgery-related	
Surgical approach	
Transhiatal	26 (8%)
Thoracoabdominal	309 (92%)
Reconstruction	
Gastric tube	321 (96%)
Colon interposition	14 (4%)
Duration of surgery (hours)	7.0 (2.2)
Blood loss (ml)	700 (600)
Anesthesia-related	
Average Norepinephrine (μg/kg/min)	0.03 (0.07)
Crystalloids (ml)	5500 (3000)
FFP (ml)	136 ± 760
PRBC (ml)	426 ± 1188
Colloids (ml)	1000 (500)
TEA	286 (85%)
TIVA/Gas	94 (28%) / 240 (72%)
Isoflurane	188 (56%)
Desflurane	50 (15%)
Sevoflurane	2 (0.6%)
Hospital stay (days)	22 (19)
ICU stay (days)	8 (7)
30-days-mortality overall	17 (5%)
90-days-mortality overall	37 (11%)
Pneumonia	114 (34%)
Pleural effusion	104 (31%)
New postoperative thoracic drainage	51 (15%)
Chylothorax	23 (7%)
Pleural empyema	18 (5%)
Re-intubation	66 (20%)

Table 1 Baseline patient-specific and procedural characteristics of the entire cohort (Continued)

	Entire cohort ($n = 335$)
Tracheostomy	39 (12%)
Re-intubation followed by tracheostomy	37 (11%)
PPCs	175 (52%)
90-days-mortality with PPCs	26 (8%)

Data are presented as number of patients (percentage), median (interquartile range) or mean (standard deviation)
RCT Radio–/Chemotherapy, *ASA* American Society of Anesthesiology, *BMI* Body mass index, *UICC* Union Internationale Contre Cancer, *FFP* Fresh frozen plasma, *PRBC* Packed red blood cell, *TEA* Thoracic epidural anesthesia, *TIVA* Total intravenous anesthesia, *ICU* Intensive care unit, *PPCs* Postoperative pulmonary complications

(PRBCs) and less often TEA. To assess the importance of epidural analgesia among high risk patients with an ASA score ≥ 3 an additional analysis on this study cohort was conducted. Among patients with an ASA score ≥ 3 24 patients had no epidural analgesia. Of these, 8/24 patients developed PPCs and died within 90 days after surgery compared to 10 out of 118 patients who received preoperative epidural analgesia ($P < 0.001$).

The pain level at rest for the first three postoperative days did not show a difference between patients with and without PPCs. As a consequence patients with PPCs had a longer hospital and ICU stay. A total of 251 (75%) patients were postoperatively transferred to ICU with a retained one-lumen endotracheal tube. There was no difference with respect to the incidence of PPCs. There were 141 patients with a retained endotracheal tube in the PPC group (141/177, 80%) versus 110 patients (110/157, 70%) in the group without PPCs ($P = 0.5$).

Table 4 highlights the multivariate stepwise logistic regression analysis with respect to the incidence of PPCs.

Table 2 Univariate analysis of patient-specific parameters of patients with and without PPCs

	No PPC ($n = 157$)	PPC ($n = 178$)	P Value
Patient-specific parameters			
Age (years)	61 ± 10	62 ± 10	0.1
Gender (male/female)	137 (87)/21 (13)	153 (86)/24 (13)	1
Alcohol abuse (n)	52 (33)	65 (37)	0.5
Smoking (n)	74 (47)	96 (54)	0.2
Neoadjuvant RCT (n)	124 (79)	138 (78)	1
ASA ≥ 3 (n)	55 (35)	87 (49)	**0.01**
BMI (kg/m^2)	25 (22–27)	24 (22–28)	0.8
UICC ≥ 3 (n)	41 (26)	43 (24)	0.8
Hb before surgery (mg/dl)	12.7 (11.6–13.6)	12.6 (11.3–14)	0.65

Data are presented as number of patients (percentage), median (interquartile range) or mean (standard deviation)
RCT Radio–/Chemotherapy, *ASA* American Society of Anesthesiology, *BMI* Body mass index, *UICC* Union Internationale Contre Cancer, *Hb* Hemoglobin, *PPCs* Postoperative pulmonary complications

Table 3 Univariate analysis of procedural parameters (surgery-related and anesthesia-related) of patients with and without PPCs

	No PPC (*n* = 157)	PPC (*n* = 178)	*P* Value
Procedural parameters			
Surgery-related			
Surgical approach (n)			
Transhiatal	10 (6)	16 (9)	0.42
Thoracoabdominal	148 (94)	161 (91)	
Reconstruction (n)			
Gastric tube	154 (98)	167 (94)	0.18
Colon interposition	4 (2)	10 (6)	
Duration of surgery (hours)	7 (6–8.3)	7.1 (6.2–8.5)	0.19
Blood loss (ml)	600 (300–1000)	750 (500–1000)	0.12
Anesthesia-related			
Norepinephrine (μg/kg/min)	0.03 (0–0.06)	0.02 (0–0.07)	0.9
Crystalloids (ml)	1100 (880–1924)	1404 (1008–2071)	**0.007**
Colloids (ml)	752 (73–1000)	710 (263–1035)	0.7
Colloids (n)	141 (90)	158 (89)	1
FFP (n)	19 (12)	21 (12)	1
PRBC (n)	44 (28)	78 (44)	**0.002**
TEA (n)	142 (90)	144 (81)	**0.019**
TIVA / Gas (n)	49 (31) / 108 (69)	45 (25)/ 132 (74)	0.27
Hospital stay (days)	17 (15–23)	30 (20–50)	**< 0.001**
Extubation on ICU	110 (70)	141 (79)	0.5
Pleural effusion	0	104 (58)	**< 0.001**
Chylothorax	0	23 (13)	**< 0.001**
ICU stay (days)	6 (5–8)	12 (7–26)	**< 0.001**

Data are presented as number of patients (percentage) or median (interquartile range)
FFP Fresh frozen plasma, *PRBC* Packed red blood cell, *TEA* Thoracic epidural anesthesia, *TIVA* Total intravenous anesthesia, *ICU* Intensive care unit, *PPCs* Postoperative pulmonary complications

All parameters analyzed in the univariate analysis shown in Tables 2 and 3 were included in this multivariate approach. Only the significant risk factors are shown. Among the patient-specific parameters ASA score ≥ 3 was the only independent risk factor (OR: 1.7, 95% CI: 1.1–2.6; *P* = 0.025). There were two modifiable anesthesia-related risk factors for PPCs in this study cohort. Those were intraoperative PRBCs

(OR: 1.9, 95% CI: 1.2–3.0; *P* = 0.009) and TEA (OR: 2.0, 95% CI: 1.01–3.8; *P* = 0.046).

Table 5 shows the multivariate stepwise logistic regression analysis with respect to the 90-days mortality rate of patients with PPCs. All parameters analyzed in the univariate analysis shown in Tables 2 and 3 were included in this multivariate approach. Only the significant

Table 4 Multivariate stepwise logistic regression analysis of patient-specific and procedural risk factors with respect to PPCs

	OR (95% CI)	*P* Value
Patient-specific risk factors		
ASA ≥ 3	1.7 (1.1–2.6)	0.025
Procedural risk factors		
PRBC	1.9 (1.2–3)	0.009
TEA	2.0 (1.01–3.8)	0.046

ASA American Society of Anesthesiology, *PRBC* Packed red blood cell, *TEA* Thoracic epidural anesthesia

Table 5 Multivariate stepwise logistic regression analysis of patient-specific and procedural risk factors with respect to 90-days mortality of patients with PPCs

	OR (95% CI)	*P* Value
Patient-specific risk factors		
ASA ≥ 3	2.6 (1.1–6.2)	0.036
Procedural risk factors		
PRBC	5.0 (2.0–12.6)	0.001
TEA	3.9 (1.6–9.7)	0.003

ASA American Society of Anesthesiology, *PRBC* Packed red blood cell, *TEA* Thoracic epidural anesthesia

risk factors are highlighted. The results resemble those of Table 4 but with higher odds ratios for the same independent risk factors. Among the patient-specific parameters ASA score ≥ 3 was the only independent risk factor (OR: 2.6, 95% CI: 1.1–6.2; P = 0.036). There were two modifiable anesthesia-related risk factors for 90-days mortality of patients with PPCs in this study cohort. Those were intraoperative PRBCs (OR: 5.0, 95% CI: 2.0–12.6; P = 0.001) and TEA (OR: 3.9, 95% CI: 1.6–9.7; P = 0.003).

Discussion

This retrospective study including 335 patients undergoing open esophagectomy for esophageal cancer is the first study examining various modifiable risk factors with regard to mortality associated with PPCs. The multivariate stepwise logistic regression analysis was used to assess the importance of procedural and potentially modifiable risk factors in the context of existing patient-specific risk factors. The main results of this study can be summarized as follows. First, the incidence of PPCs in this study cohort was 52% (175/335) associated with a 90-days mortality rate of 8% (26/335). Second, ASA score ≥ 3 was the only independent patient-specific risk factor for PPCs and the associated mortality in this study cohort. Third, this study revealed two modifiable independent risk factors for PPCs and consecutive 90-days mortality. Both anesthesia-related risk factors, intraoperative PRBCs and TEA were ranked higher than the patient-specific one according to the highlighted Odds ratios of the multivariate analysis. Although significant in the univariate approach the total amount of crystalloids was not characterized as an independent risk factor for PPCs in the multivariate analysis. Fourth, type of general anesthesia (TIVA versus gas) did not show a difference between the groups with respect to the incidence of PPCs and mortality.

The overall 30- and 90-days-mortality rate of 5 and 11% in this study cohort is in accordance with current literature [1, 24, 25]. However, this is the first study focusing on mortality related to PPCs. PPCs after esophagectomy are the most frequent postoperative complications [1, 4, 9, 26, 27]. The majority of patients who died within 90 days after surgery suffered from PPCs 70% (26/37) in our study cohort. The number of patients with PPCs 52% (175/335) in our study cohort appears higher than described in current literature (incidences of 21 to 38%) [1, 26, 27]. One reason for this discrepancy might be the fact that the definition of PPCs is heterogenous. The following PPCs were included in this study: pneumonia, pleural effusion, re-intubation, tracheostomy, chylothorax and pleural empyema. The incidence of pleural effusion in our study cohort is quite high with an incidence of 31%. Pleural effusion is rarely described as a PPC after esophagectomy. However, due to its consecutive respiratory impairment

and possible side effects of prolonged thoracic drainage, pleural effusion was added as a PPC.

Our results with respect to patient-specific risk factors for postoperative complications are partially in accordance with current literature. The only independent patient-specific risk factor in this study cohort was ASA score ≥ 3 which was also described by several authors [8, 16, 26]. Further patient-specific risk factors like age, smoking, gender, neoadjuvant radio–/chemotherapy or preoperative anemia were not confirmed in this retrospective study [1, 5, 7, 9, 16, 19, 25].

Among the procedural parameters the surgery-related risk factors did not show any significant results, although blood loss and transthoracic approach were described as independent risk factors for adverse outcome with respect to postoperative mortality and PPCs after esophagectomy [1, 5]. A reason for this discrepancy with respect to the surgical approach might be the low number of bench mark patients who underwent transhiatal esophagectomy 8% (26/335) in this study cohort.

Among the procedural parameters the anesthesia-related risk factors are divided into three subgroups for the discussion section. These are intraoperative fluid therapy including quality and quantity of fluids, the type of general anesthesia (TIVA versus gas) and the use of perioperative TEA.

Several studies emphasized the importance of intraoperative restrictive fluid therapy during esophagectomy to reduce the incidence of PPCs [10, 11]. Although, patients of the PPC group received significantly more intraoperative crystalloid fluids, this difference was no longer obvious in the multivariate logistic regression analysis. The preoperative hemoglobin level and the intraoperative blood loss did not show a difference between patients with and without PPCs, nevertheless patients of the PPC group received PRBCs more often. This result was verified in the multivariate stepwise logistic regression analysis where the intraoperative transfusion of PRBCs was an independent risk factor for PPCs and its associated 90-days mortality. This is in accordance with current literature where liberal transfusion of PRBCs during esophagectomy was described as a risk factor for postoperative morbidity with respect to general postoperative complications, PPCs, increased 30-days mortality and worse long-term outcome [13, 28–31]. To our best knowledge there is no other study that focused on the 90-days mortality related to PPCs in esophageal cancer patients after esophagectomy. In our study the intraoperative use of colloids or fresh frozen plasma was not associated with an increased risk for PPCs or postoperative mortality. Subramanian and colleagues described the intraoperative use of FFP as an independent risk factor for major postoperative infectious complications including pneumonia after esophagectomy [32]. Data on the intraoperative use of colloids during esophagectomy and its effects on postoperative morbidity and mortality are scarce. Ahn and colleagues examined the effect of hydroxyethyl starch (HES) on postoperative renal function in thoracic surgery [33]. They concluded that HES should be administered with caution especially in high-risk patients undergoing thoracic surgery. Although this study focused on the incidence of acute kidney injury (AKI), they also mentioned an increased rate of PPCs in the group of patients with AKI who received more HES than the group without AKI. Further studies are needed to draw reliable conclusions on this topic.

Due to the fact that the type of anesthesia maintenance (intravenous versus gas) during esophagectomy influences the inflammatory cytokine production in the airway epithelium and impairs the pulmonary circulation, Zhang and colleagues hypothesized that the incidence of postoperative pneumonia is also effected [34–36]. However, there was no difference with respect to the incidence of postoperative pneumonia [36]. This is in accordance with our results. The type of general anesthesia did not show a difference between patients with and without PPCs and was not characterized as an independent risk factor for PPCs or 90-days mortality of patients with PPCs in our study cohort. Admittedly, the comparison of our results with current literature on this topic appears difficult because instead of sevoflurane which was mostly used in past studies, the majority of our patients received isoflurane or desflurane.

Data on the use of TEA to reduce the incidence of PPCs after esophagectomy are inconsistent [2, 14, 16–18, 20]. The current meta-analysis by Visser and colleagues shows no significant benefit for TEA compared to systemic analgesia with respect to PPCs or postoperative pain scores at 24 and 48 h after esophagectomy. In contrast to these results several authors published a significant reduction of the incidence of postoperative pneumonia by using TEA in patients undergoing esophagectomy [14, 15, 20]. Zingg and colleagues were not able to confirm these results with respect to postoperative pneumonia, but showed a significant decrease of postoperative respiratory failure and ARDS [16]. Esophageal cancer patients with TEA after esophagectomy showed decreased opioid consumption and reduced duration of ICU stay [19]. To our best knowledge there are no results on the positive effect of TEA with respect to the 90-days mortality related to PPCs after esophagectomy. The univariate analysis of the subgroup of patients with an ASA score ≥ 3 shows that especially high risk patients (ASA score ≥ 3) undergoing thoracotomic esophagectomy benefit from epidural analgesia.

For each patient only the daily maximum pain score at rest was used for the final analysis. For postoperative pain assessment the pain level at coughing and moving appears more valid to assess a sufficient pain therapy. Due to the retrospective character of this study, data on the pain score during respiratory therapy was not available as these data were not recorded in clinical routine. It was also not documented whether patients were able to participate sufficiently in physiotherapy with respect to their state of consciousness under opioid therapy. Therefore the comparison of pain scores at rest might appear misleading.

Our results show that the absence of TEA for patients undergoing open esophagectomy is a major risk factor for PPCs and the 90-days mortality related to PPCs.

Conclusion

In esophageal cancer patients undergoing thoracotomic esophagectomy epidural analgesia and the avoidance of intraoperative blood transfusion are significantly associated with a reduced 90-days mortality related to PPCs.

Abbreviations
AKI: Acute kidney injury; ARDS: Acute respiratory distress syndrome; ASA: American society of anesthesiology; BMI: Body-mass-index; DLCO: Diffusion capacity of the lung for carbon monoxide; FEV_1: Forced expiratory volume in 1 second; FFP: Fresh frozen plasma; HES: Hydroxyethyl starch; ICU: Intensive care unit; PPC: Postoperative pulmonary complications; PRBC: Packed red blood cells; SLV: Single-lung ventilation; TEA: Thoracic epidural anesthesia; TIVA: Total intravenous anesthesia; UICC: Union Internationale Contre Cancer

Acknowledgements
Not applicable.

Authors' contributions
Study design: KBK, WB, SH, HB, UG. Protocol design: KBK, WB, SH, UG. Advisor for study protocol and management of the study: KBK, TG, JH, SH, HB, UG Patient recruitment: KBK, WB, TG, JH, SH, UG. Data collection: KBK, WB, TG, JH, UG. Study conduct: KBK, SH, HB, UG. Study monitoring: KBK, WB, TG, JH, SH, HB, UG. Data analysis: KBK, WB, SH, UG. Data evaluation: KBK, SH, TG, HB, UG. Writing the manuscript: KBK, SH, UG. Editing and approval of the manuscript: KBK, WB, TG, JH, SH, HB, UG.

Author details
[1]Department of Anesthesiology and Critical Care Medicine, University of Freiburg, – University of Freiburg, Hugstetter Strasse 55, 79106 Freiburg, Germany. [2]Department of General and Visceral Surgery, Medical Center - University of Freiburg, Faculty of Medicine – University of Freiburg, Hugstetter Strasse 55, 79106 Freiburg, Germany.

References
1. Ferguson MK, Celauro AD, Prachand V. Prediction of major pulmonary complications after Esophagectomy. Ann Thorac Surg. 2011;91:1494–501.
2. Hughes M, Yim I, Deans DAC, Couper GW, Lamb PJ, Skipworth RJE. Systematic review and meta-analysis of epidural analgesia versus analgesic regimes following Oesophagogastric resection. World J Surg. 2018;42:204–10.
3. Munasinghe A, Markar SR, Mamidanna R, Darzi AW, Faiz OD, Hanna GB, et al. Is it time to centralize high-risk Cancer Care in the United States? Comparison of outcomes of Esophagectomy between England and the United States. Ann Surg. 2015;262:79–85.
4. Boshier PR, Marczin N, Hanna GB. Pathophysiology of acute lung injury following esophagectomy: ALI post esophagectomy. Dis Esophagus. 2015; 28:797–804.
5. Whooley BP, Law S, Murthy SC, Alexandrou A, Wong J. Analysis of reduced death and complication rates after esophageal resection. Ann Surg. 2001; 233:338–44.

6. Law S, Wong K-H, Kwok K-F, Chu K-M, Wong J. Predictive factors for postoperative pulmonary complications and mortality after esophagectomy for cancer. Ann Surg. 2004;240:791–800.

7. Avendano CE, Flume PA, Silvestri GA, King LB, Reed CE. Pulmonary complications after esophagectomy. Ann Thorac Surg. 2002;73:922–6.

8. Goense L, Meziani J, Bülbül M, Braithwaite SA, van Hillegersberg R, Ruurda JP. Pulmonary diffusion capacity predicts major complications after esophagectomy for patients with esophageal cancer. Dis Esophagus. 2018. https://doi.org/10.1093/dote/doy082.

9. Schlottmann F, Strassle PD, Patti MG. Transhiatal vs. transthoracic Esophagectomy: a NSQIP analysis of postoperative outcomes and risk factors for morbidity. J Gastrointest Surg. 2017;21:1757–63.

10. Chau EHL, Slinger P. Perioperative fluid Management for Pulmonary Resection Surgery and Esophagectomy. Semin Cardiothorac Vasc Anesth. 2014;18:36–44.

11. Casado D, López F, Martí R. Perioperative fluid management and major respiratory complications in patients undergoing esophagectomy: Esophagectomy and fluid management. Dis Esophagus. 2010;23:523–8.

12. Glatz T, Kulemann B, Marjanovic G, Bregenzer S, Makowiec F, Hoeppner J. Postoperative fluid overload is a risk factor for adverse surgical outcome in patients undergoing esophagectomy for esophageal cancer: a retrospective study in 335 patients. BMC Surg. 2017;17. https://doi.org/10.1186/s12893-016-0203-9.

13. Melis M, McLoughlin JM, Dean EM, Siegel EM, Weber JM, Shah N, et al. Correlations between neoadjuvant treatment, Anemia, and perioperative complications in patients undergoing Esophagectomy for Cancer. J Surg Res. 2009;153:114–20.

14. Cense HA, Lagarde SM, de Jong K, Omloo JMT, Busch ORC, Henny CP, et al. Association of no Epidural Analgesia with postoperative morbidity and mortality after transthoracic esophageal Cancer resection. J Am Coll Surg. 2006;202:395–400.

15. Pöpping DM. Protective effects of epidural analgesia on pulmonary complications after abdominal and thoracic surgery: a meta-analysis. Arch Surg. 2008;143:990.

16. Zingg U, Smithers BM, Gotley DC, Smith G, Aly A, Clough A, et al. Factors associated with postoperative pulmonary morbidity after Esophagectomy for Cancer. Ann Surg Oncol. 2011;18:1460–8.

17. Visser E, Marsman M, van Rossum PSN, Cheong E, Al-Naimi K, van Klei WA, et al. Postoperative pain management after esophagectomy: a systematic review and meta-analysis. Dis Esophagus. 2017;30:1–11.

18. Feltracco P, Bortolato A, Barbieri S, Michieletto E, Serra E, Ruol A, et al. Perioperative benefit and outcome of thoracic epidural in esophageal surgery: a clinical review. Dis Esophagus. 2018;31. https://doi.org/10.1093/dote/dox135.

19. Heinrich S, Janitz K, Merkel S, Klein P, Schmidt J. Short- and long term effects of epidural analgesia on morbidity and mortality of esophageal cancer surgery. Langenbecks Arch Surg. 2015;400:19–26.

20. Li W, Li Y, Huang Q, Ye S, Rong T. Short and long-term outcomes of epidural or intravenous analgesia after Esophagectomy: a propensity-matched cohort study. PLoS One. 2016;11:e0154380.

21. de la Gala F, Piñeiro P, Reyes A, Vara E, Olmedilla L, Cruz P, et al. Postoperative pulmonary complications, pulmonary and systemic inflammatory responses after lung resection surgery with prolonged one-lung ventilation. Randomized controlled trial comparing intravenous and inhalational anaesthesia. Br J Anaesth. 2017;119:655–63.

22. Vandenbroucke JP, von Elm E, Altman DG, Gøtzsche PC, Mulrow CD, Pocock SJ, et al. Strengthening the reporting of observational studies in epidemiology (STROBE): explanation and elaboration. Int J Surg Lond Engl. 2014;12:1500–24.

23. Low DE, Alderson D, Cecconello I, Chang AC, Darling GE, D'Journo XB, et al. International consensus on standardization of data collection for complications associated with Esophagectomy: Esophagectomy complications consensus group (ECCG). Ann Surg. 2015;262:286–94.

24. Boshier PR, Anderson O, Hanna GB. Transthoracic versus Transhiatal Esophagectomy for the treatment of Esophagogastric Cancer: a meta-analysis. Ann Surg. 2011;254:894–906.

25. Ferguson MK, Durkin AE. Preoperative prediction of the risk of pulmonary complications after esophagectomy for cancer. J Thorac Cardiovasc Surg. 2002;123:661–9.

26. Brown AM, Pucci MJ, Berger AC, Tatarian T, Evans NR, Rosato EL, et al. A standardized comparison of peri-operative complications after minimally invasive esophagectomy: Ivor Lewis versus McKeown. Surg Endosc. 2018;32:204–11.

27. Ohi M, Toiyama Y, Omura Y, Ichikawa T, Yasuda H, Okugawa Y, et al. Risk factors and measures of pulmonary complications after thoracoscopic esophagectomy for esophageal cancer. Surg Today. 2018. https://doi.org/10.1007/s00595-018-1721-0.

28. Towe CW, Gulack BC, Kim S, Ho VP, Perry Y, Donahue JM, et al. Restrictive transfusion practices after Esophagectomy are associated with improved outcome: a review of the Society of Thoracic Surgeons general thoracic database. Ann Surg. 2018;267:886–91.

29. Mirnezami R, Rohatgi A, Sutcliffe RP, Hamouda A, Chandrakumaran K, Botha A, et al. Multivariate analysis of clinicopathological factors influencing survival following esophagectomy for cancer. Int J Surg. 2010;8:58–63.

30. Kinugasa S, Tachibana M, Yoshimura H, Ueda S, Fujii T, Dhar DK, et al. Postoperative pulmonary complications are associated with worse short- and long-term outcomes after extended esophagectomy. J Surg Oncol. 2004;88:71–7.

31. Reeh M, Ghadban T, Dedow J, Vettorazzi E, Uzunoglu FG, Nentwich M, et al. Allogenic blood transfusion is associated with poor perioperative and long-term outcome in esophageal Cancer. World J Surg. 2017;41:208–15.

32. Subramanian A, Berbari EF, Brown MJ, Allen MS, Alsara A, Kor DJ. Plasma transfusion is associated with postoperative infectious complications following esophageal resection surgery: a retrospective cohort study. J Cardiothorac Vasc Anesth. 2012;26:569–74.

33. Ahn HJ, Kim JA, Lee AR, Yang M, Jung HJ, Heo B. The risk of acute kidney injury from fluid restriction and hydroxyethyl starch in thoracic surgery. Anesth Analg. 2016;122:186–93.

34. Xu W-Y, Wang N, Xu H-T, Yuan H-B, Sun H-J, Dun C-L, et al. Effects of sevoflurane and propofol on right ventricular function and pulmonary circulation in patients undergone esophagectomy. Int J Clin Exp Pathol. 2014;7:272–9.

35. Wakabayashi S, Yamaguchi K, Kumakura S, Murakami T, Someya A, Kajiyama Y, et al. Effects of anesthesia with sevoflurane and propofol on the cytokine/chemokine production at the airway epithelium during esophagectomy. Int J Mol Med. 2014;34:137–44.

36. Zhang G-H, Wang W. Effects of sevoflurane and propofol on the development of pneumonia after esophagectomy: a retrospective cohort study. BMC Anesthesiol. 2017;17. https://doi.org/10.1186/s12871-017-0458-4.

Permissions

The contributors of this book come from diverse backgrounds, making this book a truly international effort. This book will bring forth new frontiers with its revolutionizing research information and detailed analysis of the nascent developments around the world.

We would like to thank all the contributing authors for lending their expertise to make the book truly unique. They have played a crucial role in the development of this book. Without their invaluable contributions this book wouldn't have been possible. They have made vital efforts to compile up to date information on the varied aspects of this subject to make this book a valuable addition to the collection of many professionals and students.

This book was conceptualized with the vision of imparting up-to-date information and advanced data in this field. To ensure the same, a matchless editorial board was set up. Every individual on the board went through rigorous rounds of assessment to prove their worth. After which they invested a large part of their time researching and compiling the most relevant data for our readers.

The editorial board has been involved in producing this book since its inception. They have spent rigorous hours researching and exploring the diverse topics which have resulted in the successful publishing of this book. They have passed on their knowledge of decades through this book. To expedite this challenging task, the publisher supported the team at every step. A small team of assistant editors was also appointed to further simplify the editing procedure and attain best results for the readers.

Apart from the editorial board, the designing team has also invested a significant amount of their time in understanding the subject and creating the most relevant covers. They scrutinized every image to scout for the most suitable representation of the subject and create an appropriate cover for the book.

The publishing team has been an ardent support to the editorial, designing and production team. Their endless efforts to recruit the best for this project, has resulted in the accomplishment of this book. They are a veteran in the field of academics and their pool of knowledge is as vast as their experience in printing. Their expertise and guidance has proved useful at every step. Their uncompromising quality standards have made this book an exceptional effort. Their encouragement from time to time has been an inspiration for everyone.

The publisher and the editorial board hope that this book will prove to be a valuable piece of knowledge for researchers, students, practitioners and scholars across the globe.

List of Contributors

Anna Sellgren Engskov and Jonas Åkeson
Department of Clinical Sciences Malmö, Anaesthesiology and Intensive Care Medicine, Lund University, Skåne University Hospital, Carl Bertil Laurells gata 9, 3rd floor, SE-20502 Malmö, Sweden

Agneta Troilius Rubin
Dermatology, Lund University, Skåne University Hospital, Malmö, Sweden

Mark C. Kendall, Lucas Alves, Lauren L. Traill and Gildasio S. De Oliveira
Department of Anesthesiology, The Warren Alpert Medical School of Brown University, Providence, Rhode Island, USA

Ji-Hyun Lee, Seungeun Choi, Minkyoo Lee, Young-Eun Jang, Eun-Hee Kim, Jin-Tae Kim and Hee-Soo Kim
Department of Anaesthesiology and Pain Medicine, Seoul National University Hospital, Seoul National University College of Medicine, # 101 Daehakno, Jongnogu, Seoul 03080, Republic of Korea

Bogusław Gawęda, Janusz Bąk, Maciej Kolowca and Kazimierz Widenka
Division of Cardiovascular Surgery, St. Jadwiga Provincial Clinical Hospital, ul. Lwowska 60, 35-301 Rzeszów, Poland

Michał Borys and Miroslaw Czuczwar
Second Department of Anesthesia and Intensive Care, Medical University of Lublin, ul. Staszica 16, 20-081 Lublin, Poland

Bartłomiej Belina and Bogumiła Wołoszczuk-Gębicka
Anesthesiology and Intensive Care Department with the Center for Acute Poisoning, St. Jadwiga Provincial Clinical Hospital, ul. Lwowska 60, 35-301 Rzeszów, Poland

Jia Wang, Bin Liu and Jianfeng Chen
West China Hospital of Sichuan University, No. 37th, Guoxue Lane, Wuhou District, Chengdu City, Sichuan Province, P.R. China

Yu Cui
Chengdu Women's & Children's Central Hospital, Chengdu 610000, P.R. China

Qin Liao
Department of Anesthesiology, Third Xiangya Hospital of Central South University, Changsha, Hunan, China

Yuda Fei, Xulei Cui, Shaohui Chen and Yuguang Huang
Anesthesiology Department, Peking Union Medical College Hospital, Chinese Academy of Medical Sciences, and Peking Union Medical College, Shuaifuyuan 1#, Dongcheng District, Beijing 100730, China

Huiming Peng, Bin Feng, Wenwei Qian, Jin Lin and Xisheng Weng
Orthopaedic Department, Peking Union Medical College Hospital, Chinese Academy of Medical Sciences, and Peking Union Medical College, Shuaifuyuan 1#, Dongcheng District, Beijing 100730, China

Yu-jiao Guan, Qu-lian Guo and Zhi-gang Cheng
Department of Anesthesiology, Xiangya Hospital of Central South University, No. 87 Xiangya Road, Changsha, Hunan, China

Lai Wei
Department of Anesthesiology, Hunan Provincial People's Hospital, Changsha, Hunan, China

Qi-wu Fang
Department of Anesthesiology, Pain Medicine & Critical Care Medicine, Aviation General Hospital of China Medical University & Beijing Institute of Translational Medicine, Chinese Academy of Sciences, Beijing, China

Nong He
Department of Anesthesiology, Peking University Shougang Hospital, Beijing, China

Chong-fang Han
Department of Anesthesiology, Shanxi Academy of Medical Sciences, Shanxi Dayi Hospital, Shanxi, China

Chang-hong Miao
Department of Anesthesiology, Fudan University Shanghai Cancer Center, Shanghai, China

Gang-jian Luo
Department of Anesthesiology, Third Affiliated Hospital of Sun Yat-Sen University, Guangzhou, Guangdong, China

Han-bing Wang
Department of Anesthesiology, First People's Hospital of Foshan, Foshan, Guangdong, China

Hao Cheng
Department of Anesthesiology, Beijing Ditan Hospital Capital Medical University, Beijing, China

Fei Peng, Yanshuang Li, Yanqiu Ai, Jianjun Yang and Yanping Wang
Department of Anesthesiology, Pain and Perioperative Medicine, The First Affiliated Hospital of Zhengzhou University, No.1 Jianshe East Road, Zhengzhou 450052, China

Izumi Sato, Hajime Iwasaki, Takafumi Iida and Hirotsugu Kanda
Department of Anesthesiology and Critical Care Medicine, Asahikawa Medical University, Midorigaoka-higashi 2-1-1-1, Asahikawa, Hokkaido 078-8510, Japan

Sarah Kyuragi Luthe
Department of Anesthesiology and Critical Care Medicine, Asahikawa Medical University, Midorigaoka-higashi 2-1-1-1, Asahikawa, Hokkaido 078-8510, Japan
Department of Anesthesiology, Indiana University School of Medicine, 1130 W. Michigan Street, Fesler Hall 204, Indianapolis, IN 46202, USA

Bjoern Grosse, Stefan Eberbach and Martin Schmidt-Niemann
Department of Pediatric Anesthesiology, Altona Children's Hospital, Bleickenallee 38, 22763 Hamburg, Germany

Hans O. Pinnschmidt
Center of Experimental Medicine, Institute of Medical Biometry and Epidemiology, University Hospital Hamburg-Eppendorf, Hamburg, Germany

Konrad Reinshagen
Department of Pediatric Anesthesiology, Altona Children's Hospital, Bleickenallee 38, 22763 Hamburg, Germany
Department of Pediatric Surgery, University Hospital Hamburg-Eppendorf, Hamburg, Germany

Deirdre Vincent
Department of Pediatric Surgery, University Hospital Hamburg-Eppendorf, Hamburg, Germany

Benedikt Haager and Bernward Passlick
Department of Thoracic Surgery, Medical Center, University of Freiburg, Hugstetter Straße 55, 79106 Freiburg, Germany

Joerg Eschbach and Torsten Loop
Department of Anesthesiology and Intensive Care Medicine, Medical Center, University of Freiburg, Hugstetter Straße 55, 79106 Freiburg, Germany

Daniel Schmid
Department of Thoracic Surgery, Medical Center, University of Freiburg, Hugstetter Straße 55, 79106 Freiburg, Germany
Department of Anesthesiology and Intensive Care Medicine, Medical Center, University of Freiburg, Hugstetter Straße 55, 79106 Freiburg, Germany

Robin Raju
Department of Orthopedics and Rehabilitation, Yale New Haven Hospital/Yale University, 1 Long Wharf Drive, New Haven, CT 06511, USA

Michael Mehnert, David Stolzenberg, Jeremy Simon, Theodore Conliffe and Jeffrey Gehret
Department of Physical Medicine and Rehabilitation, Rothman Orthopaedic Institute/Thomas Jefferson University Hospital, 925 Chestnut Street, Philadelphia, PA 19107, USA

RyungA Kang, Ji Seon Jeong, Justin Sangwook Ko, Jong Hwan Lee, Soo Joo Choi, Sungrok Cha and Jeong Jin Lee
Department of Anesthesiology and Pain Medicine, Samsung Medical Center, Sungkyunkwan University School of Medicine, 81 Irwon ro, Gangnam gu, Seoul 06351, South Korea

Soo-Youn Lee
Department of Laboratory Medicine and Genetics, Samsung Medical Center, Sungkyunkwan University School of Medicine, Seoul, South Korea

M. Higashi, E. Nakamori, S. Sakurai and K. Yamaura
Department of Anesthesiology, Fukuoka University School of Medicine, 7-45-1, Nanakuma, Jonan-ku, Fukuoka 814-0180, Japan

K. Shigematsu
Operation rooms, Fukuoka University Hospital, Fukuoka, Japan

Raafat M. Reyad, Hossam Z. Ghobrial and Ehab H. Shaker
Department of Anesthesia & Pain Management, National Cancer Institute, Cairo University, Cairo, Egypt

Ehab M. Reyad
Department of Clinical Pathology, National Hepatology and Tropical Medicine Research Institute, Cairo, Egypt

Mohammed H. Shaaban and Rania H. Hashem
Department of Diagnostic & Interventional Radiology, Faculty of Medicine, Cairo University, Cairo, Egypt

Wael M. Darwish
Department of Diagnostic & Interventional Radiology, National Cancer Institute, Cairo University, Cairo, Egypt

Haiqing Chang, Shuang Li, Yansong Li, Bo Cheng, Jiwen Miao, Hui Gao, Hongli Ma, Yanfeng Gao and Qiang Wang
Department of Anesthesiology & Center for Brain Science, The First Affiliated Hospital of Xi'an Jiaotong University, Xi'an 710061, Shaanxi, China

Hao Hu
Department of Pharmacology, School of Basic Medical Sciences, Health Science Center, Xi'an Jiaotong University, Xi'an 710061, Shaanxi, China

Xiufang Xing, Yongyu Bai, Kai Sun and Min Yan
Department of Anesthesiology and Pain Medicine, Second Affiliated Hospital, Zhejiang University School of Medicine, No.88 Jiefang Road, Hangzhou 310009, China

Ozlem Sagir, Hafize Fisun Demir, Fatih Ugun and Bulent Atik
Department of Anesthesiology, Balıkesir University Health Application and Research Hospital, 10100 Balikesir, Turkey

Stefan J. Schaller, Felix P. Kappler, Claudia Hofberger, Jens Sattler, Richard Wagner, Gerhard Schneider and Manfred Blobner
Klinik für Anästhesiologie und Intensivmedizin, Klinikum rechts der Isar, School of Medicine, Technical University of Munich, Munich, Germany

Karl-Georg Kanz
Klinik für Unfallchirurgie, Klinikum rechts der Isar, School of Medicine, Technical University of Munich, Munich, Bavaria, Germany

Sasikaan Nimmaanrat, Manasanun Jongjidpranitarn, Sumidtra Prathep and Maliwan Oofuvong
Department of Anesthesiology, Faculty of Medicine, Prince of Songkla University, Hatyai, Songkhla 90110, Thailand

Jiao Huang and Jing-Chen Liu
Department of Anesthesiology, First Affiliated Hospital of Guangxi Medical University, 6 Shuangyong Road, Nanning 530021, Guangxi Zhuang Autonomous Region, People's Republic of China

Mayuko Kanazawa, Aiji Sato (Boku), Yoko Okumura, Mayumi Hashimoto, Naoko Tachi and Masahiro Okuda
Department of Anesthesiology, Aichi Gakuin University School of Dentistry, 2-11 Suemori-dori, Chikusaku, Nagoya 464-8651, Japan

Yushi Adachi
Department of Anesthesiology, Nagoya University Graduate School of Medicine, 65 Tsurumaicho, Showaku, Nagoya 466-8550, Japan

Guangyou Duan, Guiying Yang, Jing Peng, Zhenxin Duan, Jie Li, Xianglong Tang and Hong Li
Department of Anesthesiology, Xinqiao Hospital, Army Medical University, Chongqing 400037, China

Haichen Chu, He Dong and Zejun Niu
Department of Anesthesiology, The Affiliated Hospital of Qingdao University, No.16 Jiangsu Road, Shinan District, Qingdao, China

Yongjie Wang
Department of Thoracic Surgery, The Affiliated Hospital of Qingdao University, Qingdao, China

Jaesik Park, Minju Kim, Jung-Woo Shim, Hyung Mook Lee, Yong-Suk Kim, Young Eun Moon, Sang Hyun Hong and Min Suk Chae
Department of Anesthesiology and Pain Medicine, Seoul St. Mary's Hospital, College of Medicine, The Catholic University of Korea, 222, Banpo-daero Seocho-gu, Seoul 06591, Republic of Korea

Yong Hyun Park
Department of Urology, Seoul St. Mary's Hospital, College of Medicine, The Catholic University of Korea, Seoul, Republic of Korea

Misun Park
Department of Biostatistics, Clinical Research Coordinating Center, Catholic Medical Center, The Catholic University of Korea, Seoul, South Korea

Jing-li Zhu
Department of Anesthesiology, the Second Affiliated Hospital of Harbin Medical University, Harbin, Heilongjiang, China

Xue-ting Wang, Jing Gong, Hai-bin Sun and Xiao-qing Zhao
Department of Anesthesiology, the Second Affiliated Hospital of Harbin Medical University, Harbin, Heilongjiang, China

Wei Gao
Department of Anesthesiology, the Second Affiliated Hospital of Harbin Medical University, 246 Xuefu Road, Nangang District, Harbin, Heilongjiang, China

Kai B. Kaufmann, Wolfgang Baar, Hartmut Buerkle, Ulrich Goebel and Sebastian Heinrich
Department of Anesthesiology and Critical Care Medicine, University of Freiburg, – University of Freiburg, Hugstetter Strasse 55, 79106 Freiburg, Germany

Torben Glatz and Jens Hoeppner
Department of General and Visceral Surgery, Medical Center - University of Freiburg, Faculty of Medicine – University of Freiburg, Hugstetter Strasse 55, 79106 Freiburg, Germany

Index

Printed in the USA
CPSIA information can be obtained
at www.ICGtesting.com
JSHW051405091023
49903JS00006B/284

9 781646 465811